CLARK'S
POSITIONING IN RADIOGRAPHY

CLARK'S POSITIONING IN RADIOGRAPHY

13TH EDITION

A. STEWART WHITLEY • GAIL JEFFERSON • KEN HOLMES
CHARLES SLOANE • CRAIG ANDERSON • GRAHAM HOADLEY

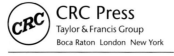

CRC Press is an imprint of the
Taylor & Francis Group, an **informa** business

CRC Press
Taylor & Francis Group
6000 Broken Sound Parkway NW, Suite 300
Boca Raton, FL 33487-2742

© 2016 by Taylor & Francis Group, LLC
CRC Press is an imprint of Taylor & Francis Group, an Informa business

No claim to original U.S. Government works

Printed and bound in India by Replika Press Pvt. Ltd.

Printed on acid-free paper
Version Date: 20150626

International Standard Book Number-13: 978-1-4441-2235-0 (Pack - Book and Ebook)

This book contains information obtained from authentic and highly regarded sources. While all reasonable efforts have been made to publish reliable data and information, neither the author[s] nor the publisher can accept any legal responsibility or liability for any errors or omissions that may be made. The publishers wish to make clear that any views or opinions expressed in this book by individual editors, authors or contributors are personal to them and do not necessarily reflect the views/opinions of the publishers. The information or guidance contained in this book is intended for use by medical, scientific or health-care professionals and is provided strictly as a supplement to the medical or other professional's own judgement, their knowledge of the patient's medical history, relevant manufacturer's instructions and the appropriate best practice guidelines. Because of the rapid advances in medical science, any information or advice on dosages, procedures or diagnoses should be independently verified. The reader is strongly urged to consult the relevant national drug formulary and the drug companies' and device or material manufacturers' printed instructions, and their websites, before administering or utilizing any of the drugs, devices or materials mentioned in this book. This book does not indicate whether a particular treatment is appropriate or suitable for a particular individual. Ultimately it is the sole responsibility of the medical professional to make his or her own professional judgements, so as to advise and treat patients appropriately. The authors and publishers have also attempted to trace the copyright holders of all material reproduced in this publication and apologize to copyright holders if permission to publish in this form has not been obtained. If any copyright material has not been acknowledged please write and let us know so we may rectify in any future reprint.

Except as permitted under U.S. Copyright Law, no part of this book may be reprinted, reproduced, transmitted, or utilized in any form by any electronic, mechanical, or other means, now known or hereafter invented, including photocopying, microfilming, and recording, or in any information storage or retrieval system, without written permission from the publishers.

For permission to photocopy or use material electronically from this work, please access www.copyright.com (http://www.copyright.com/) or contact the Copyright Clearance Center, Inc. (CCC), 222 Rosewood Drive, Danvers, MA 01923, 978-750-8400. CCC is a not-for-profit organization that provides licenses and registration for a variety of users. For organizations that have been granted a photocopy license by the CCC, a separate system of payment has been arranged.

Trademark Notice: Product or corporate names may be trademarks or registered trademarks, and are used only for identification and explanation without intent to infringe.

Visit the Taylor & Francis Web site at
http://www.taylorandfrancis.com

and the CRC Press Web site at
http://www.crcpress.com

Dedication

This volume is dedicated to the many student radiographers and radiographers in the field of Diagnostic Medical Imaging whose skills, knowledge and dedication play an important and pivotal role in modern medicine and ensuring that the patient's journey delivers the best outcomes.

We also wish to acknowledge the professional support and advice of a huge number of colleagues who have given their own time to offer advice and help in the preparation of the 13th edition. This has truly been a team effort.

Contents

Foreword ix
Authors and contributors xi
Preface xiii
Acknowledgements to the 13th edition xv
Acknowledgements to previous editions xvii
Abbreviations xix

1. Basic principles of radiography and digital technology — 1
2. Upper limb — 51
3. Shoulder — 95
4. Lower limb — 123
5. Hips, pelvis and sacro-iliac joints — 169
6. Vertebral column — 193
7. Thorax and upper airway — 227
8. Skull, facial bones and sinuses — 265
9. Dental radiography — 311
   Vivian Rushton
10. Abdomen and pelvic cavity — 365
11. Ward radiography — 385
12. Theatre radiography — 405
13. Paediatric radiography — 421
    J. Valmai Cook, Kaye Shaw and Alaa Witwit
14. Miscellaneous — 495

References/further reading 547
Index 555

Foreword

Radiography remains at the forefront of diagnosis in healthcare. Competent practitioners are required to justify and optimise exposures so that diagnostic yield is maximised and examination hazards minimised. There are a number of challenges facing educators of such practitioners including rapid technology developments, changing legal and policy contexts, increased variety of student types and greater patient reservations around radiation exposures. This text provides a wonderful core text that considers all these challenges, and will continue to be an excellent reference text for qualified personnel.

The approach used by the authors is comprehensive, current and easy to follow. The chapters for the specific body areas are presented extremely logically, each kicking off with a summary of the basic projections, followed by anatomic considerations, which in turn is followed by a detailed treatment of the relevant projections. The chapters are superbly complemented by clear and up-to-date line diagrams, photographs and X-ray images, with an easy to follow series of bullet points. The radiologic considerations are very useful and references provided are an effective reflective resource.

The preparatory sections in the text are invaluable, covering issues such as terminology, image quality, digital imaging and exposure factors. It was very reassuring to see the emphasis placed on radiation protection, which includes a mature and realistic appraisal of doses delivered, associated risk factors and the latest IRMER regulations. Increasingly patients are expecting to be examined by practitioners who can convey in the clearest way the potential dangers of diagnostic X-ray exposures; this book prepares the students well for these types of encounters.

The text has not shied away from the variety of clinical situations facing radiographers and chapters are dedicated to dental, theatre and paediatric contexts. In addition Chapter 14, *Miscellaneous*, addresses an array of important current emerging contexts including bariatrics, tomosynthesis and forensic radiography. The section on trauma radiography is particularly impressive.

It should not be a surprise that this text demonstrates excellence. Alfred Stewart Whitley FCR, HDCR, TDCR has been the driving force behind the work as well as being responsible for a number of the sections. His involvement and leadership in radiography over five decades are evident throughout this project and his achievements with, and contributions to, our profession are an inspiration for all of us. It is clear that the revision process has been lengthy with significant contributions from a dedicated team based at the University of Cumbria, and a range of other individuals including Dr. Graham Hoadley and paediatric and dental experts, who have contributed to specific sections. Stewart has steered this team of contributors to this highly successful conclusion.

In summary, this 13th edition of *Clark's Positioning* is an excellent text, which I would recommend to all my students and academic and clinical colleagues. It conveys to the reader an immense amount of easy to digest knowledge that is current, relevant and essential to modern day radiographic practice. But it does more. Increasingly as practitioners and academics we must reflect wisely on our long-established techniques and question dogma that is presented historically or by technology producers. This book encourages such reflection and questioning, and thrusts the radiographer at the centre of the justification and optimisation processes.

The patient must surely benefit by this publication.

Professor Patrick C. Brennan DCR, HDCR, PhD

Authors and contributors

A. Stewart Whitley
Radiology Advisor
UK Radiology Advisory Services
Preston, Lancashire, UK

Gail Jefferson
Senior Lecturer/Advanced Practitioner
Department of Medical and Sport Sciences, University of Cumbria
Carlisle, UK

Ken Holmes
Radiography Programme Leader
Department of Medical and Sport Sciences, University of Cumbria
Lancaster, UK

Charles Sloane
Principal Lecturer
Department of Medical and Sport Sciences, University of Cumbria
Lancaster, UK

Craig Anderson
Clinical Tutor and Reporting Radiographer
X-ray Department, Furness General Hospital
Cumbria, UK

Graham Hoadley
Consultant Radiologist
Blackpool, Fylde and Wyre Hospitals NHS Trust
Blackpool, Lancashire, UK

J. Valmai Cook
Consultant Radiologist
Queen Mary's Hospital for Sick Children, Epsom and
   St. Helier University NHS Trust Carshalton, UK

Kaye Shah
Superintendent Radiographer
Queen Mary's Hospital for Sick Children, Epsom and
   St. Helier University NHS Trust Carshalton, UK

Alaa Witwit
Consultant Radiologist
Queen Mary's Hospital for Sick Children, Epsom and
   St. Helier University NHS Trust Carshalton, UK

Viv Rushton
Lecturer in Dental & Maxillofacial Radiology
University Dental Hospital of Manchester
Manchester, UK

Andy Shaw
Group Leader Medical Physicist
North West Medical Physics, Christie Hospital
Manchester, UK

Alistair Mackenzie
Research Physicist
NCCPM, Medical Physics Department, Royal Surrey
   County Hospital
Guildford, UK

Alexander Peck
Information Systems Manager
Royal Brompton & Harefield NHS Foundation Trust
London, UK

Keith Horner
Professor
School of Dentistry, University of Manchester
Manchester, UK

Paul Charnock
Radiation Protection Adviser
Integrated Radiological Services (IRS) Ltd
Liverpool, UK

Ben Thomas
Technical Officer
Integrated Radiological Services (IRS) Ltd
Liverpool, UK

Preface

This new edition, with a newly expanded team, continues with the success of the 12th edition in containing the majority of current plain radiographic imaging techniques in a single volume. Mammography, however, is not included but is to be found in the companion volume *Clark's Procedures in Diagnostic Imaging*, where it is included in a separate chapter devoted to all the imaging modalities associated with breast imaging.

This fully revised 13th edition builds on the changes made in the 12th edition, reflecting the changing technology and demands on a modern diagnostic imaging department and the need to provide optimal images consistent with the ALARP principle.

New in Chapter 1 is the emphasis on the 'patient journey', with a focus on the needs of the patient and a reflection on the important steps in the process of delivering images of high quality.

Also introduced is the formal process of 'image evaluation', which radiographers are frequently engaged in, delivering their comments on acquired images as part of an 'initial report' in an agreed structure. Additionally, the student is further guided with the inclusion of a '10 Point Plan' which will aid in ensuring excellent diagnostic images are presented for viewing and interpretation.

The important role that 'imaging informatics' plays is added to provide a general understanding as to how it is used best, both to maximise image quality and to provide the means to administer, store and communicate images where they are needed.

For the first time recommended diagnostic reference levels (DRLs) are included within the description of a number of radiographic techniques. Those quoted are derived from the recommended references doses published in the UK in the HPA – CRCE – 034 report *Doses to patients from radiographic and fluoroscopic X-ray imaging procedures in the UK 2010 Review*. For those DRLs not included in the report DRLs are added, which are calculated on a regional basis by means of electronic X-ray examination records courtesy of Integrated Radiological Services (IRS) Ltd, Liverpool. These DRLs are meant to guide the student and to encourage them to look at the specific DRLs set in their respective health institutions. This in a small way reflects the original 'Kitty Clark' publications where guidance on exposure factors was provided. We hope that this will promote the importance of 'optimisation' and encourage practitioners and students alike to be aware of the appropriate dose for a specific patient-related examination.

The Miscellaneous chapter includes a new section on bariatric radiography reflecting the challenges in society and the need for careful pre-exposure preparation and patient care. Additionally, the tomography section is expanded to include tomosynthesis, in order to provide a wider understanding as to the capabilities of this digital technique.

Overall the book describes radiographic techniques undertaken using either computed radiography (CR) or direct digital radiography (DDR) equipment, which continues to advance both in terms of capability and detector size and weight. However, there is recognition that screen/film and chemical processing still exists and this is reflected in some of the text.

With respect to the standard template for the general radiographic technique, the familiar sub-heading 'Direction and centring of the X-ray beam' has been replaced with 'Direction and location of the X-ray beam'. This slight change is meant to focus on the fact that the beam should be collimated to the area of interest whilst still paying attention to the general guidance related to centring points.

The Paediatric chapter has been updated with a number of images included focusing on image evaluation and the Dental chapter updated to include coned beam computed tomography.

This edition contains a number of helpful references compared to previous editions with a number of suggestions for further reading.

We hope that these changes will improve the usefulness of the book and its relevance to current radiographic practice, and provide a lasting tribute to the originator, Miss K.C. Clark.

Acknowledgements to the 13th edition

We are indebted for the help and advice given by a vast range of colleagues throughout the radiological community with contributions enthusiastically given by radiographers, radiologists, physicists, lecturers from many learning institutions and colleagues in the medical imaging industry and UK government public bodies. Particular thanks go to Philips Healthcare and Agfa HealthCare for their financial support in sponsoring much of the artwork of the book.

We would particularly like to thank all of our partners and families who patiently endured the long process and the support and from many staff within the School of Medical Imaging Sciences, University of Cumbria and the X-ray Department at Blackpool Victoria Hospital who assisted with many aspects of the book.

Our thanks go to Joshua Holmes who ably undertook the majority of new positioning photographs of the book.

Thanks are also given to the many models who patiently posed for the photographs. These were drawn mainly from radiography students based at the Carlisle, Blackburn and Blackpool Hospital sites. The students include Louise Storr, Clare McFadden, Riad Harrar, Nicole Graham and Laith Hassan. Other models who we also thank include Kevin Ney, Malcolm Yeo, Amanda Spence, Simon Wilsdon and Mark Jackson and others who acted as models in the 12th edition but were not mentioned specifically.

We also would like to acknowledge the support provided by Philips Healthcare, GE Healthcare, Med Imaging UK (Liverpool) and Siemens Healthcare for their assistance in the provision of a number of diagrams, photographs and images, with thanks to Stephanie Holden, Steve Oliver, Catherine Rock and Dawn Stewart.

Thanks also go to the many departments who kindly provided images and photographs and in particular Lesley Stanney, Terry Gadallah, Elaine Scarles and Chris Lund of Blackpool Victoria Hospital, Rosemary Wilson of the Royal Lancaster Infirmary, Michael MacKenzie of the Pennine Acute Hospitals NHS Trust, Andrea Hulme of the Royal Manchester Childrens Hospital and Bill Bailey, Radiology Management Solutions Ltd, Radiology management solutions, Elite MRI Ltd.

We are particularly indebted for specific and detailed advice and illustrations to the following colleagues: Alistair Mackenzie, Research Physicist, NCCPM, Medical Physics Department, Royal Surrey County Hospital, Guildford; Andy Shaw, Group Leader Medical Physicist, North West Medical Physics, Christie Hospital, Manchester; Alexander Peck, Information Systems Manager, PACS/RIS/Agfa Cardiology, Royal Brompton & Harefield NHSFT, London; Paul Charnock, Radiation Protection Advisor and Ben Thomas, Technical Officer, Integrated Radiological Services (IRS) Ltd, Liverpool, UK; Anant Patel, Barts Health NHS Trust; Adham Nicola and Neil Barron, London North West Hospitals NHS Trust; and Keith Horner, Professor, School of Dentistry, University of Manchester, UK.

Thanks also go to Sue Edyvean, Kathlyn Slack and Sarah Peters from Public Health England for their DRL advice and providing equipment photographs and to Dr Frank Gaillard (Melbourne), founder of Radiopaedia.org, for access to images. Lastly, thanks go to Professor Maryann Hardy for her encouragement and helpful advice in a number of aspects of radiographic technique.

We also acknowledge those contributors for the 12th edition whose help and advice is still used in the 13th edition. These include: Dr Tom Kane, Mrs K. Hughes, Mrs Sue Field, Mrs R. Child, Mrs Sue Chandler, Miss Caroline Blower, Mr Nigel Kidner, Mr Sampath, Dr Vellore Govindarajan Chandrasekar and Sister Kathy Fraser, Blackpool Victoria Hospital; Dr J.R. Drummond, Dental School, University of Dundee; the International Association of Forensic Radiographers; Keith Taylor, University of Cumbria, Lancaster; and Elizabeth M. Carver (née Unett) and Barry Carver, University of Wales, Bangor.

Acknowledgements to previous editions

Miss K.C. Clark was Principal of the ILFORD Department of Radiography and Medical Photography at Tavistock House, from 1935 to 1958. She had an intense interest in the teaching and development of radiographic positioning and procedure, which resulted in an invitation by Ilford Ltd to produce *Positioning in Radiography*.

Her enthusiasm in all matters pertaining to this subject was infectious. Ably assisted by her colleagues, she was responsible for many innovations in radiography, playing a notable part in the development of mass miniature radiography. Her ability and ever active endeavor to cement teamwork between radiologist and radiographer gained worldwide respect.

At the conclusion of her term of office as President of the Society of Radiographers in 1936 she was elected to Honorary Fellowship. In 1959 she was elected to Honorary Membership of the Faculty of Radiologists and Honorary Fellowship of the Australasian Institute of Radiography.

Miss Clark died in 1968 and the Kathleen Clark Memorial Library was established by the Society of Radiographers. Today the library can be accessed by request at the Society and College of Radiographers.

The ninth edition was published in two volumes, edited and revised by James McInnes FSR, TE, FRPS, whose involvement with *Positioning in Radiography* began in 1946 when he joined Miss Clark's team at Tavistock House. He originated many techniques in radiography and in 1958 became Principal of Lecture and Technical Services at Tavistock House, which enabled him to travel as lecturer to the Radiographic Societies of Britain, Canada, America, South and West Africa.

The 10th edition, also published in two volumes, was revised and edited by Louis Kreel MD, FRCP, FRCR, a radiologist of international repute and wide experience of new imaging technologies.

The 11th edition, totally devoted to plain radiographic imaging, was edited by Alan Swallow FCR, TE and Eric Naylor FCR, TE and assisted by Dr E J Roebuck MB, BS, DMRD, FRCR and Steward Whitley FCR, TDCR. Eric and Alan were both principals of Schools of Radiography and well respected in the radiography world and champions in developing and extending radiography education to a wide radiographer and radiological community.

The 12th edition again totally devoted to plain radiographic imaging was edited by A. Stewart Whitley, FCR, TDCR, Charles Sloane MSC DCR DRI Cert CI, Graham Hoadley BSc (Hons), MB BS, FRCR, Adrian D. Moore MA, FCR, TDCR and Chrissie W. Alsop DCR. This successful team, representing both clinical and academic environments, was responsible for updating the text during the transition to digital radiography and adding a number of new features to the book.

We are indebted to these editors and the many radiographers and radiologists who contributed to previous editions for providing us with the foundations of the current edition and we hope that we have not failed to maintain their high standards.

Abbreviations

A&E	accident and emergency	IRMER	Ionising Radiation (Medical Exposure) Regulations
ACJ	acromio-clavicular joint	GCS	Glasgow Coma Scale
AEC	automatic exposure control	GIT	gastrointestinal tract
ALARP	as low as reasonably practicable	GP	general practitioner
AP	antero-posterior	HB	horizontal beam
ASIS	anterior superior iliac spine	HDU	High-dependency unit
ATLS	Advanced Trauma and Life Support	HIS	hospital information system
BSS	Basic Safety Standards	HPA	Health Protection Agency
CBCT	cone beam computed tomography	HSE	Health and Safety Executive
CCD	charge-coupled device	HTTP	hypertext transfer protocol
CCU	Coronary care unit	IAEA	International Atomic Energy Agency
CDH	congenital dislocation of the hip	ICRP	International Commission on Radiological Protection
CEC	Commission of European Communities	IRMER	Ionising Radiation (Medical Exposure) Regulations
CHD	congenital hip dysplasia	ITU	Intensive treatment unit
CID	charge-injection device	IV	intravenous
CMOS	complementary metal oxide semiconductor	IVU	intravenous urogram/urography
CPD	continued professional development	KUB	kidneys–ureters–bladder
CR	computed radiography	LAO	left anterior oblique
CSF	cerebrospinal fluid	LBD	light beam diaphragm
CSU	Cardiac surgery unit	LDR	local diagnostic reference level
CT	computed tomography	LMP	last menstrual period
CTU	computed tomography urography	LPO	left posterior oblique
CTR	cardio-thoracic ratio	LUL	left upper lobe
CXR	chest X-ray	LUT	look-up table
DAP	dose–area product	MC	metacarpal
DCS	dynamic condylar screw	MCPJ	metacarpo-phalangeal joint
DDH	developmental dysplasia of the hip	MO	mento-occipital
DDR	direct digital radiography	MPE	medical physics expert
DHS	dynamic hip screw	MPR	multiplanar reformatting/reconstruction
DICOM	digital imaging and communications in medicine	MRCP	magnetic resonance cholangiopancreatography
DNA	deoxyribonucleic acid	MRI	magnetic resonance imaging
DP	dorsi-palmar/dorsi-plantar	MRSA	methicillin resistant *Staphylococcus aureus*
DPO	dorsi-plantar oblique	MSCT	multislice computed tomography
DPT	dental panoramic tomography	MT	metatarsal
DQE	detection quantum efficiency	MTF	modulation transfer function
DRL	diagnostic reference level	MTPJ	metatarso-phalangeal joint
DTS	digital tomosynthesis	MUA	manipulation under anaesthetic
ECG	electrocardiogram	NAI	non-accidental injury
EI	exposure indicator	NGT	naso-gastric tube
EAM	external auditory meatus	NICE	National Institute for Health and Care Excellence
EPR	electronic patient record	NM	nuclear medicine
ESD	entrance skin/surface dose	NNU	Neonatal unit
ETT	endotracheal tube	NRPB	National Radiological Protection Board
FB	foreign body	OA	osteoarthritis
FFD	focus-to-film distance	OF	occipto-frontal
FO	fronto-occipital	OFD	object-to-focus distance/object-to-film distance
FOD	focus-to-object distance	OM	occipito-mental
FoV	field-of-view		
FRD	focus-to-receptor distance		
FSD	focus-to-skin distance		
II	image intensifier		

OPG	orthopantomography	SCBU	Special care baby unit
ORD	object-to-receptor distance	SD	standard deviation
ORIF	open reduction and internal fixation	SIDS	sudden infant death syndrome
PA	postero-anterior	SMV	submento-vertical
PACS	picture archiving and communication system	SOD	source-to-object distance
PAS	patient administration system	SP	storage phosphor
PCNL	percutaneous nephrolithotomy	SPR	storage phosphor radiography
PET	positron emission tomography	SS	solid state
PNS	post-nasal space	SUFE	slipped upper femoral epiphysis
PPE	personal protective equipment	SXR	skull X-ray
PPR	photostimulable phosphor radiography	TB	tuberculosis
PSL	photostimulable luminescence	TFT	thin-film transistor
PSP	photostimulable phosphor	TLD	thermoluminescent dosimeter
QA	quality assurance	TMJ	temporo-mandibular joint
RBL	radiographic baseline	TOD	table-to-object distance
RIS	Radiology information system	UAC	umbilical arterial catheter
RML	right middle lobe	US	ultrasound
RPA	Radiation Protection Advisor	UVC	umbilical venous catheter
RPS	Radiation Protection Supervisor	VNA	vendor neutral archive
SCIWORA	spinal cord injury without radiological bony injury	WHO	World Health Organization
		XDS-I	cross enterprise document sharing for imaging

Section 1

Basic Principles of Radiography and Digital Technology

CONTENTS

TERMINOLOGY	2
Introduction	2
Image evaluation – 10-point plan	8
Anatomical terminology	13
Positioning terminology	13
Projection terminology	17
THE RADIOGRAPHIC IMAGE	22
Image formation and density	22
Contrast	23
Magnification and distortion	25
Image sharpness	26
Image acquisition and display	28
DIGITAL IMAGING	29
Image acquisition	29
Factors affecting image quality	31
Imaging informatics	32
Image processing	36

EXPOSURE FACTORS	39
Introduction	39
Milliampere seconds	40
Kilovoltage	40
Focus-to-receptor distance	41
Intensifying screens	41
Digital imaging	41
Secondary radiation grids	42
Choice of exposure factors	42
SUMMARY OF FACTORS CONTRIBUTING TO OPTIMUM RADIOGRAPHIC IMAGE QUALITY	43
RADIATION PROTECTION	44
Medical exposure	44
Occupational exposure	49

1 Terminology

Introduction

The patient journey

Successful radiography is dependent on many factors but uppermost is the patient's experience during their short journey and encounter with the Diagnostic Imaging Department (see Fig. 1.3). The radiographer has a duty of care to the patient and must treat them with respect and ensure their dignity is maintained. It is essential that the radiographer establishes a rapport with the patient and carers. The radiographer must introduce themselves to the patient/carer and inform them of their role in the examination. They must make sure the request form is for the patient being examined and that the clinical details and history are accurate. The radiographer must request consent from the patient and the patient must give consent for the examination before the radiographer starts the examination.

The flow chart demonstrating a systematic way of undertaking an X-ray examination is on page 7. The purpose of the flow chart is to ensure that the patient journey is patient focussed and mistakes are eliminated. The key aspects are:

- Effective communication with patients and carers.
- The ability to follow a logical framework in order to be able to perform the X-ray examination proficiently and effectively.
- Efficient use of technology to produce diagnostic images at the first attempt.
- Evaluation of the radiographic image using the 10-point plan.

Whilst there are several 'main headings' to the algorithm it is essential to emphasise that the primary focus is the patient and their interaction within the process. Effective communications encompasses a myriad of interactions, which include being 'open and friendly' to the patient, telling them who you are, what you are intending to do, gaining consent and also inviting and answering any questions they may have about the examination.

Stages of an X-ray examination

There are 3 stages to undertaking an X-ray examination, preparation, the radiographic procedure itself and follow up from the examination undertaken. Each of these stages can be further subdivided as shown below:

Preparation for the examination:

- The request form.
- The X-ray room.
- The patient, including consent for the examination and identity checks.

Undertaking the examination:

- Patient care.
- Radiographic procedure.
- Radiation protection.

Post-examination and aftercare:

- Image quality.
- Patient aspects.
- Imaging informatics.

Preparation for the examination

The request form

- Ensure the examination requested is authorised and signed with a suitable rationale.
- Make sure the examination is justified using the IR(ME)R 2000 regulations[1] and the request card has a justifiable clinical reason for the X-ray, e.g. history of injury and pain in the metacarpal region ?fractured foot.
- Any examination using X-rays must affect the management of the patient.
- Check the protocol for the examination.
- Make sure you know which projections are required, e.g. DP and oblique foot.

Preparation of the X-ray room

- Make sure the X-ray room is clean, safe and tidy, ensure that the floor is clear and the X-ray tube is not in a position where the patient can walk into it.
- Set a preliminary exposure for the examination, i.e. X-ray tube focus size, mAs and kV.
- Have any accessory equipment available, e.g. foam pads and lead-rubber.

Preparation of the patient

- Correctly note the details on the request form ready for checking with the patient:
- Patient's full name, date of birth and address.
- Correct examination requested and reason for the X-ray.
- Is the patient fit and ambulant or have any physical needs?
- Mode of transport.

If applicable ensure the patient is undressed and dress them in a radiolucent gown.

The patient is asked:

- If they have carried out any required preparation for the examination.
- If they understand the nature of the examination and if they have any questions prior to proceeding.
- For verbal permission to proceed with the examination.
- For written consent if an examination incurs a higher risk, e.g. angiography.

To be able to give consent (adult or child) the patient should meet the following criteria. They should:

- Understand the risk versus benefit.
- Understand the nature of the examination and why it is being performed.
- Understand the consequences of not having the examination.
- Be able to make and communicate an informed decision.

If these conditions are not satisfied then other individuals may be able to give consent, e.g. parents, or in an emergency situation the examination may proceed if it is considered in the best interest of the patient (see hospital policy). Page 7 has a full page timeline.

Undertaking the examination

Patient care

At the commencement of the examination introduce yourself to the patient and ask permission to take the X-ray. If the patient has been prepared for the examination, check they have followed the instructions, e.g. undressed appropriately and in a gown, nil by mouth or any other preparation. Make a positive identity check on the patient using the details on the request form and ensure that the correct examination is indicated along with the rationale for the X-ray examination.

- Check the pregnancy status of the patient.
- Check for the patient's infection status, i.e. MRSA or other transferable diseases, to prevent cross infection by appropriate methods.
- Visibly clean hands in front of the patient before you start the procedure.
- Patient identity. Once again the patients' identity is established using the departmental protocol, which normally asks the patient to state their full name, address and date of birth. These are then cross referenced with the request form. The examination must not proceed unless the radiographer is sure of the identity of the patient.

Terminology 1

Introduction (*cont.*)

The procedure is explained to the patient in easy to understand terms.

Radiographic procedure

It is important that the department protocols are followed for the examination and that the equipment is used safely and proficiently. The preliminary exposure should be set on control panel (make sure the exposure factors are optimised for the patient body type).

As part of the procedure ensure:

- The patient is positioned accurately in relation to the examination being undertaken.
- The X-ray tube is positioned and centred to the patient and image receptor.
- The beam is collimated to the area of interest.
- Appropriate radiation protection is carried out.
- An anatomical marker is correctly applied to the image receptor.
- Instructions are effectively communicated to the patient.
- Radiographers and other staff/carers stand behind the lead glass protective control screen and exposure undertaken after the exposure factors confirmed on control panel.
- Image acquisition is correct first time.
- The patient waits whilst the image is checked.
- The image is assessed for diagnostic quality.
- You wash your hands or clean them with alcohol gel in sight of the patient.
- You consider using pads and sandbags to immobilise the patient when necessary. Distraction techniques may also be of value with paediatric patients.

1 Terminology

Introduction (cont.)

Radiation protection

Patient protection

Radiation protection and patient dose matters are discussed in depth at the end of this chapter. The following section summarises some of the important aspects of the examination, which includes before and during the procedure both in terms of the patient, staff and carers with consideration to relevant legislation.

On reviewing a request for an X-ray examination, the radiographer needs to consider carefully if the request for the examination is appropriate and has sufficient information to undertake it. In other words – is the examination justified? The radiographer should consider several questions when assessing any request for imaging:

Will the examination change the clinical management of the patient?

- While this can be a contentious area, the radiographer should consider if the requested examination will be of benefit to the patient and if the findings will affect the treatment or management of the patient. If the examination is not going to change the management of the patient the radiographer should seek further information from the referrer until they are satisfied the request is justified.
- The Radiographer has a duty of care to have a further discussion with the referrer. This must establish if the examination is justified or not under the radiation regulations and protocols of the department.

Does the completed request comply with local protocols?
For example, is the request card completed in a legible manner? Are the requested projections in line with the departmental protocol?

What are the risks/ benefits of the examination?
Even low X-ray doses can cause changes to cell DNA, leading to increased probability of cancer occurring in the years following the exposure. While in many cases the probability of this occurring is low, this risk should always be balanced against the benefits of the patient undergoing the examination. This is often acutely emphasised when a seriously ill patient or a young patient undergoes frequent X-ray examinations and the need to consider carefully each request is very important. Consultation with radiological colleagues is often required if there is any doubt over the legitimacy of any request.

Does the request comply with government legislation?
Legislation varies between countries; however, the request should comply with national legislation where applicable.

In the UK the underlying legislation is known as the Ionising Radiation (Medical Exposure) Regulations (IRMER) 2000.[1] This legislation is designed to protect patients by keeping doses 'as low as reasonably practicable' (ALARP). The regulations set out responsibilities:

- Those that refer patients for an examination (Referrers).
- Those that justify the exposure to take place (Practitioners).
- Those that undertake the exposure (Operators).

Radiographers frequently act as practitioners and operators and as such must be aware of the legislation along with the risks and benefits of the examination to be able to justify it.

Is there an alternative imaging modality?
The use of an alternative imaging modality that may provide more relevant information or the information required at a lower dose should be considered. The use of non-ionising imaging modalities, such as ultrasound and MRI should also be considered where appropriate.

Optimisation of radiographic exposure
The radiographer has a duty of care to ensure that the exposure delivered to the patient conforms to the departmental optimisation policy. This ensures that that the ALARP principle has been applied.[2]

Optimisation will involve consideration of a number of factors associated with image acquisition including:

- Exposure factors applied.
- Image detector system used.
- Patient compliance.
- Collimation and field size.

Diagnostic reference levels
Statutory dose limits do not apply to individual medical exposures. However, IRMER requires employers to establish diagnostic reference levels (DRLs) for their standard diagnostic and interventional procedures in order to assess whether these exposures are optimised. These local DRLs are based on the typical doses received by average sized patients when they undergo common procedures. DRLs have been established as a critical method in determining if a patient has been over irradiated. Contemporary practice will involve imaging departments publishing a list of DRLs for all common X-ray examinations. Patient dose must be recorded for all examinations. This will be given in different formats such as:

- Dose (kerma) area product (DAP) – Gy cm^2.
- Entrance surface (skin) dose (ESD) – mGy.
- Exposure factors/examination room.
- Fluoroscopy times.

This will be explained fully in the radiation protection section at the end of this chapter, but it is important that the radiographer ensures that the local DRL has not been exceeded.

Pregnancy

Avoiding exposure in pregnancy

All imaging departments should have written procedures for managing the small but significant radiation risk to the foetus (Fig. 1.1). Radiographers should refer to their departmental working procedures and apply them as part of their everyday working practice. The chart opposite has been constructed using joint guidance from the Health Protection Agency, the College of Radiographers and the Royal College of Radiologists (2009). Most departmental procedures will follow a similar procedure although practices may vary between departments according to specific circumstances. The procedure for pregnancy is usually applied to examinations that involve the primary beam exposing the pelvic area. Examinations of other areas can be undertaken as long as the radiographer ensures good beam collimation and employs the use of lead protection for the pelvis.

Evaluating and minimising the radiation risks in pregnancy

If a decision is made to irradiate a woman who is pregnant it will be in conjunction with the referring clinician who will have decided that there are overriding clinical reasons for the examination to take place. In such cases the relatively small radiation risk to the patient/foetus will be outweighed by the benefit of the diagnosis and subsequent treatment of potentially life-threatening or serious conditions. These could present a much greater risk to both parties if left undiagnosed.

To minimise the risks when examining pregnant women the radiographer should adopt the following strategies:

- Use of the highest imaging speed system available, e.g. 800 speed or equivalent settings for CR/DDR.
- Limit collimation to area of interest.
- Use of shielding (can the uterus be shielded without significant loss of diagnostic information?).
- Use of the minimum number of exposures to establish a diagnosis.
- Use of projections that give the lowest doses.
- Use pregnancy tests if doubt exists.

Staff and other personnel protection

Radiography is undertaken in conformance with relevant radiation legislation. This will be discussed in detail and the end of the section. The following section summarises some of the important protection aspects:

- Adherence to the local Radiation Rules.
- Monitoring of staff radiation doses.
- Staff doses conform with the ALARP principle. Adherence with the use of a controlled area both for static, mobile radiography and fluoroscopy.
- Collimation and limitation of X-ray beam.
- Use of personal protective equipment (PPE) when appropriate.
- Safe use of X-ray equipment.

Terminology 1

Introduction (*cont.*)

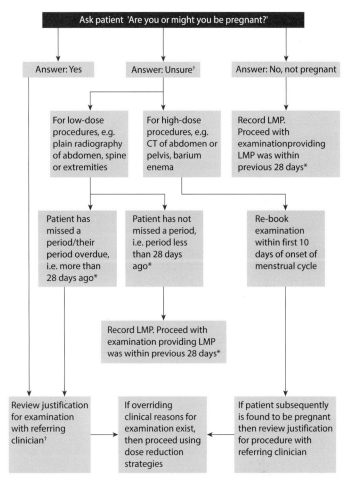

A typical 'pregnancy rule' for women of child-bearing age. *Some women have menstrual cycles of more or less than 28 days or have irregular cycles. CT, computed tomography; LMP, last menstrual period.

Fig. 1.1 Typical flow chart for 'pregnancy rule'.

Terminology

Introduction (cont.)

Post-examination and aftercare

Immediately following image acquisition the image will be reviewed to ensure it is of diagnostic quality; the patient will be managed and be given instructions as to what to do next and the examination will be completed in terms of the imaging information of the X-ray procedure.

Image quality

The image is reviewed using the '10-point plan':

1. Patient identification.
2. Area of interest is included.
3. Markers and legends.
4. Correct projection.
5. Correct exposure indicator (EI) – optimum EI and within acceptable range. Limited/no noise.
6. Optimum definition – can you see the detail of the relevant anatomy/structures, i.e. is it sharp?
7. Collimation is restricted to the area of interest.
8. Are there any artefacts and are they obscuring anatomy?
9. Any need for repeat radiographs or further projections.
10. Anatomical variations and pathological appearances.

Patient aspects

At this important stage of the procedure the Radiographer has a duty of care to ensure the patient is given and understands instructions. They need to know what to expect next in regard to the report from the examination, who will receive the report and how long this process will take. There will be local protocols to ensure the process is robust and the patient is managed effectively, e.g.:

- Go back to clinic immediately.
- The report will be posted to your GP within a certain time-frame.
- Arrange transport via porters/ambulance or ensure the patient has transport home.
- It is important that the patient takes all their belongings and valuables home with them.
- The radiographer should answer any questions the patient or carers may have on the examination /process within their scope of practice.

Imaging informatics

- It is important that the acquired images are viewed carefully using optimised conditions, e.g. ambient light conditions and the monitor is correctly adjusted. This may mean manipulating the image on the workstation monitor to demonstrate different areas of the image (Fig. 1.2).
- For extremity and axial radiography ensure an acquired image of a body part is displayed on a single monitor in order to ensure optimum display (i.e. only one image per monitor).
- Department/manufacturers' recommendations regarding any specific algorithms associated with a body part must be followed.
- Any further post processing must be carefully considered before the images are sent to picture archiving and communication system (PACS).
- Check the EI is of an optimum value to evaluate exposure to the patient and there is minimal /no noise on the image.
- The images are sent to PACS so the referring clinician can view the image and the image can be reported by the reporting radiographer or radiologist.
- The examination is completed on the Radiology information system (RIS), making sure the image is in the correct patient folder and the documentation regarding exposure details/dose reading and number of images taken is completed.
- The radiographer who is acting as the practitioner and operator must be identified on the RIS system.

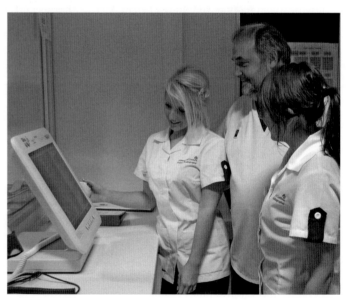

Fig. 1.2 Students and tutor at the monitor.

Terminology 1

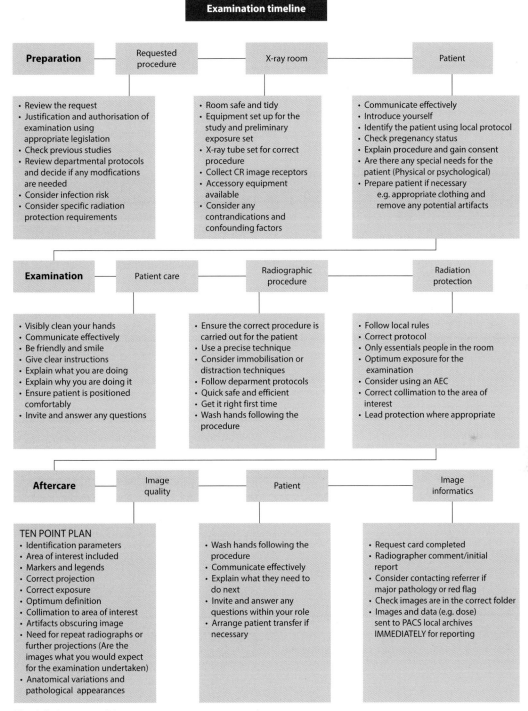

Fig. 1.3 Flow chart of the patient journey.

1 Terminology

Image evaluation – 10-point plan

It is imperative that radiographic images are properly evaluated to ensure that they are fit for purpose, i.e. they must answer the diagnostic question posed by the clinician making the request. In order to do this effectively the person undertaking the evaluation must be aware of the radiographic appearances of potential pathologies and the relevant anatomy that needs to be demonstrated by a particular projection. Points to consider when evaluating the suitability of radiographic images include:

1. Patient identification: do the details on the image match those on the request card and those of the patient who was examined? Such details will include patient name and demographics, accession number, date of examination and the name of the hospital.
2. Area of interest: does the radiograph include all the relevant areas of anatomy? The anatomy that needs to be demonstrated may vary depending on the clinical indications for the examination.
3. Markers and legends: check that the correct anatomical side markers are clearly visible in the radiation field. Ensure the marker that has been used matches the body part on the radiograph and that this in turn matches the initial request from the clinician. Ensure the correct legends have been included if not stated in the examination protocol, e.g. prone/supine. It is poor practice not to include a marker within the radiation field when making an exposure.[3]
4. Correct projections: does the acquired image follow standard radiographic technique as outlined throughout the book, with the patient being correctly positioned together with the appropriate tube angulation?

It is important to consider the pathology in question and the clinical presentation of the patient. If debating whether a projection is acceptable always consider if the 'diagnostic question' has been answered.

5. Correct exposure: the evaluation of the suitability of the exposure factors used for a radiograph will depend on the equipment and medium used to acquire and capture the image.

Conventional screen/film-based imaging

- Image density: the degree of image blackening should allow relevant anatomy to be sufficiently demonstrated, thus allowing diagnosis.
- Image contrast: the range of useful densities produced on the radiographic image should correspond to the structures within the area of interest. Each anatomical area should be of sufficient contrast to allow relevant anatomical structures to be clearly visualised.

Digital image acquisition systems

Given the wide exposure latitude of digital systems, the primary task when evaluating the image is to assess for over- or underexposure. The imaging equipment will usually give a numerical indication of the exposure used, the EI. The reading is compared with a range of exposure limits provided by the manufacturer to see if it is above or below recommended values. Unfortunately, the method used is not standardised by the different manufacturers.

Underexposure: images that are underexposed will show unacceptable levels of 'noise' or 'mottle' even though the computer screen brightness (image density) will be acceptable (Fig. 1.4a).

Overexposure: image quality will actually improve as exposure increases due to lower levels of noise. However, once a certain point is reached, further increases in exposure will result in reduced contrast. Eventually a point is reached when the image contrast becomes unacceptable (Fig. 1.4b).

NB: There is considerable scope for exposing patients to unnecessarily high doses of radiation using digital imaging technologies. When evaluating images it is important always to use the lowest dose that gives an acceptable level of image noise. The EI must be in the appropriate range and must be within the national and local DRLs.

6. Optimum definition: is the image sharp? Look at bone cortices and trabeculae to ensure movement or other factors have not caused an unacceptable degree of image unsharpness.

7. Collimation: has any of the area of interest been overlooked due to over-zealous collimation? Check relevant soft tissues have been included. Also look for signs of collimation to evaluate the success of the collimation strategy you used. This can then be used for future reference when performing similar examinations. Collimation outside the area of interest will increase both radiation dose and image noise (due to increased scattered photons).

8. Artefacts: are there any artefacts on the image? These may be from the patient, their clothing, the equipment or the imaging process. Only repeat if the artefact is interfering with diagnosis.

Terminology 1

Image evaluation – 10-point plan (*cont.*)

9. Need for repeat radiographs or further projections: a judgement is made from evaluations 1–8. If one or more factors have reduced the diagnostic quality to a point where a diagnosis cannot be made the image should be repeated. Would any additional projections enhance the diagnostic potential of the examination? For example, radial head projections for an elbow radiograph. If a repeat is required it may be appropriate to image only the area where there was uncertainty in the initial image.

10. Anatomical variations and pathological appearances: note anything unusual such as normal variants or pathology that may influence your future actions (see point 9) or aid diagnosis. For example, if an old injury is seen it may be worth questioning the patient about their medical history. This could then be recorded to aid diagnosis.

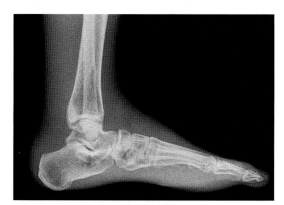

Fig. 1.4a Underexposed digital radiograph.

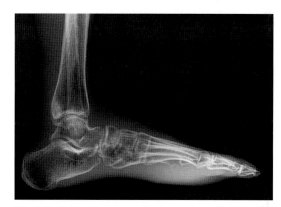

Fig. 1.4b Overexposed digital radiograph.

1 Terminology

Image evaluation – 10-point plan (cont.)

Image evaluation – Radiographer comments/initial report

As part of the image evaluation process the radiographer may also be required to provide an initial report in respect of the radiological appearances of the acquired image in order to aid prompt diagnosis. This is particularly important in the accident and emergency environment (A&E) where the experienced radiographer can make helpful comments to the referring clinician.

The methodology used is to apply an image assessment process gained via formal learning and experience to enable the radiographer to form an opinion as to whether the image is 'normal' or demonstrates a pathology/abnormality. The majority of current UK radiography degree courses include some element of 'red dot' teaching with basic image interpretation for undergraduate radiographers and there are also multiple study days for CPD of this subject area.

Radiographers due to their role have the greatest opportunity of any health professional to see a large number of 'normal' radiographs and thus have been shown to be able to identify 'abnormal' images or images with pathology with the appropriate training for this role expansion.[4] Some imaging departments operate a 'red dot' policy whereby radiographers simply flag any abnormality on an image; others use a 'Radiographer commenting' policy. Both act to enhance the radiographers' role and assist the A&E referrers to determine the appropriate treatment pathway for the patient.

The Society and College of Radiographers recognises two different levels of radiographer reporting:

Clinical reporting: carried out by advanced practitioners who have acquired a postgraduate qualification that enables them to produce a diagnostic report.

Initial reporting: where a radiographer makes a judgement based on their assessment of the image. It provides considered comments to the referrer rather than a simple 'red dot'. It should be made clear that although this may be in written form it does not constitute the equivalent of a formal report.[5]

Radiographers in the UK are encouraged to work to commenting/initial report level, but some radiographers are allowed to opt out of the process. If a 'red dot' is applied to the image but no comments added, then this may cause some confusion upon review of the image by the referrer as well as when the image is viewed for a formal clinical report.

The key points to include in the radiographers are comments are:

Abnormality	Yes / No
Description	? fracture/dislocation/other abnormality
Region of abnormality	e.g. distal radius

Suggestions for an image assessment/evaluation process

Gain an oral clinical history: obtaining a clinical history from the patient can be especially helpful for the radiographer to decide upon the correct projections required to demonstrate the injury, and a greater understanding of the area to check for injury.

Use a logical system for checking the image and any pathology: many different approaches to evaluate radiographs are suggested in the radiology literature. The 'ABCs' system provides a simple and systematic approach and has been adapted to systems other than the musculoskeletal. The ABCs stands for:

A: Adequacy; alignment. Check that the image adequately answers the clinical history/question. Are any additional projections required or repeat images needed?

B: Bones. Trace the cortical margins of all bones. Check for abnormal steps in the cortex and for any disruption in the trabecular pattern.

C: Cartilage. Alignment of all joints should be checked for signs of dislocations or subluxations. Check each joint space in an orderly fashion, looking specifically at the congruity and separation of the margins of the joint space. The bones should not overlap and the joint spaces should be uniform in width. Check for small avulsion fractures.

S: Soft tissue and foreign bodies. For example, be able to identify and recognise the significance of an elbow joint effusion or a lipohaemarthrosis (fat/blood interface within the knee or shoulder joint), all of which can be associated with an underlying fracture.

S: Satisfaction of search. If you spot one fracture, look for another. It is a common mistake to identify a fracture but miss a second by not checking the entire image. Be aware of principles such as the 'bony ring rule', which states that if a fracture or dislocation is seen within a bony ring (e.g. pelvis), then a further injury should be sought as there are frequently two fractures.

Utilise a system of pattern recognition: knowledge of normal anatomy and anatomical variants is essential. Radiographers encounter a number of 'normal' examinations and as such are well placed to use this knowledge to identify any changes in the normal 'pattern' of bones and joints. Many useful anatomical lines and measurements are used to check for abnormalities, for example 'McGrigor's three lines' for evaluating the facial bones. Whichever system is used try to apply it consistently and logically. This should reveal many subtle injuries.[6]

Pay attention to 'hot-spots': pay attention to where frequent pathology, trauma or abnormalities occur, such as the neck of the 5th metacarpal, the base of the 5th metatarsal, the dorsal aspect of the distal radius or the supracondylar region of the humerus in children. Frequently, the way the patient presents or reacts to positioning gives strong clues as to the position of the injury.[7]

The following examples of how image evaluation is applied are illustrated throughout the book using a standard template that the reader is encouraged to apply, using the basics principles of evaluating an image and providing an initial report.[8]

In these first examples comments are listed that are helpful in the checking process. In the other examples demonstrated not all correctly identified criteria are listed but only those main points to consider that may require further attention, with the assumption that the absence of comments indicates a satisfactory situation.

> Evaluation using the 10-point plan. In this example the patient has been referred for a possible fracture of the right hip.

1. Patient identification. Patient identity has been removed from the image but should include the patient name and another form of identification.
2. Area of interest. The area of interest is included and includes the top of the ilium superiorly, the lateral margins of the pelvic ring and proximal femora.
3. Markers and legends. The Left marker is applied to the left side of the patient.
4. Correct projection. The pelvis is not positioned correctly as the hips are not at the same anatomical level; however, the pelvis is not rotated and the pelvic ring is symmetrical. The right hip is not internally rotated so the femoral neck is foreshortened.
5. Image exposure. The EI is not indicated on the image; however, there is no noise in the image as the bony trabeculae can be clearly demonstrated.

Terminology

Image evaluation – 10-point plan (cont.)

6. Optimum definition. There is no blurring of the image and the structures appear to be well defined.
7. Collimation. The X-ray beam is collimated to the area of interest.
8. Artefacts. There are no artefacts obscuring the anatomy.
9. Need for repeat radiographs or further projections. Additional images are required. It is not possible to evaluate any fracture of the right hip without the hip being internally rotated. A lateral image is also required to determine the pathology.
10. Anatomical variations and pathological appearances. No significant anatomical variations. Evaluation of a fracture to the right hip needs to wait until a repeat hip X-ray and lateral is undertaken.

Radiographer Comments/Initial report

AP pelvis (Fig. 1.5)

AP pelvis demonstrating foreshortening of right femoral neck with a lateral projection required to exclude NOF #.

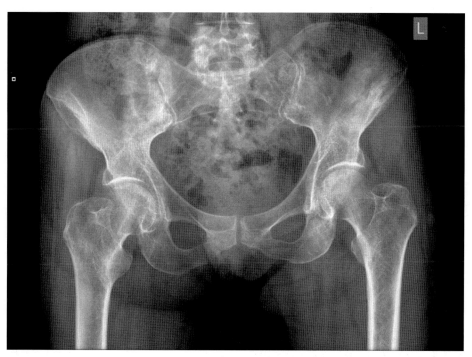

Fig. 1.5 Pelvic girdle.

1 Terminology

Image evaluation – 10-point plan

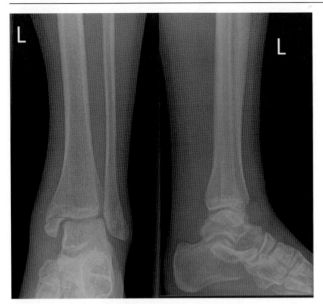

Fig. 1.6a AP and lateral ankle.

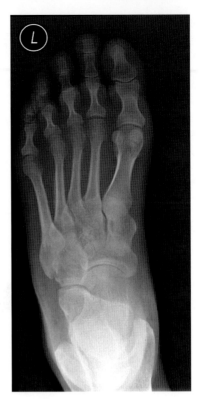

Fig. 1.6b DP foot.

In this example a 20-year-old male was referred for ankle X-ray following an injury playing football. The request was justified by the practitioner and the following images taken. Patient identification was confirmed on the RIS/PACS system.

In this example a 34-year-old female runner was referred from A&E with generalised forefoot pain, worse after exercise. The request was justified by the practitioner and the following image taken. Patient identification was confirmed on the RIS/PACS system.

IMAGE EVALUATION

AP & lateral ankle (Fig. 1.6a)

The main points to consider are:
- Images are of diagnostic quality with patient positioned optimally.
- There is an undisplaced fracture of the lateral malleolus.

Radiographer Comments/Initial report

Undisplaced fracture of the lateral malleolus.

IMAGE EVALUATION

DP foot (Fig. 1.6b)

The main points to consider are:
- Radio-opaque marker was applied post examination.
- Image is slightly over rotated.
- Image is well penetrated through the tarsal area.
- There is some early callus formation around the neck of the 3rd metatarsal (MT).

Radiographer Comments/Initial report

? Stress fracture neck of 3rd MT.

Terminology 1

The human body is a complicated structure. Errors in radiographic positioning or diagnosis can easily occur unless practitioners have a common set of rules that are used to describe the body and its movements.

This section describes terminology pertinent to radiography. It is vital that a good understanding of the terminology is attained to allow the reader to understand fully and practise the various techniques described in this text.

All the basic terminology descriptions below refer to the patient in the standard reference position, known as the anatomical position (see opposite).

Anatomical terminology

Patient aspect (Figs 1.7a–1.7e)

- Anterior aspect: that seen when viewing the patient from the front.
- Posterior (dorsal) aspect: that seen when viewing the patient from the back.
- Lateral aspect: refers to any view of the patient from the side. The side of the head would therefore be the lateral aspect of the cranium.
- Medial aspect: refers to the side of a body part closest to the midline, e.g. the inner side of a limb is the medial aspect of that limb.

Positioning terminology

Planes of the body (Fig. 1.7f)

Three planes of the body are used extensively for descriptions of positioning both in conventional radiography and in cross-sectional imaging techniques. The planes described are mutually at right-angles to each other.

- Median sagittal plane: divides the body into right and left halves. Any plane that is parallel to this but divides the body into unequal right and left portions is known simply as a sagittal plane or parasagittal plane.
- Coronal plane: divides the body into an anterior part and a posterior part.
- Transverse or axial plane: divides the body into an inferior and superior part.

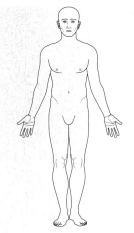

Fig. 1.7a Anatomical position.   Fig. 1.7b Anterior aspect of body.

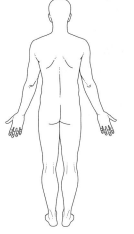
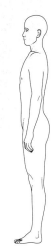

Fig. 1.7c Posterior aspect of body.   Fig. 1.7d Lateral aspect of body.

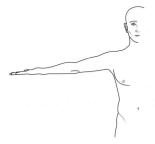

Fig. 1.7e Medial aspect of arm.

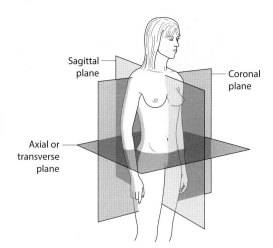

Fig. 1.7f Body planes.

1 Terminology

Positioning terminology (*cont.*) (Figs 1.8a–1.8e)

This section describes how the patient is positioned for the various radiographic projections described in the book.

Erect: the projection is taken with the patient sitting or standing. The patient may be standing or sitting when positioned erect with the:

- Posterior aspect against the image detector.
- Anterior aspect against the image detector.
- Right or left side against the image detector.

Decubitus: the patient is lying down. In the decubitus position, the patient may be lying in any of the following positions:

- Supine (dorsal decubitus): lying on the back.
- Prone (ventral decubitus): lying face-down.
- Lateral decubitus: lying on the side. Right lateral decubitus – lying on the right side. Left lateral decubitus – lying on the left side.

Semi-recumbent: reclining, part way between supine and sitting erect, with the posterior aspect of the trunk against the image detector.

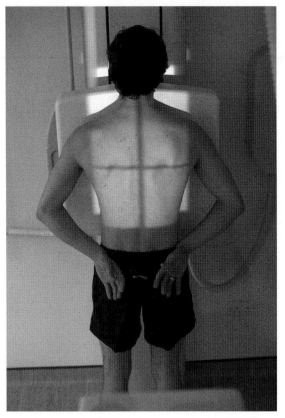

Fig. 1.8c Erect standing with the anterior aspect of the thorax against an erect detector.

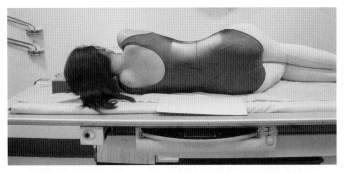

Fig. 1.8a Left lateral decubitus: the median sagittal plane is parallel to the table and the coronal plane is perpendicular to the table.

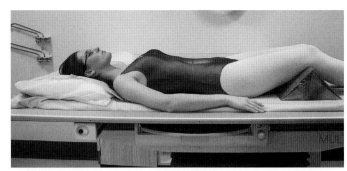

Fig. 1.8d Supine: the median sagittal plane is at right-angles to the table and the coronal plane is parallel to the table.

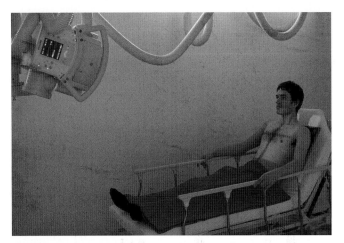

Fig. 1.8b Semi-recumbent, with posterior aspect of the thorax against the image detector and median sagittal plane perpendicular to the image detector (patient part-way between erect and supine).

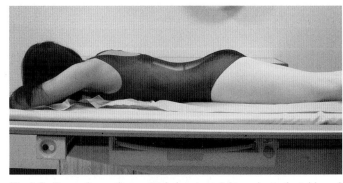

Fig. 1.8e Prone: the median sagittal plane is at right-angles to the table and the coronal plane is parallel to the table.

Terminology 1

Positioning terminology (*cont.*) (Figs 1.9a–1.9c)

All the positions may be described more precisely by reference to the planes of the body. For example, 'the patient is supine with the median sagittal plane at right-angles to the tabletop' or 'the patient is erect with the left side in contact with the image detector and the coronal plane perpendicular to the image detector'.

When describing positioning for upper limb projections, the patient will often be 'seated by the table'. The photograph below shows the correct position to be used for upper limb radiography, with the coronal plane approximately perpendicular to the short axis of the tabletop. The patient's legs will not be under the table, therefore avoiding exposure of the gonads to any primary radiation not attenuated by the image detector or the table.

When using direct digital radiography (DDR) systems radiography of the upper limb may be undertaken with the patient erect. This can reduce the time needed for the examination as the X-ray tube and detector may not need to be rotated from a previous erect examination. Careful planning can improve the throughput of patients.

CR technique may also be modified to X-ray the patient erect where their condition dictates this change. The CR cassette may be supported in an erect stand.

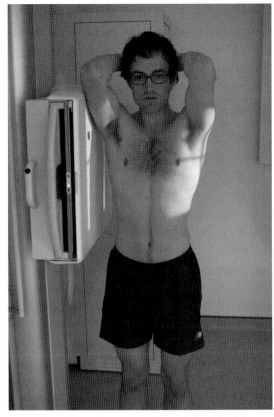

Fig. 1.9a Right lateral erect standing with the right side against the detector.

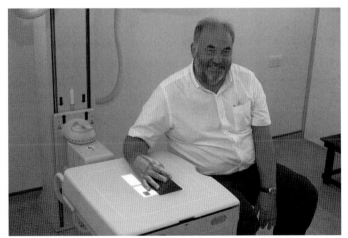

Fig. 1.9b Patient seated correctly for upper limb-radiography with the patient seated.

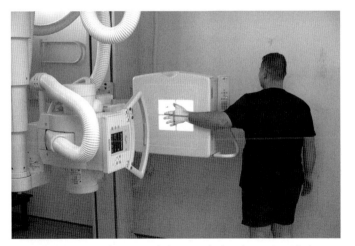

Fig. 1.9c Patient standing correctly for upper limb radiography with the patient erect.

1 Terminology

Positioning terminology (cont.) (Figs 1.10a–1.10h)

Terminology used to describe the limb position

Positioning for limb radiography may include:

- A description of the aspect of the limb in contact with the image detector.
- The direction of rotation of the limb in relation to the anatomical position, e.g. medial (internal) rotation towards the midline, or lateral (external) rotation away from the midline.
- The final angle to the image detector of a line joining two imaginary landmarks.
- The movements, and degree of movement, of the various joints concerned.

Definitions

- Extension: when the angle of the joint increases.
- Flexion: when the angle of the joint decreases.
- Abduction: refers to a movement away from the midline.
- Adduction: refers to a movement towards the midline.
- Rotation: movement of the body part around its own axis, e.g. medial (internal) rotation towards the midline or lateral (external) rotation away from the midline.
- Pronation: movement of the hand and forearm in which the palm is moved from facing anteriorly (as per anatomical position) to posteriorly.
- Supination is the reverse of pronation.

The terms applied to movement of specific body parts are illustrated in the diagrams.

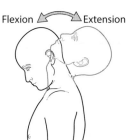

Fig. 1.10a Flexion and extension of the neck.

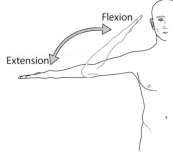

Fig. 1.10b Flexion and extension of the elbow.

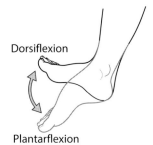

Fig. 1.10c Dorsiflexion and plantar flexion of the foot.

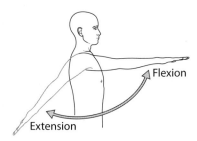

Fig. 1.10d Flexion and extension of the shoulder.

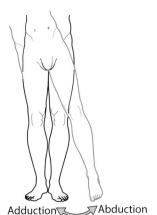

Fig. 1.10e Abduction and adduction of the hip.

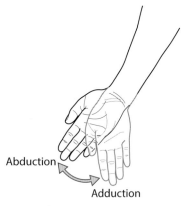

Fig. 1.10f Abduction and adduction of the wrist.

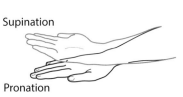

Fig. 1.10g Pronation and supination of the hand/forearm.

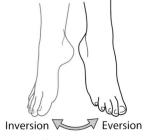

Fig. 1.10h Inversion and eversion of the foot.

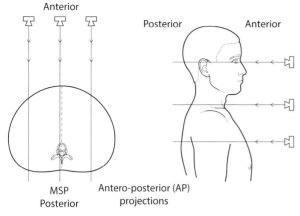

Fig. 1.11a Anterior-posterior (AP) projection extension of the neck.

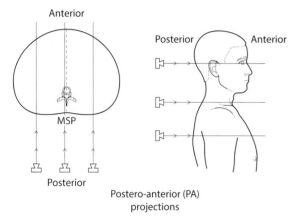

Fig. 1.11b Postero-anterior (PA) projection.

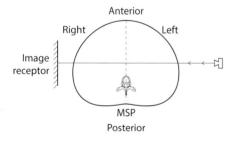

Fig. 1.11c Right lateral projection.

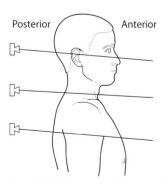

Fig. 1.11d Diagram with beam angled 15° caudal.

Terminology

Projection terminology

A projection is described by the direction and location of the collimated X-ray beam relative to aspects and planes of the body.

Antero-posterior (Fig. 1.11a)

The collimated X-ray beam is incident on the anterior aspect, passes along or parallel to the median sagittal plane and emerges from the posterior aspect of the body.

Postero-anterior (Fig. 1.11b)

The collimated X-ray beam is incident on the posterior aspect, passes along or parallel to the median sagittal plane, and emerges from the anterior aspect of the body.

Lateral (Fig. 1.11c)

The collimated X-ray beam passes from one side of the body to the other along a coronal and transverse plane. The projection is called a right lateral if the central ray enters the body on the left side and passes through to the image receptor positioned on the right side. A left lateral is achieved if the central ray enters the body on the right side and passes through to the image receptor, which will be positioned parallel to the median sagittal plane on the left side of the body.

In the case of a limb, the collimated X-ray beam is either incident on the lateral aspect and emerges from the medial aspect (latero-medial), or is incident on the medial aspect and emerges from the lateral aspect of the limb (medio-lateral). The terms 'latero-medial' and 'medio-lateral' are used where necessary to differentiate between the two projections.

Beam angulation (Fig. 1.11d)

Radiographic projections are often modified by directing the collimated X-ray beam at some angle to a transverse plane, i.e. either caudally (angled towards the feet) or cranially/cephalic angulation (angled towards the head). The projection is then described as for example below, PA with 15° caudal tilt.

1 Terminology

Projection terminology (cont.)

Oblique

The collimated X-ray beam passes through the body along a transverse plane at some angle between the median sagittal and coronal planes. For this projection the patient is usually positioned with the median sagittal plane at some angle between zero and 90° to the image receptor, with the central ray at right-angles to the image receptor. If the patient is positioned with the median sagittal plane at right-angles to or parallel to the image detector, then the projection is obtained by directing the central ray at some angle to the median sagittal plane.

Anterior oblique (Figs 1.12a, 1.12b)

The central ray enters the posterior aspect, passes along a transverse plane at some angle to the median sagittal plane, and emerges from the anterior aspect. The projection is also described by the side of the torso closest to the image detector. In the diagram below, the left side is closest to the image detector, and therefore the projection is a described as a left anterior oblique (LAO).

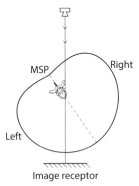

Left anterior oblique projection

Fig. 1.12a Left anterior oblique (LAO) projection.

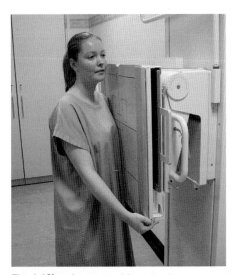

Fig. 1.12b Left anterior oblique (LAO) projection with patient erect.

Posterior oblique (Figs 1.12c, 1.12d)

The collimated X-ray beam enters the anterior aspect, passes along a transverse plane at some angle to the median sagittal plane, and emerges from the posterior aspect. Again, the projection is described by the side of the torso closest to the image receptor. The diagram below shows a left posterior oblique (LPO).

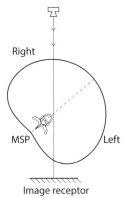

Left posterior oblique projection

Fig. 1.12c Left posterior oblique (LAO) projection.

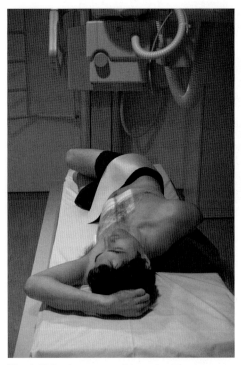

Fig. 1.12d Left posterior oblique (LPO) projection.

Oblique using beam angulation (Figs 1.13a, 1.13b)

When the median sagittal plane is at right-angles to the image receptor, right and left anterior or posterior oblique projections may be obtained by angling the central ray to the median sagittal plane.

Note: this cannot be done if using a grid, unless the grid lines are parallel to the central ray.

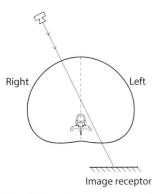

Fig. 1.13a LPO projection using beam angulation.

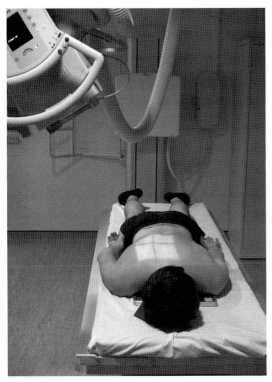

Fig. 1.13b LAO projection using beam angulation.

Terminology

Projection terminology (*cont.*)

Lateral oblique (Figs 1.13c, 1.13d)

The collimated X-ray beam enters one lateral aspect, passes along a transverse plane at an angle to the coronal plane, and emerges from the opposite lateral aspect. With the coronal plane at right-angles to the image receptor, lateral oblique projections can also be obtained by angling the central ray to the coronal plane.

Note: this cannot be done if using a grid, unless the grid lines are parallel to the central ray.

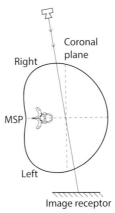

Left lateral oblique projection

Fig. 1.13c Lateral oblique projection obtained using beam angulation.

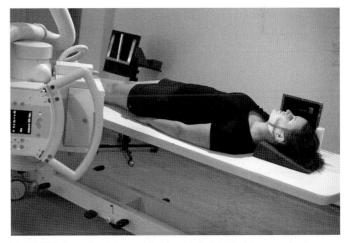

Fig. 1.13d Example of the position for a right lateral oblique projection.

1 Terminology

Projection terminology (cont.) (Figs 1.14a–1.14d)

The following sections describe the radiographic projections by reference to the following criteria:

- The position of the patient relative to the image receptor.
- The direction, location and centring of the collimated X-ray beam: this is given by reference to an imaginary central ray of the X-ray beam.
- Beam angulation relative to horizontal or vertical.

Examples of these are given below.

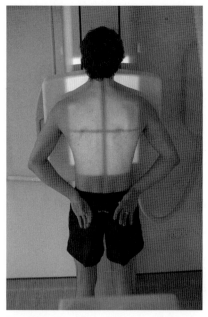

Fig. 1.14a Projection: PA.

Position: erect anterior aspect facing the image receptor with median sagittal plane at right-angles to the receptor.

Direction and location of the X-ray beam: the collimated horizontal beam is directed at right-angles to the receptor and centred at the level of the eighth thoracic vertebrae (i.e. spinous process of T7), which is coincident with the lung midpoint.

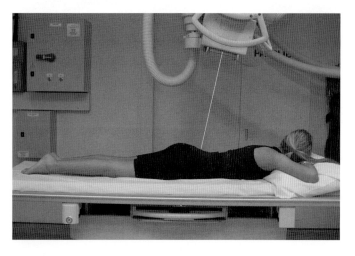

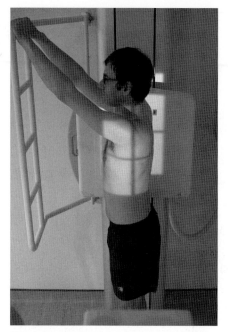

Fig. 1.14c Projection: left lateral.

Position: erect; median sagittal plane parallel to the image receptor placed in a vertical Bucky against the patient's left side.

Direction and location of the X-ray beam: the collimated horizontal central ray is directed at right-angles to the median sagittal plane and centred to the axilla in the mid-axillary line.

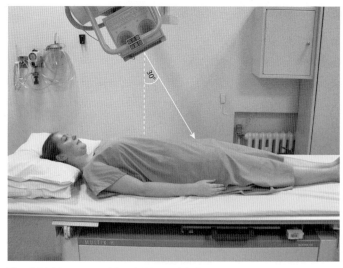

Fig. 1.14d Projection: AP with 30° caudal tilt.

Position: supine; median sagittal plane at right-angles to the table.

Direction and location of the X-ray beam: from the vertical, the central ray is angled 30° caudally and directed to a point 2.5 cm superior to the symphysis pubis.

Fig. 1.14b Projection: PA of the sacro-iliac joints with caudal tilt.

Position: prone, anterior aspect facing the image receptor, median sagittal plane perpendicular to the table and at right-angles to the image receptor.

Direction and location of the X-ray beam: the collimated vertical beam is angled 15° caudally at the level of the posterior superior iliac spines.

Terminology 1

Projection terminology (*cont.*) (Figs 1.15a–1.15d)

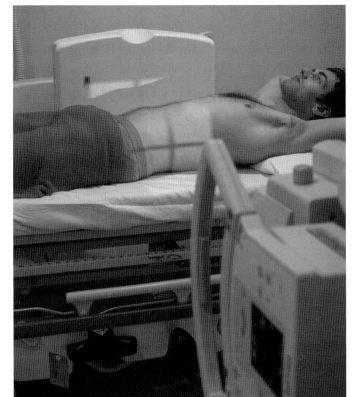

Fig. 1.15a Right lateral.

Projection: right lateral.

Position: supine; median sagittal plane parallel to the image receptor placed in a vertical Bucky against the patient's left side.

Direction and location of X-ray beam: the collimated horizontal central ray is directed at right-angles to the median sagittal plane to the lower costal margin in the mid-axillary line.

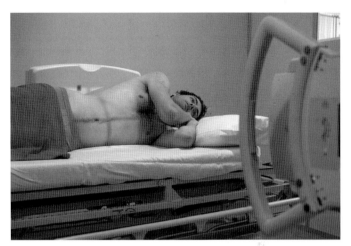

Fig. 1.15c Left lateral decubitus.

Projection: antero-posterior.

Position: left lateral decubitus. The median sagittal plane is parallel to the couch and right-angles to the image receptor, which is vertically against the patient's posterior aspect.

Direction and location of X-ray beam: the collimated horizontal X-ray beam is directed at right-angles to the anterior aspect of the patient in the midline and passes along the median plane at the level of the 3rd lumbar vertebra.

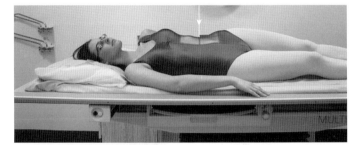

Fig. 1.15b Right posterior oblique.

Projection: right posterior oblique.

Position: supine and then rotated so that the left side is moved away from the table to bring the median sagittal plane at 45° to the table.

Direction and location of X-ray beam: the vertical beam central ray is directed to a point 2.5 cm to the right of the midline at the level of the 3rd lumbar vertebra.

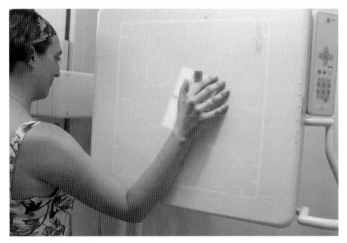

Fig 1.15d Lateral thumb.

Projection: lateral.

Position: patient erect adjacent to and facing the image receptor, with the arm extended and in contact with the vertical DDR detector. The thumb is flexed slightly and the palm of the hand is placed on the image receptor. The palm of the hand is raised slightly with the fingers partially flexed and may be supported on a non-opaque pad, such that the lateral aspect of the thumb is in contact with the image receptor.

Direction and location of X-ray beam: the collimated horizontal beam is centred over the 1st metacarpo-phalangeal joint.

1 The radiographic image

Image formation and density

The X-rays used in medical diagnosis are produced from a small area (focal spot) within the X-ray tube when an exposure is made. They diverge outwards from this area, travel in straight lines, and can be detected by a variety of image receptors used for medical imaging. As the X-rays pass through the body, some will be absorbed by the organs and structures within the body whilst others will pass through to the equipment used to form the image.

The term 'density' is often used in radiography. It can have different meanings depending on the context. In Fig. 1.16d the X-ray beam enters the body and then encounters various structures. The bone has a high density because it has a relatively high mass per unit volume and consequently will absorb more X-rays than the adjacent area of lung. The lung contains air, which has a relatively low mass per unit volume and therefore can be said to have a low density. When the beam emerges from the body, there will be more X-rays directly under the area of lung compared with the area directly under the bone.

The image is then captured using an image-acquisition device. When a relatively large number of X-rays are incident upon the detector (e.g. normal lung tissue), the image will appear to be quite dark and may be described as having a high density. The area under the bone will appear lighter, since fewer X-rays will come into contact with the detector. This area therefore has a lower image density.

When examining an image for radiological evidence of disease, the radiographer may refer to a small focal area of disease as a density within the image. Rather confusingly, this could be of a higher or lower image density compared with the surrounding tissues, depending on the organ or tissue involved, e.g. a tumour in the lung (higher density) or bone (lower density, depending on tumour type).

In summary, the term 'density' can be confusing.

- In the human body it refers to the mass per unit volume and is related to the attenuation properties of tissues.
- In film screen systems it refers to the 'optical density', which is a measure of the transmission of light through the film, or put crudely, 'blackening' within the image. The optical density is measured on film using a densitometer and is often referred to as the density on the film.
- Digital images viewed on a monitor: the density is represented by a greyscale and is displayed as differences in the screen brightness.
- In diagnosis: density can refer to a small defined area of pathology, e.g. a lung nodule.

Projection and view (Figs 1.16b–1.16d)

It is important to note that X-ray images are formed by projection, i.e. images of objects in the path of X-rays are projected onto a device for capturing the image, e.g. digital detector. This differs from the way in which images are formed on the retina of the eye or on the photographic film in a camera, where light travels from the object to the recording medium to produce an image that is a view of the object; a radiographic image is a projection of the object.

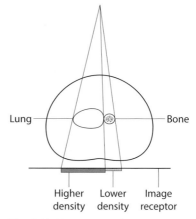

Fig. 1.16a Transmission density.

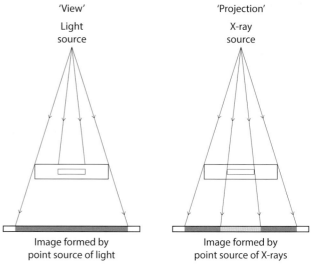

Fig. 1.16b View and projection.

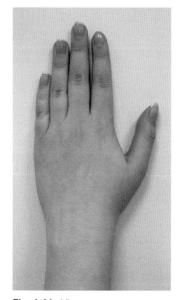

Fig. 1.16c View.

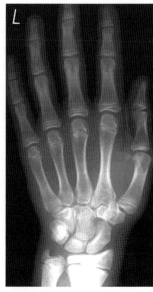

Fig. 1.16d Projection.

Photographic film

If the image is captured on a photographic emulsion, then the term 'photographic density' or 'optical density' should be used. Higher densities will be produced by greater exposures of radiation, which in turn leads to a form of silver being liberated from the photographic emulsion. This remains on the film after processing and produces the 'blackening' within the image. Photographic or optical density can be measured by determining the degree of opacity, i.e. the proportion of light absorbed by the processed film.

Digital image capture

If the image was captured by a digital system such as computed radiography (CR) or direct digital radiography (DDR), then the term 'image density' refers to the greyscale displayed on the monitor used to display the image. Put simply, it is the computer screen brightness.

The image-processing software will analyse the range of exposures that were captured by the image receptor (e.g. the CR phosphor screen). It will then assign the highest computer screen brightness to areas that have received relatively low exposures (low image density). Conversely, the lowest computer screen brightness (darkest areas) will be assigned to areas that have received a relatively high radiation exposure (high image density) (Fig. 1.17b).

Contrast

In order to detect pathology, an imaging system must be able to detect the differences in the density (patient density) of the pathology compared with that of the surrounding tissues. This must then be translated into differences in density within the final image (a digital image or film density) that are visible to the observer. Contrast is the difference in density between structures of interest within the image. A low-contrast image will show little difference in density between structures of interest, whereas a high-contrast image will show a larger difference in density between structure (Fig. 1.17a).

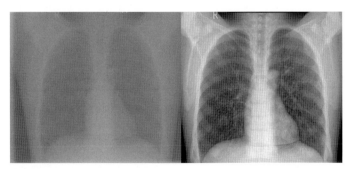

Fig. 1.17a Comparison of chest images with high and low contrast.

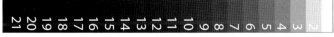

Fig. 1.17b Image of a step wedge showing a range of densities.

The radiographic image 1

Contrast

The contrast seen on a radiographic image (film) or digital display can be described in three ways:

- **Subject contrast** is a feature of the object (subject) under examination. The differences in radiation intensities emerging from the object result from the spatial distribution of X-ray attenuation within the object. At a given beam energy, the degree of beam attenuation between anatomical structures is determined by the physical density and atomic number of those structures. Differential absorption and therefore subject contrast will change if the beam energy (kV) is varied. A radiological contrast agent will also change the atomic number within an area of the object and hence subject contrast.
- **Subjective contrast** is the personal appreciation of the differences in optical density or computer screen brightness when the image is viewed. This varies with the experience and training of the viewer.
- **Radiographic contrast** is the difference in optical density on different parts of the processed film or differences in computer screen brightness recorded as a result of the range of emergent beam intensities.

Subject contrast

X-radiation passing through the body is attenuated by different amounts by the different thicknesses, densities and atomic numbers of the structures in the body. The beam emerging from the patient varies in intensity: more will emerge if the beam encounters only a small thickness of soft tissue. The difference in intensities in the emergent beam is called subject contrast or radiation contrast. Factors that influence subject contrast include the following:

- **The region of the body under examination.** There is less subject contrast if all parts of the region have a similar attenuation coefficient. Soft-tissue structures such as the breast have a low subject contrast, whereas the subject contrast increases if the region includes bone or large differences in the thickness of tissue. A good example of an area of the body that demonstrates high subject contrast is the chest.
- **Contrast media.** If high- or low-density/atomic number substances are introduced into cavities in a region, then there will be a greater difference in absorption of X-rays by different parts of that region and thus an increase in subject contrast.
- **Pathology.** If the density of a structure is changed due to pathology, then there will be a change in subject contrast; for instance, it will be reduced if the bone density reduces, as in osteoporosis.

1 The radiographic image

Contrast (*cont.*)

Subject contrast (*cont.*)

- **Kilovoltage (kV).** At lower kV, there is a greater difference in attenuation by structures of different density and atomic number than at higher kV. Therefore, at lower kV, there is a greater subject contrast. This can be used to advantage when examining areas of low subject contrast, such as the breast. Conversely, there is a high subject contrast within the chest (marked differences in patient density when comparing the lungs and the heart). A higher kV will therefore reduce this subject contrast and produce a more even image density.

Subjective contrast

When a radiographic image is viewed, the observer sees an image made up of structures of different light intensities i.e. range of densities. However, different observers might have a different/altered appreciation of the image contrast. The personal appreciation of the contrast in the image is called subjective contrast. Subjective contrast depends not only on the person but also on the viewing conditions. For example, if an image is viewed on a computer monitor and that monitor is placed near a window, then the sunlight incident upon the screen will severely impair the observer's ability to appreciate the density differences within the image. There may be good radiographic contrast but the observer cannot appreciate this because of the sunlight on the screen, so the subjective contrast will be low.

Subjective contrast depends on:

- The observer's visual perception and level of experience in viewing images. It may also depend on the time of day and how long the observer has been working.
- The viewing conditions, e.g. the type of monitor, the settings used on the monitor and ambient lighting.

Radiographic contrast

After leaving the patient, the X-radiation passes to an image-acquisition device. As it passes through the body, some of the radiation will be scattered. Scatter reduces the differences in X-ray intensity emerging from different areas of the body and thus reduces contrast. The effects of scatter can be controlled by:

- Collimating the beam or by the use of compression devices. In each of these cases, this reduces the volume of tissue irradiated and the amount of scatter produced.
- The use of a secondary radiation grid between the patient and the image receptor to reduce the scatter reaching the image receptor improves radiographic contrast.
- The use of an air gap technique will reduce the proportion of scatter photons reaching the image receptor. The scattered photons will 'miss' the detector due to their angle of deflection.

Once the image has been captured, it can be viewed either on computer monitor or in rare cases photographic film. The different patient densities are recorded either as varying photographic densities or as differences in computer screen brightness. These different densities can be measured either using densitometer or image-analysis software to give an objective measurement of contrast.

Thus, differences in measured image density between specified parts of the radiographic image may be described as radiographic or objective contrast.

The design and function of the image-acquisition device used to acquire the image can have a profound effect on contrast. In digital systems, the contrast is also influenced profoundly by the software used to process the initial image captured by the device. The contrast may also be 'post-processed' to enhance image quality. Certain types of film emulsion, intensifying screen and phosphor plate may be designed to give inherently greater contrast.

Film based systems

Contrast will also be dependent on a number of factors related to image capture using film. This will include:

- Film fog: if the image is viewed using a photographic-based system, then film fogging due to incorrect film handling or storage may reduce radiographic contrast.
- Exposure: if too much or too little radiation is used, then the film screen system may be unable to respond or may be saturated to the point that it is unable to function properly. In these examples, there may be a reduced range of densities or no difference in density visible on the image, thus radiographic contrast will be reduced or non-existent.
- Film processing/development: if a photographic emulsion is used to capture the image, then optimum radiographic contrast will be attained only if the film is developed correctly. This is achieved by careful control of factors such as developer temperature, development time and processing chemical activity. To ensure this, the film processor must be subject to a rigid quality-control regime.

Optimum radiographic image quality and contrast

In summary it is important to remember that the quality of the image perceived, i.e. subjective contrast is influenced both by the inherent *subject contrast* of the region under examination and the *radiographic contrast* related to the image acquisition system/process. These facts and some of the factors influencing them are highlighted on page 43.

The radiographic image 1

Magnification and distortion

Magnification (Fig. 1.18a, equation)

In a projected image, magnification will always be present because the X-rays continue to diverge as they pass from the object to the image receptor. The source of the X-rays is the X-ray tube focal spot. For a given focus-to-receptor distance (FRD), the greater the distance between the object and the detector, the greater will be the magnification of the image. To minimise magnification, the object under examination should be positioned in contact with the detector or as close as is reasonably possible.

If the object-to-detector distance has to be increased, e.g. in the case of a patient on a trolley, then the FRD can also be increased. This will then reduce the magnification caused by the above. (Note: an increase in exposure will be needed in this case due to the effect of the inverse square law on the beam intensity.)

Digital images

Magnification may not always apparent from the image on the monitor as the image is optimised for image viewing by the computing system and may appear 'life sized'. Measurements for the size of any object must never be taken from a monitor. If the exact size of a body structure is required, either specific software packages or imaging a known sized object, e.g. a ball bearing, within the patient image may be used to calculate the size of the object.

Image distortion (Figs 1.18b–1.18g)

A distorted image will be produced if not all parts of the image are magnified by the same amount. Considering a thin, flat object, there will be constant magnification and thus no distortion when the detector is parallel to the object. When possible, the part being radiographed should be placed parallel to the detector to avoid distortion. If the object and detector are not parallel to each other, then there is a difference in magnification of different parts of the object, leading to a distorted image.

In the diagrams opposite, the object and detector are not parallel to each other. It can be seen that if the centre of the X-ray beam is directed at right-angles to the object but the object is not parallel to the image receptor, then a distorted, elongated image is produced. If the centre of the beam is directed at right-angles to the image receptor but is angled in relation to the object, then a distorted, foreshortened image will be produced.

In cases when the object and detector cannot be parallel to each other, a compromise can be made by directing the central ray at right-angles to an imaginary line bisecting the angle between the object and the film. Although distortion does occur, the net effect is neither elongation nor foreshortening of the image. This technique may be required if a patient is unable to straighten a limb to bring it parallel to the detector when imaging a long bone. The bisecting angle technique is also used in dental radiography (see diagram opposite).

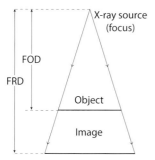

Fig. 1.18a Magnified image.

$$\text{Magnification} = \frac{\text{Image size}}{\text{Object size}} = \frac{\text{FRD}}{\text{FOD}}$$

where FOD is the focus-to-object distance.

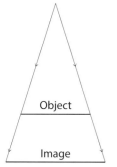

Fig. 1.18b Undistorted image.

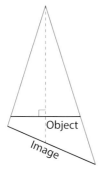

Fig. 1.18c Distortion: elongation.

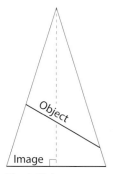

Fig. 1.18d Distortion: foreshortening.

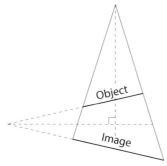

Fig. 1.18e Compromise projection: minimal distortion.

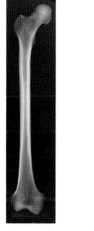

Fig. 1.18f Undistorted long bone.

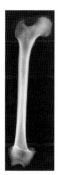

Fig. 1.18g Foreshortened long bone.

1 The radiographic image

Image sharpness

The aim in radiography is to produce images that have a minimal level of unsharpness in order to resolve fine detail within the image. This is particularly important when looking for subtle fractures or changes in bone architecture. Diagnostic images have a level of unsharpness which is not visible to the person viewing the image. This is approximately 0.3 mm and is determined by a number of factors:

- Geometry of the image production (Ug).
- Movement (Um).
- Absorption (inherent factors) (Ua).

Geometric unsharpness (Figs 1.19a, 1.19b)

If X-rays originated from a point source, then a perfectly sharp image would always be obtained. In an X-ray tube, however, the X-rays are produced from the small area of the focal spot on the anode. As can be seen from the diagram opposite, this leads to the formation of penumbra or 'partial shadows' at the edge of the object; it is this that gives rise to geometric unsharpness.

The degree of geometric unsharpness increases with an increased focal spot size and increased object-to-receptor distance:

$$\text{Geometric unsharpness (Ug)} = \frac{\text{Object-to-receptor distance (ORD)}}{\text{Focus-to-object distance (FOD)}} \times \text{focal spot size}$$

Geometric unsharpness can be a small, insignificant quantity if the object is close to the receptor and a small focal spot is used. For instance, with a PA projection of the wrist, where the maximum object-to-receptor distance is about 5 cm, and if a normal FRD of 100 cm is used, then geometric unsharpness is only 0.05 mm using a 1 mm focal spot and only 0.1 mm with a 2 mm focal spot (common focal spot sizes are 0.6 and 1.2 mm). When thicker parts of the body are being examined, which might require the use of a larger (broad) focal spot, then geometric unsharpness can make a significant contribution to total image unsharpness owing to the greater object-to-receptor distance.

Movement unsharpness (Fig. 1.19c)

This type of unsharpness is due to patient, equipment or detector vibration during the exposure. Patient movement may be involuntary, e.g. owing to heartbeat or peristalsis, or it may be the type of movement that may be controlled by immobilisation. It is important to note that any patient movement is magnified on the image because of the space between the moving object and the detector. Sharpness can be minimised by using a shorter exposure time (achieved by a lower mAs with higher kV, higher mA, or greater tube loading), by a small object-to-detector distance and particularly by immobilisation of the patient.

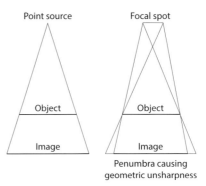

Fig. 1.19a Effect of finite focal spot.

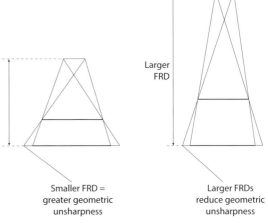

Fig. 1.19b Effect of FRD.

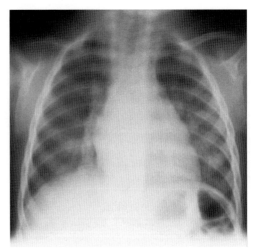

Fig. 1.19c Movement unsharpness.

Various accessories can be used for immobilisation, including non-opaque pads and sandbags to immobilise the extremities.

Distraction and immobilisation may be required to aid patients to keep still (Fig. 1.20b). Binders and Velcro straps may be used where appropriate. These accessories should be available in all examination rooms and should be used routinely. It is equally important to make the patient as comfortable as possible and to explain the procedure fully. The radiographer can also invite questions about the procedure, thus increasing the likelihood of achieving full cooperation from the patient. It may be worthwhile rehearsing respiratory manoeuvres prior to an actual exposure being made.

Absorption unsharpness (Fig. 1.20a)

This is due to the shape of the structures in the body. As illustrated, unless the structure has a particular shape, with its edges parallel to the diverging beam, then absorption of the X-ray beam will vary across the object. Considering a spherical object of uniform density, then absorption will be greatest at the centre and least at the periphery due to the difference in thickness. This gradual fall-off in absorption towards the edges leads to the image having an ill-defined boundary called absorption unsharpness. Note: most structures in the body have a round edge. Little can be done to reduce this type of unsharpness, apart from increasing image contrast or using digital edge-enhancement techniques.

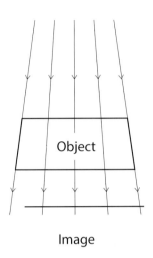
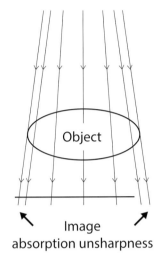

Fig. 1.20a Absorption unsharpness.

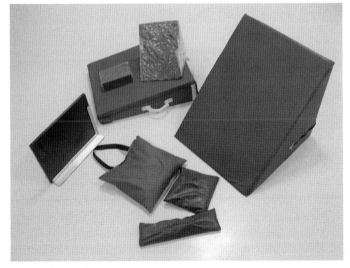

Fig. 1.20b Immobilisation devices.

The radiographic image

Image sharpness (cont.)

Geometric	Movement
Use smallest focal spot size	Patient comfort and support
Have the object being X-rayed in contact with the receptor if possible	Use short exposure times
Use a long FRD if the object is not in contact with the receptor, e.g. PA chest imaging to reduce magnification of the heart	Support/immobilise the patient when appropriate. Consider compression bands where available
	Explain the need to keep still and practise breathing techniques
	Give clear instructions and observe the patient to ensure they comply with the instructions

Table of methods to reduce unsharpness in the image

Spatial resolution

Spatial resolution refers to the ability of the imaging system to represent distinct anatomic features within the object being imaged. It may be defined as the ability of the system to distinguish neighbouring features of an image from each other and is related to sharpness. The maximum spatial resolution of a digital image is defined by pixel size and spacing. Pixel size affects the system resolution and varies between systems. Modulation transfer function (MTF) is used to fully characterise the spatial properties of an imaging system. (When MTF is combined with measurements of image noise, the overall system performance can be determined in terms of detection quantum efficiency (DQE).

Measurement of unsharpness in an image

The sharpness of the image can be measured using a test tool (resolution) or by viewing the image and determining if fine structures can be visualised (definition). The limiting resolution can be determined by measuring the ability of the imaging system to resolve the smallest object of the test tool and is expressed in line pairs per millimetre (lp mm^{-1}). This is an objective means to measure sharpness; however, from a subjective perspective sharpness can be determined by the naked eye by asking the question 'can I see the bony trabeculae?'.

Again however, definition within the image is subjective and depends on a number of factors including the resolution of the monitor, viewing conditions and the experience of the practitioner viewing the image.

1 The radiographic image

Image acquisition and display

Images can be acquired in using different systems depending on the equipment available in a particular imaging department. These include:

- Conventional screen/film technology.
- Fluoroscopy/fluorography.
- Digital imaging systems:
  - Computed radiography (CR).
  - Direct digital radiography (DDR).

Each of the above will be considered briefly.

Screen/film (Figs 1.21a, 1.21b)

Screen/film imaging in radiography has generally been replaced by digital imaging. There are many advantages to digital imaging; the workflow should be faster, and it allows image processing to optimise the clinical information from an image.

Photographic film is capable of storing an image alone, but the exposure required can be reduced considerably if the film is placed between intensifying screens that convert the X-ray energy into light, which in turn exposes the film. The film and cassettes are widely available in a variety of sizes and can be used with almost any piece of imaging equipment.

An image captured on photographic film will have high resolution, although it has narrower exposure latitude compared with other image-capture systems. This means that the radiographer has much less margin for error when selecting exposure factors before making an exposure.

A variety of systems are available in which the intensifying screens and film can be varied to suit a particular task. Thus, the speed and resolution can be changed in any given clinical situation by selecting a different film and screen.

X-ray film is highly portable, although a considerable amount of space is required to store the film envelopes/bags. Also X-ray film processors are required in a department using conventional imaging technology. These must be regularly cleaned, serviced and subjected to a rigorous quality-control programme in order to ensure consistency of performance. Processors also need to comply with regulations concerning the use and disposal of the chemicals used.[9]

Fluoroscopy/fluorography

This method of image acquisition employs an image intensifier/digital flat panel detector to capture images, which are then displayed in real time or as static images on a monitor. Fluoroscopy is very useful for following the progress of contrast agent around the body, but its resolution is poor on older systems when compared with that of other image-acquisition methods so it is not currently used for plain radiographic imaging. Fluorography may employ thermal film to capture the image from the image intensifier but has now been largely superseded by digital image-capture methods. Fluoroscopic

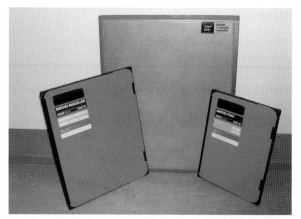

Fig. 1.21a Film screen cassettes.

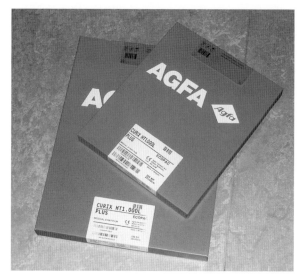

Fig. 1.21b Film boxes.

images can be transmitted directly to the PACS from theatre and ward locations around the hospital.

Automatic exposure control

When using automatic exposure control (AEC) X-rays emerging from the patient pass through a thin ionisation detector. This device contains a gas which is ionised by the X-ray beam. The ionisation process produces a signal which is proportional to the exposure received by the AEC and therefore the patient. The circuitry is pre-programmed to measure the size of this signal and once it reaches a predetermined level terminates the exposure. The chambers are typically around 5 or 6 cm long by 3–4 cm wide but only a few millimetres deep. The device simply measures the total amount of radiation passing through the sensitive area. As such, it is important that the radiographer takes into account the patient's anatomy that overlies the AEC area.

In general radiography a system of 3 chambers is normally employed; a central and two side chambers. Correct exposure can only be achieved if an appropriate chamber for the anatomy overlying is selected or there is a deliberate increase or decrease of the sensitivity of the chamber to account for an area we know will result in an over or under exposed image.

Digital imaging

Digital systems overview

These can be computed radiography (CR) or direct digital radiography (DDR) systems.

Advantages of digital systems

Digital imaging exhibits a number of advantages when compared with conventional screen/film imaging:

- Increased latitude and dynamic range.
- Images can be accessed simultaneously at any workstation.
- Viewing stations can be set up in any location.
- Ability to use digital image archives rather than film libraries.
- Images will generally be quicker to retrieve and less likely to be lost.
- Ability to post-process images to aid visualisation of anatomy and pathology.
- Availability of soft-copy reporting.
- No manual handling of cassettes for DDR systems.
- Potential patient dose reduction and less need to repeat images.
- Potential lower running costs, providing only soft-copy reporting is used.
- No handling of processing chemicals.

CR is used in all areas where screen/film systems are currently used, including mammography. DDR can be also be used in general radiography, A&E and mobile radiography. DDR is very popular in small-field mammography and is being introduced into full-field mammography. DDR detectors are now being used instead of image intensifiers in fluoroscopy.

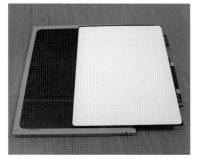

Fig. 1.22a Computed radiography plate/cassette.

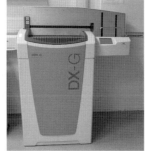

Fig. 1.22b Computed radiography reader.

Image acquisition

Computed radiography (Figs 1.22a, 1.22b)

CR is a system that produces digital radiographic images utilising imaging plates (cassettes). From a user's perspective it is very similar to film screen technology and does not generally require modifications to the X-ray equipment itself. The CR plate is in a cassette, which will fit the table and vertical Bucky trays and can be used with mobile equipment. Following an exposure, the CR imaging plate retains a latent image in a similar way to previous film screen technology and is processed in a reader.

Direct digital radiography

DDR systems are available in two formats:

- Fixed systems where the detector is fixed within the table/Bucky assembly.
- Portable systems which use wireless technology or are connected via a cable system.

The portable systems offer the same flexibility as cassettes but tend to be much larger physical size; however, at the time of writing smaller cassette sizes are being manufactured. These can be used in SCBU and smaller body part radiography. These systems offer the advantage of immediate image display without having to disturb the patient. The patient is radiographed and the image appears on the acquisition workstation in a few seconds. Here, the image can be optimised and then sent for reporting or repeated if necessary.

Computed radiography technology

The active phosphor layer of a CR plate often comprises a layer of europium-doped barium fluorobromide, which is coated on to a semi-rigid or flexible polyester base. X-ray photons are absorbed by the phosphor layer, and the phosphor electrons become 'excited' and are raised to a higher energy level, where they can stay trapped in a semi-stable higher-energy state. The trapped electrons represent a latent image in the phosphor plate in the form of 'stored energy'. The stored energy can be released by adding energy to the trapped electrons. This is done by stimulation with a laser beam. The trapped electrons then 'escape' from the traps to fall back to their equilibrium state. As they fall back, the electrons release energy in the form of light. This phenomenon is otherwise known as photostimulable luminescence (PSL). The emitted light intensity is proportional to the original X-ray intensity. The light energy is detected and the signal is digitised. These data are processed digitally to produce a visible diagnostic image on a monitor. The phosphor plate is then 'erased' with a bright white light to remove any remaining trapped electrons, and the plate is then ready for the next examination.

1 Digital imaging

Image acquisition (cont.)

Digital radiography technologies

The main detector technologies used in digital radiography are:

- X-ray scintillator bonded to a read-out array (amorphous silicon photodiode/thin-film transistor (TFT) array) or coupled to a charge-coupled device (CCD).
- X-ray detector of amorphous selenium bonded to a TFT read-out array.
- Both types can be constructed in the form of a flat panel.

Scintillator detector (Fig. 1.23a)

The X-ray detector is normally a scintillator of thallium-doped caesium iodide (CsI) (Tl) crystals, although other phosphors such as Gd_2O_2S are also used. The scintillator converts the X-rays into a light output. The CsI has a columnar crystal structure that guides the light to the read-out device, which allows the CsI to be thicker than a phosphor powder without significantly increasing unsharpness. As with phosphors in film cassettes, thinner powder phosphors (such as Gd_2O_2S) will have lower unsharpness. Gd_2O_2S phosphors are thinner than CsI scintillators, but they have higher conversion efficiency.

Scintillators are usually coupled directly to an amorphous silicon photodiode TFT flat-panel read-out array. The light from the scintillator is converted into electrical charge in a photodiode array, which stores the charge until it is read out from each of the pixels. These are commonly referred to as amorphous silicon systems.

Charge-coupled device (Fig. 1.23b)

The light output from the scintillator detector can be read out by a CCD camera. The CCD is generally smaller than the phosphor, and so it is usually coupled using a lens or fibre-optic bundles. Demagnification may be necessary, and this can result in a loss of sensitivity if the demagnification is high.

Amorphous selenium/thin-film transistor flat-panel detector (Fig. 1.23c)

The detector consists of a layer of amorphous selenium with a matrix of electrodes on each face. The X-ray energy produces electron-hole pairs in the selenium layer, which are attracted towards the electrodes by an electric field. The charge is collected and read out using a TFT array. The resolution of this type of detector is better than that using a phosphor due to the absence of light scattering.

Scanning technology

An alternative detection method for covering the full image area is to use slot-scanning technology. A linear array of detectors scans across the patient in conjunction with a narrow-fan

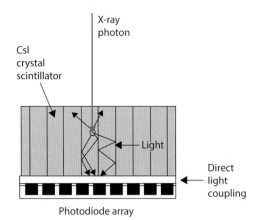

Fig. 1.23a Schematic diagram of flat-panel detector with a scintillator and an amorphous silicon photodiode thin-film transistor array.

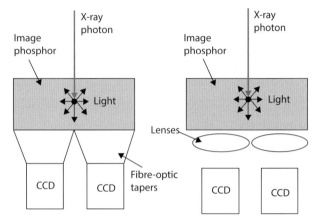

Fig. 1.23b Schematic diagrams showing a charge-coupled device coupled to a phosphor scintillator by lenses and fibre-optics.

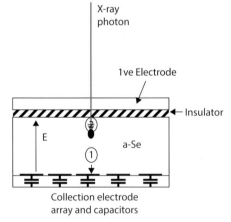

Fig. 1.23c Schematic diagram of an amorphous silicon/thin-film transistor flat-panel detector.

X-ray beam. This method may result in good scatter rejection and contrast differentiation, but it has a number of disadvantages, including a long exposure time and high tube loading. Also, the alignment of the scanning radiation beam and the detectors requires tight mechanical tolerances and mechanical stability of the scanning mechanism.

Digital imaging

There are a number of factors, both inherent in equipment design and external, that affect image quality. The following are important examples.

Fill factor (Fig. 1.24)

For flat-panel detectors, a proportion of the detector contains the read-out circuitry and will be insensitive to the incoming light photons or electrons. This leads to the concept of the fill factor (see equation below), which is the ratio of the sensitive area of the pixel to the effective area of the detector element itself.

Any improvements in resolution will require a reduced pixel pitch. The fill factor will decrease with improved resolution, as the read-out electronics will take up a larger proportion of the detector element and decrease the detector sensitivity.

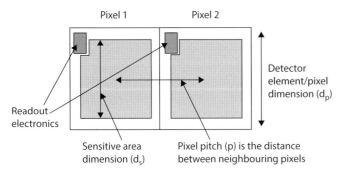

Fig. 1.24 Diagram of fill factor.

Tiling

A tiled array consists of a number of detectors butted together to sample the whole image. However, there may be small areas on read-out devices that are not sensitive; these are caused by gaps between the detectors (typically about 100 mm). There may be some image processing to compensate for this, although this may give some stitching artefacts.

Grids

Low grid strip densities can cause interference patterns in the image called Moiré patterns. This can be solved by using moving grids or high-density grids of over 60 lines/cm. When using CR, ideally the grid lines should also be perpendicular to the scan lines in the reader.

Radiation exposure (image optimisation)

Image quality is related to the radiation exposure received by the detector. Although a relatively low exposure will result in a noisy image, it may still contain sufficient information to be diagnostically acceptable. A high exposure will result in improved image quality, since quantum noise is reduced. However, image-quality improvement is not linear: it will eventually level off as the quantum noise becomes less dominant and decrease as the plate becomes overexposed. Ideally, a system should be set up to obtain adequate image quality for the lowest possible dose (optimisation).

Factors affecting image quality

Automatic exposure control response

An AEC for a screen/film system is set up by ensuring that the correct optical density is achieved across a range of kVs. This method is not practical for digital imaging, as the image will be displayed according to pre-set parameters, irrespective of the exposure used. The AEC will need to be set up in collaboration with the radiology and medical physics departments and the supplier. The level of exposure must be optimised for the selected examination and the receptor dose measured.

One other consideration is that sometimes when screen/film systems are replaced by a CR system, then for simplicity the AEC is kept at the same settings. This may not be the optimal working level, because the sensitivity and energy response of the digital system are different from those of the screen/film system it replaces. A DDR system can use the detector itself as an AEC, although currently most use a conventional AEC chamber system.

Bit depth/image size

A pixel is the smallest element of a digitised picture. A smaller pixel size will generally give an improved spatial resolution in the image. The pixel pitch is the distance between the centres of adjacent pixels.

The matrix size is the number of pixels or memory locations into which the image is divided. Thus, the total number of pixels in a 1024 × 1024 matrix is 1,048,576, defined as one megapixel.

The bit depth of the image determines the contrast resolution. The analogue value of the output from each pixel is converted to digital form, and the results are stored at a separate location in a matrix. The number of grey levels available equals two to the power of the number of bits, e.g. 2^8 or 256 levels.

Number of grey levels per bit depth

Number of bits	Grey levels
1	2
2	4
4	16
8	256
10	1024
12	4096

Clinical radiographic images require good contrast resolution, which is difficult to achieve due to the noise inherent in a radiographic image. In order to achieve good contrast resolution, high bit depths are required. The number of bits required depends on the noise level: the lower the level of noise, the higher the number of bits that can be used.

1 Digital imaging

Imaging informatics

What is imaging informatics?

As found with many other areas in healthcare institutions, radiology services have become increasingly dependent on computers. Imaging informatics is the collective name given to the field of work and combination of technologies that provide the features of a paper-less or paper-light department. In particular, imaging informatics is concerned as a specialty with the electronic acquisition, storage and distribution of the text and image data produced and utilised within a radiology department for the wider provision of care and benefit of patients.

History

For almost a century, film was the primary method of handling radiological imaging, with transferring and filing being a manual clerical process. From the early 2000s onwards, recent years have seen the move away from film-producing departments towards the integration of more modern electronic methods. In the UK this was in part due to national incentives and modernisation projects carried out under the umbrella of the previous National Programme for Information Technology, under which it was ensured that every acute NHS hospital had deployed a PACS, RIS as well as other electronic health applications.

Similarly, paper records of studies and reports have also had their processes modernised, with imaging requests being generated through eRequesting systems, and reports published as part of each patient's electronic patient record (EPR).

With financial and efficiency-based advantages in modernising radiological departments away from the traditional film, chemical and paper based practices, the field of imaging informatics continues to grow rapidly.

Components and connections (Fig. 1.25b)

Whilst local set-up is determined by necessity and services offered, the typical methods of connection and communication between the various systems and applications found in a Radiology department can be seen in Fig. 1.25b.

Picture archiving and communication system

PACS is the generic name for a set of components forming a method for receiving, storing and displaying radiological imaging. Generically, a PACS comprises a hierarchical database into which details of all image files stored are entered; a fast short-term storage device (the 'cache'); a longer-term storage device (the 'archive') and a viewing application or web-based client. Beyond these core components, additional items may include dedicated reporting workstations (high quality computer hardware with a tailored viewer application and specialist display monitors, described later), laser film printers, semi-automated robotic CD/DVD producers and backup devices.

A PACS differs from a standard storage device in that it attempts to maintain the hierarchical structure of the data and information which it holds. This hierarchical structure is based on the premise that each patient may attend on multiple occasions, have multiple studies during each of these attendances, with multiple image files per study. Fig. 1.25a illustrates this typical database structure for an individual patient. The PACS database maintains this order in such a way to allow for easy presentation and reviewing by authorised users (for example, radiographers and clinicians).

Being a technology under development for several decades, there are now a wide number of commercial PACS manufacturers on the market along with a handful of open-source developments; many of these have so far developed a distinctly proprietary arrangement of receiving, storing and disseminating the images sent to them. This proprietary arrangement requires a complex process of migration when software manufacturers are changed; in order to mitigate this, many newer PACS deployments are utilising vendor neutral archives (VNAs), which store imaging using non-proprietary standards, methods and devices. As of 2015, there is debate on whether VNAs are beneficial in the long-term, as migrations will still be required when the storage hardware ages, or becomes no longer suitable for the system.

PACS are highly customisable, and whilst off-the-shelf packages are available, systems in place in the UK are usually tailored to the particular needs of each healthcare institution. For example, some sites implement varying levels of data compression – where radiological image files are compressed to reduce their storage size and increase their speed of display. The retention period, volume and type of imaging stored to each PACS is likewise unique to each site, and a decision made jointly by radiologists, imaging staff and facility management.

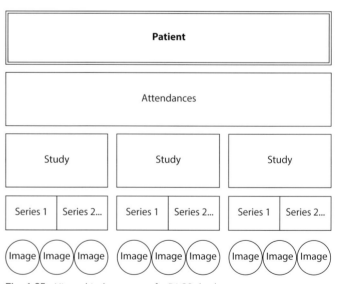

Fig. 1.25a Hierarchical structure of a PACS database.

Digital imaging 1

Imaging informatics (*cont.*)

Overview of imaging informatics applications

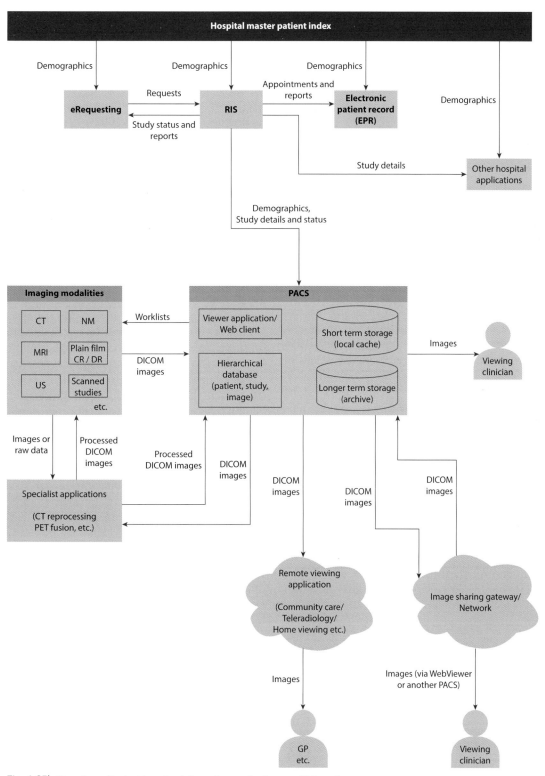

Fig. 1.25b Overview of typical imaging informatics applications and interactions.

Digital imaging

Imaging informatics (cont.)

Radiology information system (RIS)

This is the generic name for an application or group of applications used to handle the textual data related to imaging procedures – for example examination details, the attendance lists, appointment diaries, reports and billing data, as well as data required under IR(ME)R 2000[1] (e.g. radiation dose, referrer and operator details), IRR99[2] (radioisotope data) as well as the Medicines Act 1968 (any prescription-only pharmaceuticals administered as part of the imaging exam, such as contrast in intravenous urograms [IVUs] or glyceryl trinitrate in computed tomography [CT] imaging).

In the UK aggregated statistics from the RIS are also provided by NHS hospitals to a body of the Department of Health (currently the Health and Social Care Information Centre) for payments and performance monitoring. Whilst being primarily designed for use in a radiology imaging department, other areas of the hospital may in addition use RIS in locally agreed ways.

Other systems that interact with elements of the imaging informatics suite but are traditionally maintained by those outside of the radiology department:

Master patient index: also commonly known as the hospital information system (HIS) or patient administration system (PAS), the master patient index is a database application that primarily stores the demographic and contact details of patients, as well as any national identifiers ('NHS Number' in England and Wales; 'Community Health Index' [CHI Number'] in Scotland). It is common practice for demographic changes in this master database, including the addition of new patients, to be passed down to the other imaging informatics and hospital systems.

This 'cascade' update process ensures that the records on other systems each match the primary details recorded in the master patient index. Communication between the master patient index and other text-based imaging informatics components is usually carried out using the health level 7 (HL7) standard (discussed later).

Electronic patient record: the EPR is a method of storing a patient's medical records and notes electronically. A viewer application is also included to allow for clinicians and other authorised healthcare staff (and in some instances the patient themselves) to read and add to the records, just as if they were paper based. EPR applications are expected gradually to include PACS images and RIS data over the coming years.

eRequesting: eRequesting systems allow referrers to place requests for a range of diagnostic tests (including Radiology examinations) into a single online application, which then directly sends the request to the relevant department (for Radiology examinations, this would be via the RIS). In addition, eRequesting systems typically offer a range of tracking functions to allow clinicians to view the status of their request, as well as the report when available.[10] eRequesting is popular within healthcare institutions as it removes the need for a paper request form to be conveyed physically to a collection point and also provides higher quality audit data.

Other hospital applications: larger healthcare institutions in particular will have a range of other medical informatics applications, which will be required to interface with elements of the imaging informatics suite. For example, dedicated research databases, cardiology or echocardiography information systems or backup devices may well have some degree of interaction with the RIS or PACS.

Modalities: an imaging 'modality' is a term given to a particular type of image acquisition method, such as CR, DDR, ultrasound (US), CT, magnetic resonance imaging (MRI), nuclear medicine (NM) and molecular imaging. The majority of the image acquisition methods communicate images electronically into the PACS using the Digital Imaging and Communications in Medicine (DICOM) standards after the operator has post-processed them.

Specialist applications: with 'simple' imaging modalities such as CR, DDR and US, the post-acquisition processing functions may be incorporated into a workstation at the acquiring device. Multi-slice modalities that produce complex raw data imaging sets have separate workstations and applications to allow for the intricate and detailed post-acquisition processing to take place. This is commonly found with CT, MRI and NM imaging modalities, where the acquired imaging is reprocessed to allow for the clinical question to be answered. The reprocessed data are then stored to PACS for future reference, with some sites choosing not to store permanently the originally acquired raw data.

Remote viewing applications: in recent years, great emphasis has been placed upon allowing 24/7 access to diagnostics. To facilitate this, remote viewing applications allow for the secure and reliable viewing of radiological images beyond the traditional boundaries of PACS, whether this is an offsite night reporting facility or a Radiologist on-call at home.

Image sharing gateways or networks: with increased instances of collaborative care and the geographical mobility of patients, the sharing of radiological image files and textual data between healthcare institutions has become more and more of a necessity. Whereas removable media (CDs and DVDs) were initially used, direct peer-to-peer transfers and hub-and-spoke systems are now available.

Digital imaging

Imaging informatics (cont.)

Communication

The various components and applications within the realm of imaging informatics use well-developed international standards to communicate with each other. The key standards used are described below, and are complimentary to others, which together provide the ability for software from different manufacturers to communicate without significant difficulty or expense.

DICOM

DICOM is an international standard designed and implemented worldwide for the storage and exchange of medical imaging data.[11] Released in 1993 and supported universally by manufacturers of imaging equipment, new updates are backwards compatible, meaning several billion medical images can be reliably viewed and transferred today.[12] DICOM allows radiographers to be sure that the digital images they produce will store to a PACS and be viewable for the foreseeable future.

Unlike photographs taken with a digital camera or smartphone, medical imaging utilises high resolution greyscale images and is required to have some patient or clinical data attached to it. For this, the DICOM file format (.DCM extension) is used to store medical images. In a similar manner to the common JPEG file format being designed to offer a balance between size of file, quality and speed of display for domestic photographs, the DICOM file storage format was developed to meet the needs of the medical imaging community and provides similar benefits.

A DICOM file consists of multiple components, including a preamble (identifying the file type and components), a block of data (comprising patient demographics, technical information about the image, the study, its acquisition parameters and acquisition device together with many other listed attributes), and the image data. The DICOM standard also describes methods for the transmission of data across networks, and between imaging devices.

HL7 messaging

Almost all communication between modern text-based applications such as RIS, EPR, eRequesting and the patient master index will use the HL7 format. HL7 is a long-standing supplier neutral group of standards, named after their position (the seventh 'layer') on the International Organization for Standardization Open Systems Interconnection Model[13] – in the same manner as hypertext transfer protocol (HTTP) is for internet usage. The HL7 standards[14] define specified methods for healthcare systems to communicate data between each other, again allowing interoperability between software vendors. HL7 messaging (part of the standards) is a specified format for communication between different text-based systems, including EPR and RIS. HL7 version 2.x is routinely used by healthcare systems with version 3.x becoming more prevalent in other areas. Put concisely, HL7 standards are primarily concerned with text-based communications, whereas DICOM is utilised when handling image data.

Networks

Networks in this context refer to the physical connections between pieces of image acquisition equipment, storage and display devices. Whilst important to be aware of the methods of software communicating amongst each other, a physical network connection is required between each of the components, including to any workstations upon which the viewing applications are being utilised in order to allow this to happen. Networks are customarily maintained by a healthcare institutions information technology department, and must be of suitable quality to ensure fast and reliable transmissions between the imaging informatics components. Modern fibre-based networks (an optical transmission technology) are inherently faster than traditional copper-based networks (where data are transmitted electrically). Fast fibre connections are commonly used between servers, network switches and routers, with copper connecting the 'final hop' to individual computers and devices. Wireless networking is preferred in some applications, such as for theatre fluoroscopy equipment, wireless digital mobile units and handheld image display devices (tablets).

Onward transfers of radiological data to external institutions

Increasingly, with PACS archives now containing potentially around a decade of digitally stored prior imaging for each patient, there is a need to forward this data and imaging onwards to other healthcare institutions, either for immediate on-going care or for historical comparisons. With the advent of numerous electronic transfer methods now available via the internet or the intra-NHS (N3) network, this is possible without the need to create hard copies, CDs or DVDs. Networked image sharing can be one of three types – mailbox, cloud or direct:

Mailbox-based methods allow an upload into a specific virtual mailbox, either one for an entire healthcare institution, a service group or a specific clinician.

Cloud-based services provide an off-site storage of imaging data and allow for the images to be exchanged in a portal or other web-based application.

The approach taken for direct sharing varies and can involve creating a remote connection to a PACS or by utilising new technical architectures such as cross enterprise document sharing for imaging (XDS-I).

Data protection

There are legal considerations in any such transfers, whether electronic or physical, mainly stemming from the rights and principles enshrined by the Data Protection Act 1998. Along with the duties surrounding keeping patient data confidential, it is good practice to ensure that all radiological data transfers are necessary, justified and proportionate, together with records being kept to allow for audit of each individual transfer.

1 Digital imaging

Image processing

One of the drawbacks to the historic film-based imaging process was the comparative lack of ability to alter the image easily once chemically developed; if, for example, a film was significantly overexposed, there were few options other than repeating the image with corrected exposure factors. Now, with digital acquisition and post processing, more options are possible, even for the manifestly undiagnostic image.

Post processing

Acquisition workstations which are part of the acquiring modalities are used to enhance the images obtained and produce a superior quality image set for transmission to PACS. Functions provided on these workstations typically include the ability to correct demographics, place electronic markers, apply secondary collimation (shuttering), add informational text, adjust window width/level values and edit any look-up table (LUT) applied to the image. It is cautioned that good radiographic technique still needs to be followed – the principles of dose minimisation (ALARP) should not be depreciated due to the relative ease with which modern imaging modalities allow enhancement.

Look-up tables

Each digital radiological image is comprised of individual units, called pixels (or voxels for three-dimensional imaging – see opposite) (Fig. 1.26b). LUTs convert the greyscale values of each of these units to another, based on a pre-set conversion table (Fig. 1.26a). This creates a new image, intended to be of better diagnostic quality than the original. A demonstration of this effect can be seen in Fig. 1.26c. LUTs are used either to reduce the dynamic range of an acquired image (where an acquisition device acquires a wider range of data than can be displayed), or where it is known that it is clinically more appropriate to reallocate specified densities within an image to other shades of grey, such as for specifically viewing particular types of tissue or bone.

Colours may be artificially added to an image, perhaps to highlight flow rates in ultrasound Doppler imaging, or radioisotope activity levels in fused positron emission tomography (PET)–CT imaging.

Window width/window level (Fig. 1.26d)

The human eye has a non-linear response to greyscale values – not every graduation from one greyscale value to another in an image is as perceivable as others. In order to visualise the required anatomy better within radiological images, changes to the window width and level can be made either during post processing, or during later viewing. Briefly simplified, changing the window width has the effect of altering the contrast ratio of the image, whereas adjusting the window level has the effect of altering the average brightness of the image. Combinations of the two adjustments are used to enhance imaging, particularly those obtained with suboptimal exposures (Fig. 1.27).

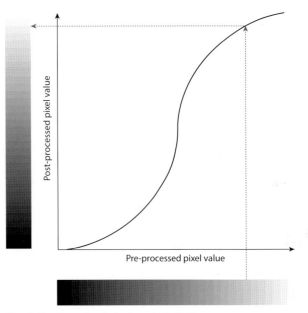

Fig. 1.26a Example of a look-up table (LUT).

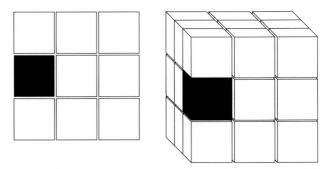

Fig. 1.26b Pixel vs. Voxel (both highly enlarged for illustration). Left: black two-dimensional square illustrating one pixel in a larger image. Right: black three-dimensional cube illustrating one voxel.

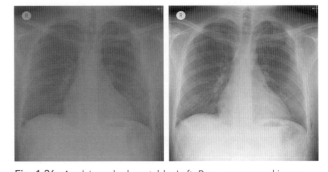

Fig. 1.26c Applying a look-up table. Left: Raw unprocessed image. Right: suitable LUT applied to the same image.

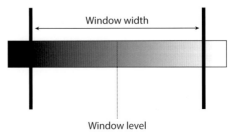

Fig. 1.26d Diagram showing the relationship between window level and window width.

Digital imaging

Image processing (cont.)

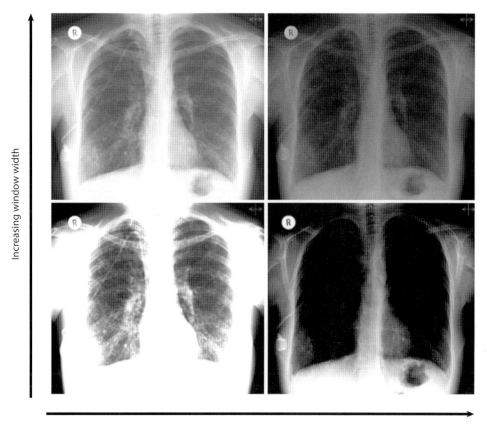

Fig. 1.27 Examples of the effect of window width and window level changes on a direct digital PA chest radiograph.

Hanging protocols

Hanging protocols determine the order and precedence of imaging displayed to clinicians and reporting staff, much like determining the order of films in a film packet. For example, common practice dictates that when a chest radiograph is displayed for reporting, the most recent prior chest radiograph is displayed on any secondary monitor, and the next most recent (in descending date order) on the 3rd monitor, and so on. With fixed hanging protocols, it is important to ensure that these are updated as needed for new acquisition modalities in order that those reviewing imaging are presented with the most appropriate prior images for easy comparison.

Quality assurance

Quality assurance (QA) in radiology departments has been commonplace for many years – most departments have a routine of checking tube output, collimation/light beam accuracy, exposure duration and contrast phantom tests in X-ray generating equipment, together with wider standard clerical procedures to ensure film packets were correctly stored and located. Imaging informatics equipment requires similar attention; IPEM reports[15] provide a fuller account, common QA actions are:

Housekeeping tasks: each part of the imaging informatics environment involves some degree of human interaction. Errors introduced in data need to be identified and corrected on a daily basis in order to ensure the datasets stored are as complete and current as possible. Housekeeping tasks vary per system, but may include matching up incorrectly identified images on the PACS, removal of missed appointments from the RIS, to managing disk space demands on servers.

1 Digital imaging

Image processing (cont.)

Display monitor calibration: with electronic acquisition, distribution and display now being standard, modern day radiology services are heavily dependent on properly functioning display devices. Most widely used display devices are flat panel monitors with images composed of a grid formed by millions of pixels, which are backlit by light emitting diodes (or now less commonly, cold cathode fluorescent tubes). Both the pixels and backlights within flat panel monitors degrade with age and use and should be regularly checked. For workstations used to report on diagnostic images, calibration to a DICOM response curve should be carried out (if not built in and automated) utilising a manual 'puck' test device and software, at least annually.

Display monitor environment: the physical surroundings and environment in healthcare institutions changes over time; lights around display devices can be altered, walls painted more brightly and windows uncovered. The suitability of viewing locations should be assessed as required, taking note of advice from medical physics personnel. Fingerprints, which accumulate on medical displays, should be cleaned away on a regular basis with care taken not to damage the screen surface.

Database integrity checks: it must be possible to guarantee that all databases and connections within an imaging informatics suite are operating correctly. These can be tested by analysing a sample of the data held on each system and ensuring results are in line with expectations. Integrity checks are typically performed before and after any changes or upgrades are carried out to the informatics equipment.

System availability: high expectations are placed on availability of imaging informatics systems; for business continuity purposes the regular testing of the redundancy of the systems and processes that surround them is important. These should be documented and might form part of a larger, institution-wide, disaster recovery programme.

Artefacts (Figs 1.28a–1.28d)

Just as found with film/chemistry-based radiography, artefacts in radiographic imaging have existed from the inception of the technology. These require guarding against as much as practicable to avoid reducing the diagnostic accuracy of the imaging, or the need to repeat any radiation exposure. Artefacts are specific to the modalities and equipment utilised; radiographers should be aware of the possible types of image degradation and their causes from the equipment that they are using. The images opposite demonstrate a small sample of common artefacts from CR and DDR systems; a wider range can be found in investigative studies such as Honey & Mackenzie and Shetty et al.[16,17]

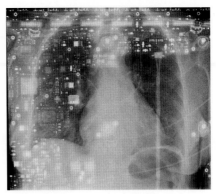

Fig. 1.28a Electronics overlaying image, due to exposure through reverse of DDR plate.

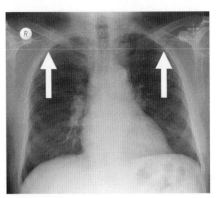

Fig. 1.28b Linear artefact caused by particle of dust obstructing portion of CR reader light guide during readout.

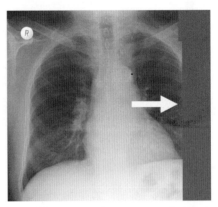

Fig. 1.28c Data transfer error – partial network communication loss during image data transmission.

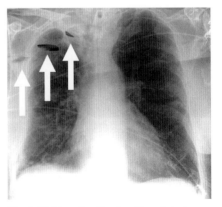

Fig. 1.28d Localised backscatter artefacts caused by damaged lead backing on a CR cassette.

Exposure factors 1

Introduction

The radiation output from an X-ray tube is a product of the current applied to the X-ray tube (measured in milliamps, mA), the duration of the exposure (measured in seconds, s) and also the voltage applied to the X-ray tube (measured in kilovoltage, kV).

Radiation output is normally known as the intensity of the X-ray beam and needs to be varied to enable different body parts to be imaged. Other factors affect the intensity of the radiation beam reaching the detector. These are:

- The medium through which the beam passes.
- The distances between the X-ray source, the patient and the detector.
- If a grid or Bucky is used to eliminate scattered radiation.
- The filtration applied to the X-ray tube.

When the radiographic technique needs to be modified either to change the distances between the elements or if the exposure time needs to be reduced, then a new exposure may need to be calculated. This can be done by using the following formula:

$$\frac{mAs \times kV^4}{grid\ factor \times FRD^2} = \frac{mAs \times kV^4}{grid\ factor \times FRD^2}$$

The mAs and kV, use of a grid and distance for the initial examination are put into the left hand side of the equation and the new ones into the right hand side. Changing the mAs is straightforward as the intensity of the beam is directly proportional to the mAs. Changing the kV is more complex and the calculation should be performed with the kV to the 4th power, i.e. kV^4. If no grid is used the grid factor is 1.

With screen/film imaging the exposure determines the 'film blackening' of the image. Exposures in digital imaging are a more complex process as digital systems have a much great 'exposure latitude' and dynamic range. Image processing can convert an under- or overexposed image into a diagnostic image by altering the grey scale into the optimum range. Underexposed may appear noisy and have mottle on the image, which may detract from the image quality. Overexposure up to 20 times the norm may look identical to the image with the correct exposure (see Fig. 1.29).[18]

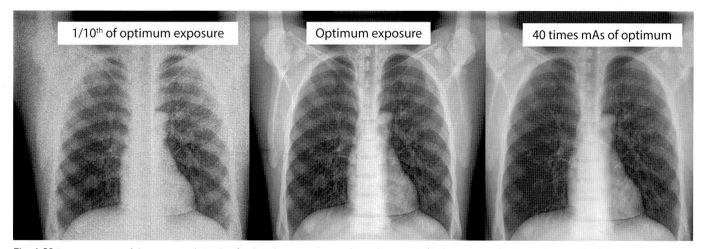

Fig. 1.29 Demonstration of the exposure latitude of a digital system using a chest phantom. Left: The image underexposed at 1/10th of the optimum exposure (mAs) demonstrates unacceptable noise; Right: 40 times the optimum mAs (Middle) demonstrates the effect of overexposed pixel values, which merge with surrounding pixels and lose anatomical definition.

1 Exposure factors

Milliampere seconds

This is the intensity of the X-ray beam being used to produce the image. Any radiation which has enough energy to penetrate the body part will impact on the image detector.

The mA determines the number of X-rays being produced; the quantity of X-rays produced is proportional to the mAs. Therefore:

Doubling the mAs will double the intensity of the X-ray beam.
Halving the mAs will result in a reduction of intensity of 50%.
The mAs is the product of mA (tube current) and exposure time:

$$mA \times time.$$

The anatomically programmed generator will automatically set the highest mA and shortest time for an examination, e.g. 1 mAs may be 1,000 mA and 0.001 s.

The radiographer does, however, have the option of increasing this tube loading to give a shorter time and higher mA should the clinical situation demand this, e.g. in the case of a restless patient. Altering the mAs only affects the intensity of the beam and not the quality, i.e. it increases the number of photons produced but not the range of intensities.

Kilovoltage

This indicates how the X-ray beam will penetrate the body. The range of kVs used in diagnostic radiography is normally between 50 and 125 kV, although a kV as low as 25 kV may be used for certain soft-tissue examinations, such as mammography. High-kV techniques, such as those used in chest radiography, employ a kV of approximately 125 kV.

As the kV increases, the X-rays produced have a higher energy and more photons have the energy therefore to be able to penetrate the body and be detected by the image detector. With film screen detectors kV is an important factor in the control of contrast of the radiographic image and should therefore be chosen carefully. Applying different LUTs can compensate for changes in kV and this issue is not as critical in digital imaging; however, the basic principles of absorption and scattering of the X-ray beam will not change (Fig. 1.30).

The kV should be such that the radiation has enough energy to penetrate the body part and reach the image-acquisition device. At lower kVs dense structures within the body (e.g. bone) will absorb low-energy X-rays, but structures of lower density (e.g. soft tissue) will absorb relatively few X-rays. As the kV increases, proportionately more radiation will be able to penetrate the denser body part compared with the less dense part, which results in a lower contrast image.

If there is a very wide range of patient densities within the region being examined (e.g. the chest), then the image may show excessive contrast and it might be necessary to reduce the contrast within the image to allow a diagnostic image density to be attained throughout the region of interest. This can be achieved by increasing the kV and is commonly undertaken in chest radiography.

Another reason for increasing the kV is to allow the mAs, and therefore the exposure time, to be reduced. As kV is increased, not only does the radiation have more energy but also more radiation is produced, thus allowing the reduction in mAs.

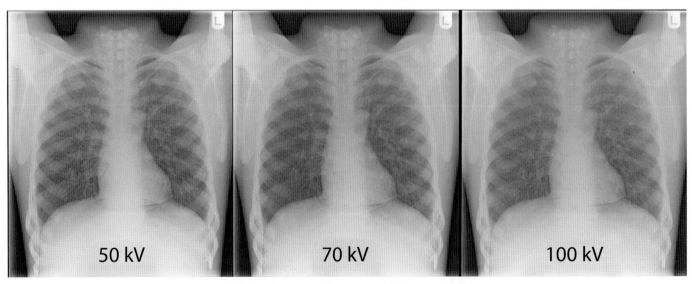

Fig. 1.30 Digital image set demonstrating image quality at different kVs (all images are of diagnostic quality).

Focus-to-receptor distance (Figs 1.31a, 1.31b)

For a given kV and mAs, the greater the FRD, the lower the intensity of radiation reaching the image receptor. Therefore, to obtain the same intensity, if the FRD is increased the mAs must also be increased.

When choosing the FRD, the following factors are taken into consideration:

- The X-ray tube must not be too close to the patient's skin, otherwise radiation damage could be caused.[19]
- Short FRDs could give unacceptable geometric unsharpness.

Most extremity and table radiographic examinations are carried out with an FRD of 100–110 cm, which gives acceptable focus-to-skin distance and geometrical unsharpness. The FRD used may have an impact on the type of grids used. Focused grids need to be purchased which fit the FRD used in your department.

If there is a large object-to-receptor distance, FRD is sometimes increased to reduce geometrical unsharpness and magnification. To calculate the new exposure at the changed distance, the following formula can be used:

$$\text{New mAs} = \frac{\text{New distance}^2}{\text{Old distance}^2} \times \text{Original mAs}$$

For example, if at 100 cm FRD an exposure of 60 kV and 20 mAs produced a satisfactory result, then at 200 cm FRD, the new mAs would be calculated as follows:

$$\text{New mAs} = \frac{200^2}{100^2} \times 20$$

Therefore, the exposure factors required at an FRD of 200 cm will be 60 kV and 80 mAs.

Exposure factors

Intensifying screens

Intensifying screens used in conjunction with photographic film are usually in pairs, with the film sandwiched between them and contained in a rigid, light-tight container, i.e. a cassette.

Different types of intensifying screen emit different intensities and different colours of light when irradiated by X-rays. It is important to ensure that the type of film used with a particular type of screen is matched in terms of the colour of light to which it is most sensitive.

'Fast' or regular screens require less radiation to produce the same film blackening than the 'slow' screens used for extremity radiography. When changing from slow to fast screens, the exposure must be reduced. This has the advantage that a lower radiation dose is received by the patient; however, greater screen speed will result in greater photographic unsharpness, with a resultant decrease in image quality. It is important to consult the screen manufacturers' guidelines to become aware of the difference in speed of the particular screens used in a particular department.

Digital imaging

When a digital method of image acquisition is being used then a wide range of exposures will produce a diagnostic image. If the equipment does not receive an exposure within the dynamic range, then the image may show noise or mottle and will not be suitable for diagnosis. Exposures over a given optimum will still produce an acceptable image up to a point (approximately 20 times more), but the patient will have been exposed to a radiation dose that is unjustifiable.

The equipment used for digital image acquisition should have an exposure index (EI) that displays how much exposure was used for a particular examination. The radiographer should check the exposure is within the correct value recommended by the manufacturer. All manufacturers use different EIs, therefore the radiographer must be familiar with the values for each piece of digital equipment they use.

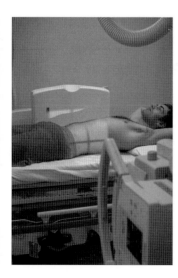

Fig. 1.31a FRD increased to reduce increased geometric unsharpness from a large OFD.

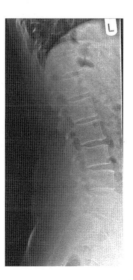

Fig. 1.31b Radiographic image with excessive noise from underexposure.

1 Exposure factors

Secondary radiation grids

Grids are used when the thicker or denser parts of the body are being examined, where scattered radiation is likely to reduce/degrade significantly the contrast of the image. Bucky assemblies/antiscatter grids are the most commonly used method to reduce noise and thus improve contrast in an X-ray image in large body parts, e.g. the spine and pelvis. This is achieved by absorbing scattered radiation that exits the patient before it reaches the image receptor. The grid allows the majority of the primary X-rays to be transmitted and the majority of the scattered X-rays to be absorbed. It is constructed from lead strips (that absorb the scatter) that are separated by radiolucent aluminium material or fibre.

The grid, however, also absorbs some of the primary beam and the radiation exposure to the patient must be increased by a factor of 2–3 to compensate for the loss of primary and scattered X-rays removed by the grid.

Grids can be stationary and simply placed between the patient and the image receptor or inserted into a Bucky mechanism where they move in a reciprocating manner to absorb the scattered photons.

If the grid remains stationary during the exposure, then the grid pattern may be seen on the radiograph. This is usually the case when a stationary grid is used, e.g. for ward and some trauma radiography. In the imaging department, the grid is attached to a mechanism in the X-ray table or vertical stand that gives it an oscillatory movement, so that the grid pattern is not seen. If the grid has a lattice of 50 lines or more per centimetre, then it can be used stationary without the grid lines being visible on the resultant image.

The Bucky mechanism is located under the X-ray table or vertical-stand. The specifications of different grids can vary based on:

- The number of strips over the length of the grid (numbers of strips per centimetre).
- The grid ratio (height of the lead strips to the interspace distance) (Fig. 1.32a).
- Whether the grid is focused or parallel (alignment of the lead strips). A focused grid allows more useful photons to reach the image detector but has restrictions of the FRD used. Focused grids are available that are manufactured for a range of specific FRDs, and care must be taken to select the relevant grid for the FRD employed.
- The pattern of the lead strips or orientation.

The grid frequency and ratio can range from 25 to 45 lines/cm and from a ratio of 4:1 to 16:1, respectively. The higher the frequency the more effective the removal of scatter. The grid pattern can be linear (strips running in one direction) or crossed (strips running perpendicular to one another), where crossed grids are associated with higher scatter reduction.

The higher the grid capability to absorb scattered radiation (i.e. higher frequency or ratio or grid with crossed pattern),

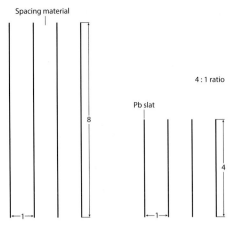

Fig. 1.32a Grid ratio.

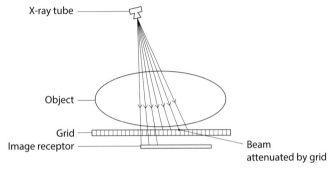

Fig. 1.32b One cause of grid cut-off: beam angulation across gridlines.

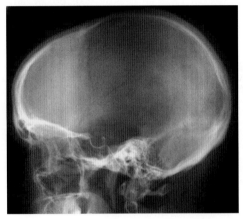

Fig. 1.32c Grid cut-off due to focused grid being upside down.

the more it absorbs useful X-ray photons and the more increase in dose is needed. It is also important to note that grid misalignment may result in grid 'cut-off' where a large number of useful X-ray photons are absorbed by the grid, thus causing a substantial loss of image density (Figs 1.32b, 1.32c).

Choice of exposure factors

Exposure factors must be optimised according to the ALARP principle. The appropriate kV is selected to give the required penetration and subject contrast. The mAs is selected to give the correct incident intensity. The magnitude of the exposure depends on:

- The type of image-acquisition device, e.g. the relative speed of intensifying screens.
- The FRD.
- The grid factor (if a grid is used).

Measures used to reduce the exposure time should be considered if movement unsharpness is likely to be a problem by increasing the kV and using a shorter exposure time.

Summary of factors contributing to optimum radiographic image quality

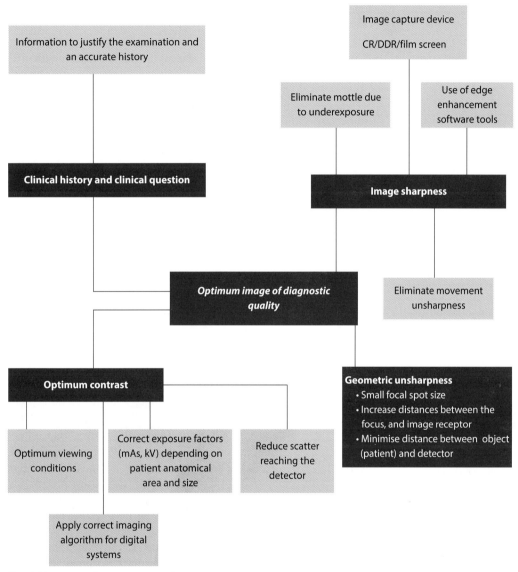

Fig. 1.33 Factors affecting image quality.

1 Radiation protection

Although imaging with X-rays offers great benefits to patients, the risks associated with using ionising radiation require the implementation of robust systems of radiation protection for patients, staff and members of the public. In the UK the requirements for protection of staff and the public are set out in the Ionising Radiations Regulations 1999 (IRR99),[2] while protection of patients is mainly covered by the Ionising Radiations (Medical Exposures) Regulations. Both sets of regulations follow accepted international principles for radiation protection: that all exposures are justified taking the risks and benefits into account; exposures are optimised so that they are as low as practicable given the intended purpose; and that doses do not exceed statutory limits where these apply.

The radiographer has a duty of care to undertake radiography within an environment that takes into account legislation that specifically relates to medical exposures. Legislation is specific to the use of equipment generating ionising radiation. This section will deal with these issues in detail taking into consideration the radiographer, patient, carers and other healthcare professionals.

Medical exposure

The Ionising Radiation (Medical Exposure) Regulations (IRMER) 2000 and IR(ME)R Amendment Regulations 2006/2011

These regulations are intended to protect individuals against the dangers of ionising radiation while undergoing medical exposures. These include diagnostic procedures such as X-rays, CT scans and NM examinations, as well as treatment such as radiotherapy, irrespective of where they are undertaken, e.g. hospital department, dental practice, chiropractic clinic. Medical exposures undertaken for research purposes are also covered by these Regulations.

The Regulations define the duty-holders who carry responsibility under IR(ME)R 2000. These are:

- The employer (normally a NHS Trust or regulated private sector provider of the hospital-based environment) is the body responsible for putting all of the necessary procedures and protocols in place to ensure that the IR(ME)R 2000 regulations can be fully applied.
- The referrer, a registered healthcare professional (e.g. a medical or dental practitioner, radiographer, chiropodist, physiotherapist) who is entitled in accordance with the employer's procedures to refer patients for medical exposures.
- The practitioner, a registered healthcare professional who is entitled in accordance with the employer's procedures and whose primary responsibility is justification of the individual medical exposure (e.g. the radiographer or radiologist).
- The operator, a person who is entitled in accordance with the employer's procedures to undertake the medical exposure (e.g. a radiographer, radiologist, clinical scientist, technologist or an assistant practitioner). Operators are also involved in other aspects of medical exposures, such as equipment calibration or quality control. Student radiographers may undertake imaging procedures under strict protocols and with supervision by a practitioner.

Justification

The regulations state that no person shall carry out a medical exposure unless it has been justified by the practitioner as showing a sufficient net benefit to the individual. As part of the justification a risk–benefit analysis must be undertaken.

Risk–benefit

Risk–benefit analysis is one of the best tools for managing risk on a daily basis and is still a part of the process of protecting radiation workers, patients and carers. The use of X-rays for diagnosis has associated dangers or risks, yet distinct benefits for mankind (can you imagine a 21st century hospital providing its services without using X-rays in either a diagnostic or therapeutic capacity?). It therefore follows that it is necessary to use a process that assesses risks and benefits when using X-rays.

Radiation legislation in the UK requires that those patients referred as part of their own medical diagnosis or treatment should not be irradiated intentionally unless there is a valid clinical indication. In making this judgement, the clinician must determine that the benefit to the patient in having the examination will outweigh the risk. This is the process of justification; if the result of having the X-ray examination will change the clinical management of the patient then that examination can be said to be justified.

We have to be aware however, that requesting an X-ray to exclude an injury or a disease process can be perfectly justifiable also, providing it is not possible to be reasonably sure of the outcome by other, 'less risky' means. An example of 'less risky' in this case might be a thorough clinical examination.

So justification is the first step in a radiation protection strategy because the best way to reduce the radiation dose to the patient is not to undertake the examination in the first place, if this is considered to be an appropriate course of action. The justification of an X-ray examination is a two-stage process and should be the responsibility of both the referring clinician along with the radiographer responsible for undertaking the request. Determining whether an examination is justified will vary depending on factors such as the age of the individual, the pregnancy status or the availability of other diagnostic procedures.

Benefits of X-ray examinations

The benefits of having X-ray procedures are associated with managing the treatment and or diagnosis of the patient. These may include:

- Saving the person's life by providing the correct diagnosis that may not be able to be made without the use of X-rays, e.g. chest X-ray to demonstrate extent of pathology.
- Giving the patient the correct treatment as a result of the correct diagnosis.
- Eliminating disease/disorders that affect the management of the patient, e.g. determining if a patient has a fracture and how best to manage the patient's fracture.
- Managing the treatment of a patient by imaging the response to treatment, e.g. images to determine the effect of radiotherapy.
- Making a diagnosis with an examination that has less morbidity and mortality than an alternative test, e.g. CT rather than invasive surgery.[19]

Radiation dose quantities

Dose quantity	Unit	Definition
Absorbed dose	Gy	Energy absorbed in known mass of tissue
Organ dose	mGy	Average dose to specific tissue
Effective dose	mSv	Overall dose weighted for sensitivity of different organs; indicates risk
Entrance surface dose	mGy	Dose measured at entrance surface; used to monitor doses and set DRLs for radiographs
Dose–area product	Gy cm^2	Product of dose (in air) and beam area; used to monitor doses and set DRLs for examinations

DRL, dose reference level.

Radiation risk for X-ray examinations to an average adult

Examination	Typical effective dose (mSv)	Risk*
Chest	0.02	1 in 1 000 000
Mammography	0.06	1 in 300 000
Abdomen	0.7	1 in 30 000
Lumbar spine	1.3	1 in 15 000
CT head	2	1 in 10 000
Barium enema	7.2	1 in 2800
CT body	9	1 in 2200

* Additional lifetime risk of fatal cancer.

Radiation protection

Medical exposure (*cont.*)

Dose quantities

In order to assess potential harm caused by ionising radiation, quantification of the radiation used is essential.

The likelihood and severity of harm depends on the amount of X-ray energy absorbed in the patient. Radiation dose (expressed in joules/kilogram. J/kg or Gray, Gy) is used to quantify the amount of energy absorbed within a known mass of tissue. Some types of radiation cause more harm than others for the same absorbed dose. The equivalent dose (expressed in Sieverts, Sv) is found by multiplying the absorbed dose by the quality factor assigned to specific types of radiation. For diagnostic X-rays, the quality factor is one, so that absorbed dose and equivalent dose have the same value. The risk also depends on which organs and tissues are irradiated. To take account of this, the tissues are given a weighting factor according to their susceptibility to harm from radiation. Organ dose multiplied by the tissue-weighting factor gives the weighted equivalent dose for that organ. The effective dose for an examination (expressed in Sv) is found by adding up the weighted equivalent doses for tissues or organs that have been irradiated. Effective dose indicates the detriment to health of an X-ray, allowing for the site of the examination and the exposure conditions.

For most tissues, it is not feasible to measure organ doses directly. However, they can be derived using mathematical models of the dose distributions within simulated patients for different examinations and exposure conditions. The models are used to convert patient dose–area product readings (DAP, expressed in Gy cm^2) or entrance skin dose measurements (ESD, expressed in mGy) into organ doses. Combining the weighted organ doses gives the effective dose for the given examination conditions. Skin doses are usually measured using thermoluminescent dosimeters (TLDs) or are calculated indirectly from tube output and back-scatter data.

For monitoring the relative patient dose levels for different types of examination performed using a variety of equipment, it is usually sufficient to analyse DAP readings or skin dose data without deriving effective doses. National and local DRLs will also be set in terms of these quantities and are discussed on page 48.

1 Radiation protection

Medical exposure (*cont.*)

Radiation risks

There is no safe dose limit and all exposures carry some risk. The purpose of a risk–benefit discussion should therefore be to justify the examination to the patient, discuss the need for the examination and quantify the risk. The Health Protection Agency produces an excellent leaflet called *X-rays: how safe are they?*, which outlines the common imaging procedures and levels of risk for common X-ray and isotope procedures. To quote them:

"You will be glad to know that the radiation doses used for X-ray examinations or isotope scans are many thousands of times too low to produce immediate harmful effects, such as skin burns or radiation sickness. The only effect on the patient that is known to be possible at these low doses is a very slight increase in the chance of cancer occurring many years or even decades after the exposure.".[20]

It also gives approximate estimates of the chance or risk that a particular examination or scan might result in a radiation-induced cancer later in the lifetime of the patient are shown in the table opposite.

There are a number of ways of describing the risk.[18] These include:

- Equivalent background dose, expressed in equivalent period of natural background radiation, e.g. a few days to several years.
- Statistical risk expressed in numbers, such as minimal risk of cancer of 1 in 1,000,000 to 1 in 100,000.
- Comparisons to general risks of cancer, i.e. the population have a 1 in 3 chance of getting cancer.
- Comparison to everyday activities: e.g. airline flights are very safe with the risk of a crash being well below 1 in 1,000,000.

A 4-hour plane flight exposes you to the same radiation dose (from cosmic rays) as a chest X-ray.

The purpose of managing radiation dose in diagnostic procedures using X-ray is to avoid predictable (deterministic) health effects and to reduce the probability of randomly determined (stochastic) health effects of ionising radiation.

Referrers and practitioners must be educated in the risks and benefits and the radiation dose given from different X-ray procedures and how to communicate them effectively to patients and carers. Whichever comparison you decide to use, make sure that the correct information is at hand and always discuss risk verses benefit. The principles of justification and optimisation can be used to inform the patient that X-rays are not undertaken without a valid clinical reason. Any examinations will use the lowest dose compatible with making a diagnosis (ALARP principle) and the exposure will be optimised. It must also be remembered that the patient always has the right to decide not to have the examination.

Optimisation

The IRMER regulations states that "The practitioner and the operator, to the extent of their respective involvement in a medical exposure, shall ensure that doses arising from the exposure are kept as low as reasonably practicable consistent with the intended purpose."

Additionally the regulations also state that that the operator shall select equipment and methods to ensure that for each medical exposure the dose of ionising radiation to the individual undergoing the exposure is as low as reasonably practicable and consistent with the intended diagnostic or therapeutic purpose, and in doing so shall pay special attention to:

- Careful/precise technique to minimise repeat examinations.
- QA of equipment.
- Optimisation of exposure factors to provide a diagnostic image within the DRLs set for each procedure.
- Agreed exposure charts.
- Clinical audit of procedures and exposures.

It is important therefore, that special attention is paid to these relevant issues to ensure that patient doses are kept to a minimum.[1]

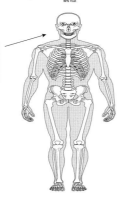

Fig. 1.34a Exposure chart.

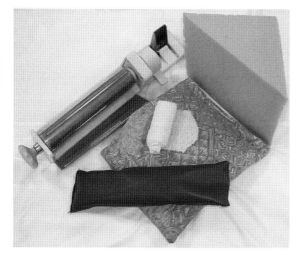

Fig. 1.34b Immobilisation devices.

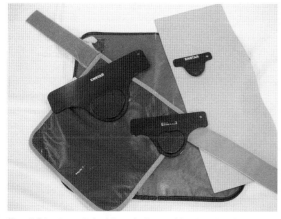

Fig. 1.34c Gonad shields with sheet of lead rubber for gonad protection.

Radiation protection 1

Medical exposure (*cont.*)

Exposure charts

Modern X-ray generators have an anatomically programmed generator. When selecting a body part to be examined the generator will also set preliminary exposure factors, the tube focus, any AECs and chambers for the examination. These can be moderated and adjusted by the radiographer but are generally used for a standard protocol. Variations on the pre-set factors for bariatric or paediatric patients and modified techniques may find an exposure chart useful if these examinations are performed infrequently (Fig. 1.34a). Carrying a pocket notebook with notes on agreed departmental exposures is another option, as well as providing a record of agreed exposure factors and DRLs for standard examinations.

Immobilisation

Ensuring the patient is comfortable and understands the need to keep still is often all that is required to eliminate movement unsharpness. However, when the patient is in pain or uncomfortable and there is a possibility of involuntary movement accessories may be useful.

Radiolucent foam pads and sandbags come in a variety of shapes and sizes and may be useful to immobilise the patient. Compression bands may also reduce the volume of tissue irradiated and reduce the production of scattered radiation (Fig. 1.34b).

Patient holding

In rare cases a patient may require to be held in position during the exposure. Such holding should be undertaken in accordance with the Local Rules with appropriate personal protective equipment (PPE) worn by the carer and a record kept of the examination undertaken and the person doing the holding. Under no circumstances should a radiographer undertake this task.

Aprons and shields

Fig. 1.34c demonstrates a selection of lead-rubber aprons, strips and shields that may be useful to restrict the primary and secondary radiation beam from reaching the patient and or detector. Together with precise collimation, radiation shields can reduce the radiation dose to the patient and improve image quality by reducing noise (scattered radiation).

Training

IRMER states that no practitioner or operator shall carry out a medical exposure or any practical aspect without having been adequately trained. Additionally those engaged in medical exposures have a requirement to undertake continuing education and training after qualification including, in the case of new techniques, training related to these techniques and the relevant radiation protection requirements.

1 Radiation protection

Medical exposure (cont.)

Diagnostic reference levels and dose monitoring

Employers have a duty under IRMER to establish DRLs for radiodiagnostic examinations.[21] European reference levels should be considered when setting DRLs. For the UK, such levels have been based on a series of national patient dose surveys conducted over the years with the latest Doses to patients from radiographic and fluoroscopic X-ray imaging procedures in the UK 2010 Review, HPA–CRCE - 034 published in June 2012.[21]

The recommended DRLs for the procedures published are based on rounded 3rd quartile values of the mean patient doses observed for common X-ray examinations in a nationally representative sample of X-ray rooms.

The doses are expressed as either ESD (mGy) or DAP (Gy cm^2), or both. In the main, the focus is on the most frequent or relatively higher dose examinations. The table summaries the content of Table 28 of the report in respect of plain radiographic examinations. The report also includes recommended national DRLs for fluoroscopic and interventional procedures.

The DRLs quoted should be used as a reference for comparison with local diagnostic reference levels (LDRs). These should be regularly reviewed in light of national guidance or changes in technique and procedures. Additionally there is a requirement for the employer to undertake appropriate reviews whenever diagnostic levels are consistently exceeded and ensure that corrective action is taken where appropriate. This means that there should be a regular review of patient doses. The operator, i.e. the radiographer, has a legal requirement to optimise the radiation dose and although individual exposures may vary around the DRL, the average for standard patients should comply with the established level. This is within the overall framework of ensuring that for each medical exposure the dose of ionising radiation to the individual undergoing the exposure conforms to the ALARP principle.

This edition quotes DRLs (highlighted in red) for those adult individual radiographs described using the current recommended UK national DRLs (see table),[21] and for those not included, DRLs are added (highlighted in grey) calculated on a regional basis by means of electronic X-ray examination records, findings courtesy of Integrated Radiological Services (IRS) Ltd Liverpool, which are based on calculated weighted averages.

Paediatric DRLs are addressed in the Paediatric chapter. These DRLs are given as a guide and readers are referred to their local protocols and procedures where relevant LDRs should be in place.

Dose monitoring on a national level enables the establishment of DRLs as well as enabling calculation of the dose burden to the population as a whole.

Working with the practitioners and operators, medical physics experts (MPEs) assist with patient dosimetry and dose optimisation. In some cases the employer may be able to justify use of higher doses if there are aspects of the examination that are justifiably non-standard.

Note. The Basic Safety Standards (BSS) Directive (2013/59/Euratom), was adopted on the 5th December 2013[22] with the UK Government having to implement the Directive into UK law by the 6 February 2018. The new BSS Directive incorporates the latest recommendations from the International Commission on Radiological Protection (ICRP) published in 2007, and harmonises the EU regime with the BSS of the International Atomic Energy Agency (IAEA). The new directive introduces stronger requirements on DRLs with a greater emphasis on regular review and use of DRLs. It is important therefore, that all patient doses are recorded.

Investigation and notification of overexposure (IRMER)

Although individual patient doses will vary around the local DRL, occasionally an incident will occur where the exposure is much greater than intended. The regulations indicate that where an employer knows or has reason to believe that an incident has or may have occurred in which a person, while undergoing a medical exposure was, otherwise than as a result of a malfunction or defect in equipment, exposed to an extent 'much greater than intended', a preliminary investigation to determine the magnitude of the exposure must be undertaken. If an overexposure of a patient is confirmed then the employer has a duty to report the incident to the appropriate authority and arrange an investigation of the circumstances and assessment of the dose received.

In England this is reported to the Care Quality Commission within a set period of time and will involve the appointed radiation protection advisor (RPA) and MPE.

Recommended national reference doses for individual radiographs on adult patients

Radiograph	ESD per radiograph (mGy)	No. of rooms	DAP per radiograph (Gy cm^2)
Abdomen AP	4	167	2.5
Chest AP	0.2	53	0.15
Chest LAT	0.5	47	
Chest PA	0.15	285	0.1
Cervical spine AP			0.15
Cervical spine LAT			0.15
Knee AP	0.3	40	
Knee LAT	0.3	32	
Lumbar spine AP	5.7	192	1.5
Lumbar spine LAT	10	185	2.5
Pelvis AP	4	204	2.2
Shoulder AP	0.5	34	
Skull AP/PA	1.8	21	
Skull LAT	1.1	21	
Thoracic spine AP	3.5	104	1.0
Thoracic spine LAT	7	104	1.5

The reporting of such incidents takes a different pathway compared with overexposures due to malfunction of equipment, which are covered under the Ionising Radiation Regulations 1999 as discussed in the next page.

The Health and Safety Executive (HSE) specific guidance in determining dose overexposure, as addressed in the next sections, is employed in determining the dose.

Patients, who undergo a procedure that was not intended, as a result of mistaken identification or other procedural failure, and consequently have been exposed to an ionising radiation dose, should be considered as having an unintended exposure.

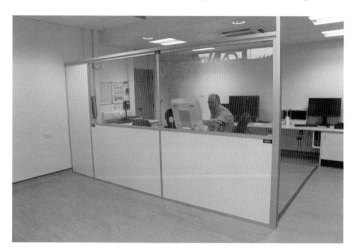

Fig. 1.35a Controlled area.

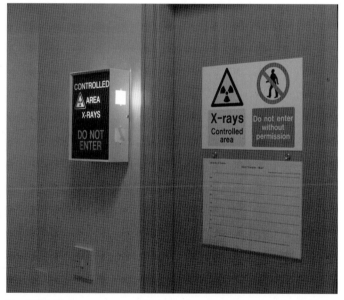

Fig. 1.35b Entrance to a controlled area showing warning signs and lights.

Adult employees – 20 mSv
Trainees under 18 – 6 mSv
Others – 1 mSv
Comforters and carers (5 years) – 5 mSv
Dose to foetus during pregnancy – 1mSv
Dose to abdomen of woman of reproductive capacity in 3 month period – 13 mSv

Fig. 1.35c The application of the Dose Equivalent Limits for different categories of workers.

Radiation protection 1

Occupational exposure

Ionising Radiations Regulation 1999 (IRR99)

Whereas the IR(ME)R regulations deal specifically with medical exposure to patients, the IRR99 regulations and associated guidance notes facilitate the protection of staff and the public when using ionising radiation, including equipment generating X-rays. This next section highlights some of the important aspects of occupational exposure.

A key requirement of IRR99 is that there must always be prior risk assessments of all work involving ionising radiation and that these are reviewed regularly and whenever there is a change of practice. Employers are required to apply a range of regulations in order to restrict the exposures to their employees and other persons so far as is reasonably practicable (ALARP). These include individual dose limitation (Fig. 1.35c), ensuring the safe design, installation and assessment of radiation equipment and employing a hierarchy of control measures. Engineered means of controlling exposures, such as fixed shielding, interlocks and warning devices are preferred, backed up by supporting systems of work described in local rules, and with provision of PPE to restrict exposure further where practicable.

In order to restrict doses, employers are required to designate the areas where staff or the public could exceed the dose limits that apply to them. X-ray rooms are usually controlled areas (Figs 1.35a, 1.35b), requiring staff to be classified or to follow strict systems of work when they work in them. Sometimes, other areas where the public could exceed their lower dose limit are designated as supervised. Designated areas must be clearly marked, with systems to control entry and require supervision by radiation protection supervisors (RPSs). The areas, systems of work and supervision must be documented in local rules and there may be additional requirements for dose monitoring of an area. Contingency arrangements in the event of an accident or incident are also a requirement.

A system of personal dose monitoring is required to ensure that staff do not exceed the relevant dose limits. In situations where staff could exceed 3/10ths of a dose limit, these staff must be classified, which will entail closer monitoring of their doses and health. Classification is rare when using X-rays in diagnostic radiology though is occasionally needed for those performing interventional procedures.

Employers must have sound management arrangements in place, to ensure that they meet the requirements of IRR99. Normally they will have to consult a RPA to advise them on compliance. The employer must also inform, instruct and train all categories of staff involved in work with ionising radiation so that they follow the specified systems of work.

Radiation protection

Occupational exposure (cont.)

The protection of staff is largely controlled through the application of IRR99. The legislation makes stringent requirements of employers to protect their staff and also patients and members of the general public. Practical aspects of the regulations that will be encountered will include:

- Staff dose and environmental monitoring.
- The selection, installation, maintenance, calibration and replacement of equipment.
- Criteria of acceptability of both new and older equipment.
- QA programmes, including adoption of suspension levels.
- The investigation of incidents involving a malfunction or defect in radiation equipment that results in an exposure much greater than intended.

The following section expands on some of the important protection elements of the legislation.

Designation of classified persons

This is defined as those employees who are likely to receive an effective dose in excess of 6mSv per year or an equivalent dose which exceeds 3/10ths of any relevant dose limit.

Investigation and notification of incidents resulting in much greater than intended exposure

This applies to both patients and staff where the overexposure is related to *a malfunction or defect in equipment*.

An overexposure may be defined as an exposure in excess of a relevant dose limit (employee or member of the public). This is an exposure much greater than intended, therefore the dose to a patient that exceeds the guideline multiplying factors in HSE publication Guidance Note PM77 (3rd edition) Appendix 2 should be investigated and notified to the appropriate Authority.

The notification guidelines are broadly representative of patient exposure, i.e. effective dose or mean glandular dose. Suitable measurements for determining these quantities are:

- DAP.
- Duration of exposure.
- Product of tube current and time (mAs) and/or
- Volume of tissue irradiated.
- Radiography of extremities, skull, dentition, shoulder, chest, elbow and knee, with intended dose of 0.5mSv must notify the HSE if the dose is 20 times more than intended.

ALARP principle

ALARP refers to the radiation doses that may be absorbed by operators of equipment generating ionising radiation.

Applying the ALARP principle is one of the main considerations when staff operate X-ray equipment to ensure that any dose that they might receive is kept to the minimum. This must be applied not only to the patient but to visitors and other staff.

Optimisation of the exposure factors and simple measures such as ensuring that all X-ray room doors are closed and all non-essential staff are excluded during X-ray examinations and that the X-ray tube is directed away from staff areas are important considerations.

Designated areas

The X-ray room is a controlled area and warning signs must be present and lit when an exposure is taking place. Entry/exit doors must be closed during exposure and staff must not enter (Fig. 1.35b).

Radiation protection of staff

Staff must ensure they are not accidentally exposed to radiation and have a legal requirement to protect themselves from risk. This can be achieved in a number of ways:

- X-ray and gamma camera rooms are designed to minimise the dose to staff.
- Only staff necessary should be present when an exposure is made.
- The use of time, distance and shielding principles:
  - Time: staff should minimise the amount of time spent in fluoroscopy.
  - Distance: use the inverse square law to stand far enough away from the X-ray or radiation source. NB: There is a 2 metre controlled area from the image intensifier in which the staff MUST wear appropriate PPE.
  - Shielding:
    - Stand behind a protective screen when an exposure is made (Fig. 1.35a).
    - Wear PPE when undertaking fluoroscopy.
    - Staff may also be monitored to ensure they do not exceed the legal dose limits for workers.

Section 2
Upper Limb

CONTENTS

RECOMMENDED PROJECTIONS	52	Lateral method 2	72
		Oblique (anterior oblique)	73
POSITION OF PATIENT IN RELATION TO THE IMAGE DETECTOR	53	Image evaluation – 10-point plan	74
		FOREARM	75
HAND	54	Antero-posterior	75
Basic projections	55	Lateral	76
Dorsi-palmar	55		
Anterior oblique (DP oblique)	56	ELBOW	77
Image evaluation – 10-point plan	57	Lateral	77
Lateral	57	Antero-posterior	78
Dorsi-palmar both hands	58	Antero-posterior – partial flexion	78
Antero-posterior oblique both hands (ball catcher's or Norgaard projection)	59	Antero-posterior – forearm in contact	79
		Antero-posterior – upper arm in contact	79
FINGERS	60	Full flexion	80
Basic projections	60	Axial – upper arm in contact	80
Dorsi-palmar (DP)	60	Axial – forearm in contact	81
Lateral index and middle fingers	60	Image evaluation – 10-point plan	81
Lateral ring and little fingers	61	Lateral head of radius	82
		Proximal radio-ulnar joint – oblique	83
THUMB	62	Ulnar groove – axial	83
Basic projections	62	Radiological considerations	84
Lateral	62	Image evaluation – 10-point plan	85
Antero-posterior	62		
Postero-anterior foreign body	63	HUMERUS – SUPRACONDYLAR FRACTURE	86
		Lateral	86
SCAPHOID (CARPAL BONES)	64	Antero-posterior	87
Postero-anterior – ulnar deviation	64		
Anterior oblique – ulnar deviation	65	HUMERUS – SHAFT	88
Posterior oblique	66	Antero-posterior – erect	88
Lateral	67	Lateral – erect	88
Postero-anterior – ulnar deviation and 30° cranial angle	68	Antero-posterior – supine	89
		Lateral – supine	89
CARPAL TUNNEL	69	HUMERUS – INTERTUBEROUS SULCUS (BICIPITAL GROOVE)	90
Axial – method 1	69	Axial	90
Axial – method 2	69	Alternative axial projection	90
WRIST	70	HUMERUS – NECK	91
Basic projections	70	Antero-posterior	91
Method 1	70	Axial	92
Method 2	70	Supero-inferior (axial)	92
Postero-anterior	71	Infero-superior (reverse axial)	93
Lateral method 1	71	Lateral oblique (lateral)	93
		Image evaluation – 10-point plan	94

2 Recommended projections

Area	Indication	Projection
Hand	Fractures and dislocation of metacarpals	Postero-anterior (basic) Anterior oblique (basic)
	Serious injury or foreign bodies	Lateral (basic) Antero-posterior (alternate)
	Pathology e.g. rheumatoid arthritis	Postero-anterior – both hands Postero-oblique – both hands (ball catcher's)
Fingers	Fractures and dislocation/foreign bodies	Postero-anterior (basic) Lateral (basic)
Thumb	Fractures and dislocation of phalanges	Antero-posterior (basic) Lateral (basic)
	Injury to base of first metacarpal e.g. Bennett's fracture	Antero-posterior (basic) Lateral (basic)
Carpal bones	e.g. Scaphoid	Postero-anterior with hand adducted (ulnar deviation) Anterior oblique (basic) Posterior oblique Lateral (basic) PA ulnar deviation and 30° cranial angle
Carpal tunnel syndrome		Axial Postero-anterior
Distal end radius and ulna	Trauma or pathology	Postero-anterior (basic) Lateral (basic) Oblique
Forearm	Trauma or pathology	Antero-posterior (basic) Lateral (basic)
	Serious injury	Antero-posterior (modified) Lateral (modified)
Elbow joint	Trauma or pathology	Lateral (basic) Antero-posterior (basic)
	Elbow cannot be extended	Lateral (basic) Antero-posterior Axial
	Trauma or pathology head of radius	Antero-posterior (basic) Lateral with rotation of radius Axial (2)
	Proximal radio-ulnar joint	Lateral (basic) Antero-posterior – oblique
	Ulnar groove	Antero-posterior (basic) Axial
	Supracondylar fracture	Antero-posterior (modified) Lateral (modified)
Humerus	Trauma or pathology	Antero-posterior (erect) Lateral (erect)
	Intertuberous sulcus (bicipital groove)	Antero-posterior (basic) Axial
Neck of humerus	Fracture	Antero-posterior Lateral oblique Lateral – supero-superior Lateral – infero-superior

Position of patient in relation to the image detector

2

Although radiographic examinations of the upper limb are routine a high standard of radiography must be maintained. The best possible radiographs are essential as decisions about injuries especially of elbow and wrist affect future dexterity, employment and earnings of the patient.

The importance of registering the correct right or left marker at the time of the exposure cannot be overemphasised nor can the importance of recording the correct patient identification and date of the examination.

To ensure maximum radiation protection when using computed radiography (CR) cassettes, the patient should be seated at the side or end of the table with the lower limbs and gonads away from the primary beam, i.e. with the legs to the side of the table not under it and the beam should be collimated within the margins of the image receptor (Figs 2.1a, 2.1b).

The limb should be immobilised by the use of non-opaque pads within the radiation field and sandbags outside the field. It is important to remember that the patient will only be able to keep the limb still if it is in a comfortable relaxed position. When the hand or wrist is being examined the patient's forearm and hand can rest on the table. For examination of the forearm, elbow and humerus, the shoulder, elbow and wrist should be in a plane parallel to the image receptor. This means that the shoulder, elbow and wrist will be at the same horizontal level, i.e. the upper arm, elbow and forearm should be in contact with the digital receptor.

Direct digital radiography (DDR) allows more flexibility for the examination as the detector can be positioned:

- Similar to a CR procedure with the detector used like a table procedure.
- Erect, which allows the extremity to be positioned with the patient standing and reduces examination times (see Section 1 page 15; a patient standing adjacent to the DDR detector positioned for a DP thumb).

DDR detectors have, in the main, a large receptive field (normally 43 cm × 43 cm) and the limb can be positioned anywhere within that field for upper-limb examinations.

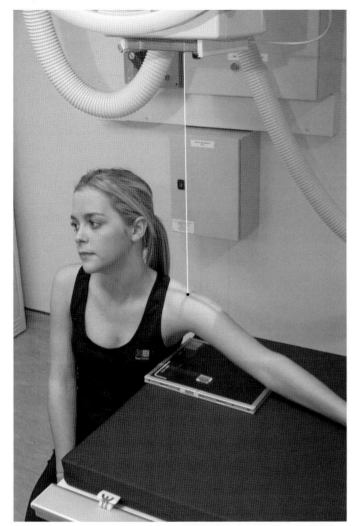

Fig. 2.1a Patient position for an upper limb examination using CR.

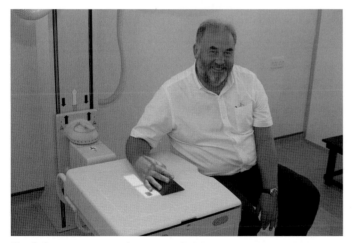

Fig. 2.1b Patient position for an upper limb examination using DR.

2 Hand

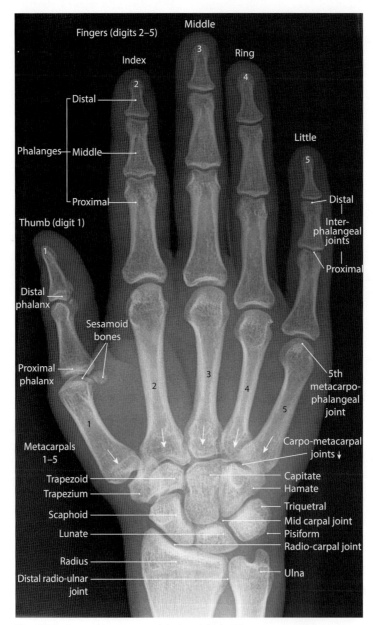

Fig. 2.2 Radiographic anatomy of the hand; Right PA.

Hand 2

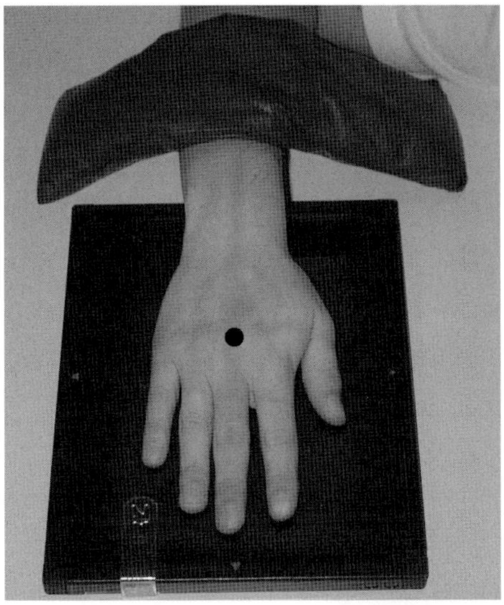

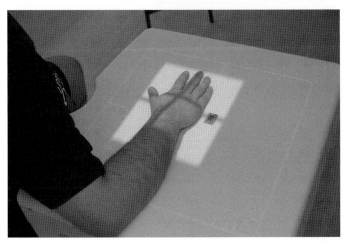

Fig. 2.3a Positioning for dorsi-palmar (DP) hand for CR imaging.

Fig. 2.3b Positioning for DP hand for DDR imaging.

Basic projections

Two projections are routinely taken, a dorsi-palmar (DP) and an anterior oblique (DP oblique). Each image is acquired using a CR image receptor or alternatively within the field of view of a DDR detector. An 18 cm × 24 cm size cassette is used for CR imaging.

Dorsi-palmar (Figs 2.3a, 2.3b)

Position of patient and image receptor

The patient is seated alongside the table with the affected arm nearest to the table.

- The forearm is pronated and placed on the table with the palmer surface of the hand in contact with the image receptor.
- The fingers are separated and extended but relaxed to ensure that they remain in contact with the image receptor.
- The wrist is adjusted so that the radial and ulna styloid processes are equidistant from the image receptor.
- A sandbag is placed over the lower forearm for immobilisation.

Direction and location of X-ray beam

- The collimated vertical beam is centred over the head of the 3rd metacarpal.

Essential image characteristics (Figs 2.3c, 2.3d)

- The image should demonstrate all the phalanges, including the soft tissue of the fingertips, the carpal and metacarpal bones and the distal end of the radius and ulna.
- The interphalangeal and metacarpo-phalangeal and carpo-metacarpal joints should be demonstrated clearly.
- No rotation of the hand.

Radiation protection/dose

- Careful technique and close collimation will assist in reducing the patient dose.

Expected DRL: ESD 0.058 mGy.

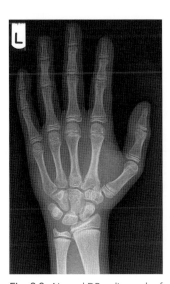

Fig. 2.3c Normal DP radiograph of the left hand.

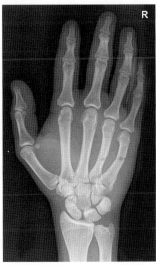

Fig. 2.3d DP radiograph showing fracture of the 4th and 5th metacarpals.

2 Hand

Anterior oblique (DP oblique) (Fig. 2.4a)

Position of patient and image receptor

- From the basic postero-anterior position, the hand is externally rotated 45° with the fingers extended.
- The fingers should be separated slightly and the hand supported on a 45° non-opaque pad.
- A sandbag is placed over the lower end of the forearm for immobilisation.

Direction and location of the X-ray beam

- The collimated vertical beam is centred over the head of the 5th metacarpal.
- The tube is then angled so that the central ray passes through the head of the 3rd metacarpal, enabling a reduction in the size of the field.

Essential image characteristics (Figs 2.4b, 2.4c)

- The image should demonstrate all the phalanges, including the soft tissue of the fingertips, the carpal and metacarpal bones and the distal end of the radius and ulna.
- The correct degree of rotation has been achieved when the heads of the 1st and 2nd metacarpals are seen separated whilst those of the 4th and 5th are just superimposed.

Common faults and remedies

- Over rotation will project the metacarpals and digits on top of each other (Fig 2.4c).
- Under rotation will fail to open out the metacarpals.

Notes

- The exposure should provide adequate penetration too visualise the metacarpal bones and fall within the exposure indicator (EI).

Radiological considerations

There are numerous possible accessory ossicles around the hand (see radiographic anatomy page 54)

Expected DRL: ESD 0.060 mGy.

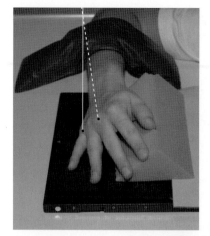

Fig. 2.4a Patient positioning for the DP oblique hand.

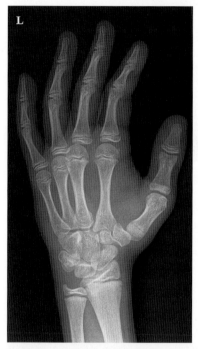

Fig. 2.4b Normal DP oblique radiograph of the hand.

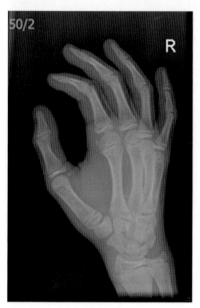

Fig. 2.4c Over-rotation of the hand.

Image evaluation – 10-point plan

IMAGE EVALUATION

DP oblique (Fig. 2.4c)

The main points to consider are: over-rotated hand.
1. Patient demographics have been removed for confidentiality reasons.
2. Area of interest is included.
3. Correct anatomical marker (Right).
4. Hand over-rotated with 3rd, 4th and 5th metacarpals superimposed.
5. Correct image exposure – EI correct and no noise.
6. Optimum resolution – good bony trabeculae and soft-tissue resolution.
7. Collimated to area of interest.
8. No artefacts.
9. Repeat required demonstrating 3rd to 5th metacarpals not superimposed.
10. Paediatric hand so epiphyses not fused.

Radiographer Comments/Initial report

DP oblique hand

DP oblique hand demonstrating over-rotation. The 3rd, 4th and 5th metacarpals are superimposed. A repeat X-ray is required.

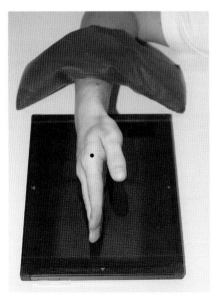

Fig. 2.5a Patient positioning for lateral radiograph.

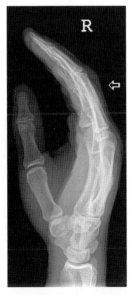

Fig. 2.5b Lateral radiograph of the hand demonstrating a foreign body. There is an old fracture of the 5th metacarpal.

Hand 2

Lateral (Fig. 2.5a)

In the lateral position the metacarpals overshadow and obscure each other. However, this projection is essential to demonstrate anterior or posterior displacements of fracture fragments. This projection is also used to determine the position of foreign bodies in the palmar or dorsal aspect of the hand.

Position of patient and image receptor

- From the postero-anterior (DP) position, the hand is externally rotated 90°.
- The palm of the hand is perpendicular to the image receptor, with the fingers extended and the thumb abducted and supported parallel to the image receptor on a non-opaque pad.
- The radial and ulnar styloid processes are superimposed.

Direction and location of the X-ray beam

- The collimated vertical beam is centred over the head of the 2nd metacarpal.

Essential image characteristics (Fig. 2.5b)

- The image should include the fingertips, including soft tissue, and the radial and ulnar styloid processes.
- The heads of the metacarpals should be superimposed. The thumb should be demonstrated clearly without superimposition of other structures.

Radiological considerations

- The hand and wrist (like the ankle and foot) have many accessory ossicles, which may trap the unwary into a false diagnosis of pathology.
- 'Boxer's fracture' of the neck of the 5th metacarpal is seen easily, but conspicuity of fractures of the bases of the metacarpals is reduced by over-rotation and underexposure.

Notes

- If the projection is undertaken to identify the position of a foreign body when using screen/film systems, the kilovoltage (kV) should be reduced to improve radiographic contrast.
- A metal marker is used to demonstrate the site of entry of the foreign body.

Radiation protection/dose

- Careful technique and close collimation will assist in reducing the patient dose.

Expected DRL: ESD 0.081 mGy.

2 Hand

Dorsi-palmar both hands (Figs 2.6a, 2.6b)

This projection is often used to demonstrate subtle radiographic changes associated with early rheumatoid arthritis and to monitor the progress of the disease.

Position of patient and image receptor

- Ideally, the patient is seated alongside the table. However, if this is not possible due to the patient's condition, the patient may be seated facing the table (see Radiation protection, page 15).
- Both forearms are pronated and placed on the table with the palmer surface of the hands in contact with the image receptor.
- The fingers are separated and extended but relaxed to ensure that they remain in contact with the image receptor.
- The wrists are adjusted so that the radial and ulna styloid processes are equidistant from the image receptor.
- A sandbag is placed over the lower forearms for immobilisation.

Direction and location of the X-ray beam

- The collimated vertical beam is centred over a point midway between the interphalangeal joints of both thumbs.

Essential image characteristics (Figs 2.6c, 2.6d)

- The image should demonstrate all the phalanges, including the soft tissue of the fingertips, the carpal and metacarpal bones and the distal end of the radius and ulna.
- The exposure factors selected must produce an accurate EI and optimally demonstrate joint detail

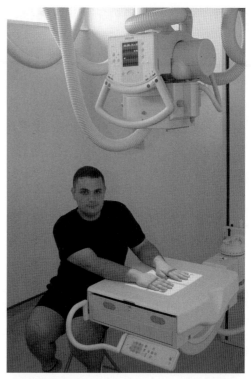

Fig. 2.6a Patient positioning for postero-anterior (DP) radiograph, both hands.

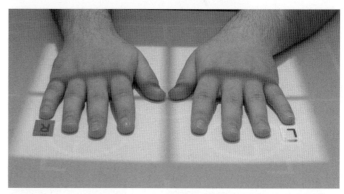

Fig. 2.6b Patient position for both hands.

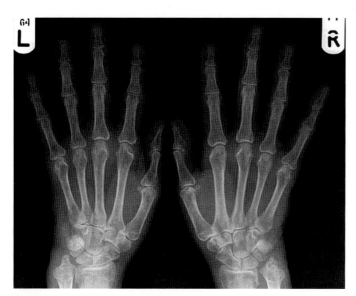

Fig. 2.6c Normal postero-anterior (DP) radiograph, both hands on an elderly patient.

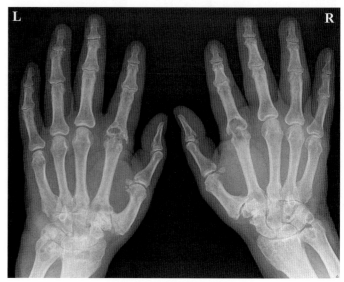

Fig. 2.6d Postero-anterior (DP) radiograph of both hands showing severe erosive disease.

Hand 2

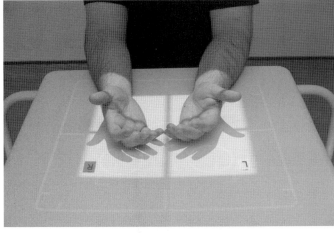

Fig. 2.7a Patient positioning in ball catcher's position.

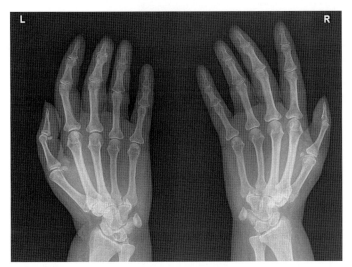

Fig. 2.7b Normal radiograph of hands in 'ball catcher's' position.

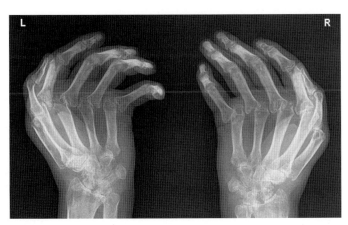

Fig. 2.7c Radiograph of hand in ball catcher's position showing severe erosive disease.

Antero-posterior oblique both hands (ball catcher's or Norgaard projection) (Fig. 2.7a)

This projection may be used in the diagnosis of rheumatoid arthritis. It can also be used to demonstrate fractures of the base of the 5th metacarpals. For CR a 24 × 30 cm cassette is employed.

Position of the patient and image receptor

- Ideally the patient is seated alongside the table. However, if this is not possible, due to the patient's condition, the patient may be seated facing the table (see Radiation protection, page 15).
- Both forearms are supinated and placed on the table with the dorsal surface of the hands in contact with the image receptor.
- From this position both hands are rotated internally (medially) 45° into a 'ball catching' position.
- The fingers and thumbs are separated and extended but relaxed to ensure that they remain in contact with the image receptor.
- The hands may be supported using 45° non-opaque pads.
- A sandbag is placed over the lower forearms for immobilisation.

Direction and location of X-ray beam

- The collimated vertical beam is centred to a point midway between the hands at the level of the 5th metacarpophalangeal joints (MCPJ).

Essential image characteristics (Figs 2.7b, 2.7c)

- The image should demonstrate all the phalanges, including the soft tissue of the finger tips, the carpal and metacarpal bones and the distal end of the radius and ulna.
- The exposure factors selected must produce an accurate EI and optimally demonstrate joint detail.
- The heads of the metacarpals should not be superimposed.

Radiation protection

If it has been necessary to position the patient facing the table it is essential to provide radiation protection for the lower limbs and gonads. This may be achieved by placing a lead-rubber sheet on the table underneath the image receptor to attenuate the primary beam.

2 Fingers

Basic projections

Two projections are routinely taken, a postero-anterior and a lateral. The adjacent finger is routinely imaged unless the injury is very localised, e.g. a crush injury to the distal phalanx. Each image is acquired using an 18 × 24 CR cassette or alternatively within the field of view of a DDR detector.

Dorsi-palmar (DP) (Figs 2.8a, 2.8b)

Position of patient and image receptor

- The patient is positioned seated alongside the table as for a postero-anterior projection of the hand.
- The forearm is pronated with the anterior (palmer) aspect of the finger(s) in contact with the image receptor.
- The finger(s) are extended and separated.
- A sandbag may be placed across the dorsal surface of the wrist for immobilisation.

Direction and location of X-ray beam

- The collimated vertical beam is centred over the proximal interphalangeal joint of the affected and adjacent finger.

Essential image characteristics (Fig. 2.8b)

- The image should include the fingertips, including soft tissue, and distal 3rd of the metacarpal bone(s).
- It is necessary to include adjacent finger(s), i.e. the 2nd and 3rd or 4th and 5th to aid in identifying the relevant anatomy. If this is the case, then care should be taken to avoid superimposition, particularly in the lateral projection, by fully extending one finger and partly flexing the other.

Radiological considerations

- The image should include the fingertip and the distal 3rd of the metacarpal bone.

Lateral index and middle fingers (Fig. 2.8d)

Position of patient and image receptor

- The patient is seated alongside the table with the arm abducted and medially rotated to bring the lateral aspect of the index finger into contact with the image detector.
- The raised forearm is supported.
- The index finger is fully extended and the middle finger slightly flexed to avoid superimposition.
- The middle finger is supported on a non-opaque pad.
- The remaining fingers are fully flexed into the palm of the hand and held there by the thumb.

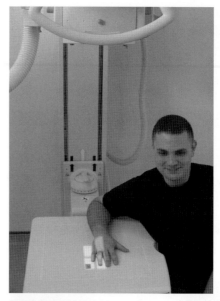

Fig. 2.8a Patient positioning for postero-anterior radiograph of fingers.

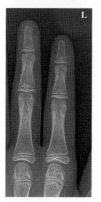

Fig. 2.8b Postero-anterior radiograph of the index and middle fingers.

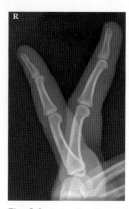

Fig. 2.8c Lateral radiograph of index and middle fingers.

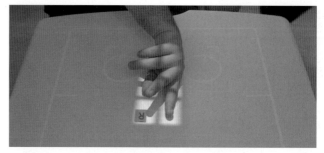

Fig. 2.8d Patient positioning for lateral radiograph of index and middle fingers.

Direction and location of X-ray beam

- The collimated vertical central ray is centred over the proximal interphalangeal joint of the affected finger.

Essential image characteristics (Fig. 2.8c)

- The image should include the fingertip and the distal 3rd of the metacarpal bone.

Expected DRL:
- DP – ESD 0.054 mGy.
- Lateral – ESD 0.054 mGy.

Fingers 2

Lateral ring and little fingers (Fig. 2.9a)

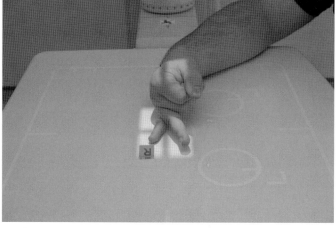

Fig. 2.9a Patient positioning for lateral ring and little fingers.

Position of patient and image receptor

- The patient is seated alongside the table with the palm of the hand at right-angles to the table and the medial aspect of the little finger in contact with the image receptor.
- The affected finger is extended and the remaining fingers are fully flexed into the palm of the hand and held there by the thumb in order to prevent superimposition.
- It may be necessary to support the ring finger on a non-opaque pad to ensure that it is parallel to the image receptor

Direction and location of X-ray beam

- The collimated vertical beam is centred over the proximal interphalangeal joint of the affected finger.

Essential image characteristics (Figs 2.9b–2.9d)

- The image should include the tip of the finger and the distal 3rd of the metacarpal bone.

Radiological considerations

- Scleroderma (one cause of Raynaud's disease) causes wasting and calcification of the soft tissue of the finger pulp.
- Chip fracture of the base of the dorsal aspect of the distal phalanx is associated with avulsion of the insertion of the extensor digitorum tendon, leading to the mallet finger deformity.

Radiation protection/dose

Careful technique and close collimation will assist in reducing the patient dose.

Expected DRL: ESD 0.054 mGy.

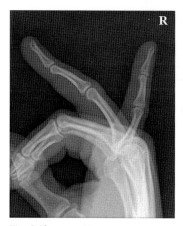

Fig. 2.9b Normal lateral radiograph of ring and little fingers.

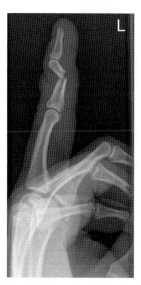

Fig. 2.9c Lateral radiograph of middle finger showing a fracture of the middle phalanx.

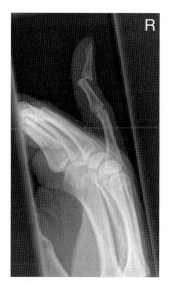

Fig. 2.9d Lateral radiograph of little finger showing dislocation of the distal interphalangeal joint.

2 Thumb

Basic projections

Two projections are routinely taken, a lateral and an antero-posterior. Occasionally a postero-anterior may be undertaken if the patient is unable to get into position because of a painful fracture. Each image is acquired using an 18 × 24 CR cassette or alternatively within the field of view of a DDR detector.

Lateral (Fig. 2.10a)

Position of patient and image receptor

- The patient is seated alongside the table with the arm abducted, the elbow flexed and the anterior aspect of the forearm resting on the table.
- The thumb is flexed slightly and the palm of the hand is placed on the image receptor.
- The palm of the hand is raised slightly with the fingers partially flexed and may be supported on a non-opaque pad, such that the lateral aspect of the thumb is in contact with the image receptor.

Direction and location of X-ray beam

The collimated vertical beam is centred over the 1st MCPJ.

Essential image characteristics (Figs 2.10b, 2.10d, 2.10e)

- The image should include the fingertip and the distal 1/3 of the metacarpal bone.
- Where there is a possibility of injury to the base of the 1st metacarpal, the carpo-metacarpal joint must be included on the image.

Expected DRL: ESD 0.067 mGy.

Antero-posterior (AP) (Fig. 2.10c)

Position of patient and image receptor

- The patient is seated facing away from the table with the arm extended backwards and medially rotated at the shoulder. The hand may be slightly rotated to ensure that the 2nd, 3rd and 4rth metacarpals are not superimposed on the base of the 1st metacarpal.
- The patient leans forward, lowering the shoulder so that the 1st metacarpal is parallel to the tabletop.
- The image receptor is placed under the wrist and thumb and oriented to the long axis of the metacarpal.

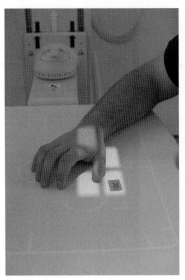

Fig. 2.10a Patient positioning for lateral radiograph of the thumb.

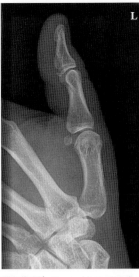

Fig. 2.10b Normal lateral radiograph of the thumb.

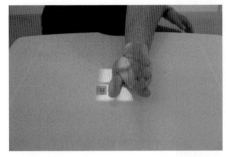

Fig. 2.10c Patient positioning for antero-posterior (AP) radiograph of the thumb.

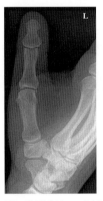

Fig. 2.10d Normal AP radiograph of the thumb.

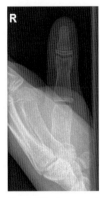

Fig. 2.10e Incorrectly positioned AP radiograph of thumb.

Direction and location of X-ray beam

- The collimated vertical central ray is centred over the 1st MCPJ.

Radiation protection/dose

Expected DRL: ESD 0.064 mGy.

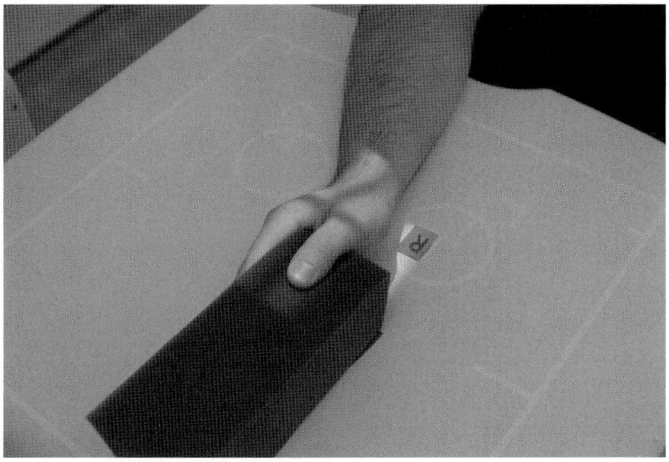

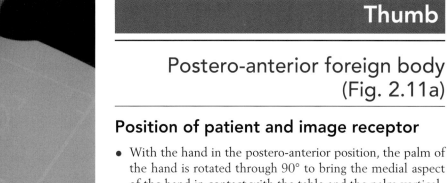

Fig. 2.11a Patient positioning for postero-anterior (PA) thumb.

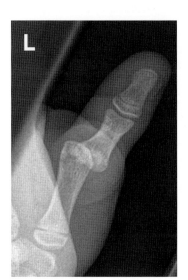

Fig. 2.11b PA radiograph thumb demonstrating dislocation of the 1st MCPJ.

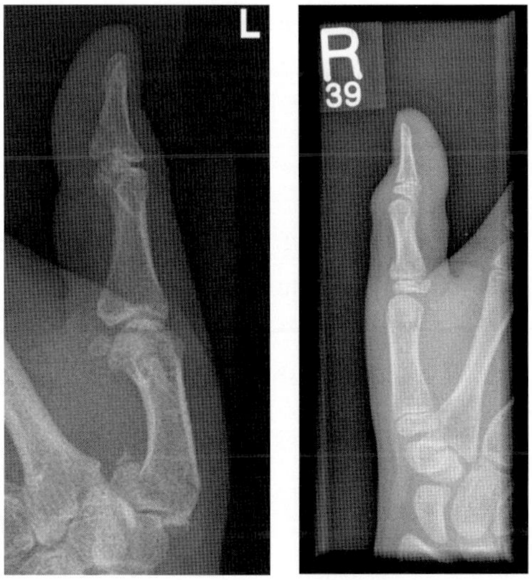

Figs. 2.11c and d Radiograph of lateral thumb with Bennett's fracture (left) and radiograph of fracture proximal phalanx (right).

Thumb 2

Postero-anterior foreign body (Fig. 2.11a)

Position of patient and image receptor

- With the hand in the postero-anterior position, the palm of the hand is rotated through 90° to bring the medial aspect of the hand in contact with the table and the palm vertical.
- The image receptor is placed under the hand and wrist, with its long axis along the line of the thumb.
- The fingers are extended and the hand is rotated slightly forwards until the anterior aspect of the thumb is parallel to the image receptor.
- The thumb is supported in position on a non-opaque pad.

Direction and location of X-ray beam

- The collimated vertical beam is centred over the base of the 1st metacarpal.

Notes

- The use of the postero-anterior projection maintains the relationship of the adjacent bones, i.e. the radius and ulna, which is essential in cases of suspected foreign body in the thenar eminence.
- When undertaking a PA projection there is an increased object to detector distance. This will lead to magnification of the image and any associated unsharpness. To prevent this, increase the focus receptor distance.

Radiological considerations (Figs 2.11b–2.11d)

- Fracture of the base of the 1st metacarpal through the joint surface may be associated with dislocation due to the pull of the abductor and extensor tendons of the thumb. This is known as Bennett's fracture and may cause functional impairment and early degenerative disease if not corrected. In contrast, a fracture that does not transgress the articular surface does not dislocate and does not have the same significance (Rolando fracture).

Radiation protection/dose

Careful technique and close collimation will assist in reducing the patient dose.

Expected DRL: ESD 0.064 mGy.

2 Scaphoid (carpal bones)

Postero-anterior – ulnar deviation (Figs 2.12b, 2.12c)

Imaging of the carpal bones is most commonly undertaken to demonstrate the scaphoid. The projections may also be used to demonstrate other carpal bones, as indicated below. Five projections (depending on departmental protocol) may be taken to demonstrate all the carpal bones, with each acquired using the smallest CR image receptor, i.e. 18 × 24 cm cassette or alternatively within the field of view of a DDR detector.

Position of patient and image receptor

- The patient is positioned seated alongside the table with the affected side nearest the table (CR) or adjacent to the DDR detector either seated or standing.
- The arm is extended across the table with the elbow flexed and the forearm pronated.
- If possible, the shoulder, elbow and wrist should be at the level of the tabletop.
- The wrist is positioned over the centre of the image receptor and the hand is adducted (ulnar deviation).
- Ensure that the radial and ulnar styloid processes are equidistant from the image receptor.
- The hand and lower forearm may be immobilised using a sandbag.

Direction and location of X-ray beam

- The collimated vertical beam is centred midway between the radial and ulnar styloid processes.

Essential image characteristics (Figs 2.12a, 2.12d)

- The image should include the distal end of the radius and ulna and the proximal end of the metacarpals.
- The joint space around the scaphoid should be demonstrated clearly.

Expected DRL: ESD 0.072 mGy.

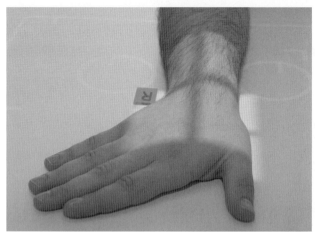

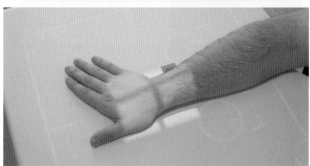

Figs. 2.12b and c Patient positioning for postero-anterior (PA) scaphoid with ulnar deviation.

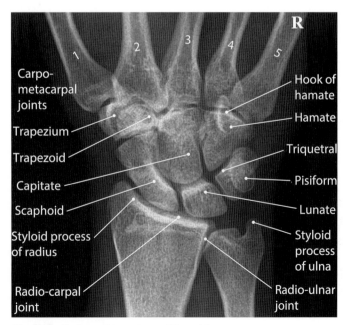

Fig. 2.12a Radiographic anatomy of the wrist.

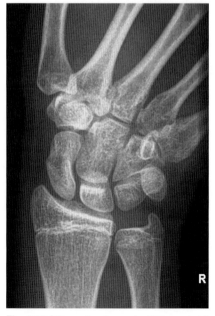

Fig. 2.12d Normal radiograph of PA scaphoid with ulnar deviation.

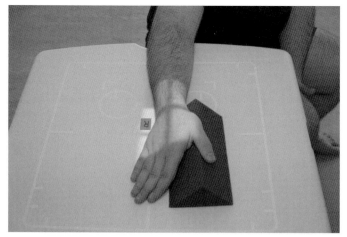

Fig. 2.13a Patient positioning for anterior oblique with ulnar deviation.

Scaphoid (carpal bones) 2

Anterior oblique – ulnar deviation (Fig. 2.13a)

Position of patient and image receptor

- From the postero-anterior position, the hand and wrist are rotated 45° externally and placed over the image detector.
- The hand should remain adducted in ulnar deviation.
- The hand is supported in position, with a non-opaque pad placed under the thumb.
- The forearm may be immobilised using a sandbag.

Direction and location of X-ray beam

- The collimated vertical beam is centred midway between the radial and ulnar styloid processes.

Essential image characteristics (Figs 2.13b, 2.13c)

- The image should include the distal end of the radius and ulna and the proximal end of the metacarpals.
- The scaphoid should be seen clearly, with its long axis parallel to the detector.

Expected DRL: ESD 0.072 mGy.

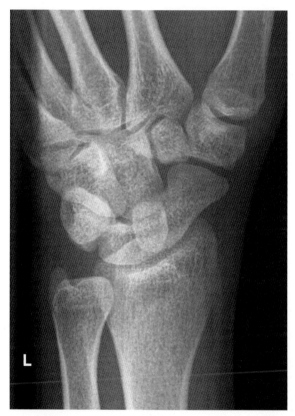

Fig. 2.13b Radiograph of anterior oblique with ulnar deviation.

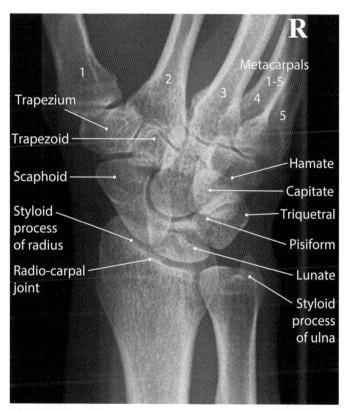

Fig. 2.13c Normal radiograph of anterior oblique with ulnar deviation, demonstrating anatomy.

2 Scaphoid (carpal bones)

Posterior oblique (Fig. 2.14a)

Position of patient and image receptor

- From the anterior oblique position, the hand and wrist are rotated externally through 90°, such that the posterior aspect of the hand and wrist are at 45° to the image detector.
- The wrist is placed over the centre of the detector with the wrist and hand supported on a 45° non-opaque foam pad.
- The forearm may be immobilised using a sandbag.

Direction and location of X-ray beam

- The collimated vertical beam is centred over the styloid process of the ulna.

Essential image characteristics (Figs 2.14b, 2.14c)

- The image should include the distal end of the radius and ulna and the proximal end of the metacarpals.
- The pisiform should be seen clearly in profile situated anterior to the triquetral.
- The long axis of the scaphoid should be seen perpendicular to the long edge of the image detector.

Expected DRL: ESD 0.072 mGy.

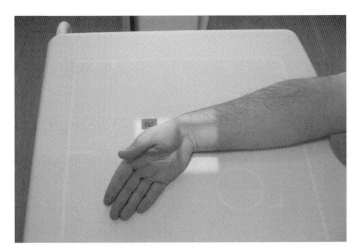

Fig. 2.14a Patient positioning for posterior oblique scaphoid.

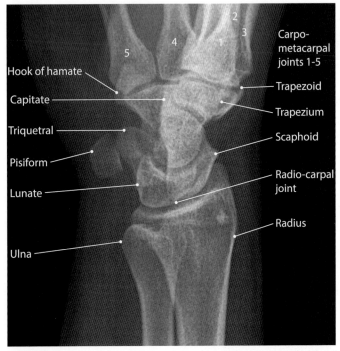

Fig. 2.14b Radiograph of posterior oblique scaphoid demonstrating anatomy.

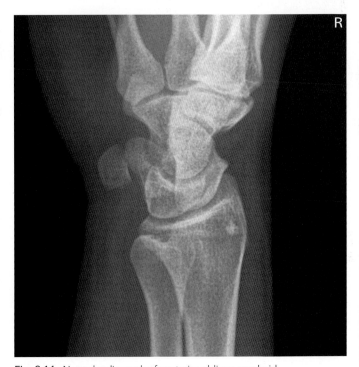

Fig. 2.14c Normal radiograph of posterior oblique scaphoid.

Scaphoid (carpal bones) 2

Lateral (Fig. 2.15a)

Position of patient and image receptor

- From the posterior oblique position, the hand and wrist are rotated internally through 45°, such that the medial aspect of the wrist is in contact with the image detector.
- The hand is adjusted to ensure that the radial and ulnar styloid processes are superimposed.
- The hand and wrist may be immobilised using non-opaque pads and sandbags.

Direction and location of the X-ray beam

- The collimated vertical beam is centred over the radial styloid process.

Essential image characteristics (Figs 2.15b–2.15d)

- The image should include the distal end of the radius and ulna and the proximal end of the metacarpals.
- The image should demonstrate clearly any subluxation or dislocation of the carpal bones.

Radiological considerations

- Fracture of the waist of the scaphoid may be very poorly visualised, or may go unnoticed, at presentation.
- These fractures carry a high risk of delayed avascular necrosis of the distal pole, which can cause severe disability. If suspected clinically, the patient may be re-examined after 10 days of immobilisation, otherwise a magnetic resonance imaging scan (MRI) may offer immediate diagnosis or alternatively digital tomosynthesis.

Expected DRL: ESD 0.082 mGy.

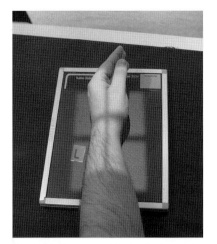

Fig. 2.15a Patient positioning for lateral scaphoid.

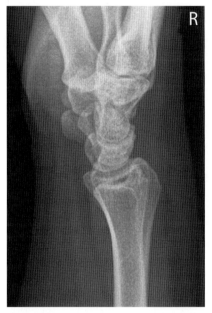

Fig. 2.15b Normal lateral radiograph of wrist.

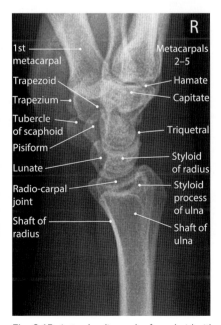

Fig. 2.15c Lateral radiograph of scaphoid with anatomy annotated.

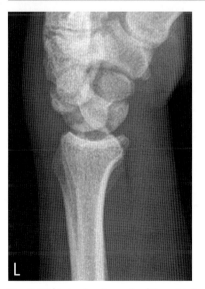

Fig. 2.15d Lateral radiograph of the wrist demonstrating dislocation of the lunate. The lunate bone is rotated and anteriorly displaced.

2 Scaphoid (carpal bones)

Postero-anterior – ulnar deviation and 30° cranial angle (Figs 2.16a, 2.16b)

Position of patient and image receptor

- The patient and image receptor are positioned as for the postero-anterior scaphoid with ulnar deviation. The wrist must be positioned to allow the X-ray tube to be angled at 30° along the long axis of the scaphoid.

Direction and location of X-ray beam

- The collimated vertical beam is angled 30° and centred to the scaphoid.

Essential image characteristics (Fig. 2.16c)

- This projection elongates the scaphoid and with ulnar deviation demonstrates the space surrounding the scaphoid.

Notes

- As the X-ray beam is directed towards the patient's trunk radiation protection of the gonads should be administered.

Radiological considerations

- For scaphoid fractures, three or more projections may be taken: These normally include the postero-anterior (with ulnar deviation), and lateral (wrist projections). Plus one or more of the three projections described in this book.
- A carpal fracture is a break of one of the eight small bones of the carpus. These bones are the scaphoid, lunate, capitate, triquetrum, hamate, pisiform, trapezium, and trapezoid. Fractures of the other carpal bones do occur but the scaphoid is accountable for 60–70% of fractures of the carpal bones.

Radiation protection/dose

Careful technique and close collimation will assist in reducing the patient dose.

Expected DRL: ESD 0.072 mGy.

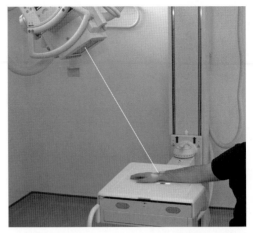

Fig. 2.16a Patient positioning for a postero-anterior (PA) scaphoid with ulnar deviation and 30° cranial angle.

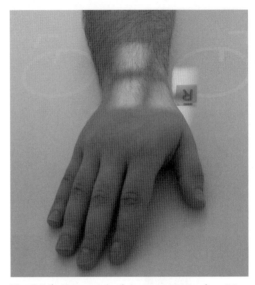

Fig. 2.16b Photograph of close-up position for a PA scaphoid projection with ulnar deviation and 30° cranial angle.

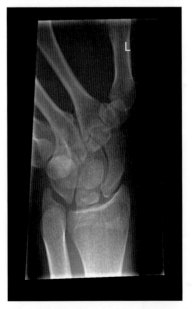

Fig. 2.16c Radiograph of PA with ulnar deviation and 30° cranial angle.

The carpal bones form a shallow concavity, which, with the bridging flexor retinaculum, forms the carpal tunnel. The flexor retinaculum is attached to the two medial prominences (the pisiform and the hook of the hamate) and to the two lateral prominences (the tubercle of the scaphoid and the tubercle of the trapezium). The median nerve along with the flexor tendons pass through the tunnel and any swelling here can cause compression of the median nerve, giving rise to the carpal tunnel syndrome. Radiographic examination of the bony part of the tunnel is by an axial projection to demonstrate the medial and lateral prominences and the concavity.

Carpal tunnel 2

This examination is requested less often nowadays due to improved electrophysiological techniques and the advent of MRI, which gives far better anatomical information.

Two alternative positions using a 18 × 24 cm CR cassette are described, depending on the condition of the patient. These techniques may be modified with DDR detectors and the patient X-rayed erect.

Axial – method 1 (Fig. 2.17a)

Position of patient and image receptor

- The patient is standing facing away from the table.
- The detector is placed level with the edge of the tabletop.
- The palm of the hand is pressed onto the detector, with the wrist joint dorsiflexed to approximately 135°.
- The fingers are curled around under the table to assist in immobilisation.

Direction and location of X-ray beam

- The collimated vertical beam is centred between the pisiform and the hook of the hamate medially and the tubercle of the scaphoid and the ridge of the trapezium laterally.

Essential image characteristics (Figs 2.17c, 2.17d)

- The image should include the distal end of the radius and ulna and the proximal end of the metacarpals.
- The joint space around the scaphoid should be demonstrated clearly.

Axial – method 2 (Fig. 2.17b)

Position of patient and image receptor

- The patient is seated alongside the table.
- The detector is placed on top of a plastic block approximately 8 cm high.
- The lower end of the forearm rests against the edge of the block, with the wrist adducted and dorsiflexed to 135°.
- This position is assisted using a traction bandage held by the patient's other hand.

Direction and location of X-ray beam

- The collimated vertical central ray is centred between the pisiform and the hook of the hamate medially and the tubercle of the scaphoid and the ridge of the trapezium laterally.

Essential image characteristics

- The image should demonstrate clearly the pisiform and the hook of the hamate medially and the tubercle of the scaphoid and the tubercle of the trapezium laterally.

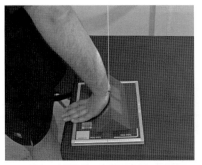
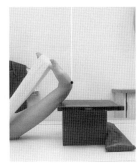

Figs. 2.17a and b Patient positioning for axial projection of carpal tunnel; method 1 (left) method 2 (right)

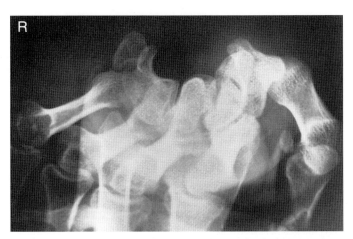

Fig. 2.17c Normal radiograph of carpal tunnel, viewed as looking straight at the palm of the outstretched hand with the wrist dorsiflexed.

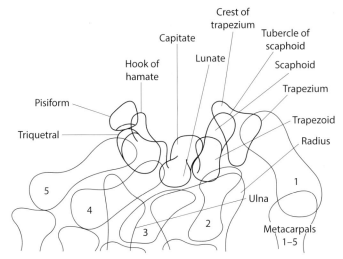

Fig. 2.17d Line diagram of carpal tunnel.

2 Wrist

Basic projections

Two projections are routinely taken, a postero-anterior and a lateral, using an 18 × 24 cm high resolution cassette. A lead-rubber sheet can be used to mask the half of the cassette not in use. An additional oblique projection may also be undertaken to provide addition information.

When carrying out radiographic examinations of the radius and ulna we should bear in mind the movements that occur at the joints of the upper limb. The hand can be rotated from the palm facing the table to the palm at right-angles to the table, with little or no rotation of the ulna. In this movement the upper end of the radius rotates about its long axis while the lower end rotates around the lower end of the ulna carrying the hand with it.

The hinge formed by the trochlear surface of the humerus and the trochlear notch of the ulna prevents rotation of the ulna unless the humerus rotates. If therefore the wrist is positioned for a postero-anterior projection and then moved into the position for the lateral by simply rotating the hand we will obtain two projections of the radius but the same projection of the ulna. To obtain two projections at right-angles of both the radius and the ulna the two positions must be obtained by rotating the humerus (not simply the hand) through 90°, i.e. there should be no rotation at the radio-ulnar joints.

There are then basically two methods of positioning the wrist for a radiographic examination of the lower end of radius and ulna but only one of these will give two projections of both the radius and ulna.

Method 1 (Figs 2.18a, 2.18b)

The forearm remains pronated and the change in position from that for the postero-anterior projection to that for the lateral is achieved by rotation of the hand. In this movement the radius only rotates, not the ulna, giving two projections at right-angles to each other of the radius but the same projection each time for the ulna (Figs 2.18d, 2.18e).

Of the two bones the radius is the more frequently injured so this positioning method can be used to demonstrate the injury providing the patient can rotate the hand. Very often the patient cannot so the second method must be used.

Method 2 (Fig. 2.18c)

The change in position is achieved by rotation of the humerus and because the humerus rotates so does the ulna. This method therefore gives us two projections at right-angles to each other of the radius and ulna.

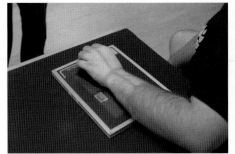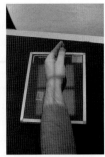

Fig. 2.18a and b Method 1 for radiography of the wrist.

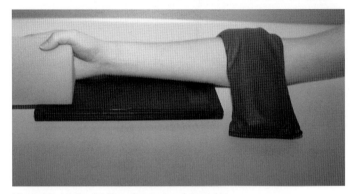

Fig. 2.18c Method 2 for radiography of the wrist.

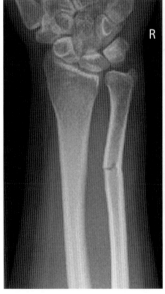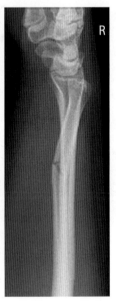

Figs. 2.18d and e Almost identical projections of the ulna produced by using the PA projection, and method 1 for the lateral projection. Note the orientation of the fracture of the distal ulna remains the same.

Radiation protection/dose

Careful technique and close collimation will assist in reducing the patient dose.

Expected DRL:
- PA wrist – ESD 0.072 mGy.
- Lateral wrist – ESD 0.082 mGy.

Position of patient and image receptor

- The patient is seated alongside the table with the affected side nearest to the table.
- The elbow joint is flexed to 90° and the arm abducted such that the anterior aspect of the forearm and the palm of the hand rest on the image receptor.

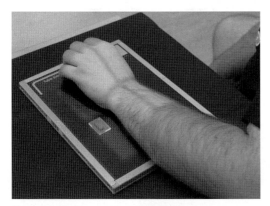

Fig. 2.19a Patient positioning for wrist.

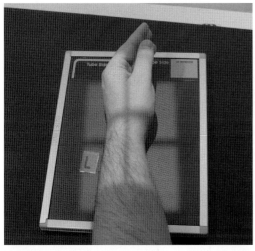

Fig. 2.19b Patient positioning for lateral wrist.

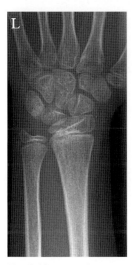

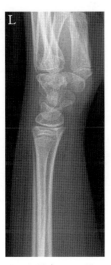

Fig. 2.19c Normal postero-anterior radiograph of wrist.

Fig. 2.19d Normal lateral radiograph of wrist, method 1.

Wrist 2

Postero-anterior (Fig. 2.19a)

- If the mobility of the patient permits, the shoulder joint should be at the same height as the forearm.
- The wrist joint is placed on one half of the cassette and adjusted to include the lower part of the radius and ulna and the proximal 2/3 of the metacarpals.
- The fingers are slightly flexed to bring the anterior aspect of the wrist into contact with the image receptor.
- The wrist joint is adjusted to ensure that the radial and ulnar styloid processes are equidistant from the image receptor and the forearm is immobilised using a sandbag.

Direction and centring of the X-ray beam

- The vertical central ray is centred to a point midway between the radial and ulnar styloid processes.

Essential image characteristics (Fig. 2.19c)

- The image should demonstrate the proximal 2/3 of the metacarpals, the carpal bones, and the distal 1/3 of the radius and ulna.
- There should be no rotation of the wrist joint.

Note

- When undertaken for scaphoid projection, ulnar deviation should be applied.

Lateral method 1 (Fig. 2.19b)

Position of patient and image receptor

- From the postero-anterior position the wrist is externally rotated through 90° to bring the palm of the hand vertical.
- The wrist joint is positioned over the unexposed half of the cassette to include the lower part of the radius and ulna and the proximal 2/3 of the metacarpals.
- The hand is rotated externally slightly further to ensure that the radial and styloid processes are superimposed.
- The forearm is immobilised using a sandbag.

Direction and location of X-ray beam

The vertical central ray is centred over the styloid process of the radius.

Essential image characteristics (Fig. 2.19d)

- The exposure should provide adequate penetration to visualise the carpal bones.
- The radial and ulnar styloid processes should be superimposed.
- The image should demonstrate the proximal 2/3 of the metacarpals, the carpal bones and the distal 1/3 of the radius and ulna.

2 Wrist

Lateral method 2 (Fig. 2.20a)

This projection will ensure that both the radius and ulna will be at right-angles compared with the postero-anterior projection.

Position of patient and image receptor

- From the postero-anterior position the humerus is externally rotated through 90°.
- The elbow joint is extended to bring the medial aspect of the forearm, wrist and hand into contact with the table.
- The wrist joint is positioned over the unexposed 1/2 of the cassette to include the lower part of the radius and ulna and the proximal 2/3 of the metacarpals.
- The hand is rotated externally slightly further to ensure that the radial and styloid processes are superimposed.
- The forearm is immobilised using a sandbag.

Direction and location of X-ray beam

The vertical central ray is centred over the styloid process of the radius.

Essential image characteristics (Fig. 2.20b)

- The exposure should provide adequate penetration to visualise the carpal bones.
- The radial and ulnar styloid processes should be superimposed.
- The image should demonstrate the proximal 2/3 of the metacarpals, the carpal bones and the distal 1/3 of the radius and ulna.

Notes (Figs 2.20c, 2.20d)

- If the patient's limb is immobilised in plaster of Paris it may be necessary to modify the positioning of patient to obtain an accurate postero-anterior and lateral projections. Increased exposure factors will be necessary to penetrate the plaster and the resultant image will be of reduced contrast.
- Light-weight plasters constructed with a polyester knit fabric are radiolucent and require exposure factors similar for uncasted areas.

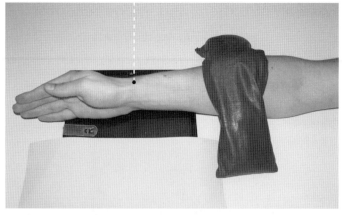

Fig. 2.20a Patient positioning for lateral radiography method 2.

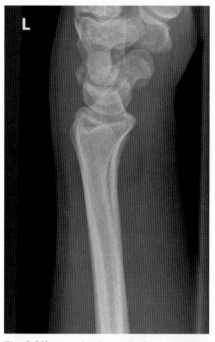

Fig. 2.20b Lateral radiograph of wrist, method 2.

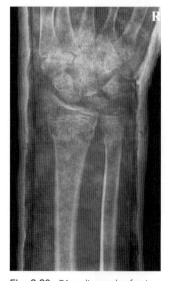

Fig. 2.20c PA radiograph of wrist through normal plaster.

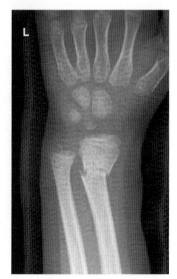

Fig. 2.20d PA radiograph of wrist through lightweight plaster.

Wrist 2

Oblique (anterior oblique) (Fig. 2.21a)

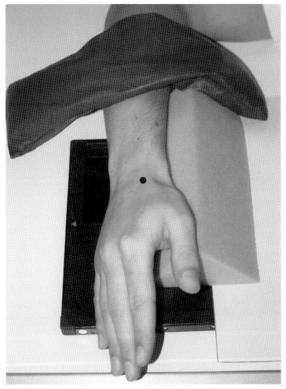

Fig. 2.21a Patient positioning for anterior oblique radiography of the wrist.

This is an additional projection that may be necessary to confirm the presence of a suspected fracture not demonstrated in the postero-anterior and lateral projections.

Position of patient and image receptor

- The patient is seated alongside the table, with the affected side nearest to the table.
- The elbow joint is flexed to 90° and the arm is abducted, such that the anterior aspect of the forearm and the palm of the hand rest on the tabletop.
- If the mobility of the patient permits, then the shoulder joint should be at the same height as the forearm.
- The wrist joint is placed on the image receptor and adjusted to include the lower part of the radius and ulna and the proximal 2/3 of the metacarpals.
- The hand is externally rotated through 45° and supported in this position using a non-opaque pad.
- The forearm may be immobilised using a sandbag.

Direction and location of X-ray beam

- The collimated vertical beam is centred midway between the radial and ulnar styloid processes.

Essential image characteristics (Fig. 2.21b)

- The exposure should provide adequate penetration to visualise the carpal bones.
- The image should demonstrate the proximal 2/3 of the metacarpals, the carpal bones and the distal 1/3 of the radius and ulna.

Note

- This projection results in an additional oblique projection of the metacarpals, the carpal bones and lower end of the radius. To obtain an additional projection of the lower end of the ulna, it is necessary to rotate the humerus (see Wrist, lateral method 2, page 72).

Radiological considerations

- Fracture of the distal radius can be undisplaced, dorsally angulated (Colles' fracture) or ventrally angulated (Smith's fracture). The importance of Smith's fracture lies in the fact that it is less stable than Colles' fracture.
- Dislocations of the carpus are uncommon, but again they carry potential for serious disability.
- One manifestation of lunate dislocation is an increased gap between it and the scaphoid, which will be missed if the wrist is rotated on the postero-anterior projection.

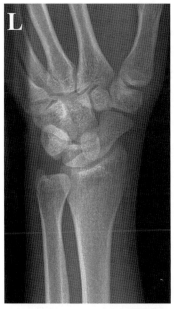

Fig. 2.21b Normal radiograph of anterior oblique wrist.

2 Wrist

Image evaluation – 10-point plan

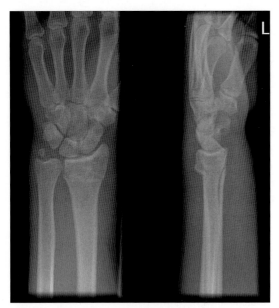

Fig. 2.22a Optimal radiographic examination.

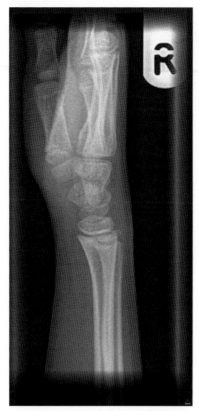

Fig. 2.22b Suboptimal lateral radiograph.

IMAGE EVALUATION

Wrist PA & lateral (Fig. 2.22a)

The main points to consider are:
1. Patient demographics have been removed for confidentiality reasons.
2. The area of interest is included:
   - Distal part of the radius and ulna.
   - The proximal 2/3 of the metacarpals.
   - Skin surfaces.
3. Correct anatomical marker is applied post processing.
4. The wrist is correctly positioned:
   - DP fingers raised and no rotation.
   - Lateral the styloid processes are superimposed.
5. The image displays optimum density and contrast.
6. Good bony trabecular seen.
7. Collimated to the area of interest.
8. No artefacts obscuring the image.
9. No repeats necessary as the image is correctly positioned and diagnostic.

Radiographer Comments/Initial report

The image demonstrates a fracture of the distal radius and lateral styloid process.

IMAGE EVALUATION

Lateral wrist (Fig. 2.22b)

The main points to consider are:
1. Patient demographics have been removed for confidentiality reasons.
2. The area of interest is included:
   - Distal part of the radius and ulna.
   - The proximal 2/3 of the metacarpals.
   - Anterior and posterior skin surfaces.
3. Correct anatomical marker is applied during exposure.
4. The wrist is underrotated and needs to be rotated further so the styloid processes are superimposed.
5. The image displays the correct density and contrast but has some image noise, which indicates the image is underexposed.
6. Good bony trabecular seen.
7. Collimated to the area of interest.
8. No artefacts obscuring the image.
9. Needs to be repeated to get a true lateral.
10. The image is a child so the epiphysis is demonstrated on the radius and ulna.

Radiographer Comments/Initial report

No clinical report can be made until the image is repeated.

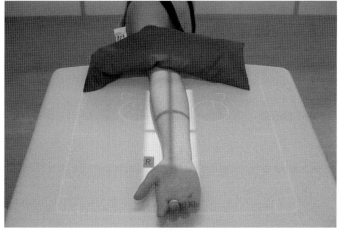

Fig. 2.23a Patient positioning for an antero-posterior (AP) forearm.

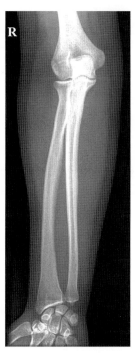

Fig. 2.23b Normal AP radiograph of forearm

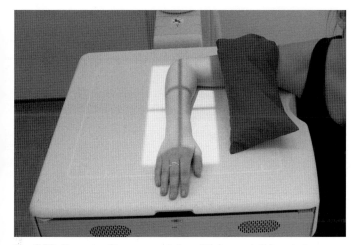

Fig. 2.23c Example of incorrect technique (PA forearm). This technique will superimpose the radius and ulna. (**Note:** Anatomical marker has been excluded.)

Forearm 2

Two projections are routinely taken, an antero-posterior and lateral. The projections must be at right-angles to each other and demonstrate the full length of the radius and ulna including both the elbow and the wrist joint.

The antero-posterior projection with the forearm supinated demonstrates the radius and ulna lying side by side. Poor quality images have superimposition of the radius and ulna and this may obscure pathology.

Each image is acquired using a CR image receptor or alternatively within the field of view of a DDR detector. The smallest image detector is used for CR imaging, i.e. 24 × 30 cm CR cassette.

Antero-posterior (Fig. 2.23a)

Position of patient and image receptor

- The patient is seated alongside the table, with the affected side nearest to the table.
- The arm is abducted and the elbow joint is fully extended, with the supinated forearm resting on the table.
- The shoulder is lowered to the same level as the elbow joint.
- The image receptor is placed under the forearm to include the wrist joint and the elbow joint.
- The arm is adjusted such that the radial and ulnar styloid processes and the medial and lateral epicondyles are equidistant from the image receptor.
- The lower end of the humerus and the hand may be immobilised using sandbags.

Direction and location of X-ray beam

- The collimated vertical beam is centred in the midline of the forearm to a point midway between the wrist and elbow joints.

Essential image characteristics (Fig. 2.23b)

- Both the elbow and the wrist joint must be demonstrated on the radiograph.
- Both joints should be seen in the true antero-posterior position, with the radial and ulnar styloid processes and the epicondyles of the humerus equidistant from the image receptor.

Note

- The postero-anterior projection of the forearm with the wrist pronated is not satisfactory because, in this projection, the radius is superimposed over the ulna for part of its length (Fig. 2.23c).

Radiation protection/dose

Careful technique and close collimation will assist in reducing the patient dose.

Expected DRL: ESD 0.13 mGy.

2 Forearm

Lateral (Fig. 2.24a)

Position of patient and image receptor

- From the antero-posterior position, the elbow is flexed to 90°.
- The humerus is internally rotated to 90° to bring the medial aspect of the upper arm, elbow, forearm, wrist and hand into contact with the table.
- The image receptor is placed under the forearm to include the wrist joint and the elbow joint.
- The arm is adjusted such that the radial and ulnar styloid processes and the medial and lateral epicondyles are superimposed.
- The lower end of the humerus and the hand may be immobilised using sandbags.

Direction and location of X-ray beam

- The collimated vertical beam is centred in the midline of the forearm to a point midway between the wrist and elbow joints.

Essential image characteristics (Fig. 2.24b)

- Both the elbow and the wrist joint must be demonstrated on the image.
- Both joints should be seen in the true lateral position, with the radial and ulnar styloid processes and the epicondyles of the humerus superimposed.

Notes

- In trauma cases, it may be impossible to move the arm into the positions described, and a modified technique may need to be employed to ensure that diagnostic images are obtained.
- If the limb cannot be moved through 90°, then a horizontal beam should be used (Fig. 2.24c).
- Both joints should be included on each image.
- No attempt should be made to rotate the patient's hand.

Radiological considerations (Figs 2.24d, 2.24e)

- When two or more bones such as the radius and ulna form a ring, fracture of one of the bones is often associated with fracture or dislocation elsewhere in the ring, especially if the fracture is displaced or the bone ends overlap.
- In Galeazzi fracture there is a fracture of the radius with dislocation of the distal ulna, while in Monteggia fracture there is fracture of the ulna with dislocation of the head of the radius. In forearm fracture, therefore, both ends of both bones, as well as the proximal and distal radio-ulnar joints, must be demonstrated.
- Basic forearm projections do not give adequate views of the elbow and should not be relied upon for diagnosis of radial head injury.
- If an elbow joint effusion is shown, formal projections of the elbow joint will be required.

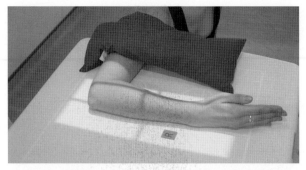

Fig. 2.24a Patient positioning for lateral radiography of the forearm.

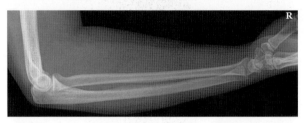

Fig. 2.24b Normal lateral radiograph of the forearm.

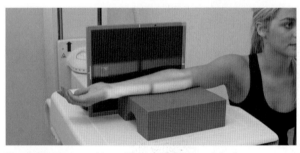

Fig. 2.24c Horizontal lateral beam projection of the forearm.

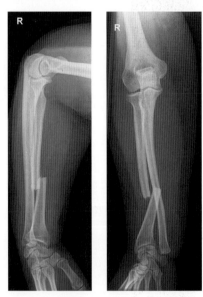

Fig. 2.24d and e Radiographs of lateral (left) and AP (right) projections showing a Galeazzi fracture.

Radiation protection/dose

Careful technique and close collimation will assist in reducing the patient dose.

Expected DRL: ESD 0.13 mGy.

Each image is acquired using a CR image receptor or alternatively within the field of view of a DDR detector. The smallest image detector is used for CR imaging, i.e. 18 × 24 cm or 24 × 30 cm, depending on the size if the patient.

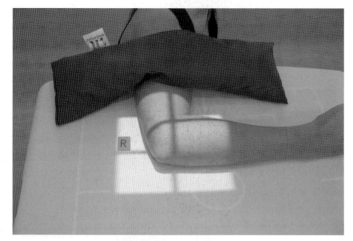

Fig. 2.25a Patient positioning for lateral radiography of the elbow.

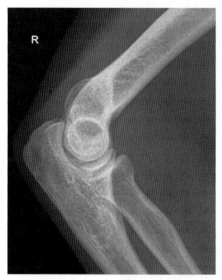

Fig. 2.25b Normal lateral radiograph of the elbow.

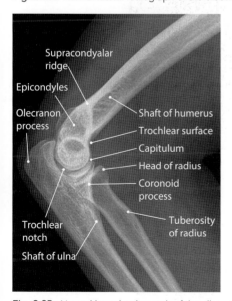

Fig. 2.25c Normal lateral radiograph of the elbow (annotated with anatomy).

Elbow 2

Optimum projections of the elbow joint are obtained when the upper arm is in the same plane as the forearm. For many examinations, the patient will be seated at the table with the shoulder lowered, so that the upper arm, elbow and forearm are on the same horizontal level.

- To gain the patient's confidence, the lateral projection is taken first, because the patient will find it easier to adopt this position.
- The humerus must be rotated through 90° to make sure that two projections at right-angles are obtained of the humerus as well as the ulna and radius. Alternatively, if the limb cannot be moved, two projections at right-angles to each other can be taken by keeping the limb in the same position and moving the tube through 90° between projections.
- If the patient cannot extend the elbow fully, modified positioning is necessary for the antero-posterior projection.

Note

Special care should be taken with a child suspected of having a supracondylar fracture of the humerus. Modified projections must be obtained without moving the arm from the collar and cuff that should be used to immobilise the arm.

Lateral (Fig. 2.25a)

Position of patient and image receptor

- The patient is seated alongside the table, with the affected side nearest to the table.
- The elbow is flexed to 90° and the palm of the hand is rotated so that it is at 90° to the tabletop.
- The shoulder is lowered or the height of the table increased so that it is on the same plane as the elbow and wrist, such that the medial aspect of the entire arm is in contact with the tabletop.
- The image receptor is placed under the patient's elbow, with its centre to the elbow joint and its short axis parallel to the forearm.
- The limb may be immobilised using sandbags.

Direction and location of X-ray beam

- The collimated vertical beam is centred over the lateral epicondyle of the humerus.

Essential image characteristics (Figs 2.25b, 2.25c)

- The central ray must pass through the joint space at 90° to the humerus, i.e. the epicondyles should be superimposed.
- The image should demonstrate the distal 1/3 of humerus and the proximal 1/3 of the radius and ulna.

Expected DRL: ESD 0.13 mGy.

2 Elbow

Antero-posterior (Fig. 2.26a)

Position of patient and image receptor

- From the lateral position, the patient's arm is externally rotated.
- The arm is then extended fully, such that the posterior aspect of the entire limb is in contact with the tabletop and the palm of the hand is facing upwards.
- The image receptor is positioned under the elbow joint, with its short axis parallel to the forearm.
- The arm is adjusted such that the medial and lateral epicondyles are equidistant from the image receptor.
- The limb is may be immobilised using sandbags.

Direction and location of X-ray beam

- The collimated vertical beam is centred through the joint space 2.5 cm distal to the point midway between the medial and lateral epicondyles of the humerus.

Essential image characteristics (Figs 2.26b, 2.26c)

- The central ray must pass through the joint space at 90° to the humerus to provide a satisfactory view of the joint space.
- The image should demonstrate the distal 1/3 of humerus and the proximal 1/3 of the radius and ulna.

Notes

- When the patient is unable to extend the elbow to 90°, a modified technique is used for the AP projection.
- If the limb cannot be moved, two projections at right-angles to each other can be taken by keeping the limb in the same position and rotating the X-ray tube through 90°.

Expected DRL: ESD 0.12 mGy.

Antero-posterior – partial flexion

Adaptation of technique

If the patient is unable to extend the elbow fully, the positioning for the AP projection may be modified.

- For a general survey of the elbow, or if the main area of interest is the proximal end of the radius and ulna, then the posterior aspect of the forearm should be in contact with the image detector.
- If the main area of interest is the distal end of the humerus, however, then the posterior aspect of the humerus should be in contact with the image detector.
- If the elbow is immobilised in the fully flexed position, then an axial projection must be used instead of the AP projection.

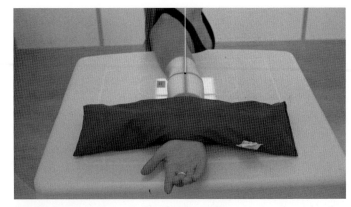

Fig. 2.26a Patient positioning for an antero-posterior (AP) radiography of the elbow.

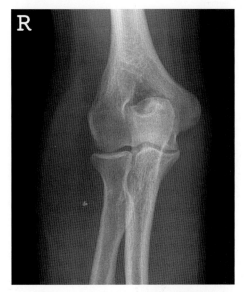

Fig. 2.26b Normal AP radiograph of elbow.

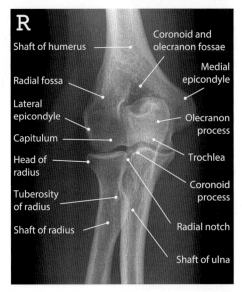

Fig. 2.26c Radiograph of AP elbow (annotated with anatomy).

Notes

In both of the above cases, some superimposition of the bones will occur. However, gross injury and general alignment can be demonstrated.

Elbow 2

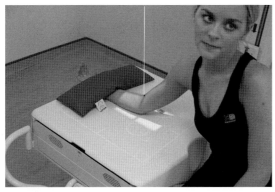

Fig. 2.27a Patient positioning for radiography of the elbow, forearm in contact with image receptor.

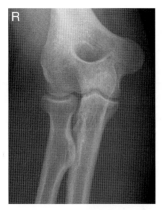

Fig. 2.27b Radiograph of AP elbow in partial flexion.

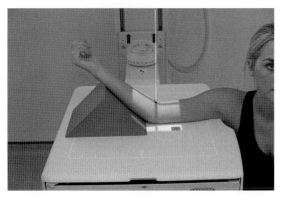

Fig. 2.27c Patient positioning for radiography of the elbow, upper arm in contact with image receptor.

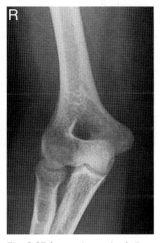

Fig. 2.27d AP radiograph of elbow upper arm in contact with image receptior.

Antero-posterior – forearm in contact (Fig. 2.27a)

Position of patient and image receptor

- The patient is seated alongside the table, with the affected side nearest to the table.
- The posterior aspect of the forearm is placed on the table, with the palm of the hand facing upwards.
- The image receptor is placed under the forearm, with its centre under the elbow joint.
- The arm is adjusted such that the medial and lateral epicondyles of the humerus are equidistant from the image receptor.
- The limb may be supported and immobilised in this position.

Direction and location of X-ray beam

- The collimated vertical beam is centred in the midline of the forearm 2.5 cm distal to the crease of the elbow.

Essential image characteristics (Fig. 2.27b)

- The image should demonstrate the distal 1/3 of humerus and the proximal 1/3 of the radius and ulna.

Antero-posterior – upper arm in contact (Fig. 2.27c)

Position of patient and imaging receptor

- The patient is seated alongside the table, with the affected side nearest to the table.
- The posterior aspect of the humerus is placed on the table, with the palm of the hand facing upwards.
- The image receptor is placed under the forearm, with its centre under the elbow joint.
- The arm is adjusted such that the medial and lateral epicondyles of the humerus are equidistant from the image receptor.
- The limb may be supported and immobilised in this position.

Direction and location of X-ray beam

- The collimated vertical beam is centred midway between the epicondyles of the humerus.

Essential image characteristics (Fig. 2.27d)

- The image should demonstrate the distal 1/3 of humerus and the proximal 1/3 of the radius and ulna.

2 Elbow

Full flexion

When the patient's elbow is immobilised in full flexion, an axial projection may be substituted for the AP projection. It is preferable for the patient's upper arm to be in contact with the image receptor for examination of the distal end of the humerus and olecranon process of the ulna, and for the forearm to be in contact with the image receptor if the proximal ends of the radius and ulna are to be examined.

In either of these cases, the bones of the forearm will be superimposed on the humerus. However, gross injury and general alignment can be demonstrated.

Axial – upper arm in contact (Fig. 2.28a)

Position of patient and image receptor

- The patient is seated alongside the table, with the affected side nearest to the table.
- The elbow is fully flexed, and the palm of the hand is facing the shoulder.
- The posterior aspect of the upper arm is placed on the image receptor, with the arm parallel to the long axis of the image detector.
- The patient's trunk is adjusted in order to bring the medial and lateral epicondyles of the humerus equidistant to the image detector.

Direction and location of X-ray beam

- The collimated vertical beam is centred:
  - For the lower end of the humerus and the olecranon process of ulna, the vertical central ray is centred 5 cm distal to the olecranon process.
  - For the proximal ends of the radius and ulna, including the radio-humeral joint, the central ray is directed at right-angles to the forearm and centred 5 cm distal to the olecranon process.

Essential image characteristics (Figs 2.28b, 2.28c)

- The image will include the olecranon process and the proximal 1/3 of the radius and ulna superimposed on the lower 1/3 of the humerus.
- The exposure should be adequate to visualise all three bones.

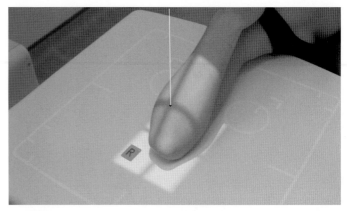

Fig. 2.28a Patient positioning for axial radiography of elbow, upper arm in contact.

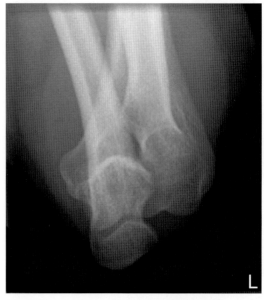

Fig. 2.28b Axial radiograph of elbow, upper arm in contact.

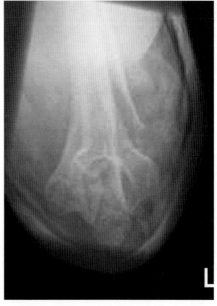

Fig. 2.28c Axial radiograph of elbow–arm in plaster, with the upper arm in contact.

Elbow 2

Axial – forearm in contact (Figs 2.29a, 2.29b)

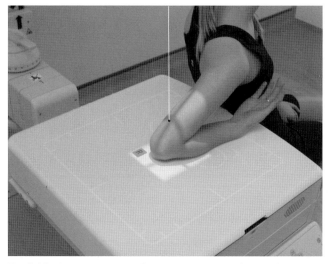

Fig. 2.29a Patient positioning for axial radiography of elbow, forearm arm in contact.

Position of patient and image receptor

- The patient is seated alongside the table, with the affected side nearest to the table.
- The elbow is fully flexed, and the palm of the hand is facing the upwards.
- The forearm is fully supinated, with the posterior aspect of the forearm resting on the image detector and the arm parallel to the long axis of the image detector.
- The patient's trunk is adjusted in order to bring the medial and lateral epicondyles of the humerus equidistant to the image detector.

Direction and location of X-ray beam

The collimated vertical beam is centred:
- For the proximal ends of the radius and ulna and the radiohumeral joint to a point on the posterior aspect of the upper arm 5 cm proximal to the olecranon process.
- For the lower end of the humerus and the olecranon process of the ulna to a point at right-angles to the upper arm 5 cm proximal to the olecranon process.

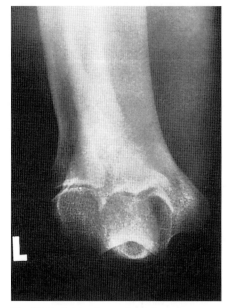

Fig. 2.29b Axial radiograph of elbow, forearm in contact.

Image evaluation – 10-point plan

IMAGE EVALUATION

Axial radiograph with forearm in contact (Fig. 2.29b)

The main points to consider are:
1. Patient demographics have been removed for confidentiality reasons.
2. Area of interest – included:
   - Distal 1/3 of humerus.
   - Proximal 1/3 of radius and ulna.
   - Lateral margins of the elbow.
3. Correct anatomical marker (Left).
4. No rotation of bones.
5. Correct image exposure. EI correct and no noise.
6. Good resolution – good bony trabeculae but poor soft tissue resolution.
7. Collimated to area of interest (as in 2 above).
8. No artefacts present.
9. No repeat required as alignment demonstrated and no fracture seen.
10. Lateral required for full evaluation of the patient.

Radiographer Comments/Initial report

No fracture seen.

2 Elbow

Lateral head of radius (Figs 2.30a–2.30c)

Each image is acquired using a CR image receptor or alternatively within the field of view of a DDR detector. The smallest image detector is used for CR imaging, i.e. 18 × 24 cm CR cassette.

The elbow is positioned as for the lateral elbow. The hand is then moved through different degrees of rotation, enabling visualisation of small fissure fractures through the head of the radius.

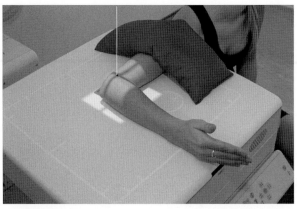

Fig. 2.30a Patient position 1.

Position of patient and image receptor

- For the first projection, the patient is positioned as for a lateral elbow projection, with the palm of the hand vertical. The forearm may be immobilised using a sandbag.
- For the second exposure, the upper arm and elbow are maintained in the same position, whilst the hand is rotated medially until the palm of the hand rests on the table. The forearm may be immobilised using a sandbag.
- For the third exposure, the upper arm and elbow are maintained in the same position, whilst the hand is rotated further medially, until the palm of the hand is vertical, facing away from the body. The forearm may be immobilised using a sandbag.

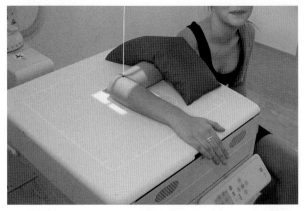

Fig. 2.30b Patient position 2.

Direction and location of X-ray beam

- The collimated vertical beam is centred to the lateral epicondyle of the humerus for all projections.

Essential image characteristics (Figs 2.30d–2.30f)

- The elbow joint should be seen in the true lateral position in each projection.
- Sufficient detail of bony trabeculae should be demonstrated to enable fine fractures to be detected.

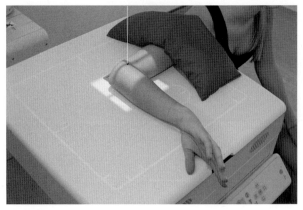

Fig. 2.30c Patient position 3.

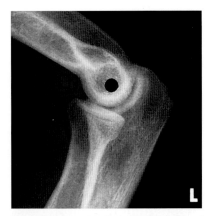

Fig. 2.30d Lateral radiograph of the elbow for head of radius, palm at right-angles to the table.

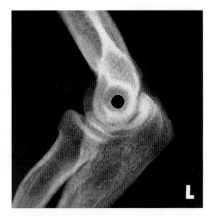

Fig. 2.30e Lateral radiograph of the elbow for head of radius, palm in contact with the table.

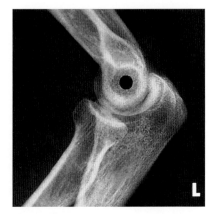

Fig. 2.30f Lateral radiograph of the elbow for head of radius, palm facing away from the trunk.

Each image is acquired using a CR image receptor or alternatively within the field of view of a DDR detector. The smallest image detector is used for CR imaging, i.e. 18 × 24 cm CR cassette.

Position of patient and image receptor

- The patient is positioned for an anterior projection of the elbow joint.
- The image receptor is positioned under the elbow joint, with the long axis parallel to the forearm.

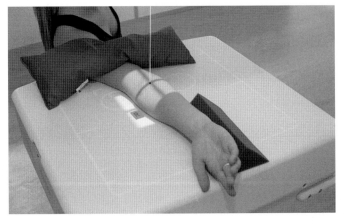

Fig. 2.31a Patient positioning for proximal oblique radiography of radio-ulnar joint.

Elbow 2

Proximal radio-ulnar joint – oblique (Fig. 2.31a)

- The humerus is then rotated laterally (or the patient leans towards the side under examination) until the line between the epicondyles is approximately 20° to the image receptor.
- The forearm may be immobilised using a sandbag.

Direction and location of X-ray beam

The collimated vertical beam is centred 2.5 cm distal to a midpoint between the epicondyles.

Essential image characteristics (Figs 2.31b, 2.31c)

- The image should demonstrate clearly the joint space between the radius and the ulna.

Ulnar groove – axial (Fig. 2.31d)

The ulnar groove through which the ulnar nerve passes lies between the medial epicondyle and the medial lip of the trochlear of the humerus and is a possible site for ulnar nerve compression. A modified axial projection with the elbow joint fully flexed demonstrates the groove and any lateral shift of the ulna, which would lead to tightening of the ligaments overlying the ulnar nerve.

A 18 × 24 cm CR cassette is used or alternatively within the field of view of a DDR detector.

Position of patient and image receptor

- The patient is seated alongside the X-ray table, with the affected side nearest the table.
- The elbow is fully flexed, and the posterior aspect of the upper arm is placed in contact with the tabletop.
- The image detector is positioned under the lower end of the humerus, with its centre midway between the epicondyles of the humerus.
- With the elbow still fully flexed, the arm is externally rotated through 45° and supported in this position.

Direction and location of X-ray beam

- The collimated vertical beam is centred over the medial epicondyle of the humerus.

Essential image characteristics (Fig. 2.31e)

- The image should be exposed to show the ulnar groove.

Note

- A well-collimated beam is used to reduce degradation of the image by scattered radiation.

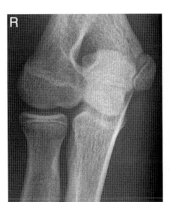 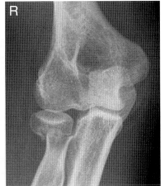

Figs. 2.31b and c Oblique radiographs of elbow to show proximal radio-ulnar joint (left, normal; right, fracture of radial head).

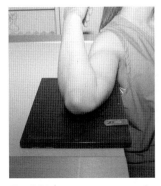 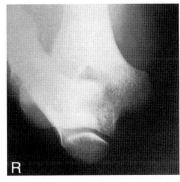

Fig. 2.31d Patient positioning for axial radiography of elbow ulnar groove.

Fig. 2.31e Radiograph of elbow for ulnar groove.

2 Elbow

Radiological considerations (Figs 2.32a–2.32e)

- An effusion is a useful marker of pathology and may be demonstrated in trauma, infection and inflammatory conditions. It is seen as an elevation of the fat pads anteriorly and posteriorly (see below) and requires a good lateral projection with no rotation. It may be an important clue to otherwise occult fracture of the radial head or a supracondylar fracture of the humerus.
- Radial head fracture may be nearly or completely occult, showing as the slightest cortical infraction or trabecular irregularity at the neck or just a joint effusion.
- Avulsion of one of the epicondyles of the humerus may be missed if the avulsed bone is hidden over other bone or in the olecranon or coronoid fossae. Recognition of their absence requires knowledge of when and where they should be seen.

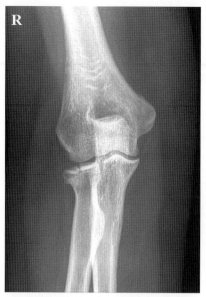

Fig. 2.32c Antero-posterior radiograph of elbow showing vertical fracture of the head of radius.

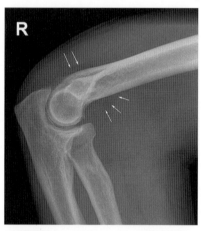

Fig. 2.32a Lateral radiograph of elbow showing elevation of anterior and posterior fat pads.

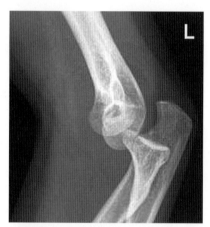

Fig. 2.32d Lateral radiograph showing dislocation of the elbow.

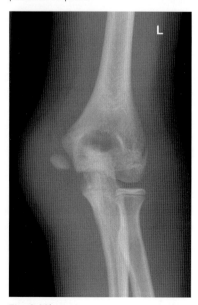

Fig. 2.32b Avulsion injury of the medial epicondyle. With adjacent soft tissue swelling in a paediatric elbow.

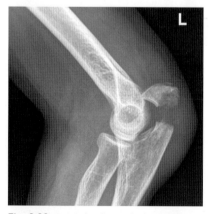

Fig. 2.32e Lateral radiograph showing fracture through the olecranon process, with displacement due to the pull of the triceps.

Elbow 2

Image evaluation – 10-point plan

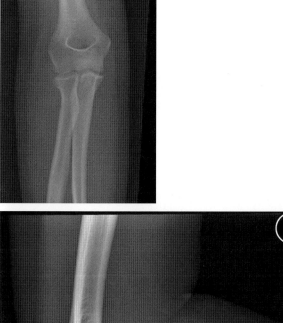

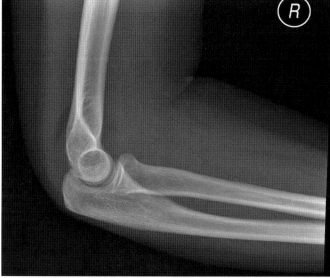

Fig. 2.33a and b Optimal radiographic examination.

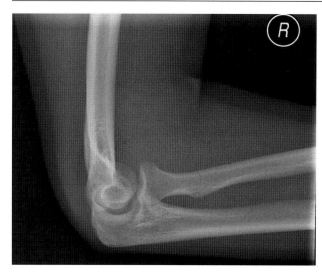

Fig. 2.33c Suboptimal radiograph.

IMAGE EVALUATION

AP & lateral elbow (Figs 2.33a, 2.33b)

The main points to consider are:
1. Optimum quality images.
2. Area of interest – included:
   - Distal 1/3 of humerus.
   - Proximal 1/3 of radius and ulna.
   - Skin margins of the elbow.
3. Correct anatomical marker (Right applied digitally).
4. Correct image exposure. EI correct and no noise.
5. No artefacts present.
6. No repeat required as alignment demonstrated and no fracture seen.

Radiographer Comments/Initial report

No fracture seen.

IMAGE EVALUATION

Lateral elbow (Fig. 2.33c)

The main points to consider are:
1. Area of interest – included:
   - Distal 1/3 of humerus.
   - Proximal 1/3 of radius and ulna.
   - Skin margins of the elbow.
2. Correct anatomical marker (Right applied digitally).
3. Poor patient positioning with humerus, radius and ulna not in the same plane, i.e. humerus is elevated in relation to the forearm.
4. Good demonstration of bony trabeculae and soft tissue effusion.
5. No artefacts present.

Radiographer Comments/Initial report

- Sub optimal lateral projection; however, together with the AP projection the images are diagnostic.
- Elbow joint effusion. Probable radial head fracture.

Humerus – supracondylar fracture

A common type of injury found in children is a fracture of the lower end of the humerus just proximal to the condyles. The injury is very painful and even small movements of the limb can exacerbate the injury, causing further damage to adjacent nerves and blood vessels.

Any supporting sling should not be removed, and the patient should not be asked to extend the elbow joint or to rotate the arm or forearm.

A 18 × 24 cm CR cassette is used or alternatively within the field of view of a DDR detector.

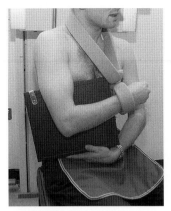 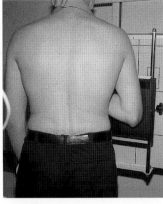

Fig. 2.34a Patient positioning method 1.   Fig. 2.34b Patient positioning 2.

Lateral

Position of patient and image receptor

Method 1 (Fig. 2.34a)

- The patient sits or stands facing the X-ray tube.
- An image receptor is supported between the patient's trunk and elbow, with the medial aspect of the elbow in contact with the image detector.
- A lead-rubber sheet or other radiation protection device is positioned to protect the patient's trunk from the primary beam.

Method 2 (Fig. 2.34b)

The patient stands sideways, with the elbow flexed and the lateral aspect of the injured elbow in contact with a vertical DDR receptor. The arm is gently extended backwards from the shoulder. The patient is rotated forwards until the elbow is clear of the rib cage but still in contact with the receptor, with the line joining the epicondyles of the humerus at right-angles to the receptor.

Direction and location of X-ray beam

Method 1

The collimated beam is angled so that the beam is directed perpendicular to the shaft of the humerus and centred to the lateral epicondyle.

Method 2

The collimated horizontal beam is angled so that the beam is directed perpendicular to the shaft of the humerus and centred to the medial epicondyle.

Essential image characteristics (Figs 2.34c, 2.34d)

- The image should include the lower end of the humerus and the upper 1/3 of the radius and ulna.

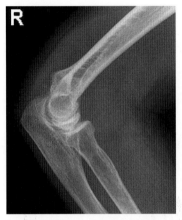

Fig. 2.34c Lateral radiograph of elbow showing undisplaced supracondylar fracture.

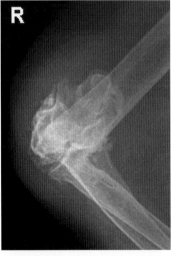

Fig. 2.34d Lateral radiograph of elbow showing supracondylar fracture with displacement and bone disruption.

Notes

- The patient should be made as comfortable as possible to assist immobilisation.
- An erect cassette holder, or similar device, may be used to assist the patient in supporting a CR cassette is used.
- The X-ray beam should be collimated carefully to ensure that the primary beam does not extend beyond the area of the image detector.

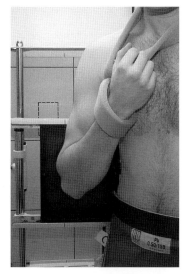

Fig. 2.35a Patient positioning for antero-posterior (AP) radiography of the humerus, patient facing tube.

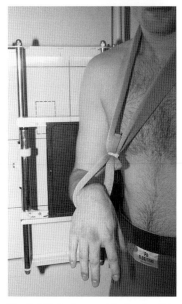

Fig. 2.35b Patient positioning for AP radiography of humerus, patient facing tube.

Humerus – supracondylar fracture 2

Antero-posterior (Figs 2.35a, 2.35b)

As in the lateral projection, the CR cassette can be held in a vertical cassette holder with the patient either standing or sitting during the procedure. Alternatively a vertical DDR receptor is selected.

Position of patient and image receptor

- From the lateral position, the patient's upper body is rotated towards the affected side.
- The CR cassette is placed in an erect cassette holder, and the patient's position is adjusted so that the posterior aspect of the upper arm is in contact with the image detector.

Direction and location of X-ray beam

The collimated X-ray beam:

- If the elbow joint is fully flexed, the central beam is directed at right-angles to the humerus to pass through the forearm to a point midway between the epicondyles of the humerus.
- If the elbow joint is only partially flexed, the central ray is directed at right-angles to the humerus to a point midway between the epicondyles of the humerus without first passing through the forearm.

Essential image characteristics (Figs 2.35c, 2.35d)

- If the elbow joint is fully flexed, sufficient exposure must be selected to provide adequate penetration of the forearm.

Notes

- It is essential that no movement of the elbow joint occurs during positioning of the patient.
- Particular attention should be paid to radiation protection measures.

Radiological considerations

- Signs of supracondylar fracture can be very subtle. Demonstration of the position of the condyles in relation to the anterior cortical line of the humeral shaft may be crucial and demands a true lateral image.

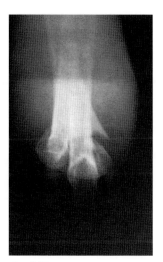

Fig. 2.35c AP radiograph in full flexion showing supracondylar fracture.

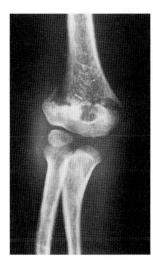

Fig. 2.35d AP radiograph in partial flexion showing supracondylar fracture.

87

2 Humerus – shaft

Antero-posterior – erect (Figs 2.36a, 2.36c, 2.36e)

When movement of the patients arm is restricted a modified technique may be required. There is always a need to assess the ability of the patient to comply with the radiographer's instructions. Positioning the patient erect allows greater flexibility than positioning the patient standing.

Position of patient and image receptor

- A 35 × 43 cm CR cassette is positioned in an erect cassette holder or alternatively a vertical DDR receptor is selected.
- The patient sits or stands with their back in contact with the image receptor.
- The patient is rotated towards the affected side to bring the posterior aspect of the shoulder, upper arm and elbow into contact with the image receptor.
- The position of the patient is adjusted to ensure that the medial and lateral epicondyles of the humerus are equidistant from the receptor.
- The forearm may be immobilised using a sandbag.

Direction and location of X-ray beam

- The vertical collimated X-ray beam is centred to a point midway between the shoulder and elbow joints at right-angles to the image receptor.

Lateral – erect (Figs 2.36b, 2.36d)

If the arm is immobilised in order to obtain a true lateral projection, i.e. one that is at right-angles to the antero-posterior, then it will be necessary to have the patient's median sagittal plane parallel to the image receptor and the lateral aspect of the injured arm in contact with the image receptor, and to direct the horizontal central ray through the thorax to the injured arm. This has the disadvantage that the ribs and lungs will be superimposed on the humerus, obscuring details of the injury and signs of healing and adding to the radiation dose to the patient. The position described, although not fully at right-angles to the antero-posterior projection, avoids this superimposition.

Position of patient and image receptor

- A 35 × 43 cm CR cassette is positioned in an erect cassette holder or alternatively a vertical DDR receptor is selected.
- From the anterior position, the patient is rotated through 90° until the lateral aspect of the injured arm is in contact with the image receptor.
- The patient is now rotated further until the arm is just clear of the rib cage but still in contact with the image receptor.

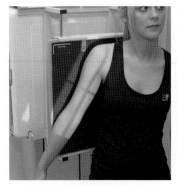

Fig. 2.36a Patient positioned erect with DDR detector AP.

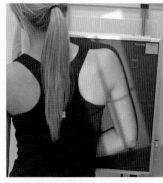

Fig. 2.36b Patient positioned erect with DDR detector lateral.

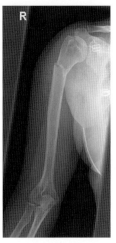

Fig. 2.36c AP radiograph of humerus showing a fracture of the proximal shaft of the humerus.

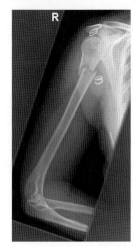

Fig. 2.36d Lateral radiograph of the same patient.

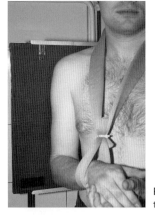

Fig. 2.36e Photograph of patient positioned for AP humerus in a sling.

Direction and location of X-ray beam

- The horizontal collimated X-ray beam is centred to a point midway between the shoulder and elbow joints at right-angles to the shaft.

Essential image characteristics

- The exposure should be optimised to ensure that the area of interest is clearly visualised.

Positioning the patient supine allows greater stability than positioning the patient standing.

Position of patient and image receptor

- The patient lies supine on the X-ray table, with the unaffected side raised and supported on pads.
- A 35 × 43 cm CR cassette is positioned under the affected limb and adjusted to include the shoulder and elbow joints.

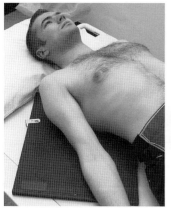
Fig. 2.37a Patient positioned supine with CR detector AP.

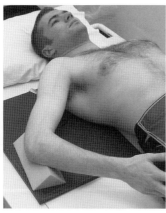
Fig. 2.37b Patient positioned supine with CR detector lateral.

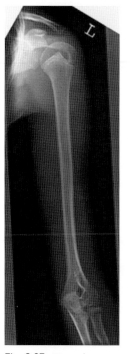
Fig. 2.37c Normal antero-posterior radiograph of humerus.

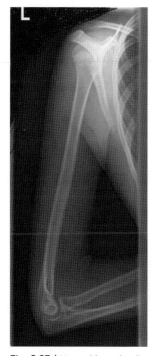
Fig. 2.37d Normal lateral radiograph of humerus.

Radiation protection/dose

- Careful technique and close collimation will assist in reducing the patient dose.

Expected DRL:
- AP – ESD 0.28 mGy.
- Lateral – ESD 0.35 mGy.

Humerus – shaft 2

Antero-posterior – supine (Figs 2.37a, 2.37c)

- The arm is slightly abducted and the elbow joint is fully extended, so that the posterior aspect of the upper arm is in contact with the image receptor.
- The arm is adjusted to ensure that the medial and lateral epicondyles are equidistant from the image detector.
- The forearm may be immobilised using a sandbag.

Direction and location of X-ray beam

- The vertical collimated X-ray beam is centred to a point midway between the shoulder and elbow joints.

Lateral – supine (Figs 2.37b, 2.37d)

Position of patient and image receptor

- From the antero-posterior position, the elbow joint is flexed to 90°.
- The arm is abducted and then medially rotated through 90° to bring the medial aspect of the arm, elbow and forearm in contact with the table.
- A 35 × 43 cm CR cassette is placed under the arm and adjusted to include both the shoulder and the elbow joints.
- The humerus is adjusted to ensure that the medial and lateral epicondyles of the humerus are superimposed.
- The forearm may be immobilised using a sandbag.

Direction and location of X-ray beam

- The vertical collimated X-ray beam is centred to a point midway between the shoulder and elbow joints.

Notes

- When rotating the humerus, it is essential to ensure that the forearm and hand rest on the tabletop and not the trunk.
- The humerus is normally examined with the patient erect and the image receptor is placed in an erect cassette holder. The radiographic technique is similar (except that a horizontal central ray is used) but additional care should be taken to ensure that the patient is immobilised adequately.

Essential image characteristics

- Both joints should be seen on the image.
- The elbow joint should be seen in the true lateral and antero-posterior positions.

Humerus – intertuberous sulcus (bicipital groove)

The intertuberous sulcus or bicipital groove is situated between the greater and lesser tuberosities of the humerus. It transmits the tendon of the long head of the biceps. An 18 × 24 cm CR cassette is selected.

Axial (Fig. 2.38a)

Position of patient and image receptor

- The patient lies supine on the X-ray table.
- The image receptor is supported vertically above the shoulder.
- The arm is rested on the tabletop with the palm of the hand facing the patient's side and the line joining the epicondyles of the humerus at 45° to the table.

Direction and location of X-ray beam

- The horizontal collimated X-ray beam is directed cranially and centred to the anterior part of the head of the humerus.

Essential image characteristics (Figs 2.38c, 2.38d)

- The sulcus should be seen in profile, and the exposure is such as to demonstrate lesions within or impingements on the sulcus.

Notes

- To reduce the risk of patient movement, the exposure is made on arrested respiration.
- The exposure is adjusted to demonstrate soft-tissue structures within the sulcus.

Alternative axial projection (Fig. 2.38b)

Position of patient and image receptor

- The patient sits with their shoulder joint against a vertical cassette holder or a vertical DDR detector.
- Ideally, this holder should be angled 15° forwards, but if this facility is not available the image detector can be supported above the shoulder.
- The arm is abducted anteriorly and supported to bring the long axis of the shaft of the humerus perpendicular to the image receptor.
- The hand is rotated 45° laterally from the prone position to bring the bicipital groove in profile with the central beam.

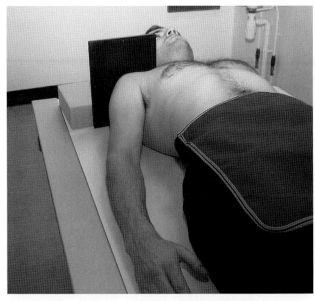

Fig. 2.38a Patient positioning for axial image (patient supine).

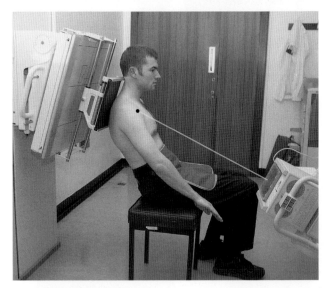

Fig. 2.38b Patient positioning for alternative axial image (patient erect).

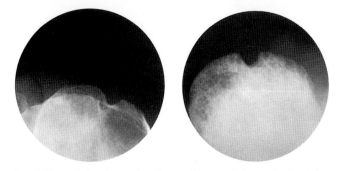

Fig. 2.38c and d Radiographs of bicipital groove (left, standard technique; right, alternative technique).

Direction and location of X-ray beam

The horizontal collimated X-ray beam is directed cranially along the long axis of the humerus and centred to the anterior part of the head of the humerus. The beam is collimated to the humeral head.

Humerus – neck 2

The most common reason for radiography of the neck of the humerus is suspected fracture, either pathological or traumatic.

Two projections at right-angles are necessary: an antero-posterior and an axial or a lateral projection. Movement of the arm may be limited, and the technique may need to be modified accordingly. Where possible, the supporting sling should be removed.

Depending on the condition of the patient, the examination may be undertaken with the patient erect, providing adequate immobilisation is used, supine on the X-ray table, or, in cases of multiple trauma, on a trolley.

The exposure is made on arrested respiration. An 18 × 24 cm CR cassette is used or alternatively within the field of view of a DDR detector.

Antero-posterior (Figs 2.39a, 2.39b)

Position of patient and image receptor

- The patient stands or lies supine facing the X-ray tube.
- The patient is rotated towards the affected side to bring the posterior aspect of the injured shoulder into contact with the midline of the image receptor.
- The image receptor is positioned to include the acromion process and the proximal 1/3 of the humerus.

Direction and location of X-ray beam

- The collimated X-ray beam is directed at right-angles to the humerus and centred to the head of the humerus.

Essential image characteristics (Fig. 2.39c)

- The image should include the acromion process and proximal head and neck of the humerus.
- The exposure should demonstrate adequately the neck of the humerus clear of the thorax.

Notes

- Exposure should be made on arrested respiration.
- The patient should immobilise the affected forearm by supporting its weight with the other arm. If the patient is supine, a sandbag may be placed over the forearm.

Radiation protection/dose

Careful technique and close collimation will assist in reducing the patient dose.

Expected DRL: ESD 0.35 mGy.

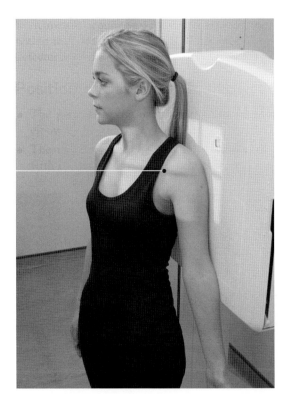

Fig. 2.39a Patient positioning for antero-posterior (AP) neck of humerus (patient erect).

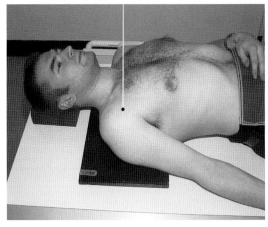

Fig. 2.39b Position for AP neck of humerus (patient supine).

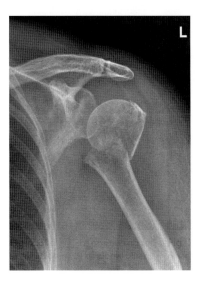

Fig. 2.39c AP radiograph of neck of humerus taken erect to demonstrate fracture of the neck of the humerus.

2 Humerus – neck

Axial

Positioning for the lateral projection will depend on how much movement of the arm is possible.

If the patient is able to abduct the arm, then a supero-inferior projection is recommended with the patient sitting at the end of the X-ray table. Alternatively, if the patient is lying on a trolley, then an infero-superior projection is acquired. If, however, the arm is fully immobilised, then an alternative lateral oblique (as for the lateral scapula) may be taken.

A small CR receptor is selected, i.e. an 18 × 24 cm CR cassette.

Supero-inferior (axial) (Fig. 2.40a)

Position of patient and image receptor

- The patient is seated at one end of the table, with the trunk leaning towards the table, the arm of the side being examined in its maximum abduction, and the elbow resting on the table.
- The height of the table is adjusted to enable the patient to adopt a comfortable position and to maximise full coverage of the neck of the humerus and the shoulder joint.
- The image receptor rests on the table between the elbow and the trunk.

Direction and location of X-ray beam

- The collimated vertical X-ray beam is directed to the acromion process of the scapula.
- Owing to increased object-to-detector distance, a small focal spot together with an increased FRD should be selected.

Essential image characteristics (Figs 2.40b, 2.40c)

- The image should include the acromion and coracoid processes, the glenoid cavity and the proximal head and neck of the humerus.
- The exposure should demonstrate adequately the neck of the humerus.

Radiation protection/dose

Careful technique and close collimation will assist in reducing the patient dose.

Expected DRL: ESD 0.58 mGy.

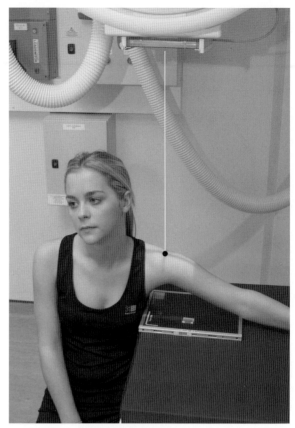

Fig. 2.40a Patient positioning for axial projection of the neck of humerus.

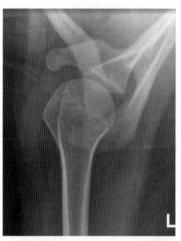

Fig. 2.40b Normal supero-inferior radiograph to show the neck of humerus.

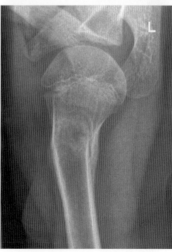

Fig. 2.40c Supero-inferior projection to show healing fracture of neck of humerus with angulation.

This projection is usually undertaken with the patient supine on a trolley or the X-ray table when the patient's condition makes it impossible for them to adopt the seated supero-inferior position.

Humerus – neck

Infero-superior (reverse axial) (Fig. 2.41a)

Position of patient and image receptor

- The patient lies supine on the trolley, with the arm of the affected side abducted as much as possible (ideally at right-angles to the trunk), the palm of the hand facing upwards and the medial and lateral epicondyles of the humerus equidistant from the tabletop.
- The shoulder and arm are raised slightly on non-opaque pads, and a 18 × 24 cm CR cassette, supported vertically against the shoulder, is pressed against the neck to include as much of the scapula as possible in the image.

Direction and location of X-ray beam

- The collimated horizontal X-ray beam is directed and centred to the patient's axilla with minimum angulation towards the trunk.

Essential image characteristics

- The image should include the acromion and coracoid processes, the glenoid cavity and the proximal head and neck of the humerus.

Notes

- Exposure should be made on arrested respiration.
- It is important that no attempt is made to abduct the arm more than the patient is able or willing to make.

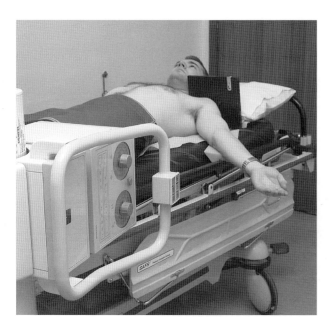

Fig. 2.41a Patient positioning for infero-superior projection on a trauma trolley.

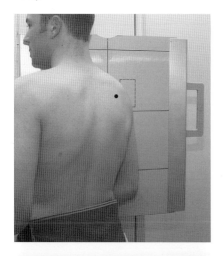

Fig. 2.41b Patient positioning for lateral oblique radiography of neck of humerus.

Lateral oblique (lateral) (Fig. 2.41b)

This projection is used when the arm is immobilised and no abduction of the arm is possible. A vertical Bucky technique may be necessary to improve image quality.

Position of patient and image receptor

- The patient stands or sits with the lateral aspect of the injured arm against the image receptor (18 × 24 CR cassette or DDR detector) /vertical Bucky.
- The patient is rotated forwards until the line joining the medial and lateral borders of the scapula is at right-angles to the image receptor.
- The image receptor is positioned to include the head of the humerus and the whole scapula.

Direction and location of X-ray beam

- The collimated horizontal X-ray beam is directed to the medial border of the scapula and centred to the head of humerus.

Essential image characteristics (Fig. 2.41c)

- The scapula and the upper end of the humerus should be demonstrated clear of the thoracic cage.

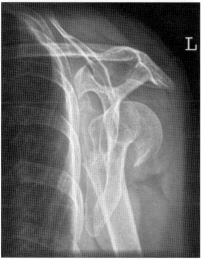

Fig. 2.41c Radiograph of lateral oblique projection showing fracture of neck of humerus.

2 Humerus – neck

Image evaluation – 10-point plan

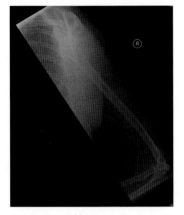 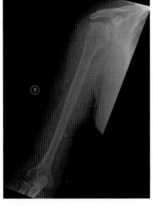

Fig. 2.42a and b Optimal radiographic examination.

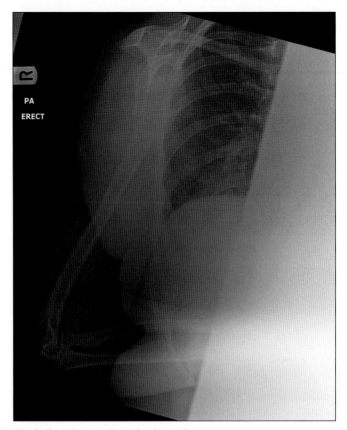

Fig. 2.42c Suboptimal lateral radiograph.

IMAGE EVALUATION

AP and lateral humerus (Figs 2.42a, 2.42b)

The main points to consider are:
1. Patient demographics have been removed for confidentiality reasons.
2. The area of interest is included:
   - The whole of the shaft of the humerus, shoulder and elbow joint.
   - Skin surfaces.
3. Correct anatomical marker is applied post processing.
4. The humerus is correctly positioned:
   - AP shoulder and elbow joint.
   - Lateral elbow and shoulder joint.
5. The image displays optimum density and contrast.
6. Good bony trabecular seen.
7. Collimated to the area of interest.
8. No artefacts obscuring the image.
9. No repeats necessary as the image is correctly positioned and diagnostic.

Radiographer Comments/Initial report

No abnormality seen.

IMAGE EVALUATION

Lateral humerus (Fig. 2.42c)

The main points to consider are:
1. Area of interest – included: shoulder joint, the whole of the humerus and elbow joint.
2. Correct anatomical marker.
3. Good patient positioning but poor collimation including the chest, forearm and abdomen.
4. Good demonstration of bony trabeculae and soft-tissue effusion.
5. No artefacts present.

Radiographer Comments/Initial report

Humerus intact with anterior subluxation of the humeral head from the glenoid fossa.

Section 3
Shoulder

CONTENTS

INTRODUCTION	96
Radiological considerations	96
RECOMMENDED PROJECTIONS	97
BASIC PROJECTIONS	98
Radiological anatomy	98
Antero-posterior (15°) erect	99
Supero-inferior (axial)	100
Infero-superior (reverse axial)	102
ALTERNATIVE PROJECTIONS FOR TRAUMA	103
Apical oblique (Garth projection)	103
Supero-inferior modified (modified axial – Wallace projection)	104
Anterior oblique ('Y' projection)	105
ADDITIONAL PROJECTIONS	106
Infero-superior modified (West Point projection)	106
Antero-posterior modified (Stryker projection)	107
GLENOHUMERAL JOINT	108
Antero-posterior modified (Grashey projection)	108
OUTLET PROJECTIONS (CALCIFIED TENDONS)	109
Antero-posterior 25°↓ (outlet projection)	109
Lateral oblique 15°↓ (outlet projection)	110
ACROMIOCLAVICULAR JOINTS	111
Antero-posterior	111
CLAVICLE	112
Postero-anterior	112
Antero-posterior – supine	113
Modified infero-superior (modified axial)	114
STERNOCLAVICULAR JOINTS	115
Postero-anterior oblique	115
Semi-prone (alternative)	115
Postero-anterior	116
Lateral	116
SCAPULA	117
Antero-posterior – erect	117
Anterior oblique (lateral)	118
Lateral (alternative)	118
CORACOID PROCESS	119
Antero-posterior shoulder (arm abducted)	119
Axial	119
SHOULDER	120
Image evaluation – 10-point plan	120

3 Introduction

The shoulder is a complex joint capable of a great range of movements. It's position close to the upper torso can make the acquisition of a second projection, perpendicular to the first, quite problematic, particularly in trauma where the patient has a limited range of movement. This has led to the development of a wide range of projections, which is reflected by the addition of a column in the recommended projections section of this chapter. The choice of the second projection in any given circumstance will be dictated by the capability of the patient and local protocols within the imaging department concerned.

Radiographic examinations of the shoulder joint and shoulder girdle can be carried out with the patient supine on the X-ray table or trolley, but in most cases it will be more comfortable for the patient to sit or stand with the back of the shoulder in contact with the image receptor. The erect position affords ease of positioning, allows the head of humerus to be assessed more accurately for potential impingement syndrome, and can sometimes demonstrate a lipohaemarthrosis where there is a subtle intra-articular fracture.

For radiation protection, particularly of the eyes, the patient's head should be rotated away from the side being examined.

The central ray can be directed caudally after centring to the coracoid process so that the primary beam can be collimated to the area under examination. Careless collimation can lead to significant breast radiation dose in a female patient.

For a general survey of the shoulder, e.g. for injury, the field size must be large enough to cover the whole of the shoulder girdle on the injured side. When localised areas are being examined, however, e.g. tendon calcifications or joint spaces, the X-ray beam should be well collimated.

To improve radiographic contrast, a secondary radiation grid should be used for large patients.

When examining the shoulder joint, it is important to check on the position of the head of the humerus by palpating and positioning the epicondyles at the distal end of the humerus. When the line joining the epicondyles is parallel to the tabletop (or vertical cassette), the humerus is in position for an antero-posterior (AP) projection of the head of the humerus. To judge the degree of rotation of the humerus by the position of the hand can be very misleading.

The image appearance is affected significantly by the posture of the patient. If the patient leans back into the image receptor, adopting a lordotic stance, then the head of humerus will overlie the acromion process. Conversely, if the patient leans forward, the head of humerus becomes projected inferiorly, appearing to be subluxed.

As in all other skeletal examinations, radiographs showing good bone detail are required to demonstrate minor fractures and bone changes associated with pathology, including injuries to tendon insertions.

Radiological considerations

The rounded humeral head articulates with a rather flat glenoid to maximise the possible range of movement at the joint. The stability of the joint is maintained by the cartilage of the glenoid labrum, ligaments and the tendons of the rotator cuff. The rotator cuff is four broad tendons encircling the glenohumeral joint. The most superior of these is the supraspinatus, which traverses the subacromial tunnel between the undersurface of the acromion and the upper surface of the humerus to reach its insertion.

Impingement is a common orthopaedic problem occurring when the subacromial space is compromised by degenerative disease and weakness of the stronger supporting muscles around the shoulder. It may be exacerbated by congenital anomalies of the acromion such as prominent inferior spurs or an unfused ossification centre at the tip of the acromion, producing an accessory ossicle called the os acromiale. The tendon of supraspinatus becomes compressed between the humerus and the acromion, causing mechanical pain, tendinitis and ultimately tendon tears. Radiological signs are non-specific, but radiographs help to assess the width of the subacromial space and the shape of the acromion. It is important that projections of the shoulder in patients with suspected impingement show the subacromial space adequately. Rotation of the patient or incorrect angulation of the beam can obscure the signs.

Tendinitis (inflammation) may cause visible calcification which is seen most frequently in the supraspinatus tendon on a good AP projection, although an outlet projection may be a useful addition. The calcification can be obscured by poor technique. The axial projection shows calcification in subscapularis and infrapinatus, which may otherwise be missed.

In the various forms of arthritis, the glenohumeral articulation is primarily affected. The width of this joint space is a marker of the severity and progression of disease, and obtaining a projection along the joint line is therefore crucial.

Posterior dislocation is uncommon. Signs on the AP image may be no more than subtle loss of the normal congruity between the glenoid and humeral articular surfaces; therefore, if this is suspected, an axial projection is particularly important.

Detailed examination of the entire shoulder mechanism would require multiple projections. The practitioner must therefore be familiar with the reasons for examination to ensure selection of the appropriate projections to address the clinical problem.

Ultrasound in experienced hands is a valuable tool for assessment of the shoulder, especially for rotator cuff tears. It may be more sensitive than plain radiography for some calcifications. It is often easier to obtain than magnetic resonance imaging (MRI), although it cannot image the glenohumeral joint.

MRI can show all the joint structures, including the rotator cuff, and will be required if there is concern regarding areas not seen well on ultrasound, if ultrasound is equivocal or if ultrasound expertise is not available.

Unenhanced computed tomography (CT) has a role in assessing the severity of complex fractures around the shoulder, and for assessing bone stock and quality prior to joint replacement.

For recurrent dislocations, accurate imaging of the bony glenoid and labrum, the capsule and glenohumeral ligaments, as well as the rotator cuff is needed. Cross-sectional imaging (MRI or CT) with arthrography is often required.

Recommended projections 3

Indication/area	Available projections	Recommended projections (may vary with local preferences)	Alternative/additional projections (to be used according to local preferences)
General survey (non-trauma)	AP (external rotation)	AP (external rotation)	AP (internal rotation)
	AP (internal rotation)	Supero-inferior (axial)	Posterior oblique (Grashey projection)
	Posterior oblique (Grashey projection)		
	Supero-inferior (axial)		
Trauma projections	AP (external rotation)	AP (external rotation)	AP (internal rotation)
	Supero-inferior (axial)	Supero-inferior (axial) or Apical oblique (Garth projection)	Super-inferior modified (modified axial – Wallace)
	Apical oblique (Garth projection)		
	Supero-inferior modified (modified axial – Wallace projection)		
	Anterior oblique (Y projection)		
	Infero-superior (axial)		Infero-superior (reverse axial)
Acromio-clavicular joints	AP	AP	
Instability/recurrent dislocation	AP (internal & external rotation)	Will depend on local protocols	Will depend on local protocols
	Supero-inferior (axial)		
	AP modified (Stryker)		
	Axillary infero-superior modified (West Point)		
Calcified tendons & impingement	AP	AP 25°↓	
	AP 25°↓ (outlet projection)	Lateral oblique modified (outlet projection)	
	Lateral oblique modified (outlet projection)	Axial	
	Supero-inferior (axial)		
Clavicle	PA	PA	AP
	AP	Modified infero-superior (modified axial)	
	Modified infero-superior (modified axial)		
Sternoclavicular joints	PA	PA	Lateral
	PA oblique	PA oblique	
	Lateral		
Scapula	AP	AP	
	Anterior oblique (lateral)	Anterior oblique (lateral)	
Coracoid process	AP (arm abducted)	AP (arm abducted)	
	Supero-inferior (axial)	Supero-inferior (axial)	

AP, antero-posterior; PA, postero-anterior.
From Goud et al. (2008)[1]; Sanders et al. (2005)[2]

3 Basic projections

Radiological anatomy

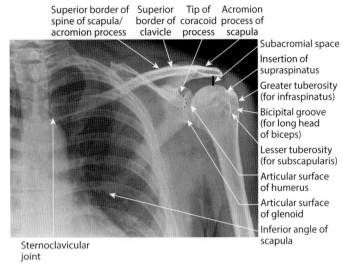

Fig. 3.1 Radiograph of antero-posterior shoulder (with anatomy labelled).

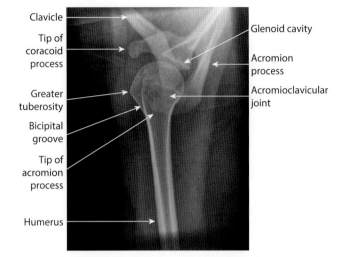

Fig. 3.2 Radiograph of axial shoulder (with anatomy labelled)

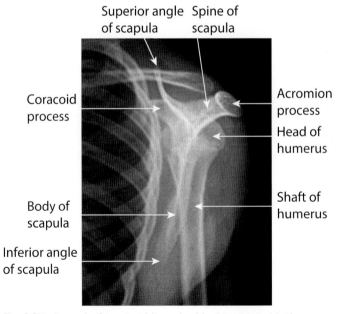

Fig. 3.3 Radiograph of anterior oblique shoulder (Y projection) (with anatomy labelled).

Basic projections 3

Antero-posterior (15°) erect (Figs 3.4a, 3.4b)

The image is acquired using a 24 × 30 cm computed radiography (CR) cassette or alternatively within the field of view of a vertical direct digital radiography (DDR) detector system.

Position of patient and image receptor

- The patient stands with the affected shoulder against the image receptor and is externally rotated 15° to bring the shoulder under examination closer to the image receptor and the plane of the acromioclavicular joint (ACJ) perpendicular to the image receptor.
- The arm is supinated and slightly abducted away from the body. A line joining the medial and lateral epicondyles of the distal humerus should be parallel to the image receptor.
- The image receptor is positioned so that its upper border is at least 5 cm above the shoulder to ensure that the oblique rays do not project the shoulder off the final image.
- The patent should be asked to rotate their head away from the side under examination to avoid superimposition of the chin over the medial end of the clavicle.
- Additionally the humerus can be internally rotated (so a line joining the epicondyles is perpendicular to the image receptor) or left in the neural position which will give a different perspective of the humeral head.

Direction and location of the X-ray beam

- The collimated horizontal beam is directed to the palpable coracoid process of the scapula and collimated to include the structures below.

Essential image characteristics (Fig. 3.4c)

- The image should demonstrate the head and proximal end of the humerus, the inferior angle of the scapula and the whole of the clavicle including the sternoclavicular joint.
- The apex of the lung should be included due to the possibility of a pancoast tumour[1].
- The head of the humerus should be seen slightly overlapping the glenoid cavity but separate from the acromion process.
- Arrested respiration aids good rib detail in acute trauma.

Common faults and remedies

- Failure to include the medial end of the clavicle and inferior border of the scapula within area of interest.
- Lung markings or body of the scapula not visible due to poor exposure or image post processing.

Radiation protection/dose

Expected DRL: ESD 0.5 mGy.

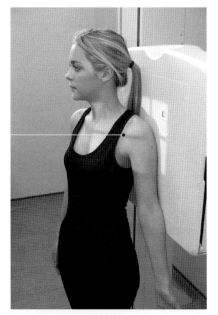

Fig. 3.4a Patient positioning for antero-posterior (AP) projection.

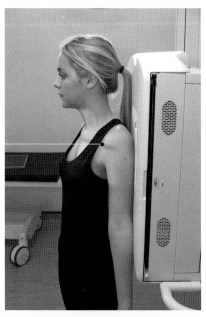

Fig. 3.4b Patient positioning for AP, lateral aspect.

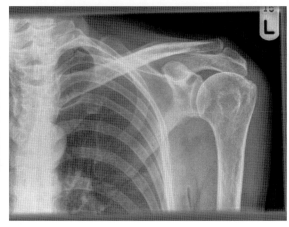

Fig. 3.4c Radiograph of AP shoulder.

3 Basic projections

Antero-posterior (15°) erect (cont.)

Radiological considerations (Fig. 3.5)

- External rotation of the humerus shows the greater tuberosity in profile and the humeral head has a 'walking stick' appearance.
- Internal rotation of the humerus demonstrates the lesser tuberosity in profile and the humeral head has a 'light bulb' appearance.
- It is easy to overlook fractures of the body scapula medial to the glenoid fossa.
- Sometimes lung pathologies are detected in shoulder radiographs so it is important to ensure that technical factors related to image quality enable lung markings to be demonstrated.
- A posterior dislocation is difficult to detect on an AP and a second projection should always be obtained in trauma.

Notes

- A compensation filter may be used to reduce the big subject contrast difference between the area over the ACJ and the body of the scapula.
- A grid should be used for obese patients.
- Do not try to move the arm if a fractured humerus is suspected.

Supero-inferior (axial) (Fig. 3.6a)

The image is acquired using an 18 × 24 cm CR cassette or alternatively within the field of view of a DDR detector.

Position of patient and image receptor

- The patient is seated with their affected side adjacent to the table, which is lowered to waist level.
- The image receptor is placed on the tabletop, and the arm under examination is abducted over the table.
- The patient leans towards the table to reduce the object-to-receptor distance (ORD) and to ensure that the glenoid cavity is included in the image. A curved cassette, if available, can be used to reduce the ORD.
- The elbow can remain flexed, but the arm should be abducted to a minimum of 45°, injury permitting. If only limited abduction is possible, the receptor may be supported on pads to reduce the OFD.

Direction and location of the X-ray beam

- The collimated vertical beam is centred over the mid-glenohumeral joint[2]. Some tube angulation, towards the palm of the hand, may be necessary to coincide with the plane of the glenoid cavity.

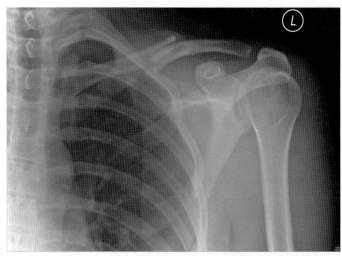

Fig. 3.5 Radiograph of AP shoulder with internal rotation. Note the 'light bulb' appearance of the head of humerus. A fractured clavicle is also present.

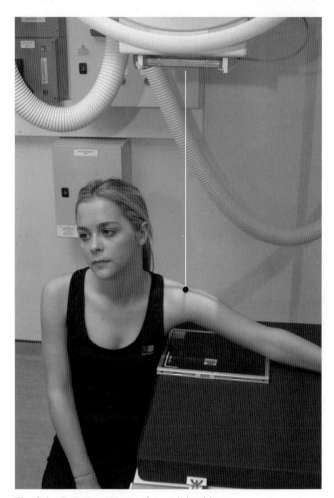

Fig. 3.6a Patient positioning for axial shoulder.

- If there is a large OFD, it may be necessary to increase the overall focus-to-receptor distance (FRD) to reduce magnification.

Basic projections 3

Supero-inferior (axial) (cont.)

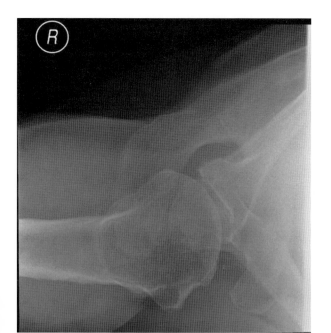

Fig. 3.6b Radiograph of axial shoulder.

Essential image characteristics (Fig. 3.6b)

- The image must demonstrate the humeral head in relation to the glenoid cavity.
- The acromion process should be visible over the neck of humerus and ideally the coracoid process will be visible.

Common faults and solutions

- Failure to demonstrate the glenoid cavity of the humerus as due to the patient not being able to abduct the arm due to trauma or failing to lean over the image receptor, thus allowing the glenoid to be included within the field of the receptor.
- A 5–10° beam angulation along the humerus whilst maintaining the centring point described above may be necessary to demonstrate the entirety of the glenohumeral joint (Fig. 3.6c).

Radiological considerations

- The lesser tuberosity will be seen in profile whilst the greater tuberosity is superimposed over the humeral head.
- The main value of the projection is in assessing subluxation or dislocation as well as Bankart lesions[1].

Note

- Trauma patients will have severe difficulty in abducting their arm and should not be forced to do so. In such cases it is recommended that the apical oblique projection is undertaken.

Radiation protection/dose

Expected DRL: ESD 0.58 mGy.

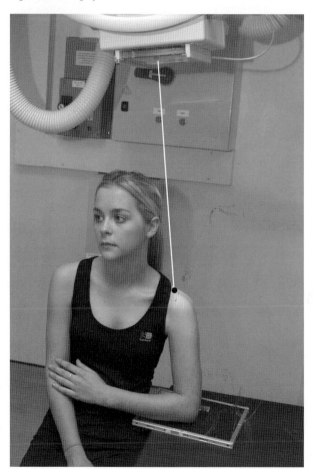

Fig. 3.6c Modifications if the patient cannot abduct the shoulder. Note tube angle and increased FRD.

3 Basic projections

Infero-superior (reverse axial) (Fig. 3.7a)

This projection may be used as an alternative to the supero-inferior projection. The image is acquired using an 18 × 24 cm CR cassette or alternatively within the field of view of a DDR detector.

Position of patient and image receptor

- The patient lies supine, with the arm of the affected side abducted and supinated without causing discomfort to the patient.
- The affected shoulder and arm are raised on non-opaque pads.
- The receptor is positioned vertically against the shoulder and is pressed against the neck to include as much as possible of the scapula within the region of interest.

Direction and location of the X-ray beam

- The collimated horizontal beam is centred towards the axilla with minimum angulation towards the trunk.
- The FRD will probably need to be increased, since the tube head will have to be positioned below the end of the trolley. Consequently, the exposure is increased compared with the supero-inferior.

Essential image characteristics (Fig. 3.7b)

- The image must demonstrate the humeral head in relation to the glenoid cavity.
- The acromion process should be visible over the neck of humerus and ideally the coracoid process will be visible.

Radiological considerations

- The lesser tuberosity will be seen in profile whilst the greater tuberosity is superimposed over the humeral head.
- The main value of the projection is in assessing subluxation or dislocation as well as Bankart lesions[1].
- The most common type of dislocation of the shoulder is an anterior dislocation, where the head of the humerus displaces below the coracoid process, anterior to the glenoid cavity.
- Much rarer is a posterior dislocation (Fig. 3.7c). Often the antero-posterior projection shows little or no evidence of a posterior dislocation; the signs may as sublte as slight loss of parallel alignment of the articular surfaces of the apposing bones. It can however, always be demonstrated in an infero-superior or supero-inferior projection of the shoulder or their alternatives.

Notes

- This projection has some advantages over the supero-inferior as the image receptor can be positioned right over the shoulder joint without interference from the torso.

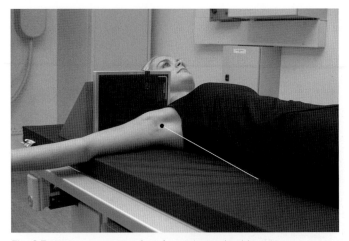

Fig. 3.7a Patient positioning for infero-superior shoulder.

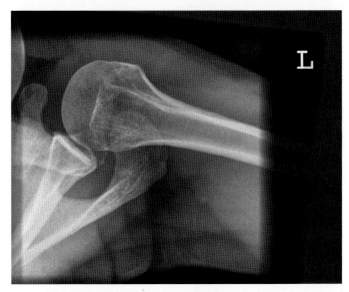

Fig. 3.7b Radiograph of infero-superior shoulder.

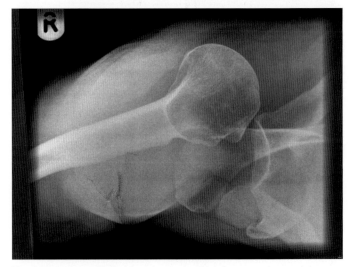

Fig. 3.7c Radiograph of infero-superior shoulder showing posterior dislocation.

An image is often obtainable when the patient can minimally abduct the arm.

- No attempt should be made to increase the amount of abduction that the patient is able and willing to make.

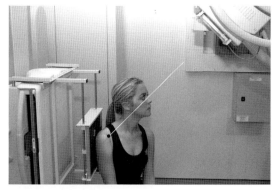

Fig. 3.8a Patient positioning for apical oblique shoulder, lateral aspect.

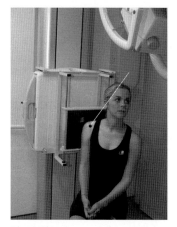

Fig. 3.8b Patient positioning for apical oblique, anterior aspect.

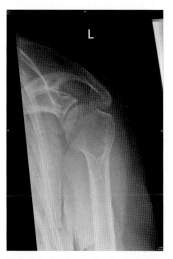

Fig. 3.8c Radiograph of apical oblique shoulder.

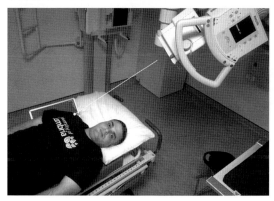

Fig. 3.8d Patient positioning on trollet for apical oblique supine.

Alternative projections for trauma

Apical oblique (Garth projection)[3–5] (Figs 3.8a, 3.8b)

This projection is recommended as the second projection, should an axial not be possible. It will more readily demonstrate Hill–Sachs lesions and glenoid rim fractures compared with the lateral oblique (Y) projection[4].

The image is acquired using a 24 × 30 cm CR cassette or alternatively within the field of view of a vertical DDR detector system.

Position of patient and image receptor

- The patient is positioned erect (either standing or seated) with their back against a vertical Bucky.
- The patient is then rotated toward the affected side so they attain a 45° posterior oblique position.
- The elbow is usually flexed with the patient's arm held across the chest.

Direction and location of the X-ray beam

- The collimated horizontal beam is centred to the image receptor and a 45° caudal tube angulation is employed.
- The central ray is located such that the centre of the glenohumeral joint is located in the middle of the image receptor. FRD 100 cm.

Essential image characteristics (Fig. 3.8c)

- The 45° oblique position allows the beam to pass through the glenohumeral joint such that the glenoid cavity and humeral head are clearly demonstrated without superimposition.
- The base of the coracoid process should appear as a ring just medial to the glenoid[3]. This is a useful reference point.

Common faults and solutions

- If using a Bucky remember not to de-centre the tube from the image receptor when positioning the patient.
- Ensure the centre of the image receptor in the Bucky is positioned at the height of the patient's shoulder and the tube is centred before the examination commences.

Notes

- The projection may also be undertaken with the patient seated with their back to an X-ray table, with the image receptor placed horizontally on the tabletop.
- The examination may also be undertaken supine on a trolley[5] (Fig. 3.8d).

3 Alternative projections for trauma

Supero-inferior modified (modified axial – Wallace projection) (Figs 3.9a, 3.9b)

The image is acquired using a 24 × 30 cm CR cassette or alternatively within the field of view of a DDR detector.

Position of patient and image receptor

- The patient sits erect with their back to the X-ray table.
- The torso is adjusted to bring the body of the scapula parallel with the table.
- The image receptor is placed flat on the tabletop immediately behind the shoulder under examination.

Direction and location of the X-ray beam

- The collimated central ray is centred to the middle of the glenohumeral joint using a 30° angulation from the vertical position.
- Collimate to include the head and neck of humerus, glenoid and the distal end of the clavicle.
- If possible use an FRD of 150 cm to reduce the degree of magnification caused by the increased object-to-receptor distance (ORD). The exposure will need to be increased due to losses of beam intensity due to the inverse square law.

Essential image characteristics (Fig. 3.9c)

- The glenohumeral joint should be demonstrated such that the glenoid cavity and humeral head should be clearly demonstrated with the minimum of superimposition from other structures.

Common faults and solutions

- It is easy to position the image receptor incorrectly and miss the region of interest. This can be avoided by ensuring the shadow of the shoulder cast by the light from the light beam diaphragm is evident on the image receptor.
- Try to avoid the patient leaning back as this will produce suboptimal results.

Radiological considerations

- The projection will more readily demonstrate Hill–Sachs lesions and glenoid rim fractures compared with the lateral oblique (Y) projection.

Notes

- This projection is similar to the apical oblique but may be easier to undertake in trauma situations, as the patient is not required to rotate the torso.
- The projection can be modified for patients on a trolley (Fig. 3.9d).

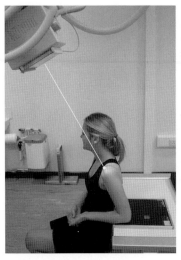
Fig. 3.9a Patient positioning for Wallace projection.

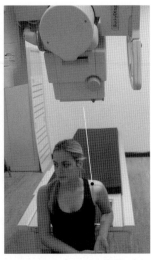
Fig. 3.9b Patient positioning for Wallace projection.

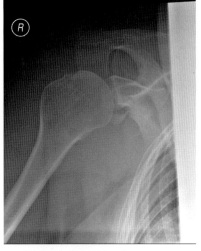
Fig. 3.9c Radiograph of Wallace projection, demonstrating a Bankhart's lesion.

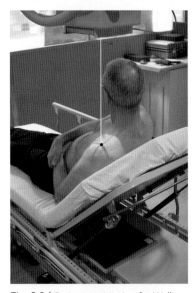
Fig. 3.9d Patient positioning for Wallace projection on a trolley.

- The image will be less distorted with the image receptor orientated horizontally rather than vertically.

Alternative projections for trauma

3

Anterior oblique ('Y' projection) (Fig. 3.10a)

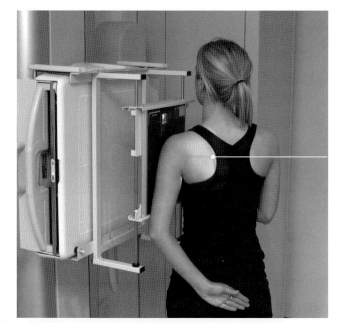

Fig. 3.10a Patient positioning for 'Y' projection.

The image is acquired using a 24 × 30 cm CR cassette or alternatively within the field of view of a vertical DDR detector system.

Position of patient and image receptor

- The patient stands or sits with the lateral aspect of the injured arm against the image receptor and is adjusted so that the axilla is in the centre of the receptor.
- The unaffected shoulder is raised to make the angle between the trunk and the receptor approximately 60°. A line joining the medial and lateral borders of the scapula is now at right-angles to the receptor.
- The image receptor is positioned to include the superior border of the scapula.

Direction and location of the X-ray beam

- The collimated horizontal beam is centred towards the medial border of the scapula and centred to the head of the humerus.
- Collimate to include the region 2 cm above the palpable acromion process superiorly; just below the inferior aspect of the scapula inferiorly; the posterior skin margin; and 2 cm of the rib cage anteriorly.

Essential image characteristics (Fig. 3.10b)

- The body of the scapula should be at right-angles to the image receptor, and thus demonstrate the scapula and the proximal end of the humerus clear of the rib cage.
- The exposure should demonstrate the position of the head of the humerus in relation to the glenoid cavity between the coracoid and acromion processes.

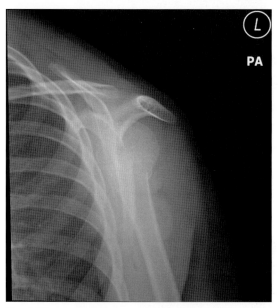

Fig. 3.10b Radiograph of 'Y' projection.

Common faults and solutions

- Over rotation or under rotation of the torso will result in superimposition of the rib cage over the region of interest.

Radiological considerations

- This is a useful projection for differentiating the direction of a dislocation but is less useful for demonstrating associated fractures.

Notes

- A 'reverse' lateral oblique may be undertaken if the patient is immobile on a trolley (Fig. 3.10c).
- This projection is very useful for the provision of a second projection in cases of fractures of the upper humerus where the patient is unable to move their arm.

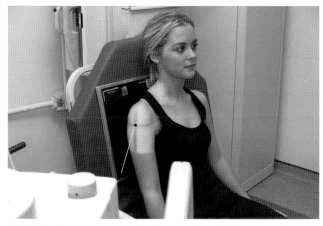

Fig. 3.10c Patient positioning for 'reverse' lateral oblique shoulder.

3 Additional projections

Infero-superior modified (West Point projection) (Figs 3.11a, 3.11b)

The image is acquired using a 24 × 30 cm CR cassette or alternatively within the field of view of a DDR detector.

Position of patient & image receptor

- The patient lies prone on the X-ray table with the head turned away from the affected side and made comfortable on a pad or small pillow.
- If the patient condition allows, the humerus is abducted 90° and a rectangular radiolucent pad placed under the affected shoulder and humerus.
- The forearm then hangs over the side of the X-ray table.
- The image receptor is positioned vertically against superior aspect of the shoulder with one end of the receptor placed against the neck.
- The receptor is supported in position with a 45° foam wedge and a large sand bag or a cassette holder.

Direction and location of the X-ray beam

- The aim is to direct the central ray through the middle of the glenohumeral joint.
- The horizontal tube is initially directed cranially along a sagittal plane passing through the upper humerus.
- The tube is then angled down 25° caudally and 25° medially.
- The beam is centred such that is passes through glenohumeral joint and exits the shoulder at a point just medial to the deltoid muscle.

Essential image characteristics (Fig. 3.11c)

- Collimate to include the head of humerus, distal 1/3 of the clavicle and the lateral 1/2 of the scapula.
- The glenohumeral joint should been seen clearly without superimposition from other structures.

Common faults and solutions

- Failure to demonstrate the glenohumeral joint without superimposition from other structures.
- Consider repeating the radiograph but varying the medial angulation.

Radiological considerations

- Demonstrates the anterior aspect of the glenoid rim and is useful for detecting Bankart lesions[1].

Notes

- Patients with acute injuries will find this projection difficult to achieve. It should only be attempted if the patient has a reasonable range of movement.
- A stationary grid is not used for this projection as a 'cut off' artefact will result.

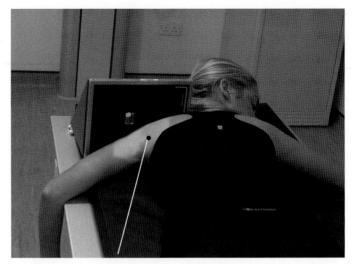

Fig. 3.11a Patient positioning for West Point projection.

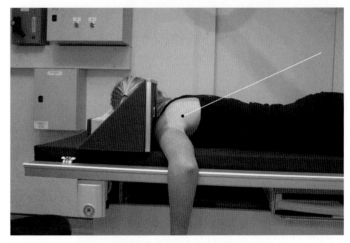

Fig. 3.11b Patient positioning for West Point projection.

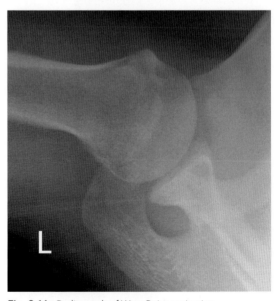

Fig. 3.11c Radiograph of West Point projection.

Additional projections 3

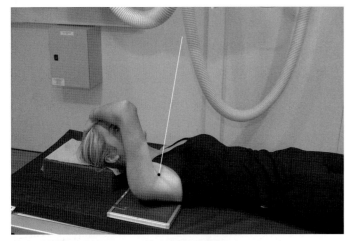

Fig. 3.12a Patient positioning for Stryker projection.

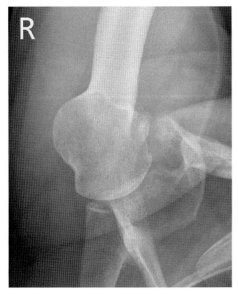

Fig. 3.12b Radiograph of Stryker projection demonstrating a Hill–Sachs lesion.

Antero-posterior modified (Stryker projection) (Fig. 3.12a)

The image is acquired using a 24 × 30 cm CR cassette or alternatively within the field of view of a vertical DDR detector system.

Position of patient and receptor

- The patient lies supine on the X-ray table.
- The arm of the affected side is extended fully and the elbow then flexed to allow the hand to rest on the patient's head.
- The line joining the epicondyles of the humerus remains parallel to the tabletop.
- The centre of the receptor is positioned 2.5 cm superior to the head of the humerus.

Direction and location of the X-ray beam

- The collimated vertical beam is angled 10° cranially and centred through the centre of the axilla to the head of the humerus and the centre of the receptor.

Essential image characteristics

- The projection should demonstrate the posterolateral aspect of the humeral head[2].

Radiological considerations (Fig. 3.12b)

- This projection is highly effective in demonstrating a Hills–Sachs deformity of the humeral head when used in conjunction with an internally rotated AP projection[1].

Note

- Ensure the exposure selected demonstrates good bony detail of the humeral head.

3 Glenohumeral joint

Antero-posterior modified (Grashey projection) (Figs 3.13a, 3.13b)

The image is acquired using a 24 × 30 cm CR cassette or alternatively within the field of view of a vertical DDR detector system.

To demonstrate the glenoid cavity and glenohumeral joint space, the body of the scapula should be parallel to the image receptor so that the glenoid cavity is at right-angles to the receptor. The horizontal central ray can now pass through the joint space parallel to the glenoid cavity of the scapula.

Position of patient and image receptor

- The patient stands with the affected shoulder against the image receptor and the torso is rotated approximately 35–45° toward the affected side to bring the plane of the glenoid fossa perpendicular to the receptor[2].
- The arm is supinated and slightly abducted away from the body.
- The receptor is positioned so that its upper border is at least 5 cm above the shoulder to ensure that the oblique rays do not project the shoulder off the receptor.

Direction and location of the X-ray beam

- The collimated horizontal beam is centred just below the palpable coracoid process of the scapula.

Essential image characteristics (Fig. 3.13c)

- The image should demonstrate a clear joint space between the head of humerus and glenoid cavity.
- The image should demonstrate the head, the greater and lesser tuberosities of the humerus, together with the lateral aspect of the scapula and the distal end of the clavicle.

Common faults and solutions

- Failure to demonstrate the clear joint space so there is no overlap of the glenoid rim and humeral head.
- This is normally due to under-rotation of the torso so try repeating the radiograph with additional rotation.

Radiological considerations

- Useful in joint instability and for narrowing seen in arthritis.

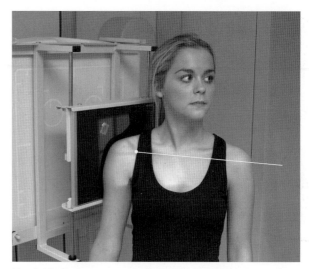

Fig. 3.13a Patient positioning for Grashey projection (antero-lateral aspect).

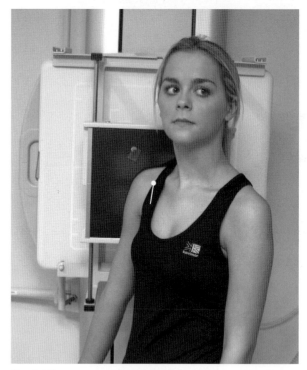

Fig. 3.13b Patient positioning for Grashey projection (anterior aspect).

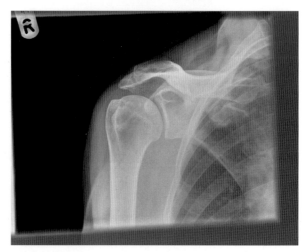

Fig. 3.13c Radiograph of Grashey projection.

Outlet projections (calcified tendons) 3

Antero-posterior 25°↓ (outlet projection) (Fig. 3.14a)

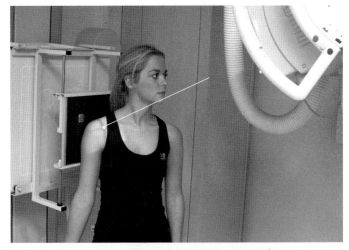

Fig. 3.14a Patient positioning for antero-posterior (AP) 25°↓ projection.

The image is acquired using a 24 × 30 cm CR cassette or alternatively within the field of view of a vertical DDR detector system.

Position of patient and image receptor

- The patient stands with the affected shoulder against a vertical cassette holder and rotated 15° to bring the plane of the scapula parallel with the image receptor.
- The arm is supinated at the patient's side, palm facing forwards, with the line joining the medial and lateral epicondyles of the humerus parallel to the image receptor.
- To allow for caudal angulation of the X-ray beam, the cassette is adjusted vertically, so that the centre of the receptor is approximately 5 cm distal to the head of the humerus.

Direction and location of the X-ray beam

- The collimated central ray is angled 25° caudally and centred to the upper border of the head of the humerus and to the centre of the receptor.

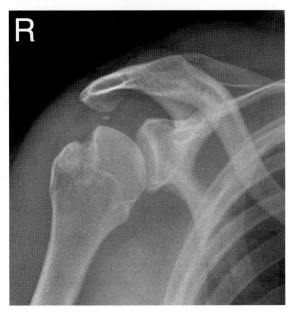

Fig. 3.14b Radiograph of AP 25°↓ projection, showing small calcification in the subacromial space.

Essential image characteristics (Fig. 3.14b)

The subacromial space should be clearly demonstrated with no overlap from the acromion process or clavicle.

Radiological considerations

- This projection is useful for demonstrating the insertion of the infraspinatus muscle and the subacromial space in cases of impingent or calcified tendons.

Note

- A similar position can be achieved if the patient leans forward as opposed to angling the tube.

3 Outlet projections (calcified tendons)

Lateral oblique 15°↓ (outlet projection) (Fig. 3.15a)

Similar to the 'Y' projection with the addition of a small caudal tube angulation[1].

The image is acquired using an 18 × 24 cm CR cassette or alternatively within the field of view of a vertical DDR detector system.

Position of patient and image receptor

- The patient stands or sits facing the image receptor, with the lateral aspect of the affected arm in contact.
- The affected arm is extended backwards, with the dorsum of the hand resting on the back of patient's waist.
- The patient is adjusted so that the head of the humerus is in the centre of the receptor.
- The patient is now rotated forward until a line joining the medial and lateral borders of the affected scapula is at right-angles to the receptor.
- The body of the scapula is now at right-angles to the receptor and the receptor is parallel to the glenoid fossa.

Direction and location of the X-ray beam

- The collimated horizontal beam is angled 10–15° caudally and centred just below the ACJ.
- The beam is collimated to include the head of humerus, acromion and medial end of the clavicle.

Essential image characteristics (Figs 3.15b, 3.15c)

- The proximal end of the humerus and scapula should be clear of the rib cage.
- The profile of acomian process should be well-demonstrated.

Common faults and solutions

- Over-rotation or under-rotation of the torso will result in superimposition of the rib cage over the region of interest.

Radiological considerations

- The projection may show subacromial abnormalities such as osteophytes, which may cause impingment[1].

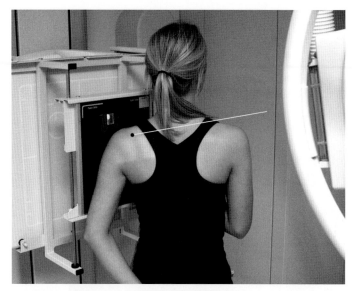

Fig. 3.15a Patient positioning for lateral oblique 15°↓ (outlet projection).

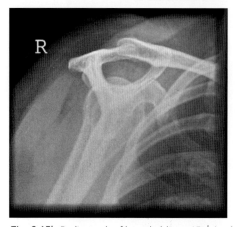

Fig. 3.15b Radiograph of lateral oblique 15°↓ (outlet projection).

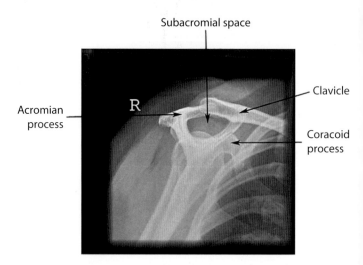

Fig. 3.15c Labelled radiograph of lateral oblique 15°↓ (outlet projection).

Antero-posterior (Figs 3.16a, 3.16b)

An antero-posterior projection of the joint in question is all that is normally required. In certain circumstances, subluxation of the joint may be confirmed with the patient holding a heavy weight.

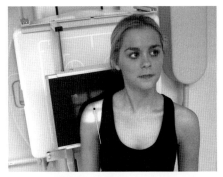

Fig. 3.16a Patient positioning for antero-posterior (AP) acromioclavicular joint (ACJ) (anterior aspect).

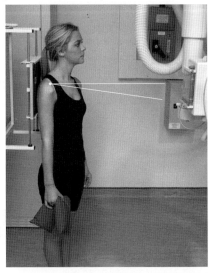

Fig. 3.16b Patient positioning for AP ACJ (oblique aspect to show beam angle and patient angulation).

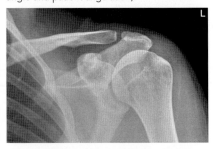

Fig. 3.16c Normal AP radiograph of ACJ.

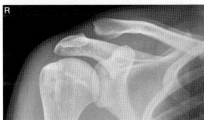

Fig. 3.16d AP radiography of ACJ showing subluxation.

Acromioclavicular joints

Position of patient and image receptor

- The patient stands facing the X-ray tube, with the arms relaxed to the side.
- The shoulder being examined is placed in contact with the receptor, and the patient is then rotated approximately 15° towards the side being examined to bring the ACJ space at right-angles to the image receptor with the acromion process central to the field.

Direction and location of the X-ray beam

- The collimated horizontal beam is centred to the palpable lateral end of the clavicle at the ACJ.
- To avoid superimposition of the joint on the spine of the scapula, the central ray can be angled 15–25° cranially before centring to the joint.

Essential image characteristics (Figs 3.16c, 3.16d)

- The image should demonstrate the acromioclavicular joint and the clavicle projected above the acromion process.
- The exposure should demonstrate soft tissue around the articulation.

Common faults and solutions

- If the joint is not clearly visible it is likely that this will have been caused by a degree of under- or over-rotation or insufficient cranial rotation.

Radiological considerations

- The normal joint is variable (3–8 mm) in width. The normal difference between the sides should be less than 2–3 mm[6].
- The inferior surfaces of the acromion and clavicle should normally be in a straight line.
- Ultrasound can also be used dynamically to assess the stability of the ACJ, as may be done during assessment of impingement.

Weight-bearing antero-posterior projection

- The ACJ has a weak joint capsule and is vulnerable to trauma. Subluxation may be difficult to diagnose in the standard antero-posterior image, because the width of the joint can be variable and may look widened in a normal joint.
- To prove subluxation, it may be necessary to do weight-bearing comparison projections of both ACJs (separate joint images).
- It is advisable to 'strap' the weights used for the procedure around the lower arms rather than getting the patient to hold on to them, as the biomechanics involved may lead to a false-negative appearance.

3 Clavicle

Postero-anterior (Fig. 3.17a)

Although the clavicle is demonstrated on the antero-posterior (AP) projection, it is desirable to have the clavicle as close to the image receptor as possible to give optimum bony detail. The postero-anterior position also reduces the radiation dose to the thyroid and eyes, an important consideration in follow-up fracture images. Alternatively, the examination may be undertaken with the patient AP or AP supine on the trolley for when immobility and movement are considerations.

The image is acquired using a 24 × 30 cm CR cassette in landscape mode or alternatively within the field of view of a vertical DDR detector system.

Position of patient and image receptor

- The patient sits or stands facing an erect image receptor.
- The patient's position is adjusted so that the middle of the clavicle is in the centre of the image receptor.
- The patient's head is turned away from the side being examined and the affected shoulder rotated slightly forward to allow the affected clavicle to be brought into close contact with the image receptor or vertical DDR Bucky system.

Direction and location of the X-ray beam

- The collimated horizontal beam is centred to the middle of the clavicle.

Essential image characteristics (Figs 3.17b, 13.17c)

- The entire length of the clavicle should be included on the image.
- The lateral end of the clavicle will be demonstrated clear of the thoracic cage.
- There should be no foreshortening of the clavicle.
- The exposure should demonstrate both the medial and the lateral ends of the clavicle.

Note

- An anti-scatter grid should be used for larger patients.
- Exposure is made on arrested respiration to reduce patient movement.

Radiation protection/dose

Expected DRL: ESD 0.099 mGy*.

* based on a small sample size

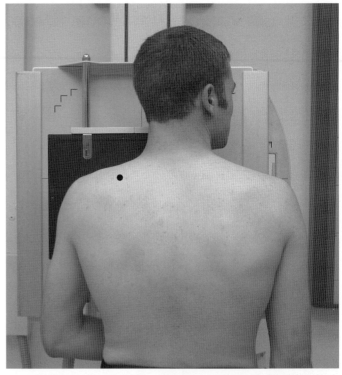

Fig. 3.17a Patient positioning for postero-anterior (PA) clavicle.

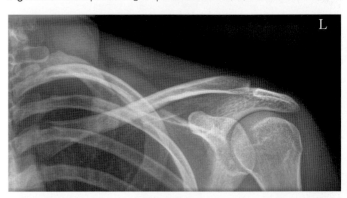

Fig. 3.17b Normal PA radiograph of clavicle.

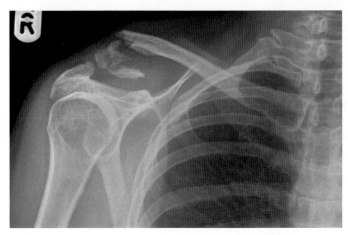

Fig. 3.17c PA radiograph of clavicle showing comminuted fracture.

Clavicle 3

Antero-posterior – supine (Fig. 3.18a)

The image is acquired using a 24 × 30 cm CR cassette in landscape mode or alternatively within the field of view of a DDR detector system.

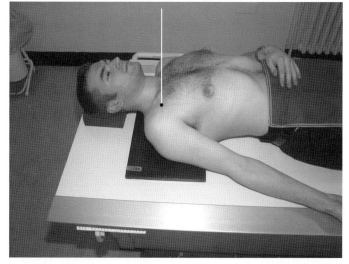

Fig. 3.18a Patient positioning for antero-posterior (AP) supine clavicle on a trolley.

Position of patient and image receptor

- The patient is supine on the X-ray trolley.
- A pad is placed under the opposite shoulder to rotate the patient slightly towards the affected side to make sure that the medial end of the clavicle is not superimposed on the vertebral column.
- The arm of the side being examined is in a relaxed position by the side of the trunk.
- The image receptor is placed transversely behind the patient's shoulder and adjusted so that the clavicle is in the middle.

Direction and location of the X-ray beam

- The collimated vertical beam is centred to the middle of the clavicle.

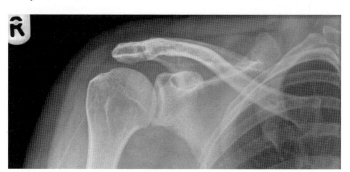

Fig. 3.18b Normal AP supine radiograph of clavicle.

Essential image characteristics (Figs 3.18b–3.18d)

- The entire length of the clavicle should be included on the image.
- The lateral end of the clavicle will be demonstrated clear of the thoracic cage.
- There should be no foreshortening of the clavicle.
- The exposure should demonstrate both the medial and the lateral ends of the clavicle.

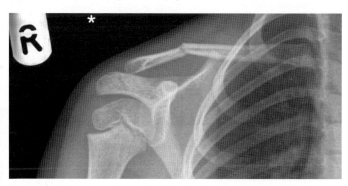

Fig. 3.18c AP supine radiograph of clavicle showing a fracture.

Notes

- The image will be more magnified compared to the PA.
- An anti-scatter grid should be used for larger patients.

Radiation protection/dose

Expected DRL: ESD 0.097 mGy.

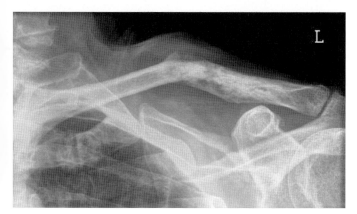

Fig. 3.18d AP supine radiograph of clavicle showing a pathological fracture through a sclerotic metastasis.

3 Clavicle

Modified infero-superior (modified axial) (Fig. 3.19a)

This projection can be very useful to confirm a possible fracture seen on the PA/AP projection, to assess the degree of any fracture displacement and to show the medial end of clavicle clear of underlying ribs.

The image is acquired using a 24 × 30 cm CR cassette in landscape mode or alternatively within the field of view of a vertical DDR detector system.

Position of patient and image receptor

- The patient sits facing the X-ray tube with resting against the image receptor. Some receptor supports allow forward-angulation of the cassette of 15° towards the shoulder. This reduces the distortion caused by the cranially projected central beam.
- The unaffected shoulder is raised slightly to bring the scapula in contact with the receptor.
- The patient's head is turned away from the affected side.
- The image receptor is displaced above the shoulder to allow the clavicle to be projected into the middle of the image.

Direction and location of the X-ray beam

- The collimated horizontal beam is angled 30° cranially and centred to the middle of the clavicle.
- The 30° needed to separate the clavicle from the underlying ribs can be achieved by a combination of patient positioning and central ray angulation.
- The medial end of the clavicle can be shown in greater detail by adding a 15° lateral angulation to the beam.

Essential image characteristics (Figs 3.19b, 3.19c)

- The image should demonstrate the entire length of the clavicle, including the sternoclavicular and ACJs.
- The entire length of the clavicle, with the exception of the medial end, should be projected clear of the thoracic cage.
- The clavicle should be horizontal.

Common faults and solutions

- Insufficient angulation leading to an image that is only marginally different to the AP.

Radiological considerations

- A clavicular fracture, especially when associated with fracture of the upper ribs, may be associated with subclavian vessel damage causing blood loss and haemothorax, or

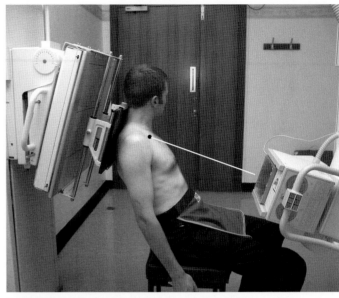

Fig. 3.19a Patient positioning for infero-superior clavicle.

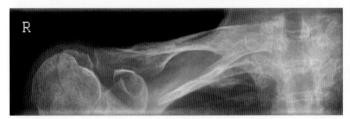

Fig. 3.19b Erect infero-superior radiograph of clavicle demonstrating fracture.

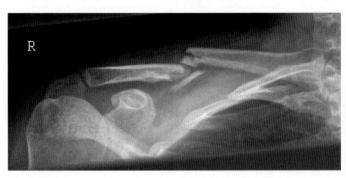

Fig. 3.19c Infero-superior radiograph of clavicle showing a fracture.

puncture of the lung and pneumothorax. Demonstration of the clavicle and upper ribs is particularly important in cases of significant thoracic trauma.

Notes

- It is not possible to undertake a lateral clavicle in addition to the AP. This projection allows the clavicle to be seen from a different aspect and will often detect abnormalities not seen on the AP.
- In cases of acute injury, it is more comfortable for the patient to be examined in the erect position.
- The projection may be undertaken supine on a trolley.

Sternoclavicular joints 3

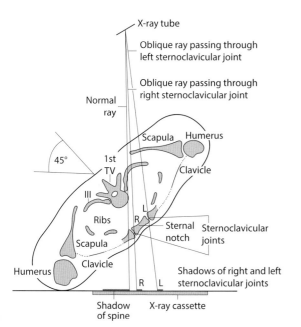

Fig. 3.20a Axial diagram showing positioning and anatomical relationships for imaging the right sternoclavicular joint.

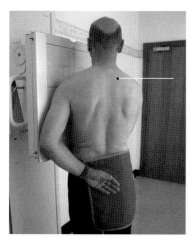

Fig. 3.20b Patient positioning for postero-anterior oblique sternoclavicular joint.

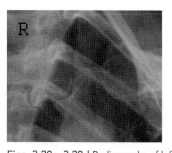 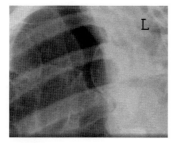

Figs. 3.20c, 3.20d Radiographs of left and right sternoclavicular joints.

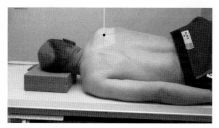

Fig. 3.20e Patient positioning for prone (alternative) sternoclavicular joint.

Postero-anterior oblique (Figs 3.20a, 3.20b)

In an antero-posterior or postero-anterior projection, the vertebral column will be superimposed on, and obscure, the sternoclavicular joints, hence an oblique projection is required to show the joint space clear of the vertebral column. An oblique projection is chosen that will bring the joint space as near as possible at right-angles to the receptor. Both sides may be imaged for comparison.

The image is acquired using an 18 × 24 cm CR cassette or alternatively within the field of view of a vertical DDR detector system.

Position of patient and image receptor

- The patient stands facing the vertical Bucky.
- The patient is then rotated through 45° so that the median sagittal plane of the body is at 45° to the receptor with the sternoclavicular joint being examined nearer the receptor and centred to it.
- The patient holds the vertical stand to help immobilisation and continues to breathe during the exposure.

Direction and location of the X-ray beam

- The collimated horizontal beam is centred at the level of the 3rd thoracic vertebra to a point 5–10 cm away from the midline on the raised side (away) from the receptor.

Essential image characteristics (Figs 3.20c, 3.20d)

- The sternoclavicular joint should be demonstrated clearly in profile away from the vertebral column.

Note

- Superimposed lung detail may be reduced by asking the patient to breathe gently during the exposure.

Semi-prone (alternative) (Fig. 3.20e)

Alternatively, the patient may be examined in the semi-prone position. Starting with the patient prone, the side not being examined is raised from the table until the median sagittal plane is at 45° to the table, with the joint being examined in the midline of the table. The centring point is to the raised side, 10 cm from the midline at the level of the fourth thoracic vertebra.

Radiological considerations

- These joints are difficult to demonstrate, even with good technique. Alternatives include ultrasound, CT (especially with three-dimensional or multiplanar reconstructions) and MRI.

3 Sternoclavicular joints

Postero-anterior (Fig. 3.21a)

Using a single-exposure technique, both joints are imaged for comparison in a case of suspected subluxation.

The image is acquired using a 24 × 30 cm CR cassette in landscape mode or alternatively within the field of view of a vertical DDR detector system.

Position of patient and image receptor

- The patient sits or stands facing an erect cassette holder with their chin resting on the top of the cassette holder.
- The patient's position is adjusted so that the median sagittal plane is at right-angles to the vertical central line of the cassette.
- The image receptor is adjusted vertically to the level of the middle of the manubrium.
- The arms are extended by the sides of the body or alternatively the patient can hold onto the vertical imaging stand.

Direction and location of the X-ray beam

- The collimated horizontal beam is centred in the midline of the thorax at the level of the head of the humerus.

Notes

- The radiographic exposure is similar to that given for an antero-posterior shoulder projection on the patient.
- The beam is collimated to the sternoclavicular joints.

Lateral (Fig. 3.21c)

Position of patient and image receptor

- The patient sits or stands sideways with the affected side adjacent to the cassette.
- The median sagittal plane is adjusted parallel to the image receptor with the upper arm in contact with it.
- The patient clasps the hands behind and pulls the shoulders well back to avoid any obscuring of the joints.
- The centre of the image receptor is adjusted to coincide with the level of the sternoclavicular joints.

Direction and location of the X-ray beam

- The horizontal central ray is centred to the palpable sternoclavicular joints just below the sternal notch.

Radiological considerations (Figs 3.21b, 3.21d)

- Ideally anterior subluxation is diagnosed clinically.
- Posterior subluxation compromises the airway.

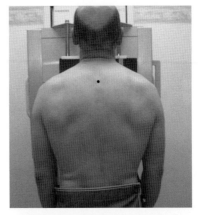

Fig. 3.21a Patient positioning for postero-anterior (PA) sternoclavicular joints.

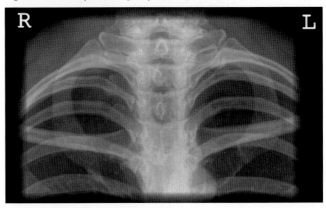

Fig. 3.21b Radiograph of normal sternoclavicular joints in PA projection.

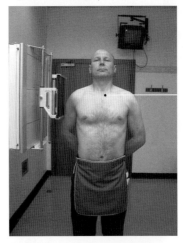

Fig. 3.21c Patient positioning for lateral sternoclavicular joints.

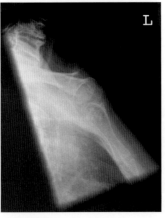

Fig. 3.21d Radiograph of normal sternoclavicular joints in lateral projection.

The position of the scapula relative to the thorax changes as the arm moves through abduction, adduction, flexion, extension and rotation. When the shoulders are pressed back, the medial borders for the scapulae are parallel to and near the vertebral column, so that most of the scapula would be superimposed on the thoracic cage in the antero-posterior projection of the scapula. With the arm in full medial rotation, the scapula glides laterally over the ribs, allowing more of the body of the scapula to be shown clearly against the rib cage.

Scapula 3

Antero-posterior – erect (Figs 3.22a, 3.22c)

The scapula can be shown on the antero-posterior basic survey projection of the shoulder but with the arm in medial rotation. It is preferable for the patient to be examined in the erect position when there is suspected injury as it is more comfortable.

The image is acquired using a 24 × 30 cm CR cassette or alternatively within the field of view of a vertical DDR detector system.

Position of patient and image receptor

- The patient stands with the affected shoulder against the vertical stand and rotated slightly to bring the plane of the scapula parallel with the receptor.
- The arm is slightly abducted away from the body and medially rotated.
- The receptor is positioned so that its upper border is at least 5 cm above the shoulder to ensure that the oblique rays do not project the shoulder off the field.

Direction and location of the X-ray beam

- The collimated horizontal beam is centred 2.5 cm inferior and medial to the head of the humerus.

Essential image characteristics (Fig. 3.22b)

- The entire scapula should be demonstrated on the image.
- The medial border of the scapula should be projected clear of the ribs.

Common faults and solutions

- Large differences in subject contrast due to differences in tissue density often lead to loss of bony detail over the neck of the scapula. Ensure the exposure is increased should this occur.

Radiological considerations

There are often underlying rib fractures in patients who have suffered trauma to the scapula. These may lead to a pneumo-thorax. It is therefore important that exposure and image processing factors are manipulated to ensure lung markings can be clearly seen.

Radiation protection/dose

Expected DRL: ESD 0.5 mGy.

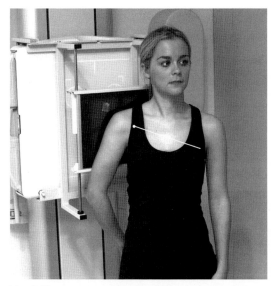

Fig. 3.22a Patient positioning for antero-posterior (AP) scapula.

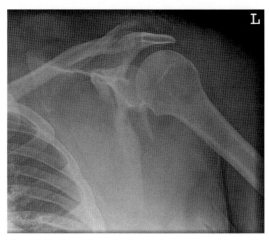

Fig. 3.22b AP radiograph of scapula showing a fracture through the neck of the glenoid.

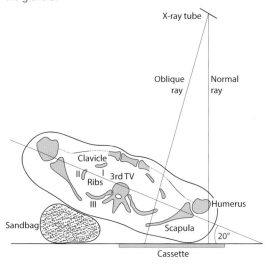

Fig. 3.22c Axial diagram showing the relationship of receptor and X-ray beam to the scapula.

3 Scapula

Anterior oblique (lateral) (Fig. 3.23a)

The image is acquired using a 24 × 30 cm CR cassette or alternatively within the field of view of a vertical DDR detector system.

Position of patient and image receptor

- The patient stands with the side being examined against a vertical Bucky.
- The patient's position is adjusted so that the centre of the scapula is at the level of the centre of the image receptor.
- The arm is either adducted across the body or abducted with the elbow flexed to allow the back of the hand to rest on the hip.
- Keeping the affected shoulder in contact with the Bucky, the patient's trunk is rotated forward until the body of the scapula is at right-angles to the receptor. This can be checked by palpating the medial and lateral borders of the scapula near the inferior angle.

Direction and location of the X-ray beam

- The collimated horizontal beam is centred to the midpoint of the medial border of the scapula and to the middle of the receptor.

Essential image characteristics (Fig. 3.23b)

- The scapula should be demonstrated clear of the ribs.
- The medial and lateral borders should be superimposed.
- The humerus should be projected clear of the area under examination.
- The exposure should demonstrate adequately the whole of the scapula.

Common faults and solutions

Over-rotation or under-rotation of the torso will result in superimposition of the rib cage over the region of interest.

Radiation protection/dose

Expected DRL: ESD 0.73 mGy.

Lateral (alternative) (Fig. 3.23c)

Position of patient and image receptor

- The patient lies prone on the X-ray table.
- The arm on the side being examined is slightly abducted and the elbow flexed.
- The unaffected side is raised until the palpable body of the scapula is at right-angles to the table and in the midline of the table.

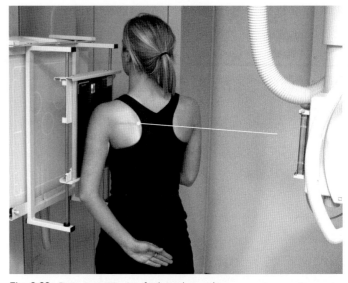

Fig. 3.23a Patient positioning for lateral scapula.

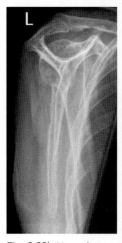

Fig. 3.23b Normal lateral radiograph of scapula.

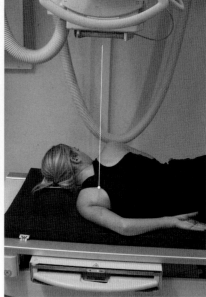

Fig. 3.23c Alternative prone positing for lateral scapula.

Direction and location of the X-ray beam

- The vertical central ray is directed just medial to the midpoint of the palpable medial border of the scapula and to the middle of the Bucky table.

Radiological considerations

- This is a very thin sheet of bone with several dense appendages overlying the upper ribs, making fractures, and their full extent, hard to assess. CT may be very useful for complete evaluation, in particular the multiplanar reconstruction, once a fracture has been detected.

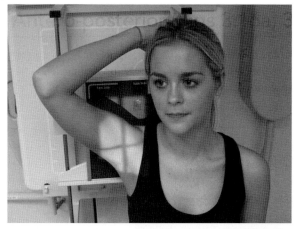

Fig. 3.24a Patient positioning for coracoid process (arm abducted).

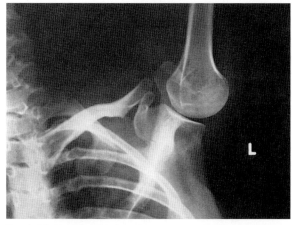

Fig. 3.24b Radiograph of coracoid process anterior aspect (shoulder flexed).

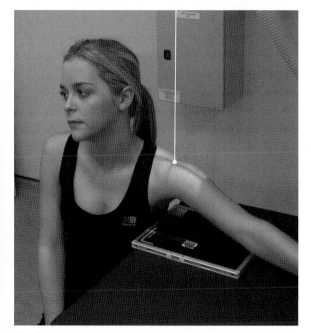

Fig. 3.24c Patient positioning for axial coracoid process projection.

Coracoid process 3

Antero-posterior shoulder (arm abducted) (Figs 3.24a, 3.24b)

The coracoid process is demonstrated more clearly in an antero-posterior projection, with the shoulder flexed to above-shoulder level. Additionally, the process is demonstrated in the axial (supero-inferior and infero-inferior) projections of the shoulder.

The image is acquired using an 18 × 24 cm CR cassette or alternatively within the field of view of a vertical DDR detector system.

Position of patient and image receptor

- The patient is supine or erect, with the posterior aspect of the affected shoulder against the receptor.
- The shoulder of the affected side is flexed to above-shoulder level and the elbow flexed, allowing the hand to rest on the patient's head.
- The patient is now rotated slightly to bring the affected side away from the image receptor.
- The position of the receptor is adjusted so that it is centred to the axilla.

Direction and location of the X-ray beam

- The collimated horizontal beam is centred at right-angles to the image receptor and centred to the axilla of the affected side.

Note

- This projection will also demonstrate the ACJ of the same side, free from overlaying structures.

Axial (Figs 3.24c, 3.24d)

A collimated axial projection as described earlier in the section provides a good second projection at right-angles to the projection described above.

The coracoid process should be clearly visible in profile. Some superimposition over the clavicle is acceptable though this should be minimised if possible.

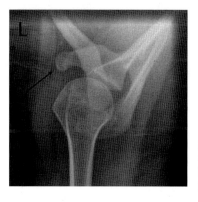

Fig. 3.24d Radiograph of coracoid process (arm abducted). (Arrow indicates the coracoid process.)

3 Shoulder

Image evaluation – 10-point plan

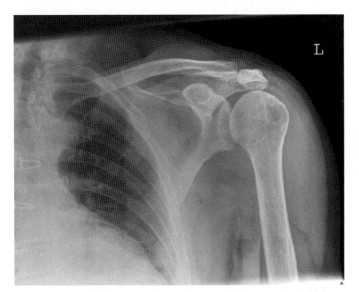

Fig. 3.25a AP shoulder.

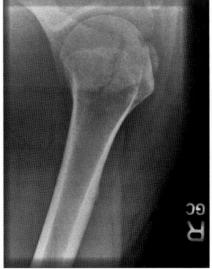

Fig. 3.25b Axial shoulder.

IMAGE EVALUATION

AP shoulder (Fig. 3.25a)

The main points to consider are:
1. Positioning adequate.
2. Technical factors such as exposure and processing are adequate.
3. The radiographic contrast is optimal. This is an area of high subject contrast as it contains tissues of many thicknesses, e.g. the region over the ACJ compared with scapula over the rib cage. The exposure and processing have produced adequate image density (screen brightness) over both these regions allowing diagnostic detail to be seen in all areas. This indicates adequate radiographic contrast.
4. Regions of interest – included:
   - Proximal 1/3 of humerus.
   - The whole of the clavicle including the sterno-clavicular joint medially.
   - The whole of the scapula including the inferior angle.
5. No need for repeats though an additional projection such as an apical oblique or lateral oblique is required to demonstrate the dislocation and possible fractures of the glenoid or humeral head.

Radiographer Comments/Initial report

Posterior dislocation of left shoulder.

IMAGE EVALUATION

Axial shoulder (Fig. 3.25b)

The main points to consider are:
1. Suboptimal demonstration of the glenoid cavity.
2. Image noisy caused by underexposure.
3. There is a normal variant present on the acromion process. This is an os acromiale, which is caused by the failure of one of the osscifation centres to fuse. This can be easily confused with a fracture.
4. Suggest repeat radiograph with an increased mAs (at least double) and repositioning to include more of the glenoid cavity and neck of scapula.

Radiographer Comments/Initial report

No fractures or dilocations. Normal variant noted (os acromiale).

Shoulder 3

Image evaluation – 10-point plan (cont.)

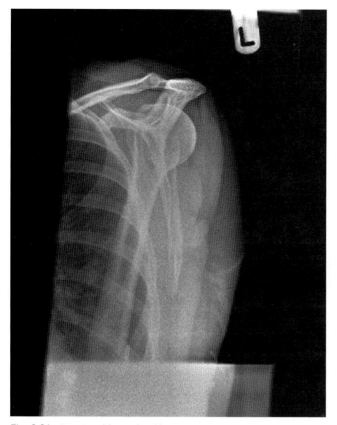

Fig. 3.26a Anterior oblique shoulder.

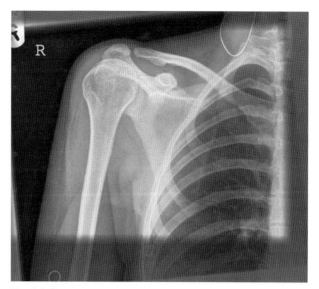

Fig. 3.26b AP shoulder.

IMAGE EVALUATION

Anterior oblique shoulder (Fig. 3.26a)

The main points to consider are:
1. Positioning optimal:
   - Proximal 1/3 of humerus.
   - All of the scapula.
   - Distal 1/3 of the clavicle.
   - The body of the scapula is well-demonstrated clear of the rib cage.
2. Technical factors within the 10-point plan are adequate apart from the exposure. The image shows noise from an underexposure.
3. A repeat would not be required if the main purpose of the examination was to exclude dislocation. If fine bony detail was needed (e.g. to show a subtle fracture or bone pathology) then the image should be repeated with a substantial increase in mAs.

Radiographer Comments/Initial report

No abnormality detected.

IMAGE EVALUATION

AP shoulder (Fig. 3.26b)

The main points to consider are:
1. Positioning poor as the patient is lordotic (leaning back) in relation to the primary beam. This is demonstrated by poor visualisation of the subacromial space and superimposition of the upper humeral head over the lower acromion.
2. The image has insufficient collimation and has been centred incorrectly (too far inferiorly and slightly too far medially)
3. Artefacts noted from metal clips on clothing and a necklace though these do not interfere with the diagnostic potential within the image.
4. Exposure and image processing factors optimal due to adequate contrast and low noise within the image.

Radiographer Comments/Initial report

No abnormality detected. Suboptimal image quality.

Section 4

Lower Limb

CONTENTS

RECOMMENDED PROJECTIONS	124
FOOT	125
Positioning terminology	125
Radiographic anatomy	126
Basic projections	127
Dorsi-plantar (Basic)	127
Dorsi-plantar oblique (DPO) (Basic)	128
Image evaluation – 10-point plan	129
Lateral	130
Lateral – erect (weight-bearing)	131
Dorsi-plantar – erect (weight-bearing)	131
TOES	132
Basic projections	132
Dorsi-plantar (Basic)	132
Dorsi-plantar oblique (Basic)	132
Lateral (Basic) (hallux)	133
METATARSAL–PHALANGEAL SESAMOID BONES	134
Basic projections	134
Lateral	134
Axial	134
ANKLE	135
Radiographic anatomy	135
Basic projections	136
Antero-posterior (AP) – mortise projection (Basic)	136
Lateral (medio-lateral) (Basic)	137
Image evaluation – 10-point plan	138
Alternative projection methods	**139**
Antero-posterior	139
Lateral (latero-medial) – horizontal beam	139
Stress projections for subluxation	**140**
Antero-posterior (stress)	140
Lateral (stress)	140
CALCANEUM	141
Basic projections	141
Lateral (Basic)	141
Axial (Basic)	142
SUBTALAR JOINTS	143
Recommended projections	143
Dorsi-plantar oblique (DPO)	144
Lateral oblique	144
Oblique medial	145
Oblique lateral	146
TIBIA AND FIBULA	147
Basic projections	147
Antero-posterior (Basic)	147
Lateral (Basic)	147
PROXIMAL TIBIO-FIBULAR JOINT	148
Basic projections	148
Lateral oblique (Basic)	148
Antero-posterior oblique (Basic)	148
KNEE JOINT	149
Radiographic anatomy	149
Basic projections	150
Antero-posterior – weight-bearing (Basic)	150
Alternative projections	**151**
Antero-posterior – supine	151
Lateral (Basic) (turned/rolled)	152
Image evaluation – 10-point plan	153
Additional projections	**154**
Lateral – horizontal beam (trauma)	154
Stress projections for subluxation	**155**
Antero-posterior – stress	155
Patella (postero-anterior, PA)	156
Skyline projections	**157**
Supero-inferior	157
Infero-superior	158
Patella – infero-superior (patient prone)	159
Postero-anterior oblique	160
Antero-posterior oblique	160
Intercondylar notch (tunnel) – antero-posterior	161
Intercondylar notch (tunnel) – posterior–anterior ('racing start')	162
FEMUR – SHAFT	163
Basic projections	163
Antero-posterior (Basic)	163
Lateral (Basic)	164
Additional projection – lateral horizontal beam	165
Image evaluation – 10-point plan	166
LEG ALIGNMENT	167
CR method	167
DDR method	168

4 Recommended projections

Area	Indication	Projection		
Foot	Fracture and dislocations of the metatarsals	DP (basic)	DP oblique (basic)	Lateral (on request)
	Fracture and dislocations of the tarsal bones	DP (basic)	DP oblique (basic)	Lateral (on request)
	Foreign bodies	DP (basic)	Lateral (basic)	
	Pathology	DP (basic)	DP oblique (basic)	
	Pes planus	Lateral – erect (both sides for comparison		
	Hallux valgus	DP – erect (both sides for comparison)		
Toes	Trauma or pathology Hallux	DP (basic)	Lateral (basic)	
	Trauma or pathology other toes	DP (basic)	DP oblique (basic)	
1st metatarso-phalangeal sesamoid bones	Trauma or pathology	Lateral	Axial	
Ankle	Trauma or pathology	AP (basic/mortise)	Lateral (basic or alternative)	AP oblique (on request)
	Subluxation (torn lateral ligaments)	AP (basic)	Lateral (basic or alternative)	
		Provided no fracture is seen, these are followed by:	AP (stress)	Lateral (stress)
Calcaneum (heel)	Trauma	Axial (basic)	Lateral (basic)	
	Pathology	Lateral (basic)	Axial on request (basic or alternative)	
Subtalar joints	Trauma or pathology	Projections on request		
Tibia and fibula	Trauma or pathology	AP (basic)	Lateral (basic or alternative)	
Proximal tibio-fibular joint	Trauma or pathology	Lateral oblique (basic) or AP oblique (alternative)		
Knee joint	Trauma	AP (basic)	Lateral horizontal beam	
	Additional trauma projections	Oblique	Skyline – infero-superior or supero- inferior	Intercondylar notch
	Loose bodies	AP (basic)	Lateral (basic)	Intercondylar notch
	Pathology	AP (erect)	Lateral (basic)	AP (supine/basic)
	Subluxation	Antero-posterior (stress)		
Femur/shaft	Trauma or pathology	AP (basic)	Lateral – basic or horizontal beam	
Lower limb	Leg alignment and measurement	AP CR method	AP DDR method	

AP, antero-posterior; CR, computed radiography; DDR, direct digital radiography; DP, dorsi-plantar.

Foot 4

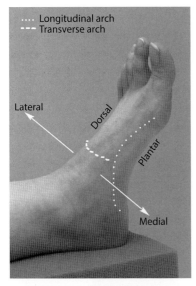

Fig. 4.3a Foot terminology.

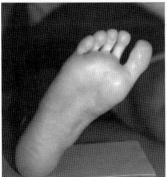

Fig. 4.3b Medial rotation.

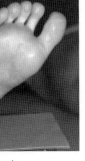

Fig. 4.3c Lateral rotation.

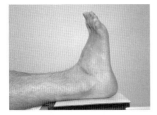

Fig. 4.3d Ankle flexion.

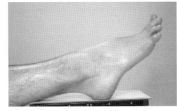

Fig. 4.3e Ankle extension.

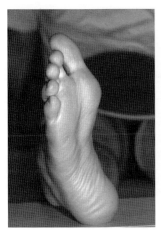

Fig. 4.3f Inversion.

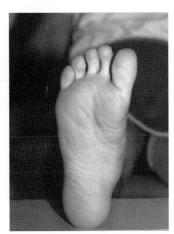

Fig. 4.3g Eversion.

Positioning terminology

Rotation of the lower limb occurs at the hip joint. The position of the foot relates to the direction of rotation.

Dorsal surface: the superior surface of the foot is known as the dorsal surface and slopes downwards, at a variable angle, from the ankle to the toes and from medial to lateral (Fig. 4.3a).

Plantar aspect: the inferior surface of the foot is known as the plantar aspect (Fig. 4.3a).

Medial aspect: the surface nearer the midline of the body is the medial aspect (Fig. 4.3a).

Lateral aspect: the surface further from the midline of the body is the lateral aspect (Fig. 4.3a).

Medial rotation: the lower limb is rotated inwards, so that the anterior surface faces medially. This will produce internal rotation of the hip joint (Fig. 4.3b).

Lateral rotation: the lower limb is rotated outwards, so that the anterior surface faces laterally. This will produce external rotation of the hip joint (Fig. 4.3c).

Ankle flexion: ('dorsiflexion') of the ankle joint occurs when the dorsal surface of the foot is moved in a superior direction (Fig. 4.3d).

Ankle extension: ('plantar flexion') of the ankle joint occurs when the plantar surface of the foot is moved in an inferior direction (Fig. 4.3e).

Inversion: inversion of the foot occurs when the plantar surface of the foot is turned to face medially – with the limb extended (Fig. 4.3f).

Eversion: eversion of the foot occurs when the plantar surface of the foot is turned to face laterally – with the limb extended (Fig. 4.3g).

Flexion of the knee joint: the degree of flexion of the knee joint relates to the angle between the axis of the tibia when the knee is extended and the angle of the axis of the tibia when the knee is flexed.

4 Foot

Radiographic anatomy (Figs 4.4a–4.4c)

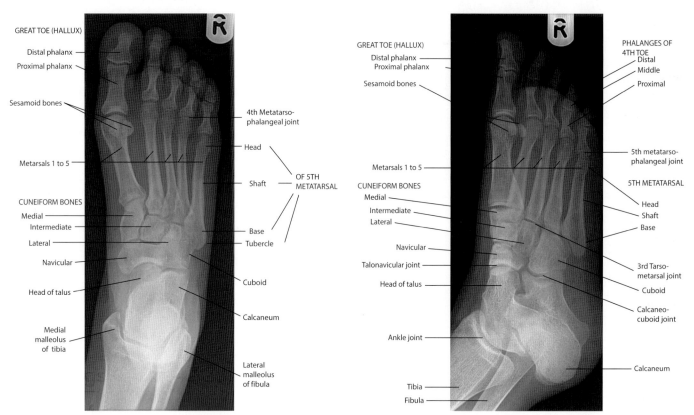

Fig. 4.4a Annotated radiograph of dorsi-plantar foot.

Fig. 4.4b Annotated radiograph of dorsi-plantar oblique foot.

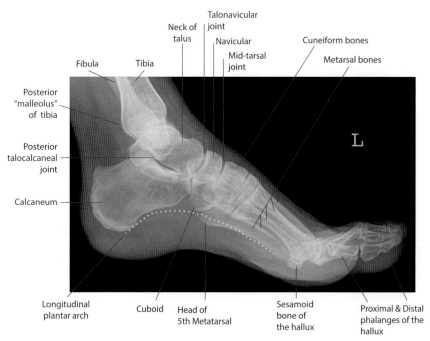

Fig. 4.4c Lateral radiograph of foot, labelled with anatomy.

Basic projections

Two projections are routinely taken, a dorsi-plantar (DP) and a DP oblique.

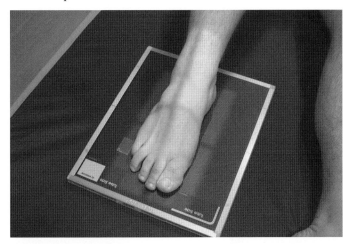

Fig. 4.5a Patient positioning for dorsi-plantar (DP) foot.

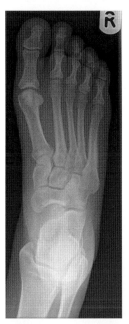

Fig. 4.5b Normal DP radiograph of foot.

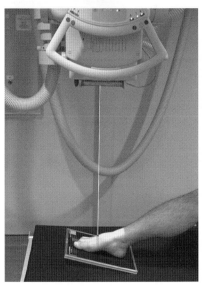

Fig. 4.5c Patient positioning for DP foot with 15° pad.

Foot 4

Each image is acquired using a computed radiography (CR) image detector or alternatively within the field of view of a direct digital radiography (DDR) detector.

Dorsi-plantar (Basic) (Figs 4.5a, 4.5c)

Position of patient and image receptor

- The patient is seated on the X-ray table, supported if necessary, with the hip and knee flexed.
- The plantar aspect of the foot is placed on the image receptor and the lower leg is supported in the vertical position by the other knee.
- The receptor can be raised by 15° to aid positioning, with a vertical central beam. This will improve the visualisation of the tarsal and tarso-metatarsal joints. This angulation compensates for the inclination of the longitudinal arch and reduces overshadowing of the tarsal bones.

Direction and location of the X-ray beam

- The collimated central beam is centred over the cuboid–navicular joint midway between the palpable navicular tuberosity and the tuberosity of the 5th metatarsal.
- The X-ray tube is angled 15° cranially when the receptor is parallel to the table.
- Alternatively, the X-ray beam is vertical if the receptor is raised by 15°.

Essential image characteristics (Fig. 4.5b)

- The tarsal bones and tarso-metatarsal joints should be demonstrated when the whole foot is examined (including lateral and medial soft tissue margins and distal toes).
- The inclusion of the medial and lateral malleoli is helpful in trauma cases to exclude bony injury to these areas.
- A wedge filter placed under the toes may be used to give a uniform range of densities, especially if the image is acquired using screen/film technology.

Notes

- For non-ambulant/wheelchair bound patients, the image receptor (CR) may be placed on a pad or stool directly in contact with the plantar aspect of the foot.
- A vertical DDR receptor may also be angled to accommodate such patients.

Radiation protection/dose

- Careful technique and close collimation will assist in reducing the patient dose.

Expected DRL: ESD 0.075 mGy.

4 Foot

Dorsi-plantar oblique (DPO) (Basic) (Fig. 4.6a)

Position of patient and image receptor

- From the basic DP position, the affected limb is leaned medially, bringing the plantar surface of the foot to approximately 30–45° to the image receptor.
- A non-opaque angled pad is placed under the foot to maintain the position, with the opposite limb acting as a support.

Direction and location of the X-ray beam

- The collimated central beam is directed over the cuboid–navicular joint.

Essential image characteristics (Fig. 4.6b)

- The exposure and processing algorithm selected should produce an image that adequately demonstrates the differences in subject contrast and density between the toes and tarsus.
- The DPO should demonstrate the intertarsal and tarso-metatarsal joints.

Common faults and solutions

- A common fault is for the foot to be slightly externally rotated on the DP projection. This obscures the detail at the base of the 5th metatarsal. Ensure both the medial and lateral aspects of the foot are in contact with the receptor.
- The DPO can easily be over internally rotated, overlapping and thus obscuring the bases of the 2nd and 3rd metatarsals. Ensure that the internal rotation does not exceed 45°.

Radiological considerations

- There are numerous possible accessory ossicles around the foot and ankle, and these must not be confused with fractures. As a general rule ossicles are in documented locations and are rounded and corticated, rather than having any sharp/straight edges as seen with fractures (Fig. 4.6c).
- The base of the 5th metatarsal ossifies from an accessory ossification centre, which is orientated parallel to the long axis of the bone. A fracture will run transversely (Fig. 4.6d).
- If the edges of an accessory ossification centre are not parallel, this may indicate an avulsion injury.
- Lisfranc fracture dislocations at the bases of the metatarsals are difficult to see, except on oblique projections. Poor positioning and underexposure may mask these important injuries.
- Weight-bearing views may be requested to assess the plantar arch and biomechanics of the foot and may also be useful in demonstrating a Lisfranc injury which may not be seen on the initial (non-weight-bearing) images, but clinical suspicion remains.[1]

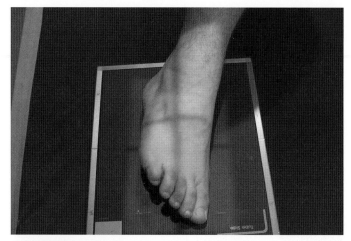

Fig. 4.6a Patient positioning for dorsi-plantar oblique (DPO) projection.

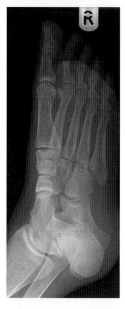

Fig. 4.6b Normal DPO foot.

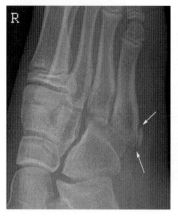 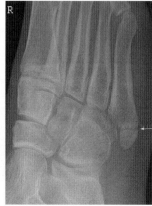

Figs 4.6c and d Radiographs showing normal 5th metatarsal ossification centre on the left, and fracture base 5th metatarsal on right (arrow).

- Ultrasound and magnetic resonance imaging (MRI) are useful to assess soft tissue abnormalities. Computed tomography (CT) has a very limited role, usually in assessment of complex fractures.

Expected DRL: ESD 0.076 mGy.

Foot 4

Image evaluation – 10-point plan

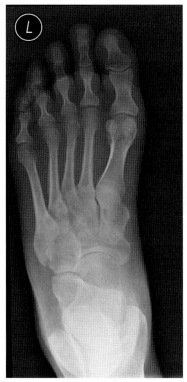

Fig. 4.7a Optimal DP radiograph.

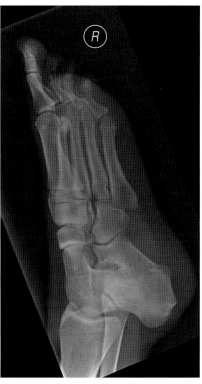

Fig. 4.7b Suboptimal DPO radiograph.

IMAGE EVALUATION

DP foot (Fig. 4.7a)

The main points to consider are:

- No radio-opaque marker was applied!
- Image is correctly positioned, with even spaces between the 2–5th metatarsals, indicating no rotation has occurred.
- Image is well penetrated through the tarsal area.
- There is some early callus formation around the neck of the 3rd metatarsal.

Radiographer Comments/Initial report

? Stress fracture neck of 3rd metatarsal.

IMAGE EVALUATION

DPO foot (Fig. 4.7b)

The main points to consider are:

- Clinical indications were: ? # 2nd metatarsal.
- No radio-opaque marker was applied!
- Evidence of over-rotation (internally) is seen, as the 2nd and 3rd metatarsals are overlapping the 1st metatarsal, the base of the 2nd metatarsal is obscured and many toes are overlapped.
- The image would not be diagnostically acceptable if the area of clinical concern was the 2nd metatarsal.
- Repeat required.

Radiographer Comments/Initial report

No fracture seen (after repeat performed).

4 Foot

Lateral (Fig. 4.8a)

This is used in addition to the routine DP projection to locate a foreign body. It may also be used to demonstrate a fracture or dislocation of the tarsal bones, or base of metatarsal fractures or dislocation.

Position of patient and image receptor

- From the DP position, the leg is rotated outwards to bring the lateral aspect of the foot in contact with the receptor.
- A pad is placed under the knee for support.
- The position of the foot is adjusted slightly to bring the plantar aspect perpendicular to the receptor.

Direction and location of the X-ray beam

- The collimated central beam is centred over the navicular–cuneiform joint if the whole foot is to be examined.
- Alternatively, if the area under question relates to a foreign body (FB) then the beam may be centred over the entry point and appropriate collimation applied to relate the FB to underlying anatomy.

Essential image characteristics (Fig. 4.8b)

- The whole of the foot, including the ankle joint, calcaneum and toes should be seen.
- If examining for a suspected FB, the contrast should be optimised to show the FB against the soft-tissue structures.

Notes

- A metal marker placed over the puncture site is commonly used to aid localisation of the FB (Fig. 4.8c).
- Where applicable, overlying wound dressings should be removed to reduce distracting artefacts.

Radiation protection/dose

- Careful technique and close collimation will assist in reducing the patient dose.

Expected DRL: ESD 0.092 mGy

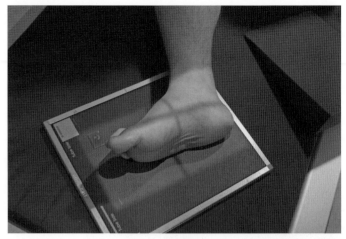

Fig. 4.8a Patient positioning for lateral foot.

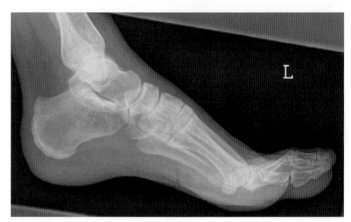

Fig. 4.8b Normal lateral radiograph of the foot.

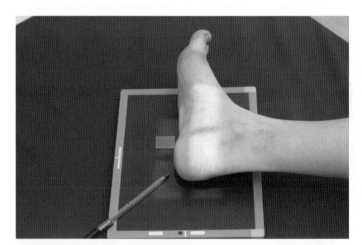

Fig. 4.8c Patient positioning for lateral foot, with pointer for potential foreign body.

Lateral – erect (weight-bearing) (Figs 4.9a, 4.9b)

This projection is used to demonstrate the condition of the longitudinal arches of the foot, usually in pes planus (flat feet).

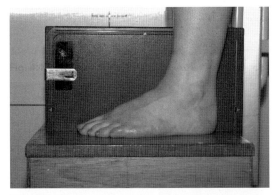

Fig. 4.9a Patient positioning for lateral erect foot.

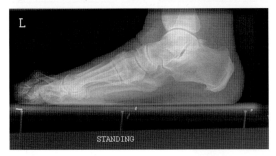

Fig. 4.9b Normal radiograph of lateral erect foot.

Both feet are examined for comparison. It is important that the full weight of the patient is placed on the feet, to allow an accurate evaluation of the effect of normal weight on the longitudinal arch and bony alignment.

Position of patient and image receptor

- The patient stands on a low platform with the receptor placed vertically between the feet.
- The feet are brought close together. The weight of the patient's body is distributed equally.
- To help maintain the position, the patient should rest their forearms on a convenient vertical support, e.g. the vertical Bucky or the platform support mechanism.

Direction and location of the X-ray beam

- The collimated central beam is centred to the tubercle of the 5th metatarsal.

Dorsi-plantar – erect (weight-bearing) (Figs 4.9c, 4.9d)

This projection can be used to show the alignment of the metatarsals and phalanges in cases of hallux valgus. Both forefeet are taken for comparison (Figs 4.9e, 4.9f).

Position of patient and image receptor

- Both feet are placed flat on the receptor adjacent to one another to be imaged together; however, often each foot is best imaged individually. This approach allows each foot to be placed flat on the receptor and minimises the risk of the feet being mildly supinated when the patient is unable to bring the knee joints close enough together. This can occur if both feet are imaged together (for example in obese patients).
- The patient stands with their foot on the receptor.
- The foot is positioned to include all the metatarsals and phalanges.
- To help maintain the position, the patient will require some support, for example by placing their hands in a supporting position onto the raised X-ray table behind the patient.

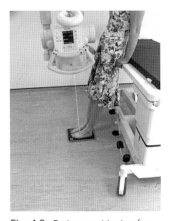

Fig. 4.9c Patient positioning for weight-bearing dorsi-plantar (DP) foot.

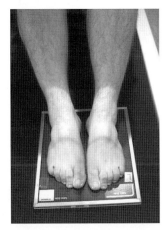

Fig. 4.9d Close up of weight-bearing DP foot.

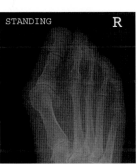

Fig. 4.9e Radiograph of weight-bearing DP foot.

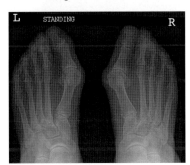

Fig. 4.9f Radiograph of DP erect projection of both feet showing hallux valgus.

Direction and location of the X-ray beam

- The collimated central beam is centred midway between the feet at the level of cuboid–navicular joints, or is centred over the specific cuboid–navicular joint if a single foot is to be examined.
- A 5° tube angulation towards the patient may be required to allow the correct centring point to be achieved, due to the close proximity of the tube housing to the patient.

4 Toes

Basic projections

It is common practice to obtain two projections, a DP and a DPO. A lateral projection is taken for fractures of the phalanges of the hallux (great toe) such as hyperflexion avulsion fractures of the distal phalanx, which could be missed on an oblique projection.

Dorsi-plantar (Basic) (Figs 4.10a, 4.10b)

Position of patient and image receptor

- The patient is seated on the X-ray table, supported if necessary, with hips and knees flexed.
- The plantar aspect of the affected foot is placed on the receptor. A CR cassette may be raised by 15°, using a pad or angling a DDR detector from the horizontal fixator (vertical DDR system).
- The leg may be supported in the vertical position by the other knee.

Direction and location of the X-ray beam

- The collimated central beam is directed over the 3rd metatarso-phalangeal joint (MTPJ), perpendicular to the receptor if all the toes are to be imaged.
- For single toes, the vertical ray is centred over the MTPJ of the individual toe and collimated to include the toe either side.

Radiation protection/dose

- Careful technique and close collimation will assist in reducing the patient dose.

Expected DRL: ESD 0.076 mGy.

Dorsi-plantar oblique (Basic) (Figs 4.10c, 4.10d)

Position of patient and image receptor

- From the basic DP position, the affected limb is allowed to lean medially to bring the plantar surface of the foot approximately 45° to the receptor.
- A 45°e non-opaque pad is placed under the side of the foot for support, with the opposite leg acting as a support.

Direction and location of the X-ray beam

- The collimated central beam is centred over the 1st MTPJ if all the toes are to be imaged and angled sufficiently to allow the central ray to pass through the 3rd MTPJ.

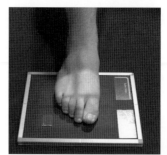

Fig. 4.10a Patient positioning for dorsi-plantar (DP) toes.

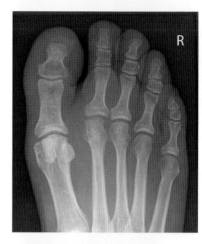

Fig. 4.10b Normal DP radiograph of all toes.

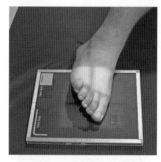

Fig. 4.10c Patient positioning for dorsi-plantar oblique (DPO) toes.

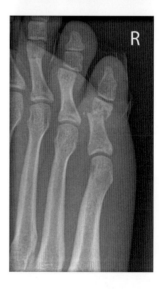

Fig. 4.10d Collimated DPO image of the 5th toe, showing fracture of the proximal phalanx.

- For single toes, the vertical ray is centred over the MTPJ of the individual toe, perpendicular to the receptor. The collimated field should include the adjacent toe(s) to the toe in question.

Expected DRL: ESD 0.076 mGy.

Toes 4

Lateral (Basic) (hallux) (Figs 4.11a, 4.11b)

Position of patient and image receptor

- From the DP position the foot is rotated medially until the medial aspect of the hallux is in contact with the receptor.
- A bandage is placed around the remaining toes (provided no injury is suspected) and they are gently pulled forwards by the patient to clear the hallux.
- Alternatively they may be pulled backwards. This shows the MTPJ more clearly.

Direction and location of the X-ray beam

- The collimated central beam is directed over the 1st MTPJ.

Essential image characteristics (Fig. 4.11c)

- The distal and proximal phalanges, together with the distal 2/3 of the 1st metatarsal should be demonstrated.
- The 1st MTPJ and interphalangeal joint should be seen clearly, with superimposition of the condyles of the head of the proximal phalanx.

Common faults and solutions

A common fault is the 2nd to 5th toes not being pulled away sufficiently, resulting in superimposition of the remaining toes on the base of the proximal phalanx. This can be an uncomfortable procedure for the patient, therefore clearly instructing the patient of the importance of maintaining the correct position and working quickly and efficiently can help reduce this problem.

Radiological considerations

The use of this projection is important for hyperflexion (stubbing) injuries, as an undisplaced avulsion fracture of the distal phalanx of the great toe can be missed on DP and DPO projections.

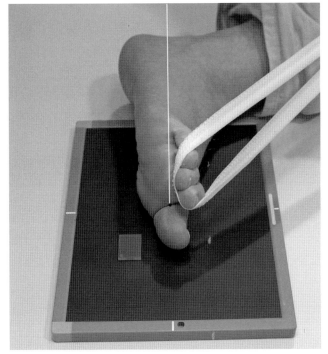

Fig. 4.11a Patient positioning for lateral basic projection of hallux (toes pulled forwards/upwards).

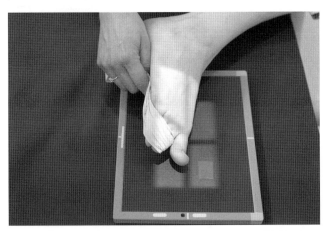

Fig. 4.11b Patient positioning for lateral basic projection of hallux (toes pulled backwards).

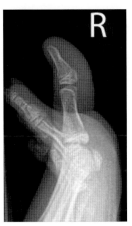

Fig. 4.11c Normal radiograph of lateral basic projection of hallux.

Metatarsal–phalangeal sesamoid bones

Basic projections

The sesamoid bones are demonstrated on the lateral foot projection but when specifically requested a modified lateral and an axial projection may be necessary for further demonstration.

Lateral (Fig. 4.12a)

Position of patient and image receptor

- The patient lies on the unaffected side and the lateral aspect of the affected leg and foot is placed in contact with the receptor.
- The foot is positioned over the receptor to include the phalanges of the hallux and the distal part of the 1st metatarsal.
- The hallux is then pulled forwards (dorsiflexed) with the aid of a bandage and held by the patient.

Direction and location of the X-ray beam

- The collimated vertical beam is centred to the receptor over the 1st MTPJ.

Axial (Figs 4.12b–4.12d)

Position of patient and image receptor

There is a choice of two positions for this projection:

1. The patient remains in the same position as for the lateral projection. The foot is raised on a support and the CR receptor is supported vertically and well into the instep. A horizontal beam is used in this case.
2. The patient sits on the X-ray table, with legs extended and knees slightly bent. The hallux is then dorsiflexed with the aid of a bandage and held by the patient. The CR receptor is raised on a support and positioned firmly against the instep. Alternatively, the patient sits on a chair with the instep of the foot against the edge of the DDR receptor and the hallux dorsiflexed. A vertical beam is used in this case.

Direction and location of the X-ray beam

Centre the collimated beam to the sesamoid bones with the central ray projected tangentially to the 1st MTPJ.

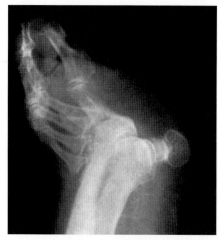

Fig. 4.12a Lateral projection of 1st metatarsal sesamoids; note exostosis on medial sesamoid.

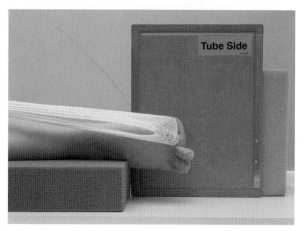

Fig. 4.12b Patient positioning for axial sesamoids.

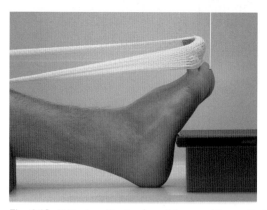

Fig. 4.12c Patient positioning for axial sesamoids – vertical method.

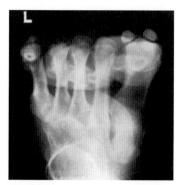

Fig. 4.12d Normal axial sesamoid radiograph.

Ankle 4

Radiographic anatomy

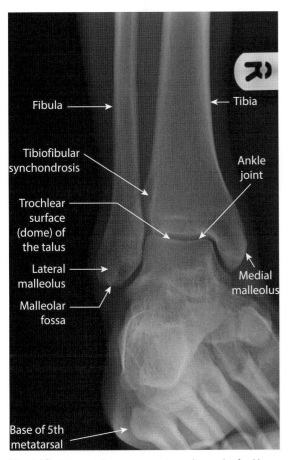

Fig. 4.13a Annotated antero-posterior radiograph of ankle.

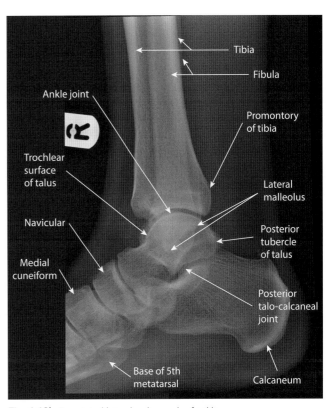

Fig. 4.13b Annotated lateral radiograph of ankle.

4 Ankle

Basic projections

Two projections are routinely taken, an antero-posterior (AP, mortise) and a lateral. Each image is acquired using a CR image detector or alternatively within the field of view of a DDR detector.

Antero-posterior (AP) – mortise projection (Basic) (Figs 4.14a, 4.14c)

Position of patient and image receptor

- The patient is either supine or seated on the X-ray table with both legs extended.
- A pad may be placed under the knee for comfort.
- The affected ankle is supported in dorsiflexion by a firm 90° pad placed against the plantar aspect of the foot. The limb is rotated medially (approximately 20°) until the medial and lateral malleoli are equidistant from the receptor.
- If the patient is unable to dorsiflex the foot sufficiently, then raising the heel on a 15° wedge or using 5–10° of cranial tube angulation can correct this problem.
- The mid-tibia may be immobilised using a sandbag.

Direction and location of the X-ray beam

- The collimated vertical beam is centred midway between the malleoli with the central ray at 90° to an imaginary line joining the malleoli.

Essential image characteristics (Fig. 4.14b)

- The lower 1/3 of the tibia and fibula should be included.
- A clear joint space between the tibia, fibula and talus should be demonstrated (commonly called the mortise view).

Common faults and solutions

- Insufficient dorsiflexion results in the calcaneum being superimposed on the lateral malleolus (Fig 4.14e)
- Insufficient medial rotation causes overshadowing of the tibio-fibular joint with the result that the joint space between the fibula and talus is not demonstrated clearly (Fig. 4.14d).
- If internal rotation of the limb is difficult, then the central ray is angled to compensate, making sure that it is still at 90°s to the imaginary line joining the malleoli.

Radiation protection/dose

- Careful technique and close collimation will assist in reducing the patient dose.

Expected DRL: ESD 0.11 mGy.

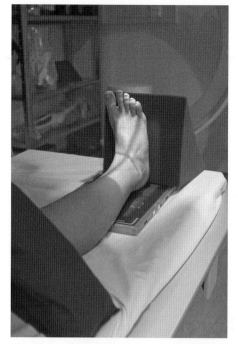

Fig. 4.14a Patient positioning for antero-posterior (AP) (mortise) ankle.

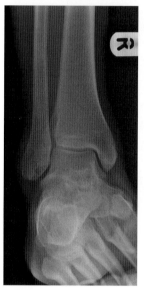

Fig. 4.14b Normal AP radiograph of ankle.

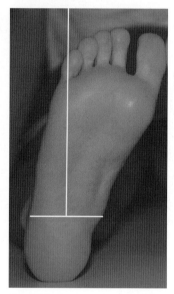

Fig. 4.14c Patient positioning for AP ankle.

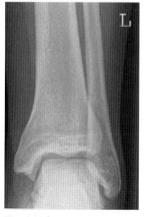

Fig. 4.14d Radiograph showing insufficient medial rotation.

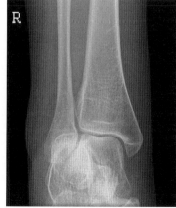

Fig. 4.14e Radiograph showing insufficient dorsiflexion.

Lateral (medio-lateral) (Basic) (Fig. 4.15a)

Position of patient and image receptor

- A 15° pad is placed under the lateral border of the forefoot and a pad is placed under the knee for support.
- From the supine position, the patient rotates on to the affected side.
- The leg is rotated until the medial and lateral malleoli are superimposed vertically.
- A 15° pad is placed under the anterior aspect of the knee and the lateral border of the forefoot for support.
- The receptor is placed with the lower edge just below the plantar aspect of the heel.

Direction and location of the X-ray beam

- The collimated vertical beam is centred over the medial malleolus, with the central ray at right-angles to the axis of the tibia.

Essential image characteristics (Fig. 4.15b)

- The lower 1/3 of the tibia and fibula, base of 5th metatarsal and calcaneum should be included.
- The medial and lateral borders of the trochlear articular surface of the talus should be superimposed on the image.

Common faults and solutions

- Over-rotation causes the fibula to be projected posterior to the tibia and the medial and lateral borders of the trochlear articulations are not superimposed (Fig. 4.15c).
- Under-rotation causes the shaft of the fibula to be superimposed on the tibia and the medial and lateral borders of the trochlear articulations are not superimposed (Fig. 4.15d).
- The base of the 5th metatarsal and the navicular bone should be included on the image to exclude fracture.

Radiological considerations

- Inversion injury of the ankle is common and may result in fracture of the lateral malleolus or the base of the 5th metatarsal. Investigation of the injury should therefore cover both areas.
- Tear of the collateral ligaments without bone fracture may make the ankle unstable, despite a normal radiograph. Stress projections may clarify this problem and ultrasound or MRI may be useful. Complex injuries may occur with fracture of both malleoli, rendering the ankle mortise very unstable, especially if associated with fracture of the posterior tibia – the so-called trimalleolar fracture – and/or disruption of the distal tibio-fibular synchondrosis. These injuries frequently require surgical fixation.
- The 'Ottawa ankle rules' are a set of guidelines which assist referrers in making the correct judgement as to when radiography of the ankle following trauma is justified. Application of the Ottawa rules have been found to reduce unnecessary radiography significantly.[2]

Expected DRL: ESD 0.11 mGy.

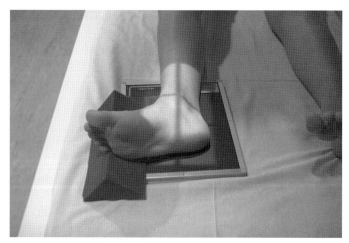

Fig. 4.15a Patient positioning for lateral ankle.

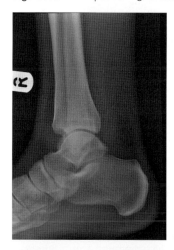

Fig. 4.15b Normal radiograph of lateral ankle, horizontal beam.

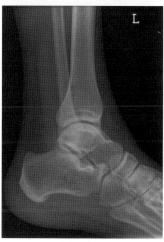

Fig. 4.15c Radiograph showing over-rotation of ankle.

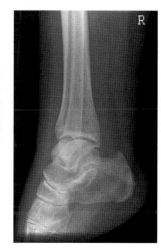

Fig. 4.15d Radiograph showing under-rotation of ankle.

4 Ankle

Image evaluation – 10-point plan

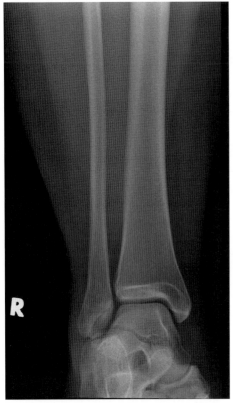

Fig. 4.16a Poor AP ankle.

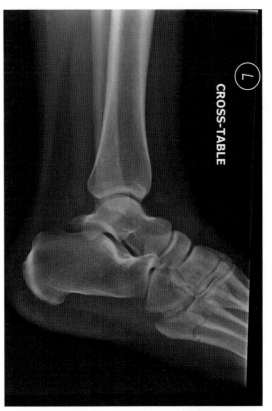

Fig. 4.16b Lateral ankle with the base of the 5th metatarsal.

IMAGE EVALUATION

AP ankle (Fig. 4.16a)

The main points to consider are:

- Correct radio-opaque marker applied.
- Ankle joint is insufficiently dorsiflexed, with the tip of the lateral malleolus partially obscured by the overlapping calcaneum.
- Ankle is sufficiently internally rotated to see the mortise joint clearly.
- The centring point appears to be too proximal, with more proximal tibia/fibula included than required.
- Repeat required.

Radiographer Comments/Initial report

No fracture seen (after repeat performed).

IMAGE EVALUATION

Lateral ankle (Fig. 4.16b)

The main points to consider are:

- No radio-opaque marker was applied!
- Positioning is just acceptable; however, the ankle is slightly externally rotated, and the joint is not quite demonstrated in the lateral position.
- Image is well-penetrated through the tarsal area.
- The base of 5th metatarsal has been included, which has revealed a fracture.

Radiographer Comments/Initial report

Transverse # base 5th metatarsal.

Ankle 4

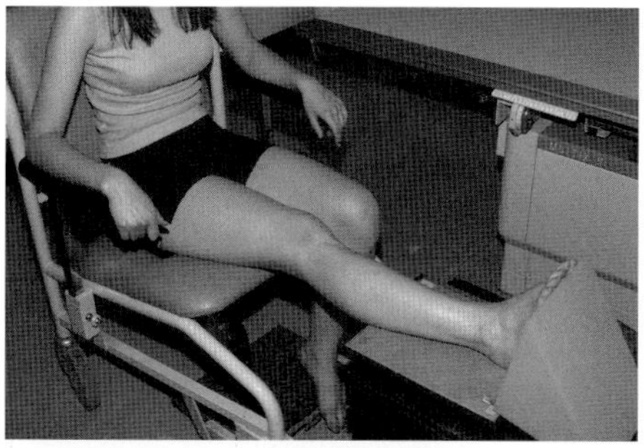

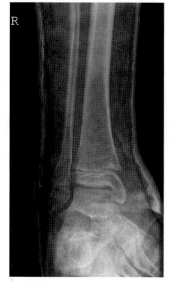

Fig. 4.17a Patient positioning for AP ankle.

Fig. 4.17b AP radiograph through plaster showing fracture of the distal fibula.

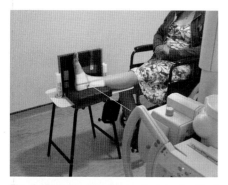

Fig. 4.17c Patient positioning for lateral ankle, horizontal beam.

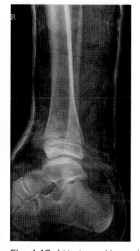

Fig. 4.17.d Horizontal beam lateral radiograph of ankle through plaster.

Alternative projection methods

In cases of trauma the techniques may be modified to obtain the basic radiographs without moving the patient from a wheelchair or turning the leg of a patient whilst lying on a trolley. This also applies to those clinic patients with below-knee plaster casts.

Antero-posterior (Figs 4.17a, 4.17b)

Position of patient and image receptor

- From the sitting position, whilst on a wheel chair, the whole limb is raised and supported on a stool and a pad is placed under the raised knee for support.
- The lower limb is rotated medially, approximately 20°, until the medial and lateral malleoli are equidistant from the receptor and a non-opaque angled pad is placed against the medial border of the foot and sandbags at each side of the leg for support.

Direction and location of the X-ray beam

- The collimated vertical beam is centred midway between the malleoli with the vertical central ray at 90° to the imaginary line joining the malleoli or compensatory angulation of the beam if the foot is straight.
- If the foot remains straight there will be overshadowing of the tibio-fibular joint combined with a vertical central ray.

Lateral (latero-medial) – horizontal beam (Figs 4.17c, 4.17d)

Position of patient and image receptor

- With the patient maintaining the sitting position or lying on the trauma trolley, the limb is raised and supported on a firm non-opaque pad.
- A receptor is placed against the medial aspect of the limb.
- The lower edge of the receptor is placed just below the plantar aspect of the heel, allowing inclusion of the base of 5th metatarsal.

Direction and location of the X-ray beam

- The collimated horizontal beam is centred to the lateral malleolus.
- If there is no internal rotation of the foot, then the distal fibula will be projected behind the distal tibia and a 'true lateral' image is not produced. If the foot cannot be rotated to superimpose the malleoli, then compensatory superior angulation (approximately 20°) can be applied to the beam.

Expected DRL: ESD 0.11 mGy.

4 Ankle

Stress projections for subluxation

Stress projections of the ankle joint are taken to demonstrate subluxation due to rupture of the lateral ligaments. Although these projections may be done in the department, they are now commonly done in theatre using a mobile image intensifier. Stress is applied to the joint by medical personnel, usually an orthopaedic surgeon.

Antero-posterior (stress) (Fig. 4.18a)

Position of patient and image receptor

- The patient and receptor are positioned for the routine AP projection.
- The doctor in charge forcibly inverts the foot without internally rotating the leg.

Direction and location of the X-ray beam

- The collimated vertical beam is centred midway between the malleoli with the central ray at right-angles to the imaginary line joining the malleoli.

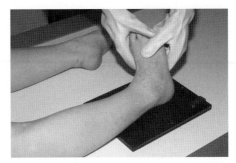

Fig. 4.18a Patient positioning for antero-posterior (AP) inversion stress projection of ankle.

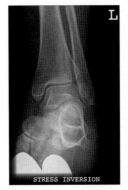 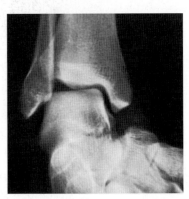

Fig. 4.18b and c Normal (left) and abnormal (subluxation, right) AP radiographs of ankle.

Lateral (stress) (Fig. 4.18d)

Position of patient and image receptor

- The patient lies supine on the table with the limb extended.
- The foot is elevated and supported on a firm pad.
- The ankle is dorsiflexed and the limb rotated medially until the malleoli are equidistant from the tabletop.
- The receptor is positioned vertically against the medial aspect of the foot.
- The doctor applies firm downward pressure on the lower leg.

Direction and location of the X-ray beam

- The collimated horizontal beam is centred to the lateral malleolus.

Notes

- The AP stress projection demonstrates widening of the joint space if the calcaneo-fibular ligament is torn (Figs 4.18b, 4.18c).
- The lateral stress projections demonstrate anterior subluxation if the anterior talo-fibular ligament is torn (Fig. 4.18e).
- Similar techniques are used in theatre with the image intensifier positioned above the ankle. The degree of stress applied is viewed and recorded.

Radiation protection/dose

- The doctor applying the stress must wear a suitable lead protective apron and gloves.

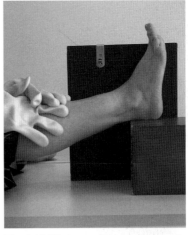

Fig. 4.18d Patient positioning for lateral projection of ankle with stress.

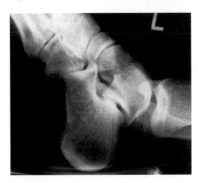

Fig. 4.18e Radiograph of lateral projection of ankle with stress, showing subluxation.

- If the technique is done using a mobile image intensifier local rules must be implemented and all staff must be provided with protective clothing.

Calcaneum 4

Basic projections

Two projections are routinely taken – a lateral and an axial. Each image is acquired using a CR image detector or alternatively within the field of view of a DDR detector.

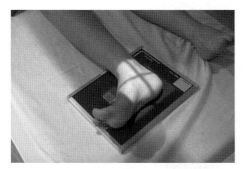

Fig. 4.19a Patient positioning for lateral calcaneum.

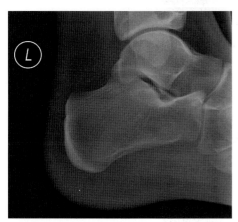

Fig. 4.19b Normal lateral radiograph of calcaneum.

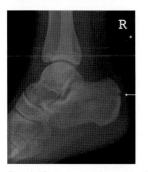

Fig. 4.19c Lateral radiograph of the calcaneum, showing fracture.

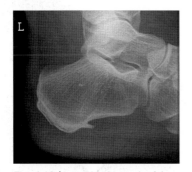

Fig. 4.19d Lateral radiograph of the calcaneum, showing a spur.

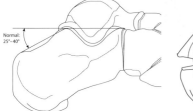
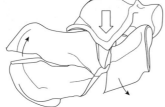

Fig. 4.19e Diagrams to show normal (left) and abnormal (right) Bohler's angle.

Lateral (Basic) (Fig. 4.19a)

Position of patient and image receptor

- From the supine position, the patient rotates on to the affected side.
- The leg is rotated until the medial and lateral malleoli are superimposed vertically.
- A 15° pad is placed under the anterior aspect of the knee and the lateral border of the forefoot for support.
- The receptor is placed with the lower edge just below the plantar aspect of the heel.

Direction and location of the X-ray beam

- The vertical collimated beam is centred 2.5 cm distal to the medial malleolus, with the central ray perpendicular to the receptor.

Essential image characteristics (Figs 4.19b–4.19d)

- The adjacent tarsal bones should be included in the lateral projection, together with the ankle joint.
- This projection is often singularly utilised to demonstrate a calcaneal spur.

Radiological considerations

- The normal juvenile calcaneal apophysis is dense and often appears fragmented. The appearance rarely obscures a fracture and should rarely, if ever, require projections of the contralateral side for assessment.
- The primary trabeculae of bones follow lines of maximum load. In the calcaneum, this results in an apparent lucency in the central area. This should not be mistaken for pathology.
- Fracture of the calcaneum due to heavy landing on the heel causes a compression injury with depression of the central area by the talus. This is seen as flattening of the Bohler's angle to less than 30°, as shown in the diagram (Fig. 4.19e).[3]
- Small spurs or 'tug' lesions at attachments of the Achilles tendon and plantar ligament are common. If significant, they are usually ill-defined and clinically tender. Ultrasound may help in their assessment.
- CT is very useful for the complete evaluation of complex calcaneal fractures, especially utilising the direct coronal plane, multiplanar and three-dimensional reconstructions.

Radiation protection/dose

- Careful technique and close collimation will assist in reducing the patient dose.

Expected DRL: ESD 0.14 mGy.

4 Calcaneum

Axial (Basic) (Figs 4.20a, 4.20b)

Position of patient and image receptor

- The patient sits or lies supine on the X-ray table with both limbs extended.
- The affected leg is rotated medially until both malleoli are equidistant from the receptor.
- The ankle is dorsiflexed.
- The position is maintained by using a bandage strapped around the forefoot and held in position by the patient.
- The receptor (CR) is positioned with its lower edge just distal to the plantar aspect of the heel.

Direction and location of the X-ray beam

- The X-ray tube is directed cranially at an angle of 40° to the plantar aspect of the heel.
- The collimated beam is centred to the plantar aspect of the heel at the level of the tubercle of the 5th metatarsal.

Essential image characteristics (Figs 4.20c–4.20e)

- The subtalar joint and sustentaculum tali should be visible on the axial projection.
- The inferior aspect of the calcaneum and soft-tissue borders should also be demonstrated.

Expected DRL: ESD 0.2 mGy.

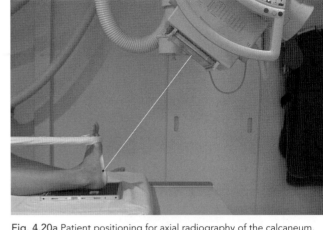

Fig. 4.20a Patient positioning for axial radiography of the calcaneum.

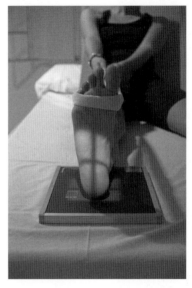

Fig. 4.20b Patient positioning for axial radiography of the calcaneum.

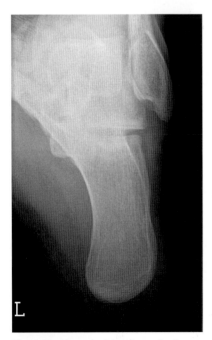

Fig. 4.20c Normal axial radiograph of calcaneum.

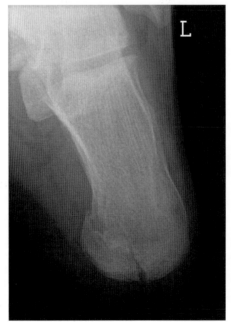

Fig. 4.20d Axial projection of calcaneum, showing a fracture.

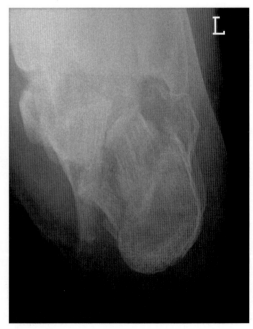

Fig. 4.20e Axial projection of calcaneum showing comminuted fracture.

Subtalar joints 4

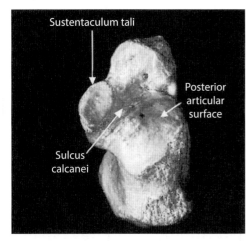

Fig. 4.21a Labelled dry bone calcaneum.

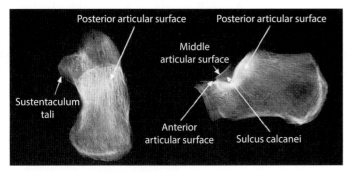

Fig. 4.21b Annotated radiograph of calcaneum, showing articular surfaces.

Recommended projections

Although an increasingly rare examination, plain radiographic imaging still has a role to play in initial diagnosis of conditions such as tarsal coalition, with CT and MRI used to provide further detailed information.[4]

There are three articular surfaces of the subtalar joint: anterior, middle and posterior. The projections undertaken with the articulations demonstrated are shown in the table below, with matching images also given (Figs 4.21a–4.21f).

Projection	Articulation
DP oblique	Anterior articulation
45° oblique – medial with 10° cranial tilt	Posterior articulation from an anterior direction
45° oblique – lateral with 15° cranial tilt	Posterior articulation from a lateral direction
Lateral oblique – 20° caudal tilt	Posterior articulation from a lateral direction

DP, dorsi-plantar.

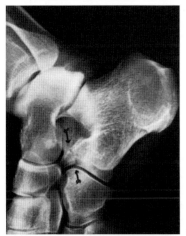

Fig. 4.21c Radiograph of DPO calcaneum, focussed on subtalar region.

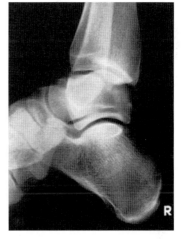

Fig. 4.21e 45°oblique lateral with 15° cranial angulation.

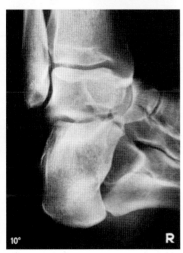

Fig. 4.21d 45°oblique lateral with 10°cranial angulation.

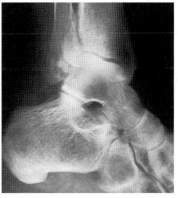

Fig. 4.21f Lateral oblique with 20° caudal angulation.

4 Subtalar joints

Dorsi-plantar oblique (DPO) (Figs 4.22a, 4.22b)

Position of patient and image receptor

- From the basic dorsi-plantar (foot) position, the affected limb is leaned medially, bringing the plantar surface of the foot to approximately 30–45° to the image receptor.

Direction and location of the X-ray beam

- The collimated vertical central beam is centred over the mid-subtalar joint region.
- The beam is collimated to include the ankle joint, calcaneum and tarso-metatarsal joints.

Lateral oblique (Figs 4.22c, 4.22d)

Position of patient and image receptor

- The patient lies on the affected side.
- The opposite limb is flexed and brought in front of the affected limb.
- The affected foot and leg are now further rotated laterally until the plantar aspect of the foot is approximately 45° to the receptor.
- The lower edge of the receptor is positioned just below the plantar aspect of the heel.

Direction and location of the X-ray beam

- The collimated beam is centred to the medial malleolus, with the central ray angled 20° caudally.
- The beam is collimated to include the ankle joint, calcaneum and tarso-metatarsal joints.

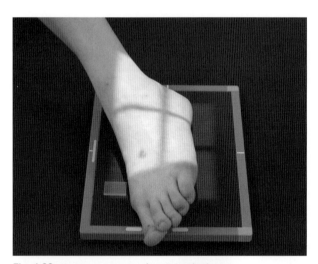

Fig. 4.22a Patient positioning for DPO subtalar joints.

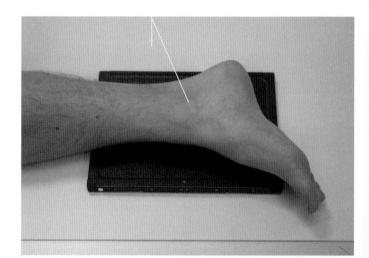

Fig. 4.22c Patient positioning for lateral oblique subtalar joints.

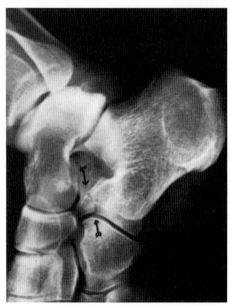

Fig. 4.22b Radiograph of DPO subtalar joints.

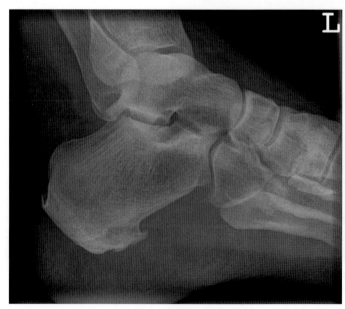

Fig. 4.22d Radiograph of lateral oblique subtalar joints.

Subtalar joints 4

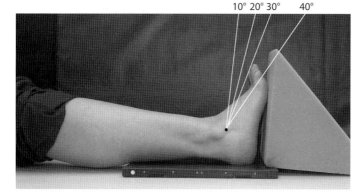

Fig. 4.23a Patient positioning for oblique medial radiography, showing position from lateral aspect with tube angulations.

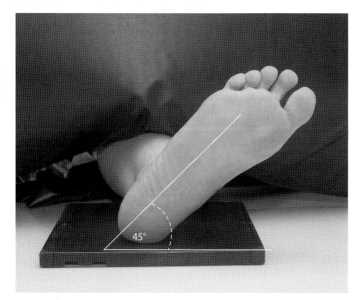

Fig. 4.23b Patient positioning for oblique medial, showing position from plantar aspect of foot.

Oblique medial (Figs 4.23a, 4.23b)

Position of patient and image receptor

- The patient lies supine on the X-ray table, with the affected limb extended.
- The ankle joint is dorsiflexed and the malleoli are equidistant from the receptor.
- The leg is internally rotated through 45°.
- A pad is placed under the knee for support.
- A non-opaque square pad and sandbag may be placed against the plantar aspect of the foot to keep the ankle joint in dorsiflexion.
- The lower edge of the receptor is placed at the level of the plantar aspect of the heel.

Direction and location of the X-ray beam

- The collimated beam is centred 2.5 cm distal to the lateral malleolus with the following cranial angulations (Figs 4.23c–4.23e):

10°	Posterior part of the posterior articulation
20–30°	Middle part of the posterior articulation and the middle articulation
40°	Anterior part of the posterior articulation

- Collimate to include the ankle mortise, calcaneum and proximal 1/3 of the metatarsals.

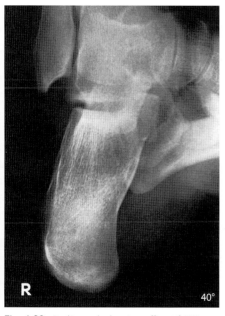

Fig. 4.23c Radiograph showing effect of 40° angulation.

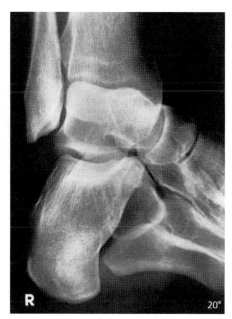

Fig. 4.23d Radiograph showing effect of 20° angulation.

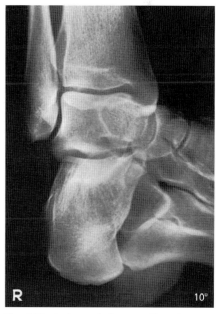

Fig. 4.23e Radiograph showing effect of 10° angulation.

4 Subtalar joints

Oblique lateral (Figs 4.24a–4.24c)

Position of patient and image receptor

- The patient lies supine on the X-ray table, with the affected limb extended.
- The ankle joint is dorsiflexed and the malleoli are equidistant from the receptor.
- The leg is externally rotated through 45°.
- A pad is placed under the knee for support.
- A non-opaque square pad and sandbag may be placed against the plantar aspect of the foot to keep the ankle joint in dorsiflexion.
- The lower edge of the receptor is placed at the level of the plantar aspect of the heel.

Direction and location of the X-ray beam

- The collimated beam is centred 2.5 cm distal to the medial malleolus, with the central ray angled 15° cranially.
- Collimate to include the ankle joint, calcaneum and midtarsal region.

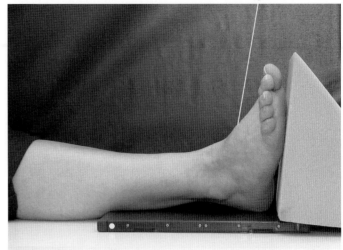

Fig. 4.24a Patient positioning for oblique lateral, lateral aspect with tube angulation.

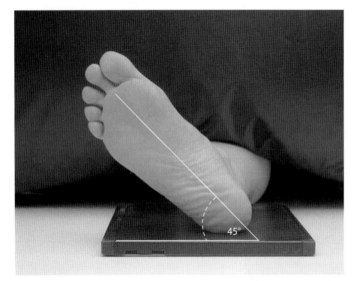

Fig. 4.24b Patient positioning for oblique lateral from plantar aspect, with 45° external rotation.

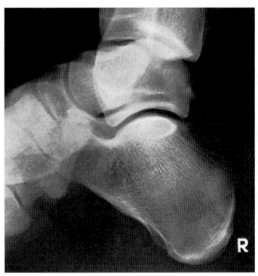

Fig. 4.24c Radiograph of oblique lateral with 15° tube angulation.

Basic projections

Two projections are taken of the full length of the lower leg. The receptor chosen should be large enough to accommodate the entire length of the tibia and fibula. This may require the leg to be positioned diagonally across the receptor to ensure the knee joint and ankle mortise is visualised on the image.

Antero-posterior (Basic) (Fig. 4.25a)

Position of patient and image receptor

- The patient is either supine or seated on the X-ray table, with both legs extended.
- The ankle is supported in dorsiflexion by a firm 90° pad placed against the plantar aspect of the foot.

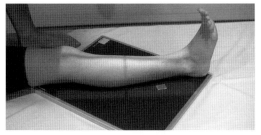

Fig. 4.25a Patient positioning for antero-posterior (AP) tibia/fibula.

Tibia and fibula 4

- The limb is rotated medially until the medial and lateral malleoli are equidistant from the receptor.
- The lower edge of the receptor is positioned just below the plantar aspect of the heel.

Direction and location of the X-ray beam

- The collimated beam is centred to the mid-shaft of the tibia with the central ray at right-angles to both the long axis of the tibia and an imaginary line joining the malleoli.

Expected DRL: ESD 0.15 mGy.

Lateral (Basic) (Fig. 4.25e)

Position of patient and image receptor

- From the supine/seated position, the patient rotates onto the affected side.
- The leg is rotated further until the malleoli are superimposed vertically.
- The tibia should be parallel to the image receptor.
- A pad is placed under the knee for support.
- The lower edge of the receptor is positioned just below the plantar aspect of the heel.

Direction and location of the X-ray beam

- The collimated beam is centred to the mid-shaft of the tibia, with the central ray at right-angles to the long axis of the tibia and parallel to an imaginary line joining the malleoli.

Essential image characteristics (Figs 4.25b–4.25d)

- The knee and ankle joints must be included, since the proximal end of the fibula may also be fractured when there is a fracture of the distal fibula/tibia or widening of the mortise joint (Maisonneuve fracture). If a fracture of one of the tibia/fibula is seen, with overlap or shortening, then the entire length of both bones must be demonstrated (bony ring rule).[5]

Notes

- If it is impossible to include both joints on one image, then two images should be exposed separately, one to include the ankle and the other to include the knee. Both images should include the middle 1/3 of the lower leg, so the general alignment of the bones may be seen.
- If it is impossible for the patient to rotate onto the affected side, then an adapted technique method should be used with the receptor supported vertically against the medial side of the leg and the beam directed horizontally to the mid-shaft of the tibia.

Expected DRL: ESD 0.16 mGy.

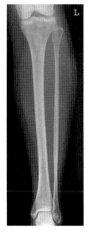

Fig. 4.25b Radiograph of AP tibia/fibula.

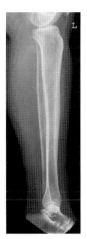

Fig. 4.25c Radiograph of lateral tibia/fibula.

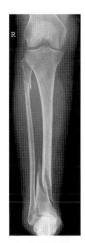

Fig. 4.25d AP radiograph, showing fracture of proximal fibula and distal tibia.

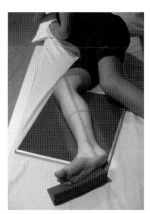

Fig. 4.25e Patient positioning for lateral tibia/fibula.

4 Proximal tibio-fibular joint

Basic projections

Either a lateral oblique or an antero-posterior oblique projection is taken to demonstrate the tibio-fibular articulation.

Lateral oblique (Basic) (Fig. 4.26a)

Position of patient and image receptor

- The patient lies on the affected side (lateral knee position), with the knee slightly flexed.
- The other limb is brought forward in front of the one being examined and supported on a sandbag.
- The head of the fibula and the lateral tibial condyle of the affected side are palpated and the limb rotated laterally to project the joint clear of the tibial condyle (approximately 45° rotation from lateral position).
- The centre of the image receptor is positioned at the level of the head of the fibula.

Direction and location of the X-ray beam

- The collimated vertical beam is centred to the head of the fibula.

Antero-posterior oblique (Basic) (Fig. 4.26c)

Position of patient and image receptor

The patient is either supine or seated on the X-ray table, with both legs extended.

- Palpate the head of fibula and the lateral tibial condyle.
- The limb is rotated medially (approximately 10–20°) to project the tibial condyle clear of the joint.
- The limb is supported by pads and sandbags.
- The centre of the image receptor is positioned at the level of the head of the fibula.

Direction and location of the X-ray beam

- The collimated vertical beam is centred to the head of the fibula.

Essential image characteristics (Figs 4.26b, 4.26d)

The collimated area should include approximately one-quarter of the proximal tibia/fibula and distal femur, with skin margins laterally and medially.

Radiological considerations

- Although these are rarely requested projections, they can be useful in the initial assessment of the proximal tibio-fibula

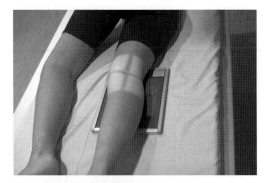

Fig. 4.26a Patient positioning for lateral oblique.

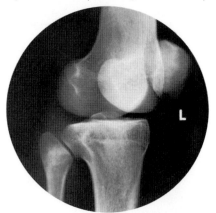

Fig. 4.26b Radiograph of lateral oblique.

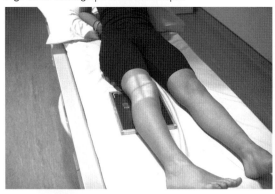

Fig. 4.26c Patient positioning for antero-posterior (AP) oblique.

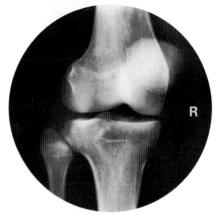

Fig. 4.26d Radiograph of AP oblique.

joint, which can be susceptible to osteoarthritis and occasionally traumatic dislocation/subluxation. However, MRI is becoming increasingly used to evaluate this joint.

Knee joint 4

Radiographic anatomy

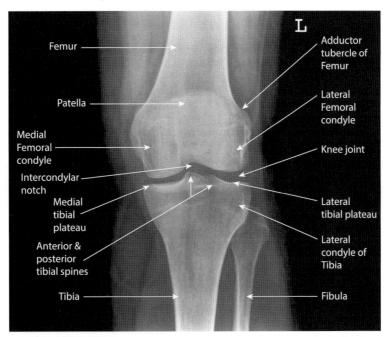

Fig. 4.27a Annotated antero-posterior radiograph of the knee.

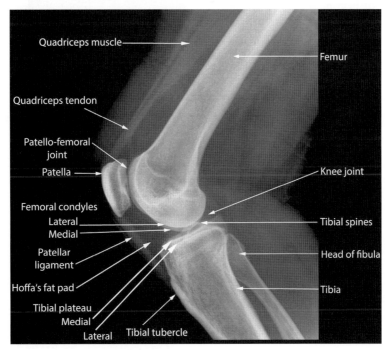

Fig. 4.27b Annotated lateral projection of the knee.

4 Knee joint

Basic projections

Two projections are taken routinely: an antero-posterior (AP) and a lateral. The AP projection is frequently obtained in the weight-bearing/standing position as it provides more meaningful information on the condition of the joint when compared to the traditional (supine) non-weight-bearing technique.[6]

Antero-posterior – weight-bearing (Basic) (Fig. 4.28a)

Position of patient and image receptor

- The patient stands with their back against the vertical Bucky or DDR receptor (grid removed) using it for support if necessary.
- The patient's weight is distributed equally.
- The knee is rotated so that the patella lies equally between the femoral condyles.
- The centre of the image receptor is level with the palpable upper borders of the tibial condyles.
- This projection is useful to demonstrate alignment of the femur and tibia in the investigation of valgus (bow-leg) or varus (knock-knee) deformity. Any such deformity will be accentuated when weight-bearing, which more closely resembles the real-life situation. It is commonly requested to assess alignment prior to joint replacement, as narrowing of one side to the joint space more than the other will produce varus or valgus tilt.

Direction and location of the X-ray beam

- The collimated horizontal beam is centred 1 cm below the apex of the patella through the joint space, with the central ray at 90° to the long axis of the tibia (midway between the palpable upper borders of the tibial condyles).
- Frequently, both knees are requested for comparison, in which case, the beam should be centred at a point midway between both knees at a level 1 cm below both patellas.
- The limb is rotated slightly medially to compensate for the obliquity of the beam when the central ray is centred midway between the knees.

Essential image characteristics (Figs 4.28b–4.28d)

- The patella must be centralised over the femur.
- The image should include the proximal 1/3 of the tibia and fibula and distal 1/3 of the femur.

Notes

- To enable correct assessment of the joint space, the central ray must be at 90° to the long axis of the tibia and, if necessary, angled slightly cranially. If the central ray is not perpendicular to the long axis of the tibia, then the anterior and posterior margins of the tibial plateau will be separated widely and assessment of the true width of the joint space will be difficult.
- If the central ray is too high, then the patella is thrown down over the joint space and the joint space appears narrower.
- If the knee joint is flexed and the patient is unable to extend the limb, then a CR cassette may be raised on pads to bring it as close as possible to the posterior aspect of the knee.
- In the AP projection, the patella is remote from the receptor. Although the relationship of the patella to the surrounding structures can be assessed, the trabecular pattern of the femur is superimposed. Therefore, this projection is not ideal for demonstrating discrete patella bony abnormalities.

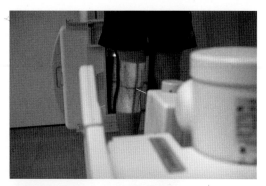

Fig. 4.28a Patient positioning for antero-posterior (AP) knee.

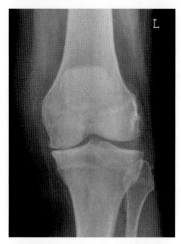

Fig. 4.28b AP radiograph of the knee (weight-bearing) with osteoarthritis.

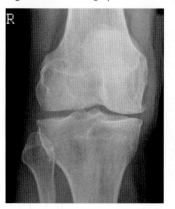

Fig. 4.28c AP radiograph showing effect of internal rotation.

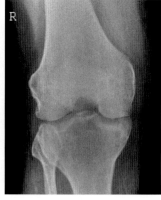

Fig. 4.28d AP radiograph showing effect of flexion of the knee.

Expected DRL: ESD 0.3 mGy.

This projection can be used when the patient is unable to stand and weight-bear, for example in the trauma situation.

Position of patient and image receptor

- The patient is either supine or seated on the X-ray table or trolley, with both legs extended.
- The affected limb is rotated to centralise the patella between the femoral condyles, and sandbags are placed against the ankle to help maintain this position.
- The image receptor, i.e. 18 × 24 CR cassette should be in close contact with the posterior aspect of the knee joint, with its centre level with the upper borders of the tibial condyles.

Direction and location of the X-ray beam

- The vertical collimated central beam is centred 1 cm below the apex of the patella through the joint space, with the central ray at 90° to the long axis of the tibia (midway between the palpable upper borders of the tibial condyles).

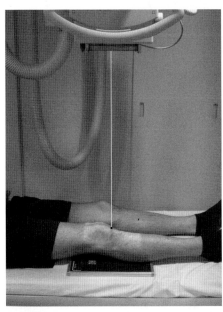

Fig. 4.29a Patient positioning for antero-posterior (AP) supine.

Knee joint 4

Alternative projections

Antero-posterior – supine (Fig. 4.29a)

Essential image characteristics (Figs 4.29b, 4.29c)

- The patella must be centralised over the femur.
- The image should include the proximal 1/3 of the tibia and fibula and distal 1/3 of the femur.

Radiological considerations

- A joint effusion is well-demonstrated on the lateral projection as an ovoid density rising above the postero-superior aspect of the patella. Its significance varies according to the clinical setting. Causes include infection, haemorrhage and arthritis, but it may also be a marker of occult fracture, e.g. tibial spine or tibial plateau fracture. Lipohaemarthrosis occurs when a fracture passes into the marrow-containing medullary space. Fat (bone marrow) leaks into the joint, producing a fluid level between fat and fluid (blood) that can be seen when a horizontal beam is used.
- Fracture of the anterior tibial spine may be subtle, with demonstration requiring attention to exposure and rotation. It is important as the attachment of the anterior cruciate ligament, avulsion of which may cause debilitating instability of the knee.
- Vertical fracture of the patella is not visible on the lateral projection and will be seen on the AP projection only if exposed properly (i.e. not underexposed). If clinically suspected, then a skyline view maybe requested.
- Tibial plateau fractures can be subtle and hard to detect, but again they are functionally very important. Good technique is the key. Full evaluation may be aided by three-dimensional CT.[7]
- The fabella is a sesamoid bone in the tendon of medial head of gastrocnemius, behind the medial femoral condyle, and should not be confused with loose body.
- Osgood–Schlatter's disease is a clinical diagnosis and does not usually require radiography for diagnosis. Ultrasound may be useful if confirmation is required. Projections of the contralateral knee should not normally be needed.

Radiation protection/dose

- Careful technique and close collimation will assist in reducing the patient dose.

Expected DRL: ESD 0.3 mGy.

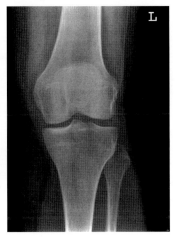

Fig. 4.29b Normal radiograph of AP supine knee.

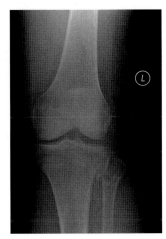

Fig. 4.29c Supine AP radiograph showing depressed tibial plateau fracture.

4 Knee joint

Lateral (Basic) (turned/rolled) (Figs 4.30a, 4.30c)

Position of patient and image receptor

- The patient lies on the side to be examined, with the knee flexed at 45° or 90°.
- The other limb is brought forward in front of the one being examined and supported on a sandbag.
- A pad is placed under the ankle of the affected side to bring the long axis of the tibia parallel to the image receptor. Dorsiflexion of the foot helps maintain this position.
- The position of the limb is now adjusted to ensure that the femoral condyles are superimposed vertically.
- The medial tibial condyle is placed level with the centre of the receptor.
- An alternative method is to keep the unaffected limb behind the knee being examined with the ankle flexed and the heel resting on the lower shaft of the unaffected leg.

Direction and location of the X-ray beam

- The collimated vertical beam is centred to the middle of the superior border of the medial tibial condyle, with the central ray at 90° to the long axis of the tibia.

Essential image characteristics (Fig. 4.30b)

- The patella should be projected clear of the femur.
- The femoral condyles should be superimposed.
- The proximal tibio-fibular joint is not clearly visible. (Approximately 1/3 of the fibula head should be superimposed behind the tibia.)

Notes

- A small cranial tube angulation of 5–7° can help superimpose the femoral condyles, which assists in patients with a wide pelvis and short femoral length.[8]
- If over-rotated, the medial femoral condyle is projected in front of the lateral condyle and the proximal tibio-fibular joint will be well-demonstrated (Fig. 4.30d).
- If under-rotated, the medial femoral condyle is projected behind the lateral condyle and the head of the fibula is superimposed on the tibia (Fig. 4.30e).
- If the central ray is not at 90° to the long axis of the tibia, the femoral condyles will not be superimposed.
- Flexion of the knee at 90° is the most easily reproducible angle and allows assessment of any degree of patella alta or patella baja (patella riding too high or too low). With the knee flexed at 90°, a patella in normal position will lie between two parallel lines drawn along the anterior and posterior surfaces of the femur.

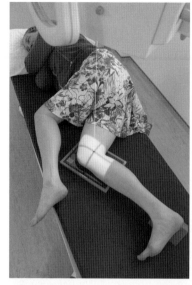

Fig. 4.30a Patient positioning for lateral knee.

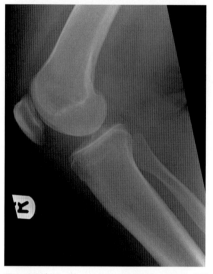

Fig. 4.30b Radiograph of lateral knee with 90° of flexion.

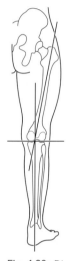

Fig. 4.30c Diagram showing central ray at 90° to tibial length.

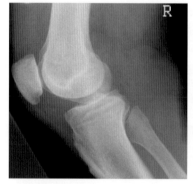

Fig. 4.30d Lateral radiograph showing effect of over-rotation.

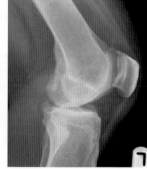

Fig. 4.30e Lateral radiograph showing effect of under-rotation.

- In patients who are unable to flex to 90°, the examination should be performed at 45° flexion. This may permit a clearer view of the patello-femoral articulation.
- This projection may also be acquired in the weight-bearing position against a vertical detector.

Expected DRL - ESD 0.3 mGy

Knee joint 4

Image evaluation – 10-point plan

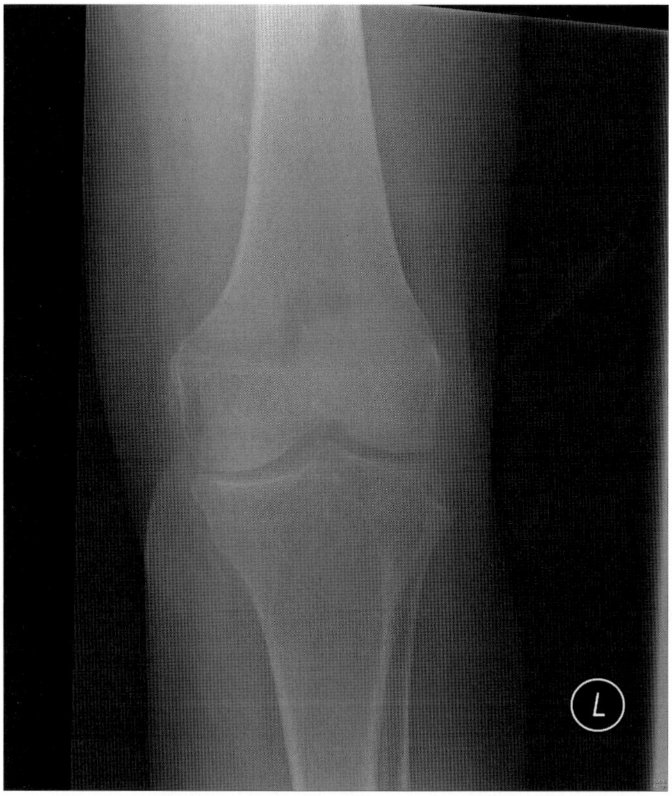

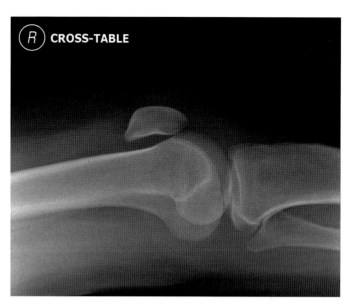

Fig. 4.31a Poor AP knee (externally rotated).

Fig. 4.31b Poor lateral knee (over rotated).

IMAGE EVALUATION

AP knee (Fig. 4.31a)

The main points to consider are:

- The knee is externally rotated and patella is not centralised.
- The fibula head is superimposed on the tibia.
- An electronic marker has been added post examination.
- Repeat required.

Radiographer Comments/Initial report

No fracture seen.

IMAGE EVALUATION

Lateral knee (horizontal beam technique) (Fig. 4.31b)

The main points to consider are:

- The knee is externally rotated and the femoral condyles are not superimposed.
- The centring point is slightly too proximal, as there is too much femur and too little of the tibia visualised.
- Repeat required – with internal rotation of the knee to superimpose the femoral condyles.

Radiographer Comments/Initial report

No fracture or lipohaemarthrosis seen (after satisfactory repeat).

4 Knee joint

Additional projections

Further projections are used to demonstrate fracture of the patella and the intercondylar notch. Stress views may also be taken in suspected ligamental tears.

A lateral projection of the knee and tibial tubercle may be useful in Osgood–Schlatter's disease, although this is primarily a clinical diagnosis and radiography is reserved for exclusion of other pathology in cases of doubt. Ultrasound may also be useful in this clinical situation

Lateral – horizontal beam (trauma) (Fig. 4.32a)

This projection replaces the conventional lateral in all cases of gross injury and suspected fracture of the patella.

Position of patient and image receptor

- The patient remains on the trolley/bed, with the limb gently raised and supported on pads.
- If possible, the leg may be rotated slightly to centralise the patella between the femoral condyles.
- The imaging receptor is supported vertically against the medial aspect of the knee.
- The centre of the receptor is level with the upper border of the tibial condyle.

Direction and location of the X-ray beam

- The collimated horizontal beam is centred to the upper border of the lateral tibial condyle, at 90° to the long axis of the tibia.

Essential image characteristics (Figs 4.32b–4.32d)

- The image should demonstrate the lower 1/3 of the femur and proximal 1/3 of the tibia. The femoral condyles should be superimposed and the soft tissues adequately demonstrated to visualise any fluid levels within the supra-patella pouch.

Notes

- No attempt must be made to either flex or extend the knee joint.
- Additional flexion may result in fragments of a transverse patellar fracture being separated by the opposing muscle pull.
- Any rotation of the limb must be from the hip, with support given to the whole leg.
- By using a horizontal beam, fluid levels may be demonstrated, indicating lipohaemarthrosis (Fig. 4.32b).[9]

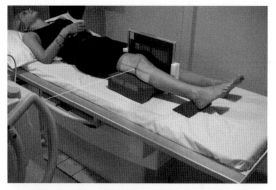

Fig. 4.32a Patient positioning for lateral knee, horizontal beam.

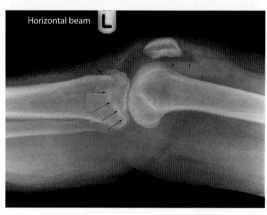

Fig. 4.32b Horizontal beam lateral knee radiograph showing depressed fracture of the tibial plateau (arrows) and lipohaemarthrosis (arrowheads).

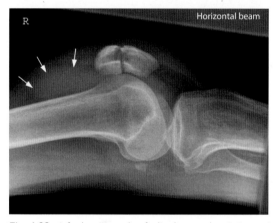

Fig. 4.32c A further example of a lipohaemarthrosis (arrows) caused by a fractured patella.

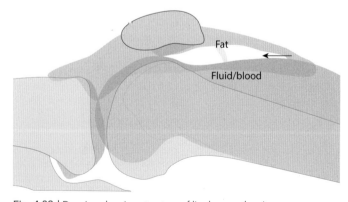

Fig. 4.32d Drawing showing structure of lipohaemarthrosis.

Knee joint 4

Stress projections for subluxation

Stress projections of the knee joint are taken to show subluxation due to rupture of the collateral ligaments. Although these projections may be done in the department using CR or DDR image acquisition, they are now commonly done in theatre using a mobile image intensifier. Stress is applied to the joint by medical personnel, usually an orthopaedic surgeon.

Antero-posterior – stress (Fig. 4.33a)

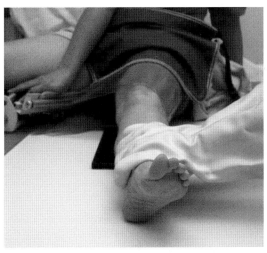

Fig. 4.33a Patient positioning for antero-posterior (AP) stress radiography of knee.

Position of patient and image receptor

- The patient and receptor are positioned for the routine antero-posterior (AP) projection.
- The doctor forcibly abducts or adducts the knee, without rotating the leg.

Direction and location of the X-ray beam

- The collimated vertical beam is centred midway between the upper borders of the tibial condyles, with the central ray at 90° to the long axis of the tibia.

Essential image characteristics (Figs 4.33b, 4.33c)

- The image should demonstrate the joint space clearly and the amount of any widening of the joint if present.

Radiation protection/dose

- The doctor applying the stress should wear a protective apron including lead gloves; discussion between the doctor and radiographer to decide how the examination will proceed may help minimise repeats and/or fluoroscopy time.
- Careful technique and close collimation will assist in reducing the patient dose.

Expected DRL: ESD 0.3 mGy.

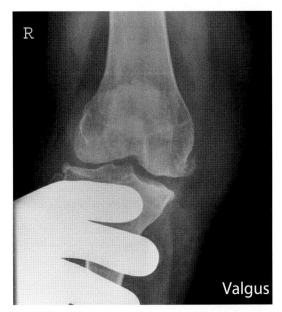

Fig. 4.33b Radiograph of AP knee with valgus stress.

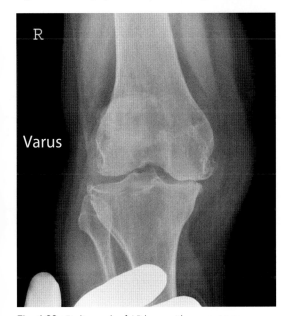

Fig. 4.33c Radiograph of AP knee with varus stress.

4 Knee joint

Patella (postero-anterior, PA) (Fig. 4.34a)

Additional projections may be necessary to demonstrate the patella adequately.

Position of patient and image receptor

- The patient lies prone on the table, with the knee slightly flexed.
- Foam pads are placed under the ankle and thigh for support.
- The limb is rotated to centralise the patella.
- The centre of the receptor is level with the crease of the knee.

Direction and location of the X-ray beam

- The collimated vertical beam is centred midway between the upper borders of the tibial condyles at the level of the crease of the knee, with the central ray at 90° to the long axis of the tibia.

Essential image characteristics (Figs 4.34b, 4.34c)

- The patella should be seen centralised over the middle of the distal femur and adequately exposed to demonstrate the bony detail.
- Approximately 1/3 of the distal femur and upper 1/3 of the tibia should be included.

Notes

- The beam may have to be angled caudally to be at right-angles to the long axis of the tibia.
- The patella may be demonstrated more clearly as it is now adjacent to the image receptor and not distant from it, as in the conventional antero-posterior projection.
- Subtle abnormalities may not be detected, as the trabecular pattern of the femur will still predominate.
- This projection depends on the fitness of the patient and must not be attempted if it results in undue discomfort or if it may exacerbate the patient's condition.
- An alternative standing PA projection could be considered if the patient is unable to tolerate lying prone on the table.

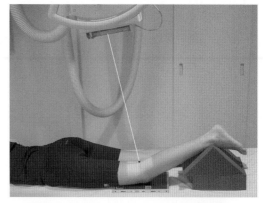

Fig. 4.34a Patient positioning for patellar projection.

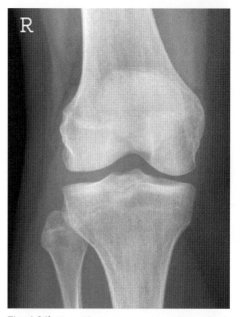

Fig. 4.34b Normal postero-anterior radiograph of patella.

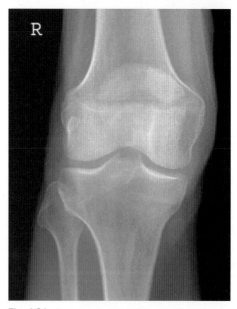

Fig. 4.34c Postero-anterior radiograph of patella, showing a transverse fracture.

Knee joint 4

Skyline projections

The skyline projection can be used to:

- Assess the retro-patellar joint space for degenerative disease.
- Determine the degree of any lateral subluxation of the patella with ligament laxity.
- Diagnose chondromalacia patellae.
- Confirm the presence of a vertical patella fracture in acute trauma.

The optimum retro-patellar joint spacing occurs when the knee is flexed approximately 30–45°. Further flexion pulls the patella into the intercondylar notch, reducing the joint spacing; as flexion increases, the patella tracks over the lateral femoral condyle. The patella moves a distance of 2 cm from full extension to full flexion.

There are three methods of achieving the skyline projection:

- Supero-inferior – beam directed downwards.
- Conventional infero-superior.
- Infero-superior – patient prone.

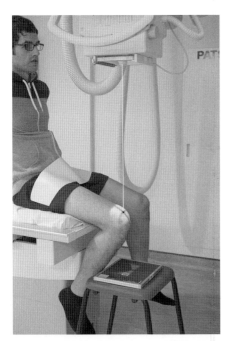

Fig. 4.35a Patient positioning for supero-inferior skyline projection.

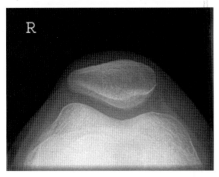

Fig. 4.35b Normal skyline radiograph of knee.

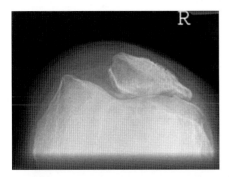

Fig. 4.35c Supero-inferior image showing advanced degenerative changes; the knee has been flexed too much, giving the appearance of lateral subluxation.

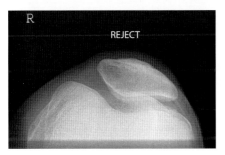

Fig. 4.35d Radiograph with too little flexion, causing the tibia to be projected over the patella.

Supero-inferior (Fig. 4.35a)

This projection has the advantage that the radiation beam is not directed towards the gonads.

Position of patient and image receptor

- The patient sits on the X-ray table, with the affected knee flexed over the side.
- Ideally, the leg should be flexed to 45° to reflect a similar knee position to the conventional skyline projection. Too much flexion reduces the retro-patellar spacing. Sitting the patient on a cushion helps to achieve the optimum position.
- The receptor is supported horizontally on a stool at the level of the inferior tibial tuberosity border.
- This method describes the use of CR equipment; however this could be adapted to be used with DDR equipment, using the erect detector placed in a horizontal position with the patient sat on a chair with the knee overhanging the detector as described above.

Direction and location of the X-ray beam

- The collimated vertical central beam is centred over the posterior aspect of the proximal border of the patella. The central ray should be parallel to the long axis of the patella.
- The beam is collimated to the patella and femoral condyles.

Essential image characteristics (Figs 4.35b, 4.35c)

- The retro-patellar space should be clearly seen without superimposition of the femur or tibia within the patella-femoral joint.

4 Knee joint

Skyline projections (cont.)

Infero-superior (Figs 4.36a–4.36d)

This procedure is undertaken using an 18 × 24 cm CR cassette.

Position of patient and image receptor

- The patient sits on the X-ray table, with the knee flexed 30–45° and supported on a pad placed below the knee.
- The image receptor is held by the patient against the anterior distal femur and supported using a non-opaque pad, which rests on the anterior aspect of the thigh.

Direction and location of the X-ray beam

- The X-ray tube is lowered into the horizontal orientation. Avoiding the feet, the central ray is directed cranially to pass through the apex of the patella parallel to the long axis. This may require a 5–10° cranial angle from horizontal.
- The beam should be closely collimated to the patella and femoral condyles to limit scattered radiation to the trunk and head.

Radiation protection/dose

- Examination of the individual single knee is recommended, rather than including both knees in one exposure when both knees are requested. This reduces the effect of the diverging beam affecting the joint space when both knees are imaged together.
- The total radiation field can be reduced, thus limiting the scattered radiation.
- A lead-rubber apron is worn for protection, with additional lead-rubber protection placed over the gonads.
- For the supero-inferior projection, radiation protection should be provided to the gonads, and the patient should lean backwards, away from the primary beam.

Notes

- Not enough flexion will cause the tibial tuberosity to overshadow the retro-patellar joint (see Fig. 4.35d).
- Too much flexion will cause the patella to track over the lateral femoral condyle.

Expected DRL: ESD 0.28 mGy.

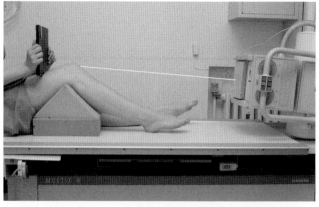

Fig. 4.36a Patient positioning for infero-superior radiograph of the knee.

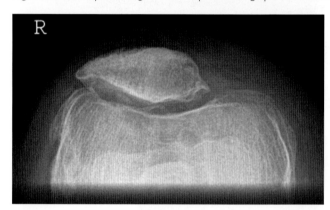

Fig. 4.36b Infero-superior radiograph demonstrating good position, showing osteophytosis affecting the retro-patellar joint.

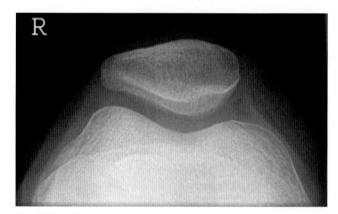

Fig. 4.36c Infero-superior projection, 30° flexion.

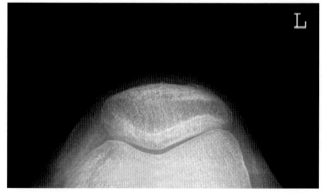

Fig. 4.36d Infero-superior projection, 60° flexion.

Knee joint 4

Patella – infero-superior (patient prone) (Figs 4.37a, 4.37b)

This projection has the advantage in that the primary beam is not directed towards the gonads, as is the case with the conventional infero-superior projection. However, the patient has to be able to adopt the prone position, which may not be suitable for all patients.

Position of patient and image receptor

- The patient lies prone on the X-ray table, with the image receptor placed under the knee joint and the knee flexed through 90°.
- A bandage placed around the ankle and either tethered to a vertical support or held by the patient may prevent unnecessary movement.
- The patient flexes the knee a further 5°, to remove any chance of superimposition of the tibia or foot on the patella-femoral joint space.

Direction and location of the X-ray beam

- The collimated vertical beam is centred behind the patella, with the vertical central ray angled approximately 15° towards the knee, avoiding the toes.

Essential image characteristics (Figs 4.37c, 4.37d)

- The patella-femoral joint space should be clearly seen.

Notes

- All of the skyline projections can be obtained with various degrees of flexion, usually 30° or 60°.

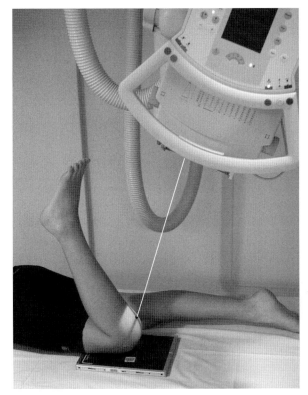

Fig. 4.37a Patient positioning for infero-superior prone projection.

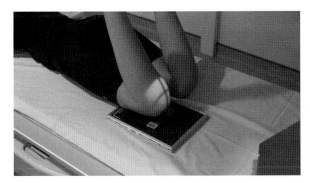

Fig. 4.37b Patient positioning for infero-superior prone projection, close-up.

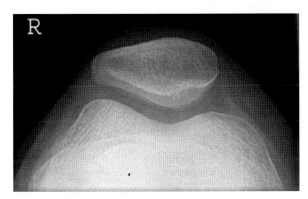

Fig. 4.37c Normal infero-posterior radiograph of patella – patient prone.

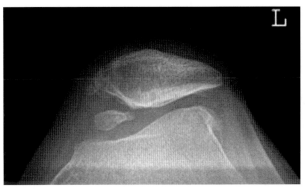

Fig. 4.37d Skyline image of knee showing degenerative changes and bony fragment.

4 Knee joint

Postero-anterior oblique (Figs 4.38a, 4.38d)

Each image is acquired using an 18 × 24 cm CR cassette or alternatively within the field of view of a DDR detector.

Position of patient and image receptor

- The patient lies prone on the X-ray table.
- The trunk is then rotated onto each side in turn to bring either the medial or the lateral aspect of the knee at an angle of approximately 45° to the image receptor.
- The knee is then flexed slightly.
- A sandbag is placed under the ankle for support.
- The centre of the image receptor is level with the uppermost tibial condyle.

Direction and location of the X-ray beam

- The collimated vertical beam is centred to the uppermost tibial condyle.

Antero-posterior oblique (Fig. 4.38e)

Position of patient and image receptor

- The patient lies supine on the X-ray table.
- The trunk is then rotated to allow rotation of the affected limb either medially or laterally through 45°.
- The knee is flexed slightly.
- A sandbag is placed under the ankle for support.
- The centre of the image receptor is level with the upper border of the uppermost tibial condyle.

Direction and location of the X-ray beam)

- The collimated vertical beam is centred to the middle of the uppermost tibial condyle.

Essential image characteristics (Figs 4.38b, 4.38c)

- The upper 1/3 of the tibia and lower 1/3 of the femur should be seen, with visualisation of the tibial spines and each half of the patella on each image clear of the femur.

Notes

- These projections may be taken in addition to the basic images to show each half of the patella clear of the femur.
- The choice of either postero-anterior oblique or antero-posterior oblique is dependent upon the condition of the patient. The postero-anterior projection will give a better quality image by placing the patella in closer proximity to the image receptor.

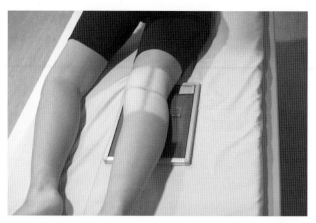

Fig. 4.38a Patient positioning for postero-anterior (PA) oblique, medial rotation.

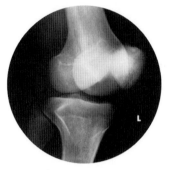 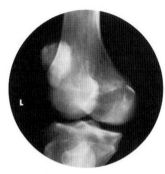

Fig. 4.38b Normal radiograph of PA oblique, medial rotation.

Fig. 4.38c Normal radiograph of PA oblique, lateral rotation.

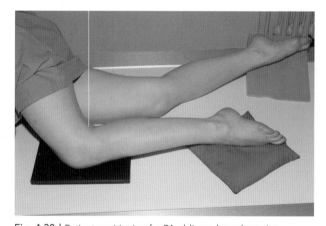

Fig. 4.38d Patient positioning for PA oblique, lateral rotation.

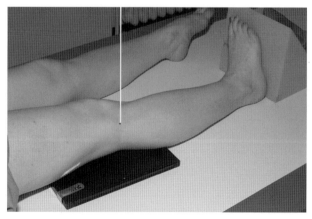

Fig. 4.38e Patient positioning for antero-posterior oblique, medial rotation.

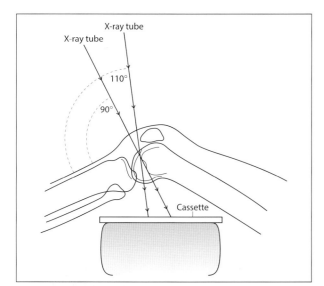

Fig. 4.39a Patient positioning for intercondylar notch projection.

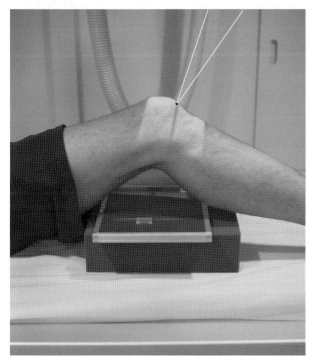

Fig. 4.39b Patient positioning for intercondylar notch projection.

Knee joint 4

Intercondylar notch (tunnel) – antero-posterior (Figs 4.39a, 4.39b)

This projection is taken to demonstrate loose bodies within the knee joint. This method is applicable to use with a small 18 × 24 cm CR receptor, which must fit behind the knee.

Position of patient and image receptor

- The patient is either supine or seated on the X-ray table, with the affected knee flexed to approximately 60°.
- A suitable pad is placed under the knee to help maintain the position.
- The limb is rotated to centralise the patella over the femur.
- The image receptor is placed on top of the pad as close as possible to the posterior aspect of the knee and displaced towards the femur.

Direction and location of the X-ray beam

- The collimated beam is centred immediately below the apex of the patella, with the following tube angulations to demonstrate either the anterior or posterior aspects of the notch:

Angulation to the long axis of the tibia	Anatomy demonstrated
110°	Anterior aspect of the notch
90°	Posterior aspect of the notch

Essential image characteristics (Figs 4.39c, 4.39d)

- The lower femur and upper tibia are demonstrated, with the intercondylar notch clearly seen.
- Commonly only the 90° angulation is used.
- This projection may be requested occasionally to demonstrate a fracture of the tibial spines, where cruciate ligaments are attached. Care must be taken when flexing the knee.

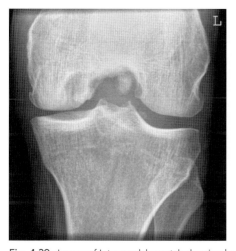

Fig. 4.39c Image of Intercondylar notch showing loose body.

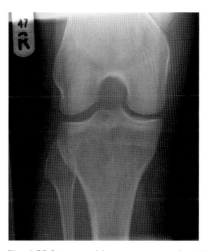

Fig. 4.39d Intercondylar image acquired at 90°.

4 Knee joint

Intercondylar notch (tunnel) – posterior–anterior ('racing start') (Figs 4.40a, 4.40b)

The advantage of this method is the reduction in magnification and increased resolution.

The image is acquired using an 18 × 24 cm CR cassette or alternatively within the field of view of a DDR detector.

Position of patient and image receptor

- The patient is placed prone on the X-ray table and sits up onto their knees with hands forwards supporting their weight (i.e. patient is 'on all fours').
- The affected lower leg is extended with the tibia parallel to the tabletop and the patient is asked to lean forwards, moving the femur into an angle of 50° from the tabletop. (The angle formed behind the knee joint between the inner thigh and lower leg is 130°.)
- The unaffected knee is moved anteriorly, thus supporting the patient. The patient is asked to support body weight on unaffected knee. The position of the patient now simulates that of a sprinter ready to start a race.
- The receptor is placed directly against the anterior aspect of the knee joint.

Direction and location of the X-ray beam

- The collimated vertical beam is centred to the middle of the knee joint/popliteal fossa (approximately over the skin crease posterior to the joint).

Essential image characteristics

- The lower femur and upper tibia are demonstrated, with the intercondylar notch clearly seen.

Note

- This method is only suitable for fairly fit patients who are able to climb onto the table and hold the position safely.

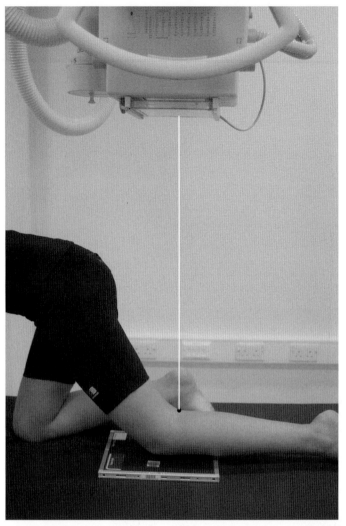

Fig. 4.40a Patient positioning for 'racing start' projection.

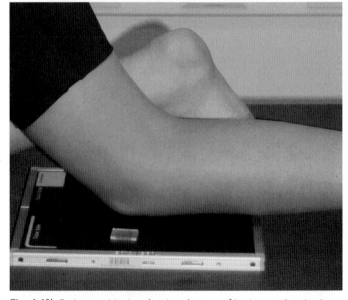

Fig. 4.40b Patient positioning showing close-up of 'racing start' projection.

Femur – shaft 4

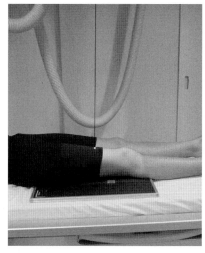

Fig. 4.41a Patient positioning for antero-posterior (AP) femur; CR cassette directly under femur.

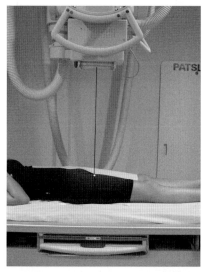

Fig. 4.41b Patient positioning for AP femur using table Bucky and DDR.

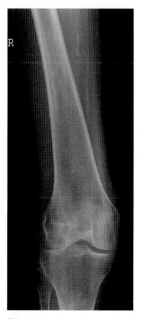

Fig. 4.41c AP radiograph of normal femur, knee up.

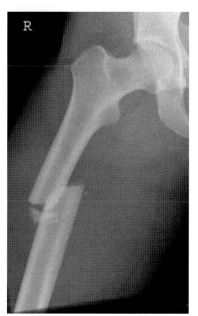

Fig. 4.41d AP radiograph of femur, hip down, showing fracture of upper femoral shaft.

Basic projections

Two projections are taken routinely, preferably with both the knee and hip joints included on the image. The images are acquired using a large 35 × 43 cm CR cassette or alternatively within the field of view of a DDR detector. If this is impossible to achieve, then the joint nearest the site of injury should be included.

A grid may be used so that the effects of scatter are reduced. However, should only an image of the distal aspect of the femur be required, ('knee up' AP) then the use of the grid can be eliminated in order to reduce patient dose.

The choice of whether a grid is employed is influenced by patient size and local protocols.

Antero-posterior (Basic) (Figs 4.41a, 4.41b)

Position of patient and image receptor

- The patient lies supine on the X-ray table, with both legs extended and the affected limb positioned to the centre line of the table.
- The affected limb is rotated to centralise the patella over the femur.
- Sandbags are placed below the knee to help maintain the position.
- The image receptor/Bucky mechanism is located directly under the posterior aspect of the thigh to include both the hip and the knee joints.
- Alternatively, a CR cassette or mobile DDR detector is positioned directly under the limb, against the posterior aspect of the thigh to include the knee and hip joints.

Direction and location of the X-ray beam

- The collimated vertical beam is centred to the mid-shaft of the femur, with the central ray at 90° to an imaginary line joining both femoral condyles.

Essential image characteristics (Figs 4.41c, 4.41d)

- Ideally, the length of the femur should be visualised, including the hip and knee joints. This may be difficult to obtain and an additional projection of the knee or hip joint may be required if coverage is not initially achieved; however, this will depend on the clinical information required.
- The patella should be centralised to indicate rotation has been minimised.

Expected DRL: ESD 1.42 mGy.

4 Femur – shaft

Lateral (Basic) (Fig. 4.42a)

Position of patient and image receptor

- From the antero-posterior position, the patient rotates on to the affected side with the knee is slightly flexed and the patient adjusted so that the thigh is positioned to the centre line of the table.
- The pelvis is rotated backwards to separate the thighs.
- The position of the limb is then adjusted to superimpose the femoral condyles vertically.
- Pads are used to support the opposite limb behind the one being examined.
- The image receptor/Bucky mechanism is located directly under the lateral aspect of the thigh to include the knee joint and as much of the femur as possible.
- Alternatively, a CR cassette or mobile DDR detector is positioned directly under the thigh to include the knee and hip joints

Direction and location of the X-ray beam

- The collimated vertical beam is centred to the middle of the femoral shaft, with the central ray parallel to the imaginary line joining the femoral condyles.

Essential image characteristics (Figs 4.42b, 4.42c)

- The length of the femur should be visualised, including the hip and knee joints.
- Often, an additional projection of the hip joint using a grid, may be required if coverage is not initially achieved or the image quality is affected by scatter and/or noise in the proximal femur; however, this will depend on the clinical information required and the patient size.

Notes

- In cases of suspected fracture, the limb must not be rotated.
- If both joints are not included on one image, then a single antero-posterior projection of the joint distal to the fracture site must be taken. This ensures that no fracture is missed and allows assessment of any rotation at the fracture site.
- Remember that the divergent beam will project the hip cranially and the knee caudally, and therefore care must be taken when positioning the patient and detector to ensure that the joint will be on the top/bottom of the image.

Radiation protection/dose

- Careful technique and close collimation will assist in reducing the patient dose.

Expected DRL: ESD 1.42 mGy.

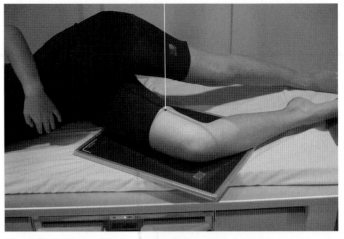

Fig. 4.42a Patient positioning for lateral femur.

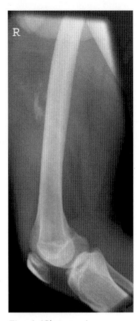

Fig. 4.42b Lateral radiograph of femur, knee up, showing an area of myositis ossificans.

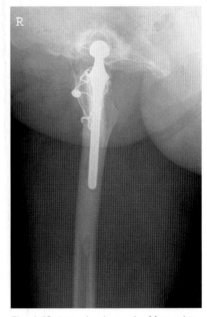

Fig. 4.42c Lateral radiograph of femur, hip down, showing a prosthetic hip.

Femur – shaft 4

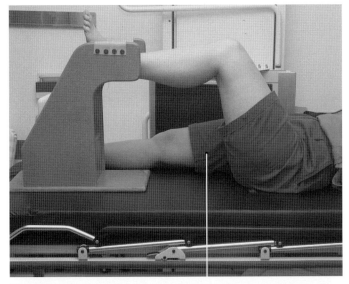

Fig. 4.43a Patient positioning for lateral horizontal beam projection.

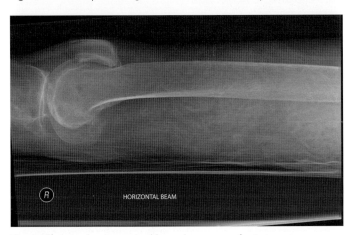

Fig. 4.43b Lateral radiograph of femur, knee up; no fracture seen.

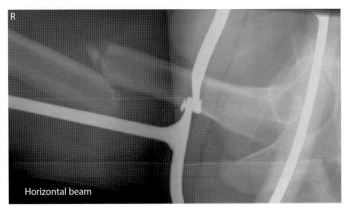

Fig. 4.43c Lateral radiograph of femur, hip down, showing a fracture of the upper femoral shaft.

Additional projection – lateral horizontal beam (Fig. 4.43a)

This projection replaces the basic lateral in all cases of gross injury and suspected fracture.

The images are acquired using a large 35 × 43 cm CR cassette or alternatively within the field of view of a DDR detector.

Position of patient and image receptor

- The patient remains on the trolley/bed. If possible, the leg may be slightly rotated to centralise the patella between the femoral condyles.
- The vertical image receptor is positioned against the lateral aspect of the thigh, with the lower border of the receptor level with the upper border of the tibial condyle.
- The unaffected limb is raised above the injured limb, with the knee flexed and the lower leg supported on a stool or specialised support.

Direction and location of the X-ray beam

- The collimated horizontal beam is directed to the mid shaft of the femur, to include as much of the proximal shaft as possible.

Essential image characteristics

- The knee joint and distal 2/3 of the femur should be included.
- The knee should be in a true lateral position, with broad superimposition of the femoral condyles.

Notes

- If the whole of the femur is required but not achieved, then a horizontal beam lateral of the neck of femur is often necessary to complete the examination. The need for this is determined by the clinical requirements in each case and should be carefully considered taking into account the increased patient dose (Fig. 4.43c).
- If the injury involves only the lower 2/3 of femur, consider placing a CR cassette vertically against the medial aspect of the thigh, directing the beam from the lateral aspect of the limb to the middle of the receptor (Fig. 4.43b).

Radiation protection/dose

- In all cases, the beam must be well collimated.
- Gonad protection must be applied in all non-trauma cases, as extra-focal radiation and scattered radiation will irradiate the gonads if not protected.
- In trauma cases, gonad protection is not used in the first instance as it may obscure injury. In subsequent follow-up radiographs, gonad protection must be used.

4 Femur – shaft

Image evaluation – 10-point plan

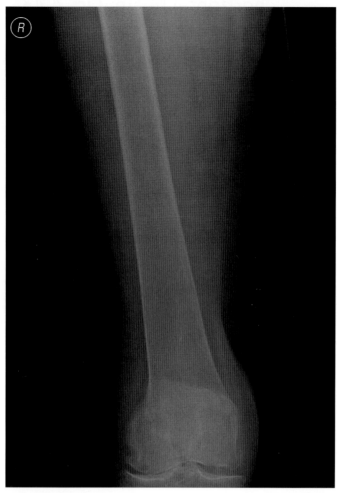

Fig. 4.44a AP femur.

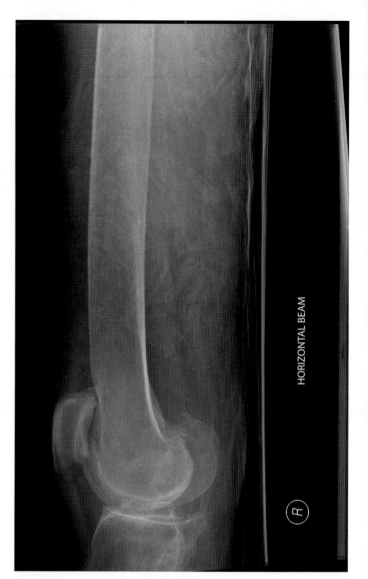

Fig. 4.44b Lateral femur.

IMAGE EVALUATION

AP femur (Fig. 4.44a)

The main points to consider are:

- The proximal femur has not been included.
- The correct marker has been applied, but electronically afterwards.
- The patella is centralised, indicating no evidence of rotation.
- An additional AP hip down projection would be required.

Radiographer comments/initial report

No fracture seen.

IMAGE EVALUATION

Lateral femur (Fig. 4.44b)

The main points to consider are:

- The proximal femur has not been included.
- There are numerous clothing artefacts, which are distracting and may disguise pathologies.
- The femoral condyles are not superimposed, indicating some rotation.
- The artefacts are significant and would require a repeat in most circumstances.
- A hip down lateral would be required to complete the full femur examination.

Radiographer comments/initial report

No fracture or Lipohaemarthrosis seen.

Composite images, seen as one single image demonstrating both lower limbs from hips to ankle joints, will enable comparison of individual leg alignment. This is undertaken for a variety of reasons, but predominately in adults before and after artificial joint replacement, and in children for bow-legs and knock-knees. The technique for children is described in the paediatric chapter (see page 467).

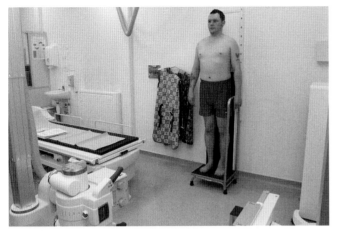

Fig. 4.45a Patient positioning for radiography for leg alignment.

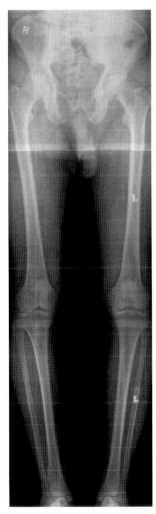

Fig. 4.45b Preoperative CR radiograph to show limb alignment.

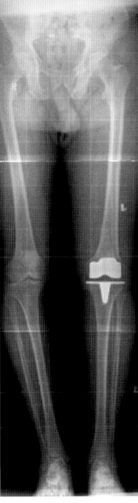

Fig. 4.45c Limb alignment on CR radiograph following total knee replacement (same patient as adjacent image).

Leg alignment

In adults, this technique is undertaken with the patient erect and therefore weight-bearing, and is described below for both digital CR and DDR.

CR method (Figs 4.45a–4.45c)

A tailored made three-cassette-holding device is secured in a vertical position to allow horizontal beam radiography using a large focus-to-receptor distance (FRD). Using this method, three individual images of the lower limbs are acquired using one exposure. These are then 'stitched together' electronically using a special imaging software package.

Position of patient and image receptor

- The patient stands on a low step, with the posterior aspect of their legs against the cassette holder. The arms are extended and supported by the side of the trunk. The anterior superior iliac spines should be equidistant from the receptors to ensure that there is no rotation. The medial sagittal plane should be vertical and coincident with the central longitudinal axis of the receptor.
- The legs should be, as far as possible, in a similar relationship to the pelvis, with the feet separated so that the distance between the ankle joints is similar to the distance between the hip joints and with the patella of each knee facing forward.
- Ideally, the knees and ankle joints should be in the anteroposterior (AP) position. However, if this impossible to achieve, it is more important that the knees, usually the subject for surgery, rather than the ankle joints are placed in the AP position.
- Foam pads and sandbags are used to stabilise the legs and maintain the position. If necessary, a block may be positioned below a shortened leg to ensure that there is no pelvic tilt and that the limbs are aligned adequately.
- The height of the cassette holder is adjusted to include the target area.

Direction and location of the X-ray beam

- The collimated horizontal central ray is directed towards a point midway between the knee joints.
- The X-ray beam is collimated to include both lower limbs from hip joints to ankle joints and inside the target field.

Notes

- A grid is selected dependant on the size of the patient.
- A large FRD is selected, i.e. 180–203 cm according to the manufacturer's recommendations.

4 Leg alignment

DDR method (Figs 4.45a–4.45c)

Image acquisition is achieved by automatic movement of the detector into two or three positions with corresponding tilting of the X-ray tube assembly.

Positioning of patient and image receptor

Positioning is similar to that described for the CR method but with the patient erect and facing the X-ray tube on the dedicated patient stand. The vertical Perspex support is positioned immediately in front of the DDR detector with sufficient distance to allow it to travel vertically without being impeded.

Direction and location of the X-ray beam

- For DDR systems using movement of the X-ray tube and DDR detector to acquire a full imaging set, with multiple exposures, the systems used vary: some manufacturers require selection of start and finishing locations while others require the collimated beam to be centred over the trunk to include the full extent of the spinal region selected. The extent of the start and finishing locations or collimation selected dictates the number of exposures taken.
- A large FRD is selected consistent with the manufacturer's recommendation.

Notes

- A vertical radiopaque ruler extending the full length of the vertical Perspex platform support may be used with some systems to aid in the electronic stitching process.
- Accurate orthopaedic measurements are facilitated by entering into the system the table-to-object distance (TOD) or source-to-object distance (SOD) used.

Essential image characteristics

Using the CR method, following exposure the cassettes are carefully identified and presented for image reading, after which post processing of the images is undertaken to correct for differences in anatomical thicknesses. The three images are then 'stitched' together following the manufacturer's protocol to produce one full-length image. This final image is correctly windowed and annotated.

Using DDR the images are presented already stitched with the opportunity to make final adjustments.

An assessment of leg alignment can then be undertaken using various post-processing tools. One technique involves drawing a line along the femur from mid-femoral head to mid-femoral condyles and a line along the length of the tibia from mid-ankle joint to mid-knee joint, which is then extended. The angle intersecting the femoral line to a continuation of the tibial line is then measured. This angle should normally be less than 3°. Alternatively, a line (the mechanical axis) can be drawn from the mid-femoral head to midpoint of the ankle; this should pass through the centre of the knee. Deflexion of the mechanical axis can be measured and the angle derived from $(m/3 +1)$ degrees, where m is the deflection measured in millimetres.[10,11]

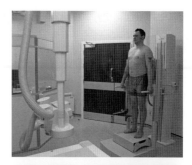
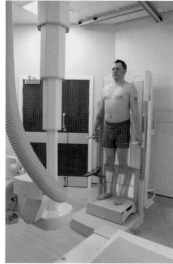

Fig. 4.45a and b DDR image acquisition with first image (top) and final image position.

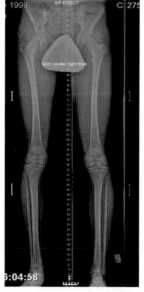

Fig. 4.45c 15-year-old boy with leg length discrepancy. Antero-posterior erect, both legs. Ruler and gonad protection in situ.

Radiological considerations

- The image must demonstrate the endpoints of the mechanical axis clearly, i.e. all three joints (hip, knee and ankle) must be exposed to gain optimum detail and contrast to assess the joints.
- Both legs must be in correct neutral anatomical position, with the patella facing forward and symmetrical.

Section 5
Hips, Pelvis and Sacro-iliac Joints

CONTENTS

RECOMMENDED PROJECTIONS	170
ANATOMY AND IMAGE APPEARANCES	171
Radiological anatomy	171
Introduction	173
EFFECT OF ROTATION AND ABDUCTION OF THE LOWER LIMB	175
HIP JOINT, UPPER THIRD OF FEMUR AND PELVIS	176
Antero-posterior – pelvis (Basic)	176
Antero-posterior – both hips (Basic)	176
HIP JOINT AND UPPER THIRD OF FEMUR	178
Antero-posterior – single hip (Basic)	178
Posterior oblique (Lauenstein's projection)	179
True lateral – neck of femur (Basic)	180
Lateral – air-gap technique	181
Lateral – single hip (alternative projection) – modified	182
Lateral – both hips ('frog's legs position')	183

ACETABULUM AND HIP JOINT	184
Anterior oblique ('Judet's' projection)	184
Posterior oblique (reverse Judet's projection)	184
PELVIS	185
Ilium	185
Posterior oblique – basic projection	185
Posterior oblique (alternative)	185
Lateral	186
Symphysis pubis	187
Postero-anterior – erect	187
SACRO-ILIAC JOINTS	188
Postero-anterior	188
Antero-posterior	189
Antero-posterior oblique	190
HIPS, PELVIS AND SACRO-ILIAC JOINTS	191
Image evaluation – 10-point plan	191

5 Recommended projections

Hip joints	Fracture proximal end of femur	AP – both hips (basic) Lateral neck of femur (basic) Lateral – single hip – air-gap technique (alternative 1 projection) Lateral – modified HB (alternative 2 projection)
	Dislocation	AP – both hips (basic) AP – single hip (post reduction) Lateral neck of femur (basic)
	Fractured acetabulum	AP (full pelvis)– both hips HB lateral hip (basic) Posterior oblique/anterior oblique (Judet's projections)
	Other pathology	AP (full pelvis) – both hips (basic) Other projections on request
	Paediatric disorders: • Development dysplasia (DDH/CHD) • Irritable hips • Postoperative for slipped upper femoral epiphysis • Trauma	See Section 13 Paediatric Radiography
Pelvis	Fractures and pathology	AP – both hips (basic) Posterior oblique (basic), Lauenstein's Posterior oblique (alternative) Lateral (FB demonstration)
	Subluxation of the symphysis pubis	PA – erect
Sacro-iliac joints	Pathology	PA (basic) with caudal angulation AP Posterior oblique on request

AP, antero-posterior; CHD, congenital hip dysplasia; DDH, developmental dysplasia of the hip; FB, foreign body; HB, horizontal beam; PA, postero-anterior.

Anatomy and image appearances 5

Radiological anatomy

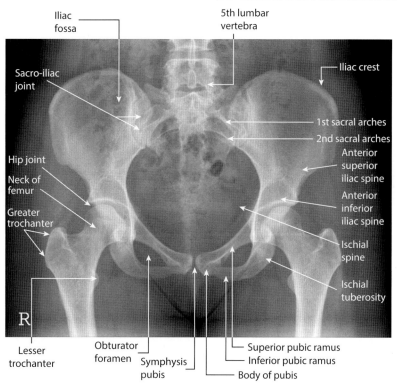

Fig. 5.3a Labelled antero-posterior radiograph of the female pelvis.

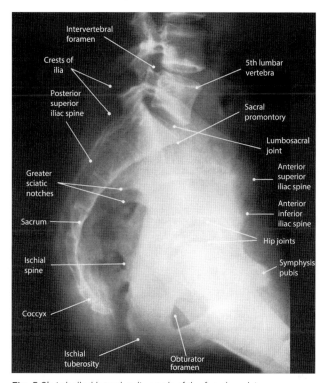

Fig. 5.3b Labelled lateral radiograph of the female pelvis.

5 Anatomy and image appearances

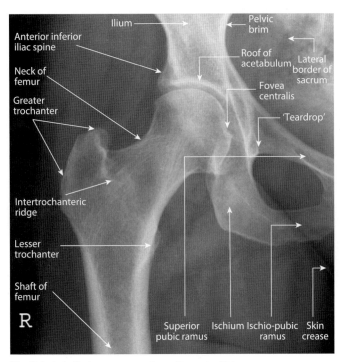

Fig. 5.4a Labelled antero-posterior radiograph of hip.

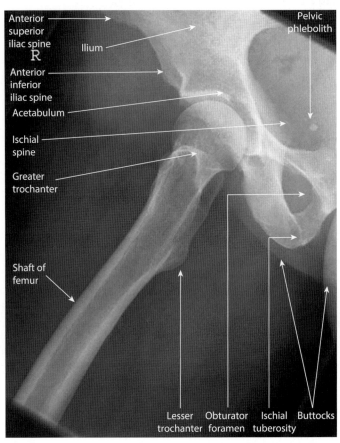

Fig. 5.4b Labelled posterior oblique (Lauenstein's) radiograph of hip (for joint).

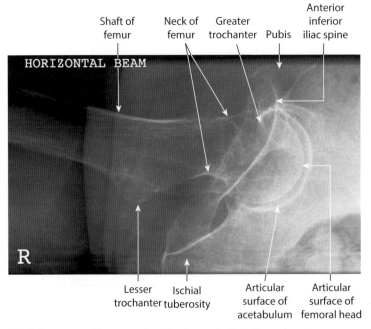

Fig. 5.4c Horizontal beam true lateral radiograph of hip (femoral neck).

Anatomy and image appearances 5

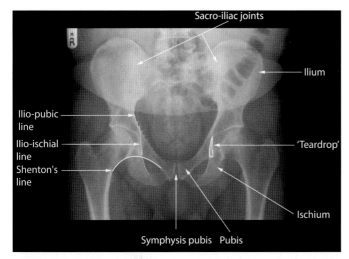

Fig. 5.5a Labelled antero-posterior radiograph of pelvis.

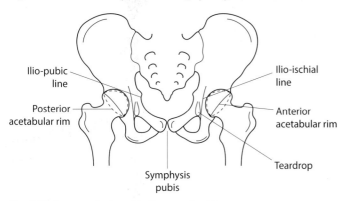

Fig. 5.5b Annotated schematic diagram of pelvis.

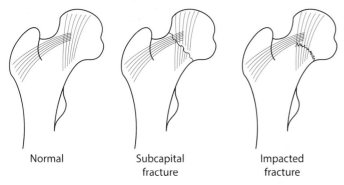

Fig. 5.5c Trabecular patterns and fracture types in the femoral neck.

Introduction

The hip joint is a ball and socket joint in which the smooth, almost spherical head of femur articulates with the acetabulum, which is formed by the three parts of the innominate bone (hemi-pelvis).

The proximal aspect of the femur consists of the head, neck and greater and lesser trochanters. The neck lies at an angle of approximately 130° with the shaft and is angulated anteriorly approximately 130° when articulated normally with the acetabulum.

The annotated images on page 172 illustrate the anatomical references used in the text.

Two principal groups of trabeculae exist within the femoral head and neck. The trabecular pattern is more obvious in the elderly and subtle fractures can cause these pattern lines to become distorted (Fig. 5.5c).[1]

The pelvis, formed by the innominate bones (ilium, ischium and pubis) and sacrum, provides a protective girdle for the pelvic organs and supports the lower limbs. The innominate bones articulate anteriorly at the symphysis pubis and posteriorly with the sacrum at the sacro-iliac joints (Fig. 5.5a). As the pelvis is a ring of bone with only slightly moveable joints, bony trauma to one side can result in a corresponding (contre-coup) injury to the opposite side.

There are several bony prominences in the pelvic region that serve as important surface landmarks in radiography. These are:

- Symphysis pubis, upper border – anterior to the bladder; aligned to the coccyx.
- Anterior superior iliac spine (ASIS) – 2nd sacral segment.
- Iliac crests – L4/5; bifurcation of the aorta.
- Posterior superior iliac spines – L5/S1; sacro-iliac joints.

There are also several anatomical radiographic lines that can be used to assess the integrity of the pelvis and hips in trauma (Fig. 5.5b):

- Shenton's line – a line following the inferior border of the femoral neck and the curve of the lower border of the superior pubic ramus. The shape of the curves on both sides of the pelvis should be the same in the absence of an acute bony injury.
- 'Teardrop' sign – floor of the acetabulum.
- Ilio-pubic line – anterior margin of the acetabulum.
- Ilio-ischial line – posterior margin of the acetabulum.

5 Anatomy and image appearances

Introduction (cont.)

Posture

When the patient is supine the pelvic brim is tilted according to the degree of angulation at the L5/S1 junction. This results in considerable variation in image appearance. A pronounced lordosis in the lower back can cause the obturator foramen to appear very elliptical and the symphysis pubis to be foreshortened. A small pad placed under the knees can reduce this lordosis and improve the image appearance.

This increased L5/S1 angulation in females when compared to the male pelvis contributes to the differing radiographic image appearance.[2]

Subject type (Figs 5.6b, 5.6c)

There is a variable difference in the breadth and depth of the pelvis according to subject type and sex. The male pelvis is narrower but has greater depth. Careful positioning is often required to include the full width of a female pelvis in the image.

Radiation protection/dose

Protection of the gonads from unnecessary X-radiation is an important factor when examining the hip joints, upper femora, pelvis and lower lumbar vertebrae. Exposure of the patient to X-radiation should be made in accordance with the ALARP principle and IR(ME)R 2000.

Primary lead protection should be applied to the gonads on patients from infancy to middle-age as appropriate. It is not recommended for initial examinations when its use may obscure anatomical information (Figs 5.6a, 5.6d).

Advice has been published from the NWRPG, based at Christie's Hospital suggesting that departments cease female gonad shielding due to unproven effectiveness. Gonad shielding for males however, is effective and should be used.

The radiation beam is restricted to the size of the receptor.

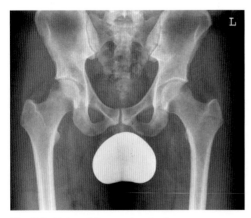

Fig. 5.6a Male pelvic gonad protection.

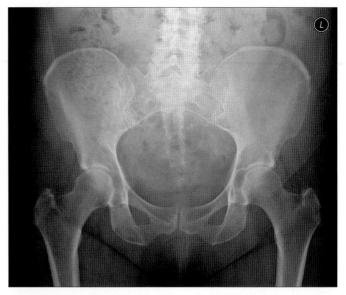

Fig. 5.6b Radiograph of female pelvis.

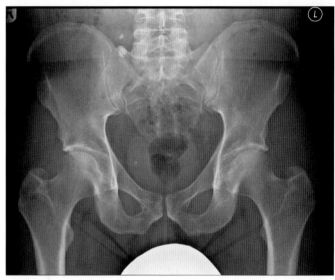

Fig. 5.6c Radiograph of male pelvis.

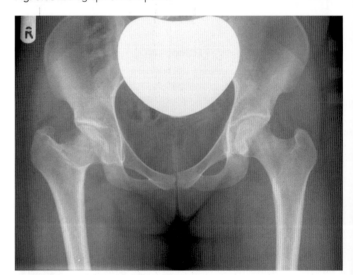

Fig. 5.6d Radiograph of female pelvis with wrongly positioned gonad protection.

Position of limb	Anatomical appearance
Neutral – long axis of foot vertical	Femoral neck oblique Lesser trochanter just visible
Internal rotation	Femoral neck elongated and lying parallel to the CR cassette/DDR receptor Lesser trochanter obscured by shaft of femur
External rotation	Femoral neck foreshortened Lesser trochanter clearly visible

Effect of rotation and abduction of the lower limb

5

Different positions of the lower limb result in different anatomical projections of the hip joint (Figs 5.7a–5.7f). The head of the femur lies anterior to the greater trochanter of the femur when articulating normally within the acetabulum. There is an approximate angulation anteriorly of 125°–130°, which is best appreciated on the true lateral projection of the hip[2].

Internal rotation of the hip joint by approximately 50° will bring the femoral neck parallel and the femoral head and trochanters on the same level (Figs 5.7b, 5.7e).

In abnormal conditions of the hip joint the position of the foot is a significant clue to the type of injury sustained. Displaced fractures involving the neck and trochanteric region will cause external rotation and usually foreshortening of the affected leg.

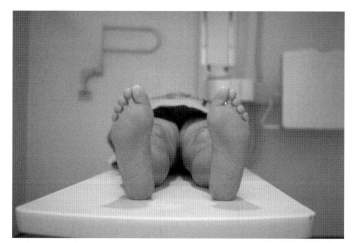

Fig. 5.7a Feet in neutral position.

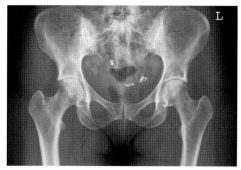

Fig. 5.7d Radiograph of pelvis, trochanters visible.

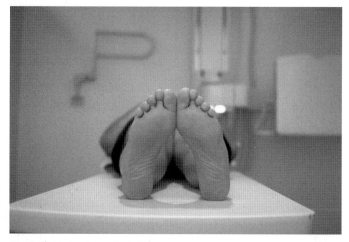

Fig. 5.7b Feet in internal rotation.

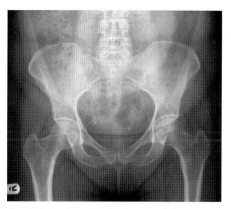

Fig. 5.7e Radiograph of pelvis; femoral neck parallel to image receptor, lesser trochanters not visible.

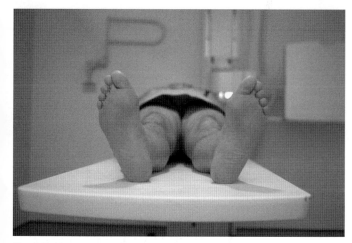

Fig. 5.7c Feet in external rotation.

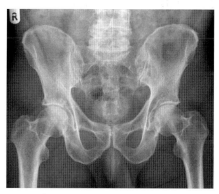

Fig. 5.7f Radiograph of pelvis, lesser trochanters clearly visible.

5 Hip joint, upper third of femur and pelvis

Antero-posterior – pelvis (Basic)

Antero-posterior – both hips (Basic) (Figs 5.8a–5.8c)

The antero-posterior (AP) projection is a general image used as a first assessment of the pelvic bones and hip joints. The position of the patient is identical for imaging both the hips and the pelvis but the centring of the beam may differ. For the hip joints and upper femora the centring may be more inferior, e.g. low centred pelvis prior to hip replacement surgery.

The AP image allows a comparison of both hips to be made and in trauma cases it ensures that a fracture to the distal pelvis is not missed, e.g. a fractured pubic ramus.

In cases of suspected fracture of the hip the injured limb is commonly externally rotated and must not be moved. If possible the opposite limb should be externally rotated to the same degree of rotation so that a more accurate comparison can be made.

A table Bucky direct digital radiography (DDR) system is employed, or alternatively a 35 × 43 cm computed radiography (CR) cassette is placed transversely in the Bucky tray using automatic exposure control (AEC).

Position of patient and image receptor

- The patient lies supine and symmetrical on the X-ray table with the median sagittal plane perpendicular to the tabletop.
- The midline of the patient must coincide with the centred primary beam and table Bucky mechanism.
- When the patient remains on a trolley, ideally they should be positioned down the midline and adjusted to achieve an optimum projection dependent on their degree of mobility.
- To avoid pelvic rotation the anterior superior iliac spines must be equidistant from the tabletop. A non-opaque pad placed under a buttock can be used to make the pelvis level. The coronal plane should now be parallel to the tabletop.
- The limbs are slightly abducted and internally rotated to bring the femoral necks parallel to the image receptor.
- Sandbags and pads are placed against the ankle region to help maintain this position.

Direction and location of the X-ray beam

- The collimated vertical beam is centred over the midline midway between the upper border of the symphysis pubis and anterior superior iliac spines for the whole of the pelvis and proximal femora.
- The upper edge of the image receptor should be 5 cm above the upper border of the iliac crest to compensate for the divergent beam and ensure the whole of the bony pelvis is included.

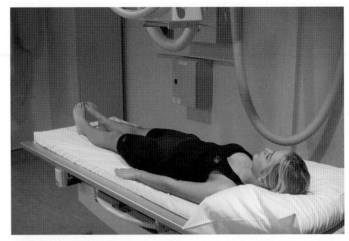

Fig. 5.8a Patient positioning for antero-posterior (AP) pelvis.

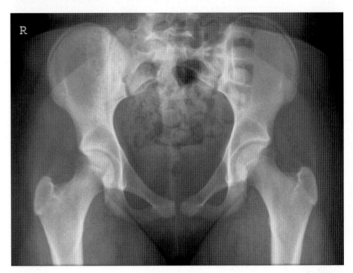

Fig. 5.8b AP projection of the full pelvis with correct internal rotation of the femora.

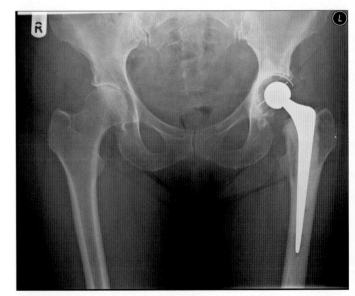

Fig. 5.8c AP radiograph of both hips and upper femora, demonstrating fully the left total hip replacement.

- The centre of the image receptor is placed level with the upper border of the symphysis pubis for the hips and upper femora (low-centred pelvis).

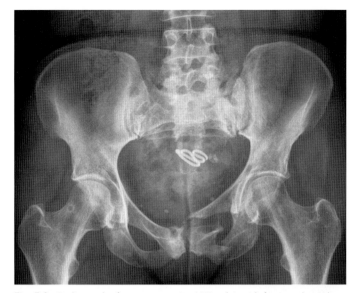

Fig. 5.9a Radiograph of antero-posterior (AP) pelvis with fracture through the left rami, i.e. the ischial and pubic bones with obvious disruption of Shenton's line.

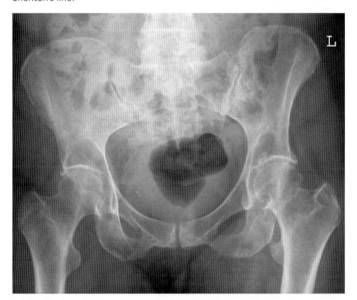

Fig. 5.9b AP pelvis with a subcapital fracture of the left femoral neck.

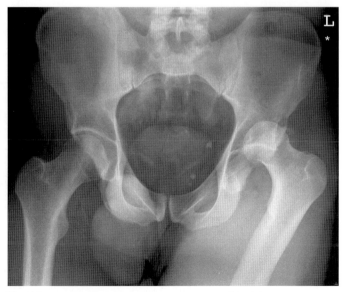

Fig. 5.9c AP pelvis showing posterior dislocation of the left hip.

Hip joint, upper third of femur and pelvis 5

Antero-posterior – both hips (Basic) (cont.)

Essential image characteristics (Figs 5.9a–5.9c)

- For the basic view of both hips, both trochanters and the upper third of the femora must be visible on the image.
- For the basic pelvis projection, both iliac crests and proximal femora, including the lesser trochanters, should be visible on the image.
- To prove there is no rotation the iliac bones should be of equal dimensions and the obturator foramina of similar size and shape.
- It should be possible to identify 'Shenton's line', which forms a continuous curve between the inferior aspect of the femoral neck and the inferior margin of the superior pubic rami. Any disruption in this curve indicates a femoral neck or superior pubic rami fracture.
- The exposure indicator (EI) reading should be adequate to visualise the bones of the posterior pelvis (sacrum and sacroiliac joints) and the proximal femora. If the EI is too low (i.e. underexposure) the superior aspect of the pelvis is not demonstrated through the lower abdomen and the image will appear 'noisy'.
- The image contrast must also allow visualisation of the trabecular patterns in the femoral necks. It is possible to use compression on appropriate bariatric patients; this can elevate and compress the abdominal apron to improve image contrast.
- No artefacts from clothing should be visible, therefore it is best practise to undress the patient.

Notes

- Internal rotation of the limb compensates for the X-ray beam divergence when centring in the midline. The resultant image will show both greater and lesser trochanters.
- At the first clinic visit and in trauma cases it is normal practice not to apply gonad protection that may obscure the pelvic bones and result in missed information.
- In follow-up visits gonad protection should be used and must be carefully positioned to avoid obscuring the region of interest resulting in an unnecessary repeat radiograph.
- The primary beam should be optimally collimated to the size of image receptor and ideally evidence of collimation should be visible on the image.
- Exposure factors and/or DAP readings should be recorded.

Radiation protection/dose

Expected DRL: DAP 2.2 Gy cm^2, ESD 4 mGy.

5 Hip joint and upper third of femur

Antero-posterior – single hip (Basic) (Figs 5.10a–5.10d)

The image is acquired using a 24 × 30 cm CR cassette placed longitudinally in the Bucky tray or alternatively within the field of view of a DDR detector system.

Position of patient and image receptor

- The patient is positioned as described for the basic pelvis and basic bilateral hip projections (see page 176).
- To avoid pelvic rotation the anterior superior iliac spines must be equidistant from the tabletop.
- The affected limb is internally rotated to bring the neck of femur parallel to the tabletop, supported by sandbags if necessary.

Direction and location of the X-ray beam

- The collimated vertical beam is centred 2.5 cm distally along the perpendicular bisector of a line joining the anterior superior iliac spine and the symphysis pubis over the femoral pulse.
- The primary beam should be collimated to the area under examination and gonad protection applied where appropriate.

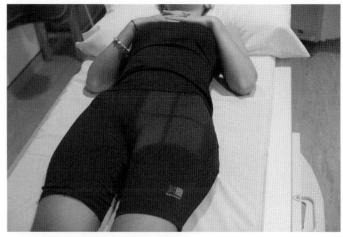

Fig. 5.10b Patient positioning for AP single hip.

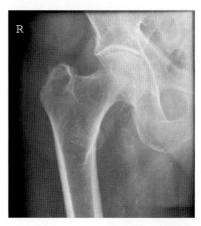

Fig. 5.10c Radiograph of AP right hip.

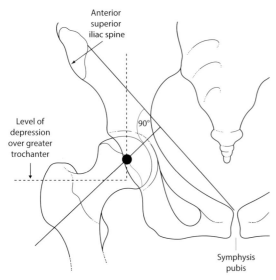

Fig. 5.10a Line diagram to illustrate positioning for antero-posterior (AP) projection of single hip.

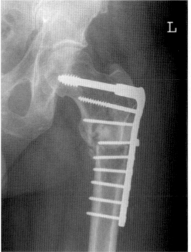

Fig. 5.10d Radiograph of AP left hip demonstrating surgical metalwork in situ.

Notes

- The image must include the proximal third of femur and when the examination is undertaken to show the positioning and integrity of an arthroplasty the whole length of the prosthesis, including the femur inferior to the cement, must be visualised.
- Over rotating the limb internally will bring the greater trochanter into profile. This may be a useful supplementary projection for a suspected avulsion fracture to this bone.
- When using conventional film/screen systems, care is needed when setting the exposure in order to optimise visualisation of the greater trochanters.

Radiation protection/dose

- Careful technique and close collimation will assist in reducing the patient dose.

Expected DRL - ESD 2.83 mGy

This projection demonstrates the upper third of femur in the lateral position and the relationship between the head of femur and the acetabulum. The posterior rim of the acetabulum is shown.[3]

The image is acquired using a 24 × 30 cm CR cassette placed longitudinally on the Bucky tray or alternatively within the field of view of a DDR detector system.

Hip joint and upper third of femur 5

Posterior oblique (Lauenstein's projection) (Fig. 5.11a)

Position of patient and image receptor

- The patient lies supine on the X-ray table, legs extended. The median sagittal plane coincides with the long axis of the table Bucky.
- The patient rotates through 45° onto the affected side with the hip abducted 45° and flexed 45° and is supported in this position by non-opaque pads.
- The knee is flexed to bring the lateral aspect of the thigh in contact with the tabletop and the knee rests on the table in the lateral position.
- The opposite limb is raised and supported.
- The image receptor is centred at the level of the femoral pulse in the groin and should include the proximal third of femur. The upper border of the image receptor should be level with the anterior superior iliac spine.

Direction and location of the X-ray beam

- The collimated vertical beam is centred to the femoral pulse in the groin of the affected side, with the central ray perpendicular to the image receptor.
- The long axis of the primary beam is adjusted by turning the light beam diaphragm (LBD) to coincide with the long axis of the femur.
- The primary beam needs to be collimated to the area under examination.

Notes

- If the unaffected side is raised greater than 45° the superior pubic ramus may be superimposed on the acetabulum.
- This projection is not used to demonstrate the neck of femur and should not be used as a first-line projection for a suspected fracture in this region.
- The patient requires a degree of mobility to be positioned satisfactorily and should not experience any great discomfort in maintaining the position.
- Used in conjunction with the AP projection it shows the satisfactory position of internal fixation pins and plates.

Radiological considerations (Figs 5.11b, 5.11c)

- The whole of the acetabular rim can be assessed when this image is used in conjunction with the anterior oblique projection (Judet's projection, see page 184).

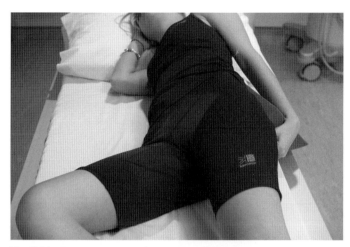

Fig. 5.11a Patient positioning for posterior oblique hip.

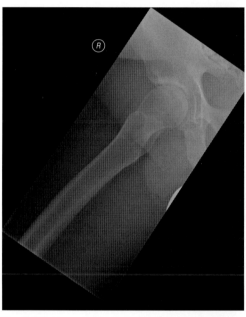

Fig. 5.11b Normal radiograph of posterior oblique hip.

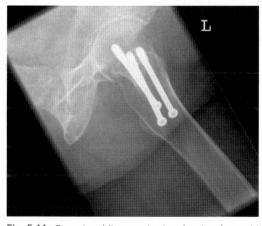

Fig. 5.11c Posterior oblique projection showing the position of surgical screws.

5 Hip joint and upper third of femur

True lateral – neck of femur (Basic) (Figs 5.12a–5.12c)

This projection is used routinely in all cases of suspected fracture of the neck of femur. It is commonly carried out with the patient remaining on a trauma trolley as it is not advisable to move patients with a clinical suspicion of a fracture (affected foot in external rotation, foreshortening of the limb and pain when moving). Patients who suffer from a fracture to the hip are often elderly and can be quite frail. It is common practice for these patients to be 'fast tracked' through A&E and for them to have received some pain relief. Care and consideration for their dignity is necessary during the examination.

Either a CR 24 × 30 grid cassette, a CR cassette and stationary grid, an erect Bucky with a DDR detector or a CR cassette placed in landscape position in the Bucky tray with AEC is used.

An air-gap technique, with or without a filter and no grid, can also be used.

Position of patient and image receptor

- The patient lies supine on the trolley or X-ray table.
- The legs are extended and the pelvis adjusted to ensure the median sagittal plane is perpendicular to the tabletop. This may not always be possible if the patient is in acute pain.
- If the patient is very slender it may be necessary to place a non-opaque pad under the buttocks so that the whole of the affected hip can be included in the image.
- The CR grid cassette is positioned vertically, with the shorter edge pressed firmly against the waist, just above the iliac crest.
- The longitudinal axis of the cassette should be parallel to the neck of femur. This can be approximated by placing a 45° foam pad between the front of the cassette and the lateral aspect of the pelvis.
- The cassette/image receptor is supported in this position by sandbags or a special cassette holder resting on the table.
- The unaffected limb is then raised until the thigh is vertical with the knee flexed. This position is maintained by supporting the lower leg on a stool or specialised equipment.

Direction and location of the X-ray beam

- The collimated vertical beam is centred through the affected groin midway between the femoral pulse and the palpable prominence of the greater trochanter, with the central ray directed horizontally and at right-angles to the cassette.
- The central beam should be adjusted vertically to pass in line with the femoral neck and collimated closely to the area to improve the image contrast.

Notes

- If the erect Bucky is used the modified 'air-gap' technique may be used as described on the following page.

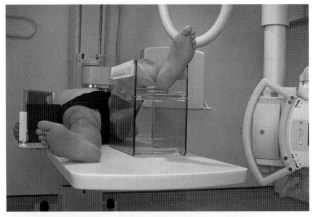

Fig. 5.12a Patient positioning for true lateral neck of femur.

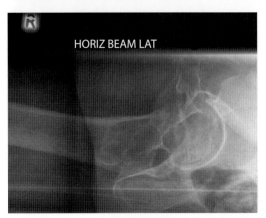

Fig. 5.12b True lateral radiograph of right hip, demonstrating undisplaced subcapital femoral neck fracture.

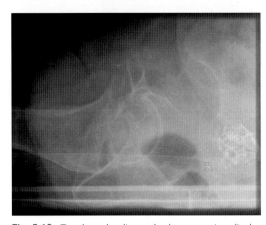

Fig. 5.12c True lateral radiograph, demonstrating displaced subcapital femoral neck fracture.

- In trauma cases, when a fracture is suspected, the limb is often externally rotated. On no account should the limb be rotated from this position. The antero-posterior and lateral projections are taken with the limb in that position.
- A relatively high kV is necessary (e.g. 100 kV) to penetrate the thigh without overexposing the trochanteric region. Using a (Ferlic) filter improves the overall optical density.
- Loss of resolution can occur when using a stationary grid and cassette due to the central X-ray beam not correctly aligned (perpendicular) to the grid lines ('grid cut-off').

Hip joint and upper third of femur 5

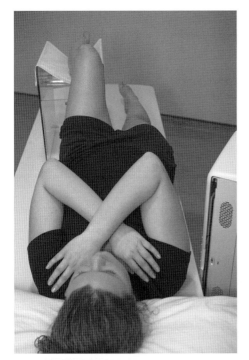

Fig. 5.13a Patient positioning for lateral air-gap technique.

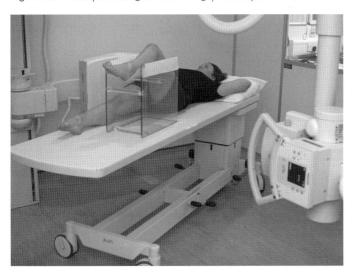

Fig. 5.13b Note the only variable is the patient on the trolley with fixed Bucky and tube parallel.

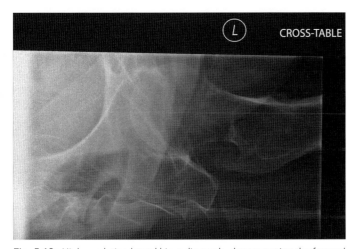

Fig. 5.13c High resolution lateral hip radiograph, demonstrating the femoral neck.

Lateral – air-gap technique (Figs 5.13a, 5.13b)

This technique is used as an alternative projection to the standard horizontal beam (HB) lateral and can produce an image with improved resolution due to the reduction in scattered radiation incident upon the CR cassette/image receptor. This projection is used on a patient with a suspicion of a femoral neck fracture.

A DDR detector in the vertical Bucky is used without a grid or alternatively a 24 × 30 cm CR cassette is used positioned vertically, in landscape position, in a vertical cassette holder or vertical Bucky without a grid.

Position of patient and image receptor

- The patient lies supine on the trolley or X-ray table with the pelvis adjusted to ensure there is no rotation.
- The unaffected limb is then raised until the thigh is vertical with the knee flexed. This position is maintained by supporting the lower leg on a stool or specialised equipment.
- The trolley is rotated to an angle of approx 45° to bring the longitudinal axis of the affected femoral neck parallel to the cassette/receptor.
- The tube is positioned with an focus-to-receptor distance (FRD) of 150 cm to compensate for the increased object-to-receptor distance (ORD) due to the patient rotation.[4]

Direction and location of the X-ray beam

- The collimated vertical beam is centred through the affected groin at the position of the groin crease with the central ray directed horizontally and at right-angles to the receptor.
- The central beam should be adjusted vertically to pass in line with the femoral neck and collimated closely to the area to improve the image contrast.

Radiological considerations (Fig. 5.13c)

- As well as being the routine projection for a suspected neck of femur fracture it should also be routine in cases where there is a suspected slipped upper femoral epiphysis or fractured acetabulum.
- Femoro-acetabular impingement is a common cause of hip pain and premature degenerative disease. For diagnosis and assessment an AP and HB lateral image will be required. Plain X-ray imaging may be all that is required after clinical examination, but magnetic resonance imaging (MRI) is useful where more detailed information is required.[5]

Radiation protection/dose

- Careful technique and close collimation will assist in reducing the patient dose.

Expected DRL: ESD 8.12 mGy

5 Hip joint and upper third of femur

Lateral – single hip (alternative projection) – modified (Figs 5.14a, 5.14b)

This projection may be used when it is impossible to either rotate the patient onto the affected side or to elevate the unaffected limb. A CR 24 × 30 grid cassette or CR cassette and stationary grid is used to acquire the image.

This projection is used if both limbs are injured or are abducted and in a plaster cast and the patient cannot be moved from the supine position.

Position of patient and image receptor

- The patient remains supine.
- The CR cassette is positioned vertically, in landscape position, against the lateral aspect of the affected hip and centred at the level of the femoral pulse.
- The CR cassette is tilted backwards through 25° and placed slightly under the affected buttock. It is supported using pads and sandbags.
- The cross-sectional diagram shows the relationship between the tube and cassette about the affected hip, enabling the two sides to be separated

Direction and location of the X-ray beam

- The collimated beam is centred to the femoral pulse with the central ray tilted 25° vertically downwards from the horizontal and at right-angles to the cassette/image receptor.
- Collimate to the area under examination.

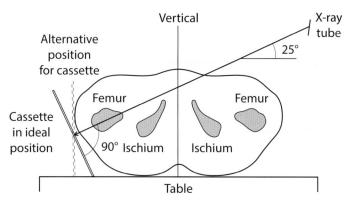

Fig. 5.14a Diagram to demonstrate position for modified lateral projection.

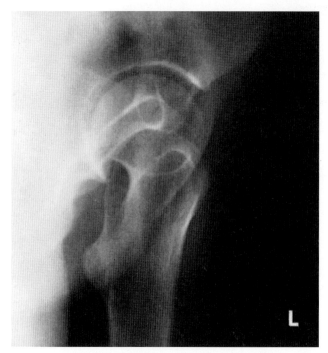

Fig. 5.14b Modified technique lateral projection of hip joint.

Radiography of the hip in children is discussed in detail in the Paediatric chapter.

When there is freedom of movement both hips can be exposed simultaneously for a general lateral projection of the femoral necks and heads. The resultant lateral hip image is similar to that obtained through the oblique lateral projection (Lauenstein's) previously described.

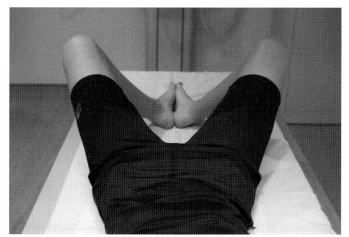

Fig. 5.15a Patient positioning for 'frog's legs' projection.

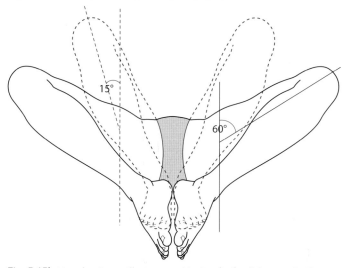

Fig. 5.15b Line drawing to illustrate positioning for frog's legs projection.

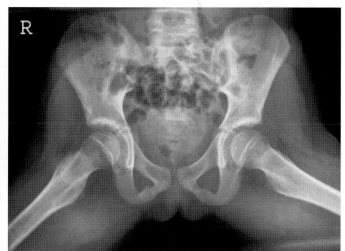

Fig. 5.15c Normal radiograph demonstrating both hips in lateral projection (frog's legs).

Hip joint and upper third of femur 5

Lateral – both hips ('frog's legs position') (Figs 5.15a–5.15c)

This projection may be used in addition to the basic antero-posterior of both hips when comparison of both hips is required. This may apply in children, for example, when diagnosing osteochondritis of the capital epiphysis (Perthe's disease) or slipped upper femoral epiphysis (SUFE). The position of the patient is often referred to as the 'frog' position.[6]

Gonad protection devices must be correctly positioned (dependant on local protocol) and firmly secured.

A DDR detector is selected in the table Bucky or alternatively a 35 × 43 cm CR cassette is selected and placed horizontally with it long axis at right-angles to the midline of the table.

Position of patient and image receptor

- The patient lies supine on the X-ray table with the anterior superior iliac spines equidistant from the tabletop to avoid rotation of the pelvis.
- The median sagittal plane is perpendicular to the table and coincident with the centre of the table Bucky mechanism.
- The hips and knees are flexed and both limbs rotated laterally through approximately 60°. This movement separates the knees and brings the plantar aspect of the feet in contact with each other.
- The limbs are supported in this position by pads and sandbags.
- The image receptor is centred at the level of the femoral pulse, to include both hip joints.

Direction and location of the X-ray beam

- The collimated vertical beam is centred in the midline at the level of the femoral pulse with the central ray perpendicular to the image receptor.

Notes

- A lateral rotation of 60° demonstrates the hip joints.
- A modified technique with the limbs rotated laterally through 15° and the plantar aspect of the feet in contact with the tabletop demonstrates the neck of femur.
- If the patient is unable to achieve 60° rotation, it is important to apply the same degree of rotation to both limbs without losing symmetry.
- In very young children a Bucky grid is not required. The child may be placed directly onto the image receptor.

Radiation protection/dose

- Gonad protection must be correctly applied according to local protocol.

Expected DRL: DAP 2.2 Gy cm², ESD 4 mGy.

5 Acetabulum and hip joint

Anterior oblique ('Judet's' projection) (Figs 5.16a, 5.16c)

This projection may be used to assess the acetabulum when a fracture is suspected. Although the acetabulum is seen on the AP pelvis, the anterior and posterior rims are superimposed over the head of femur and the ischium. If the patient is immobile or in pain a 'reverse Judet's' projection is taken.

Judet's projection demonstrates the anterior rim of the acetabulum with the patient prone. A posterior oblique projection (Lauenstein's projection) shows the posterior rim of the acetabulum with the patient supine.

A DDR detector is selected in the table Bucky or alternatively a 24 × 30 cm CR cassette is placed longitudinally in the Bucky tray.

Position of patient and image receptor

- The patient lies prone on the X-ray table.
- The trunk is then rotated approximately 45° onto the UNAFFECTED SIDE and the AFFECTED SIDE is raised and supported on non-opaque pads.
- In this position the rim of the acetabulum nearest the tabletop is approximately parallel to the image receptor.

Direction and location of the X-ray beam

- The collimated beam is centred just distal to the coccyx with the central beam directed 12° towards the head.

Posterior oblique (reverse Judet's projection) (Fig. 5.16b)

Position of patient and image receptor

- The patient lies supine on the X-ray table.
- The AFFECTED SIDE is raised approximately 45° and supported on non-opaque pads.
- The image receptor is centred at the level of the femoral pulse.

Direction and location of the X-ray beam

- The collimated vertical beam is centred to the femoral pulse on the raised side with the central ray directed 12° towards the feet.

Notes

- It is necessary in trauma cases to demonstrate adequately fractures of the pelvis and acetabulum as there is a high incident of damage to the surrounding anatomy – lower urinary tract, blood vessels and nerves. These fractures can be classified as stable/unstable depending on the position of the bony fragments.

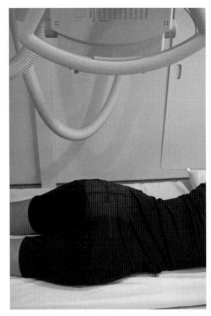

Fig. 5.16a Patient positioning for anterior oblique (Judet's) projection.

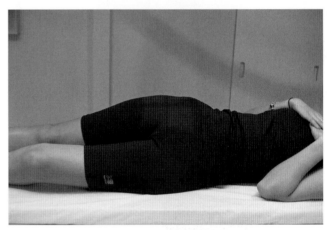

Fig. 5.16b Patient positioning for anterior oblique (Judet's) projection.

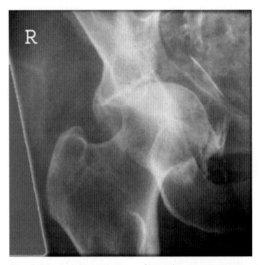

Fig. 5.16c Judet's projection of hip, showing a comminuted fracture of the acetabulum.

- Computed tomography (CT) scanning is the gold standard to assess the position of intra-articular bony fragments and soft tissue injuries in the pelvis[2].

Pelvis 5

Ilium

Although the ilium is seen on the basic pelvic projection, an oblique projection may be necessary to show the entire bone. The procedure is undertaken with the patient supine for bony trauma; however, it may not be possible to turn a badly injured patient into this position.

The posterior oblique shows the iliac wing, fossa, ischium ischial spine, the sciatic notches and acetabulum. It is a similar projection to that already described for the hip and upper femora, but with less patient rotation and centred more superiorly.

A DDR detector is selected or alternatively a 24 × 30 cm CR cassette is placed longitudinally in the Bucky tray.

Posterior oblique – basic projection (Figs 5.17a, 5.17b)

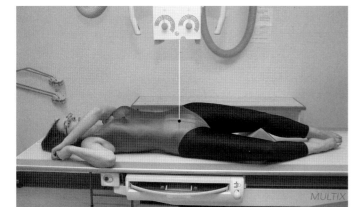

Fig. 5.17a Patient positioning for ilium.

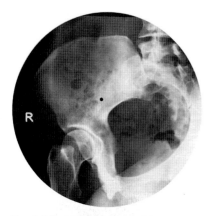

Fig. 5.17b Normal posterior oblique projection of ilium.

Position of patient and image receptor

- The patient lies supine on the Xray table and positioned for a basic AP pelvic projection.
- From this position the patient is rotated approximately 40° onto the AFFECTED side; the UNAFFECTED side is raised and supported.
- Both hips and knees are flexed and the raised limb supported on a pad.
- The iliac fossa is now parallel to the image receptor.

Direction and location of the X-ray beam

- The collimated vertical beam is centred midway between the anterior superior iliac spine of the affected side and the midline of the pelvis, with the vertical central ray perpendicular to the receptor.

Posterior oblique (alternative) (Figs 5.17c, 5.17d)

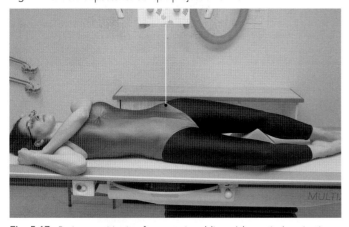

Fig. 5.17c Patient positioning for posterior oblique (alternative) projection.

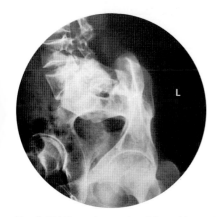

Fig. 5.17d Normal posterior oblique (alternative) projection of ilium.

This is an uncommon projection that can be used when additional information is required regarding the posterior aspect of the iliac bone.

Position of patient and image receptor

- The patient lies supine on the X-ray table.
- From this position the patient is rotated approximately 45° onto the UNAFFECTED side, with the AFFECTED SIDE raised and supported.

Direction and location of the X-ray beam

The collimated vertical beam is centred 2.5 cm behind the anterior superior iliac spine on the side being examined.

5 Pelvis

Lateral (Figs 5.18a–5.18c)

The patient may be examined in the erect or supine position. The projection is uncommon for general imaging and is primarily used for patients having gynaecological radiotherapy treatment, but may be used as part of a specific pelvimetry series for assessing the pelvic inlet and outlets.

The supine projection is described as the patient is generally heavily sedated en route from theatre for this examination.

A DDR detector is selected or alternatively a 24 × 30 cm CR cassette is placed longitudinally in the vertical Bucky.

Position of patient and image receptor (supine position)

- The patient lies supine on a trolley with either side close to the vertical Bucky, which is adjusted vertically to the pelvic level.
- Ensure that the patient is not rotated and the anterior superior iliac spines are equidistant from the trolley top.
- The median sagittal plane is parallel and coronal plane perpendicular to the image receptor.
- The arms are folded across the chest out of the way.

Direction and location of the X-ray beam

- The collimated horizontal beam is centred vertically to a depression immediately superior to the greater trochanter and collimated to the area to include the full pelvis.

Note

- A moving grid is optimal to reduce grid line artefact.

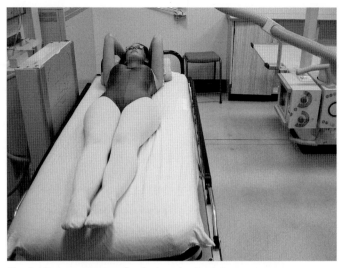

Fig. 5.18a Patient positioning for lateral pelvis – supine positioning.

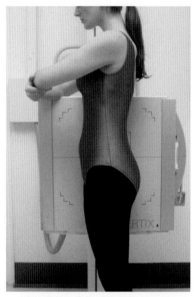

Fig. 5.18b Patient positioning for lateral pelvis – erect position.

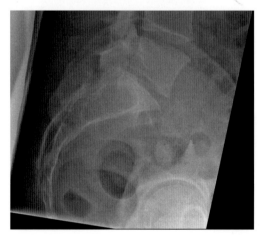

Fig. 5.18c Lateral erect radiograph of pelvis.

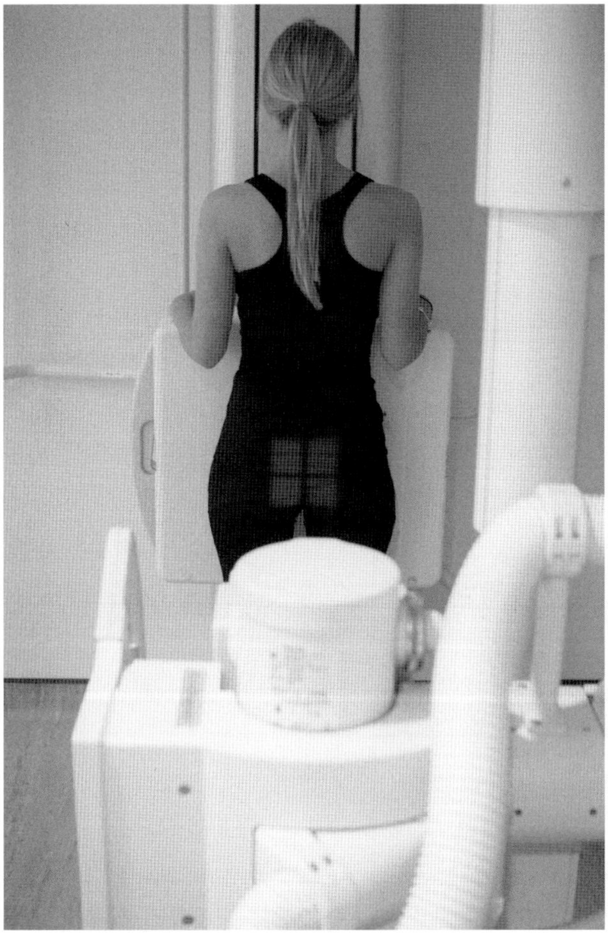

Pelvis 5

Symphysis pubis (Figs 5.19a, 5.19b)

Two postero-anterior (PA) radiographs are obtained in the erect position, with the patient transferring their full weight from one limb to the other. It is done to demonstrate widening of the symphysis pubis, usually post partum but may be post anterior compression injury.

Alternatively the procedure may be undertaken in the antero-posterior position but taking the images in the PA position reduces gonadal dose and ensures optimal resolution of the anatomy being examined.

A DDR detector is selected or alternatively a 24 × 30 cm CR cassette is placed in landscape mode in the vertical Bucky.

Postero-anterior – erect

Position of patient and image receptor

- The patient stands with the anterior aspect of the trunk against the vertical Bucky.
- The arms are folded across the chest with the feet separated, so that the patient can comfortably adopt a standing position on one foot.
- The anterior superior iliac spines should be equidistant from the image receptor with the median sagittal plane perpendicular to the vertical central line of Bucky/detector.
- The vertical Bucky is adjusted so that the horizontal central line is at the same level of symphysis pubis.
- Two exposures are taken separately with the full weight of the body on each lower limb in turn.

Direction and location of the X-ray beam

- The collimated vertical beam is centred in the midline at the level of the symphysis pubis, with the horizontal central ray perpendicular to the image receptor.

Fig. 5.19a Patient positioning for symphysis pubis projection.

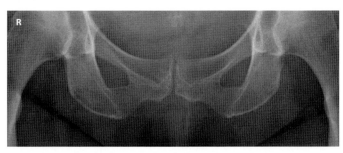

Fig. 5.19b Normal radiograph of symphysis pubis projection.

5 Sacro-iliac joints

Postero-anterior (Figs 5.20a–5.20c)

The sacrum is situated posteriorly between the two iliac bones, the adjacent surfaces forming the sacro-iliac joints. These joint surfaces are oblique in direction, sloping backward, inward and downward.

In the prone position the oblique rays coincide with the direction of the joints.

The postero-anterior (PA) projection demonstrates the joints more effectively than the antero-posterior (AP) projection. It also reduces the radiation dose to the gonads in comparison with the AP projection.

A DDR detector is selected or alternatively a 24 × 30 cm CR cassette is placed in landscape mode in the table Bucky

Position of patient and image receptor

- The patient lies prone with the median sagittal perpendicular to the tabletop.
- The posterior superior iliac spines should be equidistant from the tabletop to avoid rotation.
- The midline of the patient should coincide with the centred primary beam and table Bucky mechanism.
- The image receptor is positioned so that the central ray passes though the centre of the image receptor.

Direction and location of the X-ray beam

- The collimated vertical beam is centred in the midline at the level of the posterior superior iliac spines.
- The central ray is angled 5–15° caudally from the vertical depending on the angulation of the patient's sacrum, which is generally greater in the female due to the natural increased L5/S1 lordosis.
- The primary beam is collimated to the area of interest.

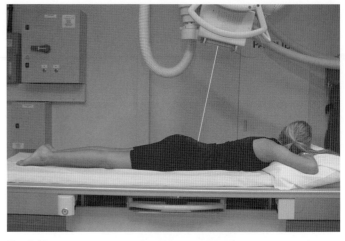

Fig. 5.20a Patient positioning for postero-anterior (PA) sacro-iliac joints.

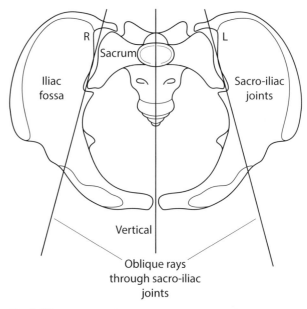

Fig. 5.20b Drawing to illustrate patient positioning for PA projection.

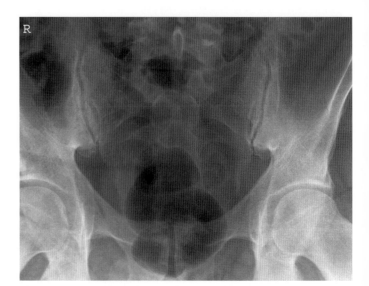

Fig. 5.20c PA radiograph demonstrating both sacro-iliac joints for comparison.

Sacro-iliac joints 5

Antero-posterior (Figs 5.21a–5.21c)

The antero-posterior (AP) projection shows both sacro-iliac joints on one image and can be done when the patient is unable to turn prone.

The position of the patient, image receptor and direction of the beam is the same as that described for the AP projection of the sacrum.

The sacro-iliac joints are routinely included on the AP projection of the lumbar spine. Additional imaging may be required as some pathologies, such as sacroiliitis, can give rise to specific sacro-iliac joint pain and require more detailed demonstration of the joints without CT/MRI imaging.

A DDR detector is selected or alternatively a 24 × 30 cm CR cassette is placed in landscape mode in the table Bucky.

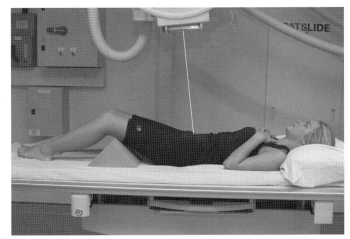

Fig. 5.21a Patient positioning for antero-posterior (AP) projection of sacro-iliac joints.

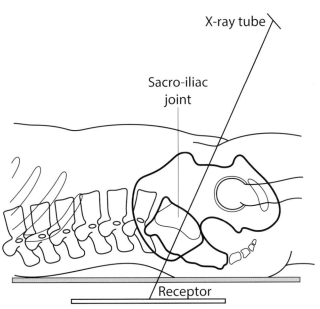

Fig. 5.21b Drawing to illustrate positioning for AP sacro-iliac.

Position of the patient and image receptor

- The patient lies supine and symmetrical on the X-ray table with the median sagittal plane perpendicular to the tabletop.
- The midline of the patient must coincide with the centred primary beam and table Bucky/detector.
- To avoid rotation the anterior superior iliac spines must be equidistant from the tabletop.
- The image receptor is positioned to coincide with the central ray.
- The shoulders are raised over a pillow to reduce the lumbar arch.
- The knees should be flexed over foam pads for comfort and to again reduce the lumbar lordosis.

Direction and location of the beam

- The collimated vertical beam is centred in the midline at a level midway between the anterior superior iliac spines and superior border of the symphysis pubis.
- The central ray is directed between 5–15° cranially depending on the sex of the patient due to the natural angulation of the male/female pelvis and lordosis of the lower lumbar spine.
- The female requires greater angulation of the beam.

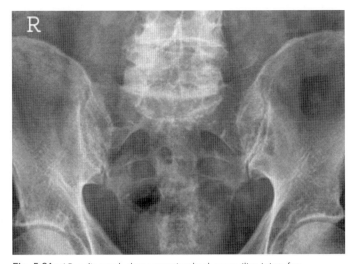

Fig. 5.21c AP radiograph demonstrating both sacro-iliac joints for comparison.

5 Sacro-iliac joints

Antero-posterior oblique (Figs 5.22a–5.22d)

Both sides are examined for comparison. This imaging technique has been primarily superseded by CT imaging.

A DDR detector is selected or alternatively a 24 × 30 cm CR cassette is placed in portrait mode in the table Bucky.

Position of patient and image receptor

- The patient lies supine on the X-ray table.
- From this position the patient is rotated 15–25° onto the side NOT being examined.
- The anterior superior iliac spine on the raised side should lie just lateral to the posterior superior iliac spine.
- The image receptor is positioned to coincide with the central ray.
- The raised side is supported with non-opaque pads.
- Pads are placed under the trunk and between the knees for comfort.

Direction and location of the X-ray beam

- The collimated vertical beam is centred 2.5 cm medial to the anterior superior iliac spine on the elevated side (side under examination) with the central ray perpendicular to the image receptor.

Note

- To demonstrate the inferior aspect of the joint more clearly, the central ray is angled 15° cranially and centred 2.5 cm medial and 5 cm inferior to the anterior superior iliac spine on the side under examination (raised side).

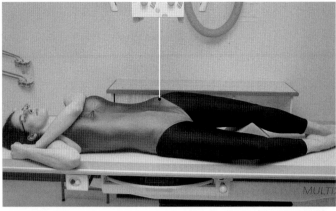

Fig. 5.22a Patient positioning for antero-posterior (AP) oblique projection of sacro-iliac joints.

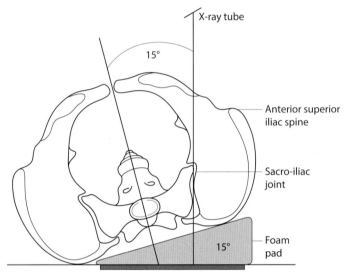

Fig. 5.22b Line drawing to illustrate positioning for AP oblique projection of sacro-iliac joints.

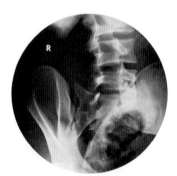

Fig. 5.22c Normal radiograph of right AP oblique sacro-iliac.

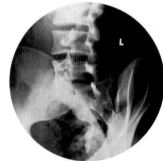

Fig. 5.22d Normal radiograph of left AP oblique sacro-iliac.

Hips, pelvis and sacro-iliac joints 5

Image evaluation – 10-point plan

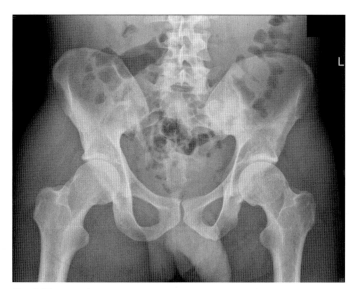

Fig. 5.23a AP pelvis.

Fig. 5.23b AP pelvis.

IMAGE EVALUATION

AP pelvis (Fig. 5.23a)

The main points to consider are:
- Radio-opaque marker was applied.
- Patient rotated – note difference in obturator foramina.
- No internal rotation of both hips.
- No gonad protection.

Radiographer Comments/Initial report

No fracture seen.

IMAGE EVALUATION

AP pelvis (Fig. 5.23b)

The main points to consider are:
- No radio-opaque marker was applied (marker digitally added post examination).
- Iliac crests and left greater trochanter not included.
- Incorrectly centred.
- High density image giving poor detail to trochanteric/crests and soft tissue.
- Both femora not fully internally rotated.
- Repeat required.

Radiographer Comments/Initial report

Fracture to right greater trochanter.

5 Hips, pelvis and sacro-iliac joints

Image evaluation – 10-point plan (*cont.*)

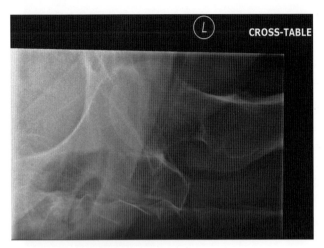

Fig. 5.24a Lateral left hip.

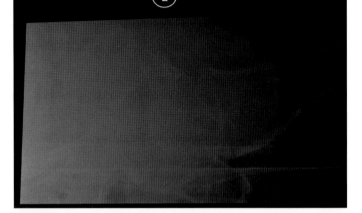

Fig. 5.24b Lateral left hip.

IMAGE EVALUATION

Lateral left hip (Fig. 5.24a)

The main points to consider are:
- Radio-opaque side marker was applied at post processing.
- Artefacts, clothing/blankets.
- Femoral neck fully demonstrated, parallel to receptor/cassette.
- Adequate contrast density.
- High resolution due to reduced scatter.

Radiographer Comments/Initial report

No fracture seen.

IMAGE EVALUATION

Lateral left hip (Fig. 5.24b)

The main points to consider are:
- Radio-opaque side marker was applied at post processing.
- Femoral neck foreshortened as not parallel to receptor/cassette.
- Incorrectly centred (too superior).
- High density and low contrast.
- Both femora not fully internally rotated.
- Repeat required.

Radiographer Comments/Initial report

Fracture to left femoral neck.

Section 6
Vertebral Column

CONTENTS

RECOMMENDED PROJECTIONS	194
VERTEBRAL CURVES	195
Important considerations in spinal radiography	195
VERTEBRAL LEVELS	196
Useful landmarks	196
CERVICAL VERTEBRAE	198
Basic projections	198
Lateral erect (Basic)	198
Lateral supine	200
Antero-posterior – first and second cervical vertebrae (open mouth)	201
Antero-posterior – third to seventh cervical vertebrae (Basic)	203
Image evaluation – 10-point plan	204
Axial – upper cervical vertebra	206
Lateral – flexion and extension	207
Right and left posterior oblique – erect	208
Right and left posterior oblique – supine	209
CERVICO-THORACIC VERTEBRAE	210
Lateral swimmers'	210
THORACIC VERTEBRAE	211
Antero-posterior (Basic)	211
Lateral (Basic)	212
Localised projections	213
Image evaluation – 10-point plan	214
LUMBAR VERTEBRAE	215
Antero-posterior (Basic)	215
Lateral (Basic)	216
Lateral horizontal beam	218
Lateral flexion and extension	219
Right or left posterior oblique	220
Image evaluation – 10-point plan	221
LUMBO-SACRAL JUNCTION	222
Lateral	222
Antero-posterior	223
Right or left posterior oblique	223
SACRUM	224
Antero-posterior/postero-anterior	224
Lateral	225
COCCYX	226
Antero-posterior	226
Lateral	226

6 Recommended projections

The projections recommended below are only a guide, as practice may vary according to local departmental protocols.

Cervical vertebrae	Severe trauma (patient on trolley with neck brace)	Lateral supine with horizontal beam (basic) AP supine (basic) AP C1/2, 'open mouth', supine (basic) Swimmers' lateral supine or oblique supine if C7/T1 not demonstrated (additional) Flexion and extension (additional), consultant request after initial images cleared
	Minor trauma (patient walking)	Lateral erect (basic) AP, erect or supine (basic) AP C1/2, 'open mouth', erect or supine (basic) Swimmers' lateral or oblique if C7/T1 not demonstrated (additional) Flexion and extension (additional), consultant request after initial images cleared
	Non-traumatic pathology	Lateral erect (basic) AP, erect or supine (basic) Flexion and extension (additional) Oblique erect (additional) Flexion and extension (additional) Swimmers' lateral if cervico-thoracic region is of particular interest (additional)
Thoracic vertebrae	Trauma (patient on trolley)	Lateral supine with HB (basic) AP supine (basic)
	Non-traumatic pathology	Lateral (basic) AP supine (basic)
Lumbar vertebrae	Trauma (patient on trolley)	Lateral supine with HB (basic) AP supine (basic)
	Non-traumatic pathology	Lateral (basic) AP supine or PA (basic) Oblique (additional) Flexion and extension (additional)
Lumbo-sacral junction	Trauma (patient on trolley)	Lateral supine with horizontal beam (basic) AP supine (basic)
	Non-traumatic pathology	Lateral (basic) AP supine (basic) Oblique (additional)
Sacrum	Trauma	Lateral (basic), HB if patient cannot turn AP supine (basic)
	Non-traumatic pathology	Lateral (basic) AP (basic) See Section 5
Coccyx	Trauma/pathology	Projections not normally performed unless patient considered for coccyxectomy Lateral (basic), AP (basic)
Scoliosis and kyphosis	See Section 13	

AP, antero-posterior; HB, horizontal beam; PA, postero-anterior.

Vertebral curves 6

At birth, the majority of the vertebral column is curved, with its concavity facing forward. As development occurs, and the child starts to lift its head and begins to walk, additional curvatures develop with the spine in response to these activities. The anterior concavity is maintained in the thoracic and sacro-coccygeal regions, hence they are given the name primary curves. The cervical and lumbar regions become convex anteriorly. These are the secondary curves.

A knowledge of vertebral curves is important in radiography as their position with respect to the direction of the X-ray beam will determine the quality of the final image in terms of ability to make an accurate diagnosis.

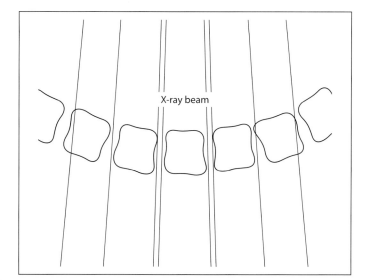

Fig. 6.1a Concavity of vertebral curve towards X-ray tube.

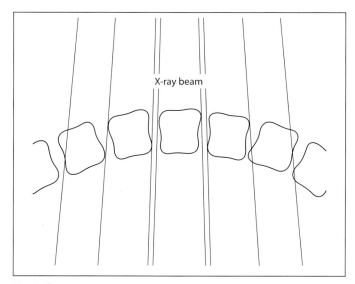

Fig. 6.1b Convexity of vertebral curve towards X-ray tube.

Important considerations in spinal radiography

- Remember that the X-ray beam diverges from the focal spot on the anode. The X-rays are not parallel to each other.
- Ideally, the vertebral bodies will not be superimposed over one another and will be separated on the image.
- Disc spaces should be demonstrated clearly, without superimposition of vertebral bodies.
- The vertebral endplates will be parallel with the X-ray beam at a given point. This will ensure that the lateral borders are superimposed and will give the typical quadrangular appearance on the final image.
- In order to achieve the above, the concavity of the part of the spine under examination should always face the X-ray tube (see Figs 6.1a, 6.1b).
- The curves are variable along the area of interest, thus making it impossible to achieve separation of individual vertebra. In this instance, it may be worth considering individual exposures, with the beam angled to achieve the required degree of separation.

6 Vertebral levels

The photographs below and Fig. 6.3 illustrate the surface markings of the vertebral levels, which are useful in radiographic positioning. The relative positions may vary according to the patient's build and posture.

Useful landmarks (Fig. 6.2)

- The easily palpated tip of the mastoid process indicates the level of C1.
- The spinous process of C7 produces a visible protuberance on the posterior aspect of the inferior part of the neck. Below this, the spinous process of the thoracic spine can be palpated. NB: the thoracic spinous processes are directed steeply downwards, so their palpable tips will be adjacent to the vertebral body below.
- The inferior angle of the scapula indicates the level of T7 when the arms are placed by the side.
- The sternal notch lies at the junction between T2 and T3.
- T4 is indicated by the sternal angle with T9 corresponding to the xiphisternal joint, although the size of this structure is variable.
- The lower costal margin indicates L3 and is located easily. This is a very useful aid to positioning in spinal radiography.
- A line joining the most superior parts of the iliac crests indicates the level of L4, whilst the tubercle of the iliac crest discloses the location of L5.
- The anterior and posterior iliac spines lie at the level of the second sacral vertebra.
- The coccyx can be palpated between the buttocks and lies at the level of the symphysis pubis.

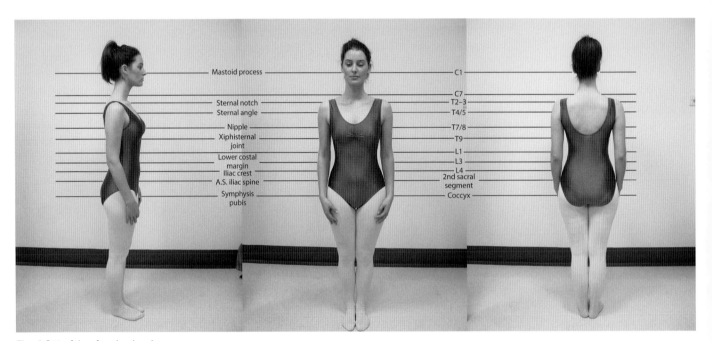

Fig. 6.2 Useful surface landmarks.

Vertebral levels 6

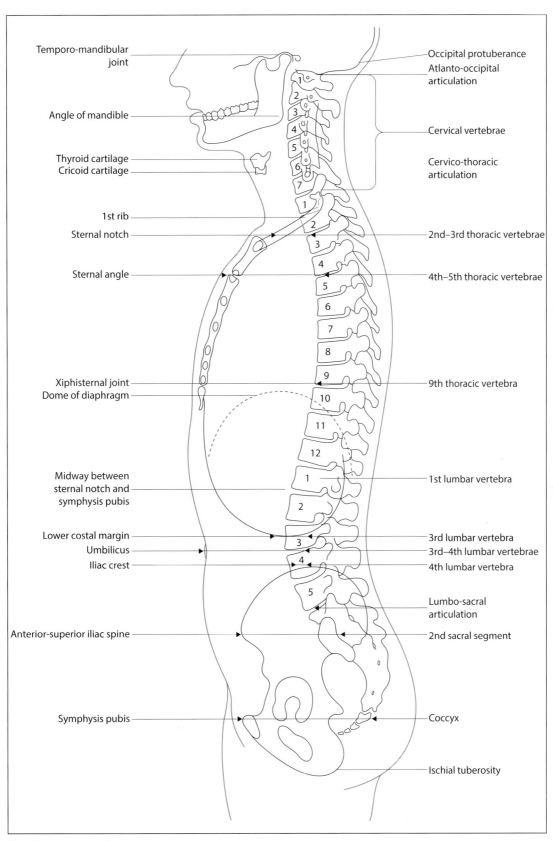

Fig. 6.3 Vertebral levels.

6 Cervical vertebrae

Basic projections

Many centres perform an antero-posterior (AP) and a lateral projection, with the addition of a further AP image to demonstrate the C1/2 region if the patient has a history of trauma.

Each image is acquired using a computed radiography (CR) image receptor or alternatively within the field of view of a direct digital radiography (DDR) detector system.

For CR, 18 × 24 cm image receptor size cassettes are employed routinely, but 24 × 30 cm cassettes are often used in difficult cases.

Lateral erect (Basic) (Figs 6.4a–6.4c)

Position of patient and image receptor

- The patient stands or sits with either shoulder against the CR cassette or vertical Bucky digital detector system (a grid may be employed dependent on department protocols).
- The median sagittal plane should be adjusted such that it is parallel with the image receptor.
- The head should be flexed or extended such that the angle of the mandible is not superimposed over the upper anterior cervical vertebra or the occipital bone does not obscure the posterior arch of the atlas.
- To aid immobilisation, the patient should stand with the feet slightly apart and with the shoulder resting against the cassette stand.
- In order to demonstrate the lower cervical vertebra, the shoulders should be depressed, as shown in the photograph. This can be achieved by asking the patient to relax their shoulders downwards. The process can be aided by asking the patient to hold a weight in each hand (if they are capable) and making the exposure on arrested expiration.

Direction and location of the X-ray beam

- The collimated horizontal beam is centred over a point vertically below the mastoid process at the level of the prominence of the thyroid cartilage.

Essential image characteristics

- The whole of the cervical spine should be included, from the atlanto-occipital joints to the top of the first thoracic vertebra.
- The mandible or occipital bone does not obscure any part of the upper vertebra.
- Angles of the mandible and the lateral portions of the floor of the posterior cranial fossa should be superimposed.
- Soft tissues of the neck should be included.
- The contrast should produce densities sufficient to demonstrate soft tissue and bony detail.

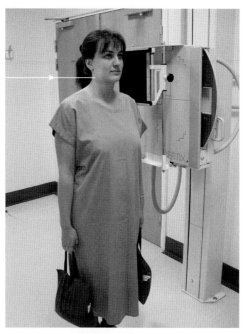

Fig. 6.4a Positioning of erect patient for cervical AP projection.

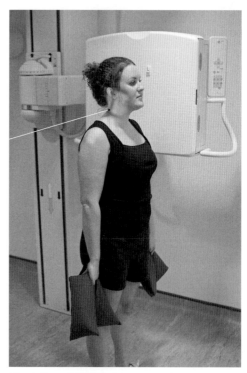

Fig. 6.4b Vertical digital detector technique.

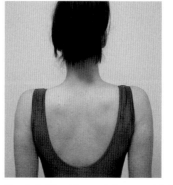 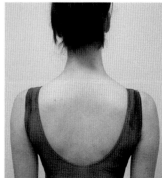

Fig. 6.4c Shoulders not depressed (left) and depressed (right).

Cervical vertebrae 6

Lateral erect (Basic) (cont.)

Radiological considerations (Figs 6.5a, 6.5b)

- Atlanto-axial subluxation is seen on the lateral projection, and is more clearly seen on flexion projection. Care is needed in making this diagnosis in children, in whom the normal space is larger (adults, 2 mm, children 3–5 mm).
- Visualisation of the margins of the foramen magnum can be difficult but is necessary for diagnosis of various skull-base abnormalities, such as basilar invagination. It will be obscured by incorrect exposure or the presence of earrings.
- A secondary sign of a vertebral injury is swelling of the soft tissues anterior to the vertebral body (normal thickness is less than the depth of a normal vertebral body). This can be mimicked by flexion of the neck – always try to obtain images in the neutral position.

Common faults and solutions

- Failure to demonstrate C7/T1: if the patient cannot depress the shoulders, even when holding weights, then a swimmers' projection should be considered.
- Care should be taken with the position of the lead name blocker if using conventional cassettes. Important anatomy may easily be obscured, especially when using a small cassette.

Notes

- The large object-to-receptor distance (ORD) will increase geometric unsharpness. This is overcome by increasing the focus-to-receptor distance (FRD) to 150 cm.
- An air gap between the neck and the receptor eliminates the need to employ a secondary radiation grid to attenuate scatter.

Radiation protection/dose

- Care should be taken when collimating to avoid including the eyes within the primary beam.

Expected DRL: DAP 0.15 Gy cm^2.

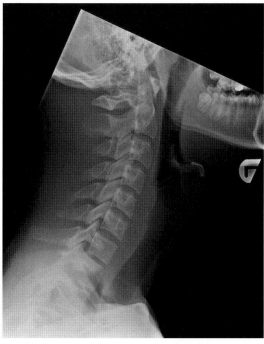

Fig. 6.5a Lateral image of cervical spine showing good technique.

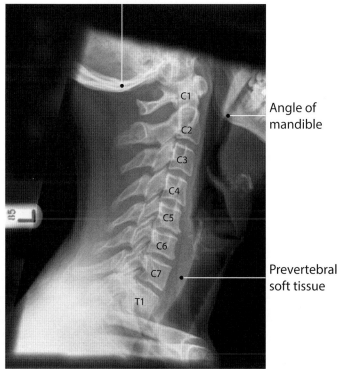

Fig. 6.5b Annotated cervical spine.

6 Cervical vertebrae

Lateral supine (Figs 6.6a, 6.6b)

For trauma cases, the patient's condition usually requires the examination to be performed on a casualty trolley. The lateral cervical spine projection is taken first, without moving the patient. The resulting radiographic image must be examined by a medical officer to establish whether the patient's neck can be moved for other projections. See Section 14 for additional information.

Position of patient and image receptor

- The patient will normally arrive in the supine position.
- It is vitally important for the patient to depress the shoulders (assuming no other injuries to the arms).
- A CR cassette can be either supported vertically or placed in the erect cassette holder, with the top of the cassette at the same level as the top of the ear or alternatively a vertical DDR system is employed which is adjusted along with the position of the trolley to ensure that the cervical spine corresponds with the central field of the detector.
- To depress the shoulders further, one or two suitably qualified individuals can apply caudal traction to the arms.

Note

- Refer to departmental local rules for staff working within a controlled area.

Common faults and solutions

- Failure to demonstrate C7/T1: if the patient's shoulders are depressed fully, then the application of traction will normally show half to one extra vertebra inferiorly. Should the cervical thoracic junction still remain undemonstrated, then a swimmers' lateral or oblique projections should be considered.

Radiological considerations (Fig. 6.6c)

- This projection is part of the Advanced Trauma and Life Support (ATLS) secondary screen.
- Clear demonstration of the C7/T1 junction is essential, as this is a common site of injury and is associated with major neurological morbidity. It is often not covered fully on the initial trauma screen and must always be demonstrated in the setting of trauma, by supplementary projections if necessary.

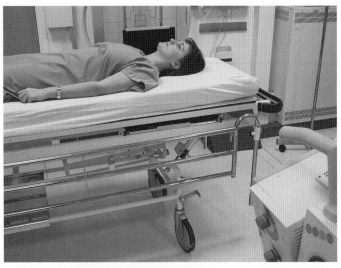

Fig. 6.6a Patient positioning on trolley using a vertical detector system.

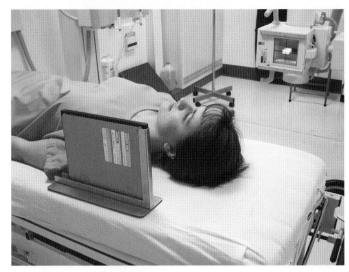

Fig. 6.6b Patient positioning for lateral supine projection.

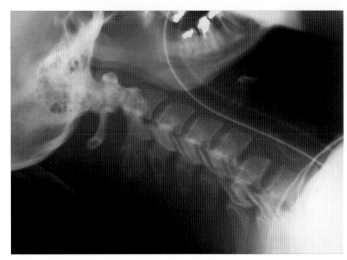

Fig. 6.6c Lateral supine projection showing fracture dislocation of C5/C6.

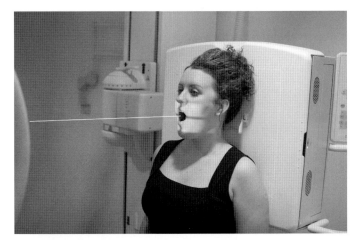

Fig. 6.7a Patient positioning for AP cervical projection.

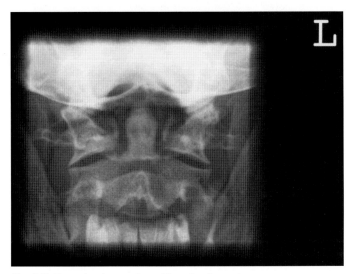

Fig. 6.7b Example of correctly positioned radiograph.

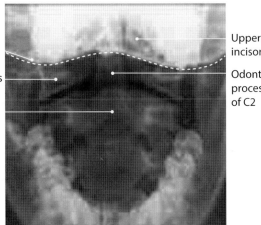

Fig. 6.7c Annotated AP cervical spine radiograph.

Cervical vertebrae 6

Antero-posterior – first and second cervical vertebrae (open mouth) (Fig. 6.7a)

Position of patient and image receptor

- The patient lies supine on the Bucky table or, if erect positioning is preferred, sits or stands with the posterior aspect of the head and shoulders against the vertical Bucky detector system.
- The medial sagittal plane is adjusted to coincide with the midline of the image receptor, such that it is at right-angles to the image receptor.
- The neck is extended, if possible, such that a line joining the tip of the mastoid process and the inferior border of the upper incisors is at right-angles to the cassette. This will superimpose the upper incisors and the occipital bone, thus allowing clear visualisation of the area of interest.
- The receptor is centred at the level of the mastoid process.

Direction and location of the X-ray beam

- The collimated beam is directed with the perpendicular central ray along the midline to the centre of the open mouth.
- If the patient is unable to flex the neck and attain the position described above, then the beam must be angled, typically 5–10° cranially or caudally, to superimpose the upper incisors on the occipital bone.
- The image receptor position will have to be altered slightly to allow the image to be centred after beam angulation.

Radiological considerations (Figs 6.7b, 6.7c, 6.8c)

- Fracture of the odontoid peg usually occurs across the base, below the suspensory ligament supporting the atlas. Optimal initial plain images are therefore essential. The base of the peg must not be obscured by any overlying structures. Failure to demonstrate the peg will lead to the need for more complex imaging, though if a patient is to have computed tomography (CT) of the head for associated trauma, scans of areas of the spine not already covered adequately are recommended in ATLS. In other patients, failure to show C1/2 either will result in the need for specific CT of the spine or will lead to protracted immobilisation, with its attendant morbidity.
- A burst (Jefferson) fracture is seen on the AP image as a loss of alignment of the margins of the lateral masses. Rotated images make this harder to appreciate (this fracture is seen very well on CT).

Widening of an interspinous interval is an indicator of instability. Flexion projections can be used to clarify in doubtful cases but should be performed under medical supervision due to the risk of spinal cord compression.

6 Cervical vertebrae

Antero-posterior – first and second cervical vertebrae (open mouth) (*cont.*)

Common faults and solutions

- Failure to open the mouth wide enough: the patient can be reminded to open their mouth as wide as possible just before the exposure.
- A small degree of rotation may result in superimposition of the lower molars over the lateral section of the joint space. Check for rotation during positioning.
- If the front teeth are superimposed over the area of interest (top left image), then the image should be repeated with the chin raised or with an increased cranial angulation of the tube (Fig. 6.8a).
- If the occipital bone is superimposed, then the chin should be lowered or a caudal angulation should be employed (Fig. 6.8b).
- It is worth noting that some individuals have a very prominent maxilla. It will be very difficult to produce an image without some degree of superimposition in these cases, so an alternative projection or modality should be considered.

Note

- A decrease in patient dose can be obtained by not using a grid. This will produce an image of lower contrast due to the increased scatter incident on the image, but it should still be of diagnostic quality. The choice of whether to use a grid will vary according to local needs and preferences.

Radiation protection/dose

- Local protocols may state that this projection is not routinely used for degenerative disease.

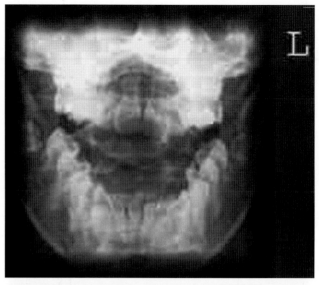

Fig. 6.8a Incorrect positioning – upper teeth superimposed.

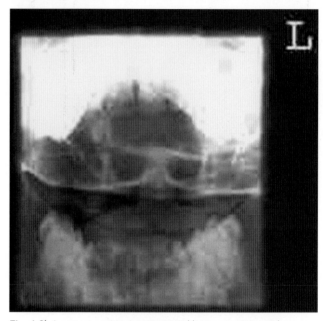

Fig. 6.8b Incorrect positioning – occipital bone superimposed.

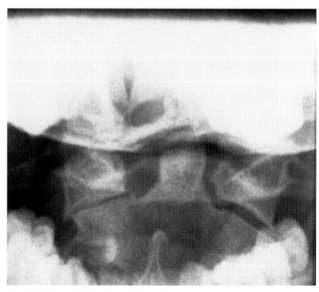

Fig. 6.8c Loss of alignment in lateral masses.

Position of patient and image receptor

- The patient lies supine on the Bucky table or, if erect positioning is preferred, sits or stands with the posterior aspect of the head and shoulders against the vertical Bucky detector system.

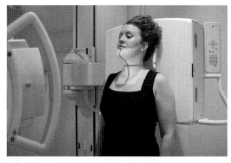

Fig. 6.9a Patient positioning for antero-posterior 3rd to 7th cervical vertebrae.

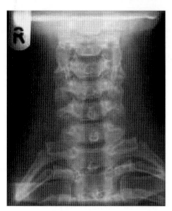

Fig. 6.9b Correctly positioned patient and x-ray tube.

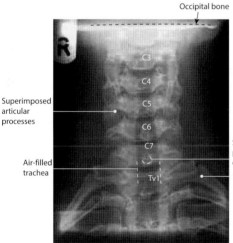

Fig. 6.9c Annotated AP cervical spine radiograph.

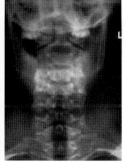

Fig. 6.9d Moving jaw technique.

Cervical vertebrae 6

Antero-posterior – third to seventh cervical vertebrae (Basic) (Figs 6.9a–6.9c)

- The median sagittal plane is adjusted to be at right-angles to the image receptor and to coincide with the midline of the table or Bucky.
- The neck is extended (if the patient's condition will allow) so that the lower part of the jaw is cleared from the upper cervical vertebra.
- The image receptor is positioned in the Bucky to coincide with the central ray. The Bucky mechanism will require some cranial displacement if the tube is angled.

Direction and location of the X-ray beam

- The collimated beam is directed with a 5–15° cranial angulation, such that the inferior border of the symphysis menti is superimposed over the occipital bone.
- The beam is centred in the midline towards a point just below the prominence of the thyroid cartilage through the fifth cervical vertebra.

Radiological considerations

- A unifacet dislocation can be diagnosed by loss of continuity of the line of spinous processes (or a line bisecting the bifid processes). This is made more difficult if the patient is rotated or the image is underexposed.

Common faults and solutions

- Failure to demonstrate the upper vertebra: an increase in the tube angle or raising the chin should provide a solution.

Notes

- Research is currently being undertaken to investigate the advantages of performing this projection postero-anteriorly. The positioning is similar to the antero-posterior projection, except that the patient faces the receptor and a 15° caudal angulation is applied to the tube. Indications suggest that this projection has the advantage of showing the disc spaces more clearly and substantially reducing the dose to the thyroid.
- The moving jaw technique uses autotomography to diffuse the image of the mandible, thus demonstrating the upper vertebra more clearly. The patient's head must be immobilised well, and an exposure time that is long enough to allow the jaw to open and close several times must be used (Fig. 6.9d).
- Linear tomography or tomosynthesis has also been used to demonstrate the cervical vertebra obscured by the mandible and facial bones (see page 516).

Radiation protection/dose

Expected DRL: DAP 0.15 Gy cm².

6 Cervical vertebrae

Image evaluation – 10-point plan

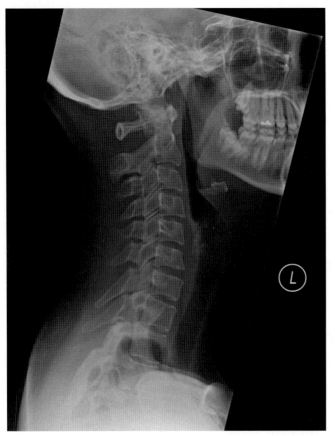

Fig. 6.10a Lateral cervical spine (optimal).

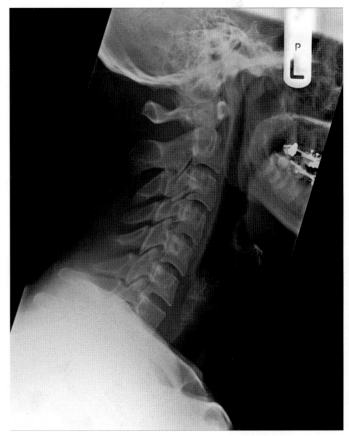

Fig. 6.10b Lateral cervical spine (suboptimal).

IMAGE EVALUATION

Lateral cervical spine (Fig. 6.10a)

Main points to consider:

- Occiput to superior aspect of T2 demonstrated.
- No rotation.
- Chin elevated sufficiently.
- Normal cervical lordosis.
- Standard soft-tissue markings.
- Side marker added post processing.

Radiographer Comments/Initial report

Diagnostic images with normal vertebral alignment and disc spaces intact.
No evidence of fracture or dislocation.

IMAGE EVALUATION

Lateral cervical spine (Fig. 6.10b)

Main points to consider:

- Occiput to superior aspect of C7 demonstrated.
- No imaging of C7/T1.
- Mandibular angle overlying vertebral body of C2.
- Slight loss of normal cervical lordosis.
- Standard soft-tissue markings.
- Additional image to demonstrate C7/T1 required.

Radiographer Comments/Initial report

No evidence of fracture or dislocation to C6, but further imaging of C7/T1 junction required.

Cervical vertebrae 6

Image evaluation – 10-point plan (cont.)

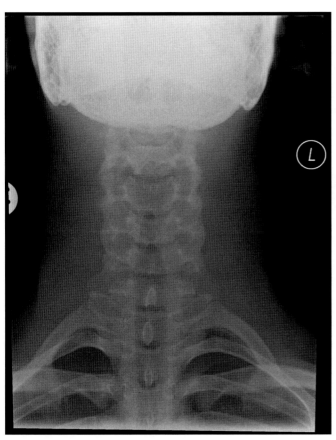

Fig. 6.11a AP cervical spine (optimal).

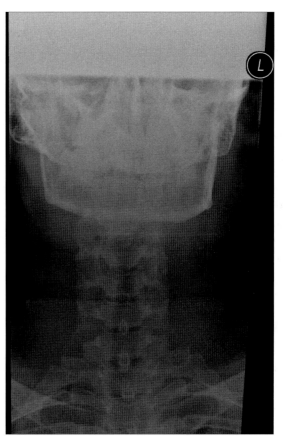

Fig. 6.11b AP cervical spine (suboptimal).

IMAGE EVALUATION

AP cervical spine (Fig. 6.11a)

Main points to consider:

- Chin elevated and inferior aspect of C2 to upper thoracic spine demonstrated.
- No rotation.
- Optimum exposure with good range of contrast.
- Side marker captured at time of exposure.
- Alignment of spinous processes with intervertebral disc space intact.

Radiographer Comments/Initial report

Diagnostic image with no abnormality seen.

IMAGE EVALUATION

AP cervical spine (Fig. 6.11b)

Main points to consider:

- Inadequate elevation of the chin, therefore mandible overlying C3 vertebral body.
- Marker applied during post processing.
- Centred correctly.
- Low contrast due to soft-tissue mass.
- Repeat needed to demonstrate from inferior aspect of C2.

Radiographer Comments/Initial report

No abnormality seen but repeat imaging required.

6 Cervical vertebrae

Axial – upper cervical vertebra (Fig. 6.12a)

This is a useful projection if the odontoid peg cannot be demonstrated using the open mouth projection. Remember that the neck must not be flexed in acute injuries.

Position of patient and image receptor

- The patient lies supine on the Bucky table, with the median sagittal plane coincident with the midline of the table and at right-angles to the image receptor.
- The neck is extended so that that the orbito-meatal baseline is at 45° to the tabletop. The head is then immobilised.
- The image receptor is displaced cranially so that its centre coincides with the central ray.

Direction and location of the X-ray beam

- The collimated beam is angled 30° cranially from the vertical and the central ray directed towards a point in the midline between the external auditory meatuses.

Essential image characteristics (Fig. 6.12b)

- The odontoid peg will be projected over the occipital bone but clear of other confusing surrounding structures.

Notes

- Additional beam angulation may be used if the patient is wearing a rigid collar.
- Linear tomography/tomosynthesis (volume rad) has also been used to demonstrate this region (Fig. 6.12c) (see also page 516).

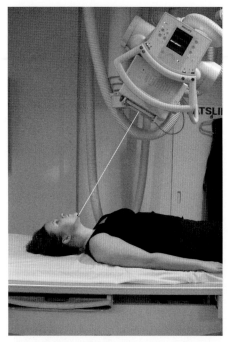

Fig. 6.12a Patient positioning and image receptor.

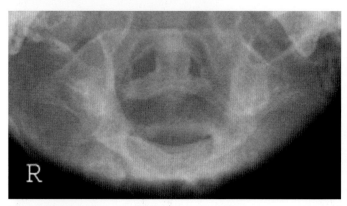

Fig. 6.12b Odontoid peg radiograph.

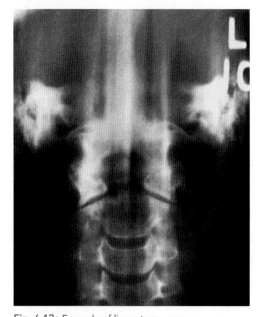

Fig. 6.12c Example of linear tomogram.

Lateral – flexion and extension (Figs 6.13a, 6.13b)

These projections may be required, but only at the request of a medical officer, to supplement the basic projections in cases of trauma, e.g. subluxation, or pathology, e.g. rheumatoid arthritis (and often before surgery to assess movement in the neck for insertion of an endotracheal tube). The degree of movement and any change in the relationship of the cervical vertebrae can also be assessed. If an injury is suspected or is being followed up, then an experienced trauma doctor must be present to supervise flexion and extension of the neck.

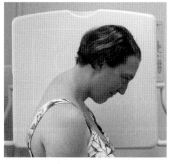 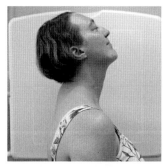

Fig. 6.13a and b Patient positioning for flexion and extension projections.

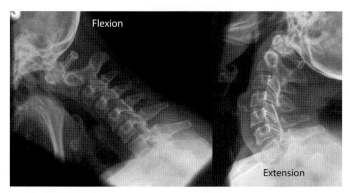

Fig. 6.13c Radiographs showing flexions and extension.

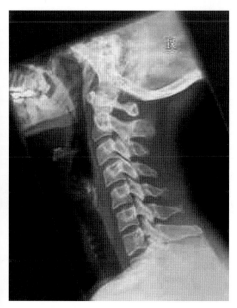

Fig. 6.13d Whiplash injury (spine in neutral position).

Cervical vertebrae 6

Position of patient and image receptor

- The patient is positioned as for the lateral basic or lateral supine projections; however, erect positioning is more convenient. The patient is asked to flex the neck and to tuck the chin in towards the chest as far as is possible.
- For the second projection, the patient is asked to extend the neck by raising the chin as far as possible.
- Immobilisation can be facilitated by asking the patient to hold on to a solid object, such as the back of a chair.
- The image receptor is centred to the mid-cervical region and if using a CR cassette this may have to be placed transversely for the lateral in flexion, depending on the degree of movement and the cassette size used.
- If imaged supine, the neck can be flexed by placing pads under the neck. Extension of the neck can be achieved by placing pillows under the patient's shoulders.

Direction and location of the X-ray beam

- The collimated horizontal beam is centred over the mid-cervical region (C4).

Essential image characteristics (Figs 6.13c, 6.13d)

- The final image should include the entire cervical vertebra, including the atlanto-occipital joints, the spinous processes and the soft tissues of the neck.

Notes

- The large ORD will increase geometric unsharpness. This is overcome by increasing the FRD to 150 cm.
- An air gap between the neck and the receptor eliminates the need to employ a secondary radiation grid to attenuate scatter.
- Refer to local protocols for the removal of immobilisation collars when undertaking these examinations.

Radiation protection/dose

Care should be taken when collimating to avoid including the eyes within the primary beam.

Expected DRL: DAP 0.15 Gy cm^2.

6 Cervical vertebrae

Right and left posterior oblique – erect (Fig. 6.14a)

Oblique projections are requested mainly to supplement the basic projections in cases of trauma. The images demonstrate the intervertebral foramina, the relationship of the facet joints in suspected dislocation or subluxation as well as the vertebral arches. Oblique projections have also been used with certain pathologies, such as degenerative disease.

Position of patient and imaging receptor

- The patient stands or sits with the posterior aspect of their head and shoulders against the vertical Bucky digital detector system (with or without a grid) or CR cassette.
- The median sagittal plane of the trunk is rotated through 45° for right and left sides in turn.
- The head can be rotated so that the median sagittal plane of the head is parallel to the receptor, thus avoiding superimposition of the mandible on the vertebra.
- The image receptor is centred at the prominence of the thyroid cartilage.

Direction and location of the X-ray beam

- The collimated beam is angled 15° cranially from the horizontal and the central ray is directed to the middle of the neck on the side nearest the tube.

Essential image characteristics (Figs 6.14b, 6.14c)

- The intervertebral foramina should be demonstrated clearly.
- C1 to T1 should be included within the image.
- The mandible and the occipital bone should be clear of the vertebrae.

Radiological considerations

- If this and the swimmers' projections are not successful, the patient may require CT).
- Complex radiographic projections are less often needed where magnetic resonance imaging (MRI) and/or CT are available as these may be the preferred method of solving difficult cases.

Notes

- Anterior oblique projections are usually undertaken on mobile patients. The position used is exactly the opposite to the posterior oblique projection, i.e. the patient faces the image receptor and a 15°caudal angulation is used. Use of this projection will reduce the radiation dose to the thyroid.
- The foraminae demonstrated on the posterior oblique are those nearest the X-ray tube.

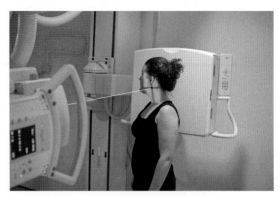

Fig. 6.14a Patient positioning for posterior oblique erect projection.

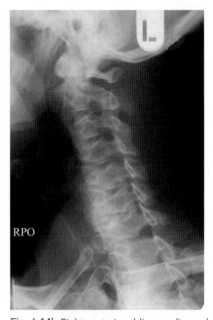

Fig. 6.14b Right posterior oblique radiograph.

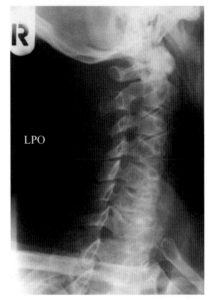

Fig. 6.14c Left posterior oblique radiograph.

Radiation protection/dose

- Care should be taken when collimating to avoid including the eyes within the primary beam.

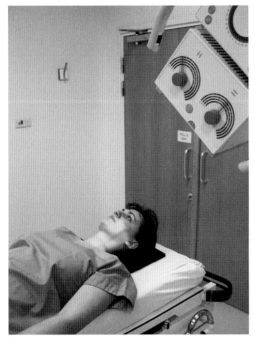

Fig. 6.15a Schematic diagram of the head and neck showing central beam angulations.

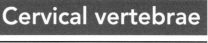

Cervical vertebrae 6

Right and left posterior oblique – supine (Figs 6.15a, 6.15b)

This positioning is often necessary in cases of severe injury, particularly if other basic projections have failed to demonstrate the lower cervical vertebrae.

Position of patient and image receptor

- The patient remains in the supine position on the casualty trolley.
- To avoid moving the neck, the CR cassette should ideally be placed in the cassette tray underneath the trolley.
- If no cassette tray is available, then the cassette can be slid carefully into position without moving the patient's neck.

Direction and location of the X-ray beam

- The collimated beam is angled 30–45° to the median sagittal plane (the degree of angulation will depend on local protocols).
- The central ray is directed towards the middle of the neck on the side nearest the tube at the level of the thyroid cartilage.

Radiological considerations

- If this and the swimmers' projections are not successful, the patient may require more complex imaging (e.g. CT).

Common faults and solutions

- Unless the equipment used allows alignment of the grid slats with the tube angle, then a grid cut-off will result.
- Grid cut-off can be prevented by not using a grid. Alternatively, the gridlines can be positioned to run transversely. This will result in suboptimal demonstration of the intervertebral foramina, but the image will be of diagnostic quality.

Fig. 6.15b Patient positioning.

6 Cervico-thoracic vertebrae

Lateral swimmers' (Figs 6.16a–6.16c)

In all trauma radiography, it is imperative that all of the cervical vertebrae and the cervico-thoracic junction are demonstrated. This is particularly important, as this area of the spine is particularly susceptible to injury. The superimposition of the shoulders over these vertebrae and subsequent failure to produce an acceptable image is a familiar problem to all radiographers. In the majority of cases, the use of the swimmers' lateral will produce an image that reveals the alignment of these vertebrae and provides an image suitable for diagnosis.

Position of patient and image receptor

- This projection is usually carried out with the patient supine on a trauma trolley. The trolley is positioned adjacent to the vertical Bucky digital detector system, with the patient's median sagittal plane parallel with the receptor.
- The arm nearest the receptor is folded over the head, with the humerus as close to the trolley top as the patient can manage. The arm and shoulder nearest the X-ray tube are depressed as far as possible.
- The shoulders are now separated vertically.
- The detector system should be raised or lowered, such that the line of the vertebrae should coincide with the middle of the receptor.
- This projection can also be undertaken with the patient erect, either standing or sitting or supine.

Direction and location of the X-ray beam

- The collimated horizontal central ray is directed to the midline of the image receptor at a level just above the shoulder remote from the receptor.

Essential image characteristics (Fig. 6.16d)

- It is imperative to ensure that the C7/T1 junction has been included on the image. It is important to include an anatomical landmark within the image that will make it possible to count down the vertebrae and ensure that the C7/T1 junction has been imaged.

Radiological considerations

- See Right and left posterior oblique – supine (previous page).

Common faults and solutions

- Failure to ensure that the raised arm is as flat as possible against the trolley may result in the head of the humerus obscuring the region of interest.

Notes

- For some patients, it may be useful to rotate the side further from the image receptor sufficiently forward to separate the shoulders transversely. This positioning will produce a lateral oblique projection of the vertebrae.

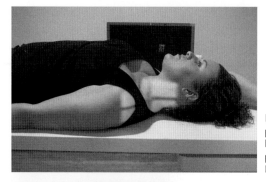

Fig. 6.16a Patient positioning for lateral swimmers' projection – supine HB.

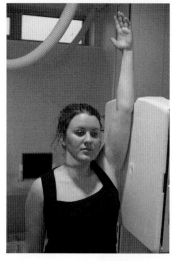

Fig. 6.16b Patient positioning for lateral swimmers' projection – erect.

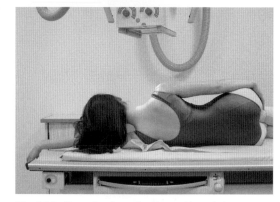

Fig. 6.16c Example of good radiographic technique.

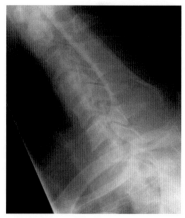

Fig. 6.16d Image of cervical spine using lateral swimmers' projection.

- Image quality will be increased if the erect Bucky is used in preference to a stationary grid. This is due to the better scatter attenuation properties of the grid within the Bucky.

A table Bucky DDR system is employed or alternatively a 35 × 43 cm CR cassette is placed in portrait mode in the Bucky tray using automatic exposure control (AEC).

Thoracic vertebrae 6

Antero-posterior (Basic) (Figs 6.17a, 6.17b)

Position of patient and image receptor

- The patient is positioned supine on the X-ray table, with the median sagittal plane perpendicular to the tabletop and coincident with the midline of the Bucky.
- The upper edge of the image detector or CR cassette (which should be at least 40 cm long for an adult), should be at a level just below the prominence of the thyroid cartilage to ensure that the upper thoracic vertebrae are included.
- Exposure is made on arrested inspiration. This will cause the diaphragm to move down over the upper lumbar vertebra, thus reducing the chance of a large density difference appearing on the image from superimposition of the lungs.

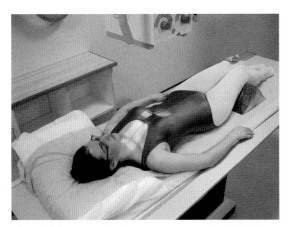

Fig. 6.17a Patient positioning.

Direction and location of the X-ray beam

- The vertical collimated beam is centred at right-angles to the image receptor and towards a point 2.5 cm below the sternal angle.
- The beam is collimated tightly to the spine.

Essential image characteristics

- The image should include the vertebrae from C7 to L1.
- The image density should be sufficient to demonstrate bony detail for the upper as well as the thoracic lower vertebrae.

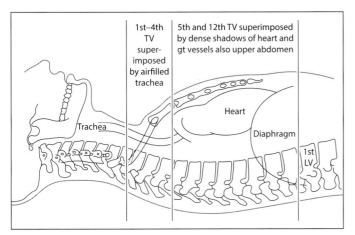

Fig. 6.17b Schematic diagram of anatomy.

Radiological considerations

- The presence of intact pedicles is an important sign in excluding metastatic disease. Pedicles are more difficult to see on an underexposed or rotated image.

Common faults and solutions

- The image receptor and beam are often centred too low, thereby excluding the upper thoracic vertebrae from the image.
- The lower vertebrae are also often not included. L1 can be identified easily by the fact that it usually will not have a rib attached to it.
- High radiographic contrast (see below) causes high density over the upper vertebrae and low density over the lower vertebra (Fig. 6.17c).

Note

- This region has an extremely high subject contrast due to the superimposition of the air-filled trachea over the upper thoracic vertebrae producing a relatively lucent area and a high density on the radiograph. The heart and liver superimposed over the lower thoracic vertebrae will attenuate more X-rays and yield a much lower image density. This can be compensated by the use of a high kV technique (Fig. 6.17d).

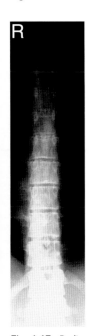

Fig. 6.17c Radiographic contrast too high.

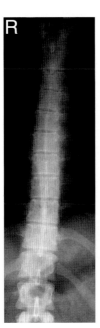

Fig. 6.17d Lower contrast producing acceptable density for upper and lower vertebrae.

Radiation protection/dose

Expected DRL: DAP 1.0 Gy cm^2, ESD 3.5 mGy.

6 Thoracic vertebrae

Lateral (Basic) (Figs 6.18a, 16.8b)

Position of patient and image receptor
- The examination is usually undertaken with the patient in the lateral decubitus position on the X-ray table, although this projection can also be performed erect.
- The median sagittal plane should be parallel to the image receptor and the midline of the axilla coincident with the midline of the table or Bucky.
- The arms should be raised well above the head.
- The head can be supported with a pillow, and pads may be placed between the knees for the patient's comfort.
- The upper edge of the image detector or cassette should be at least 40 cm in length and should be positioned 3–4 cm above the spinous process of C7.

Direction and location of the X-ray beam
- The collimated vertical beam should be at right-angles to the long axis of the thoracic vertebrae. This may require a caudal angulation.
- Centre 5 cm anterior to the spinous process of T6/7. This is usually found just below the inferior angle of the scapula (assuming the arms are raised), which is easily palpable.

Essential image characteristics
- The upper two or three vertebrae may not be demonstrated due to the superimposition of the shoulders.
- Look for the absence of a rib on L1 at the lower border of the image. This will ensure that T12 has been included within the field.
- The posterior ribs should be superimposed, thus indicating that the patient was not rotated too far forwards or backwards.
- The trabeculae of the vertebrae should be clearly visible, demonstrating an absence of movement unsharpness.
- The image density should be adequate for diagnosis for both the upper and lower thoracic vertebrae. The use of a wide-latitude imaging system/technique is therefore desirable in conventional screen/film system and an appropriate software algorithm selected for digital radiography.

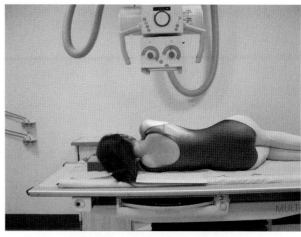

Fig. 6.18a Patient positioning.

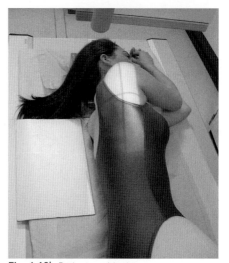

Fig. 6.18b Patient positioning.

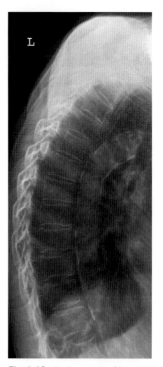

Fig 6.18c Radiograph of lateral thoracic spine.

Radiological considerations

- Mild endplate changes (e.g. early osteoporotic collapse or partial wedge fractures) are more difficult to see if the X-ray beam does not pass directly through all the disc spaces.
- 7–10% of cervical spine fractures are associated with fractures of the thoracic or lumbar vertebrae.[1]
- Radiographs of the whole spine should be considered when a cervical spine fracture is identified.

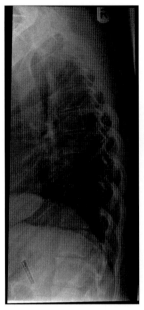
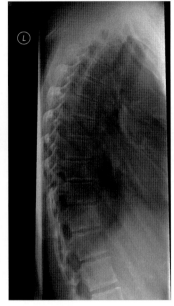

Figs. 6.19a and b The use of autotomography (6.19b) will prevent lung and rib shadows from obscuring the spine.

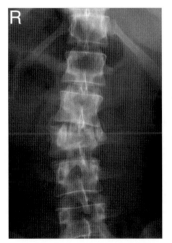
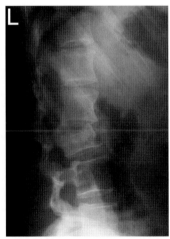

Fig. 6.19c and d Examples of localised spine projections.

Thoracic vertebrae 6

Lateral (Basic) (*cont.*)

Common faults and solutions (Figs 6.19a, 6.19b)

- If the exposure is made on arrested inspiration, then the rib shadows will be superimposed over the vertebrae and detract from the image quality. The use of autotomography (see below) should resolve this problem.

Note

- The vertebrae will be demonstrated optimally if autotomography is used to diffuse the lung and rib shadows. This involves setting a low mA (10–20 mA) and a long exposure time (3–5 s). The patient is allowed to breathe normally during the exposure.

Radiation protection/dose

Expected DRL: DAP 1.5 Gy cm², ESD 7 mGy.

Localised projections (Figs 6.19c, 6.19d)

Localised projections or tomography are requested occasionally, e.g. when following up a fracture. The centring point must be adjusted to the appropriate vertebrae. The following anterior surface markings can be used as a guide to the appropriate centring point:

- Cricoid cartilage: sixth cervical vertebra.
- Sternal notch: 2nd to 3rd thoracic vertebra.
- Sternal angle: lower border of 4th thoracic vertebra.
- Xiphisternal joint: 9th thoracic vertebra.

Posterior surface markings are more convenient for lateral projections. The level of the upper and middle thoracic vertebrae may be found by first palpating the prominent spinous process of the 7th cervical vertebrae and then counting the spinous processes downwards. The lower vertebrae can be identified by palpating the spinous process of the 3d lumbar vertebrae at the level of the lower costal margin and then counting the spinous processes upwards.

It is important to remember that the tips of the spinous processes of T5 to T10 are opposite to the bodies of the vertebrae below.

6 Thoracic vertebrae

Image evaluation – 10-point plan

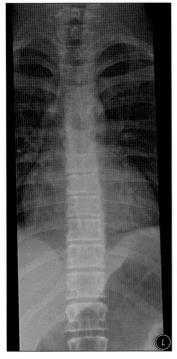

Fig. 6.20a AP thoracic spine.

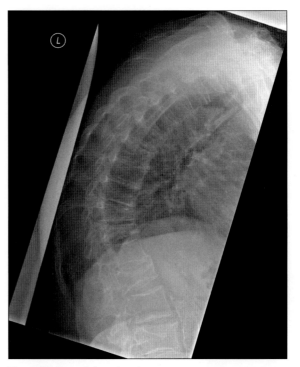

Fig. 6.20b Lateral thoracic spine.

IMAGE EVALUATION

AP thoracic spine (Fig. 6.20a)

Main points to consider:

- Inferior aspect of C7 to L2 demonstrated.
- Posterior aspect of ribs demonstrated due to collimation.
- Side markers applied at time of exposure throughout the image.
- Optimum exposure with good range of contrast.
- No repeat required.

Radiographer Comments/Initial report

Alignment of spinous processes with intervertebral disc spaces demonstrated.
No loss of vertebral body height and no abnormality seen.

IMAGE EVALUATION

Lateral thoracic spine (Fig. 6.20b)

Main points to consider:

- C7 to L2 fully demonstrated.
- Anterior rotation of the trunk.
- Longitudinal rotation in upper thoracic spine, obliquity of vertebral bodies in this region.
- Side marker added post processing.
- Diagnostic image with no repeat required as pathologies demonstrated.

Radiographer Comments/Initial report

Multiple 'crush' type fractures to vertebral bodies in lower thoracic and upper lumbar spine.
Loss of bone density and increased thoracic kyphosis.

A table Bucky DDR system is employed or alternatively a 30 × 40 cm CR cassette is placed in portrait mode in the Bucky tray using AEC.

Position of patient and image receptor

- The patient lies supine on the Bucky table, with the median sagittal plane coincident with, and at right-angles to, the midline of the table and Bucky.
- The anterior superior iliac spines should be equidistant from the tabletop.
- The hips and knees are flexed and the feet are placed with their plantar aspect on the tabletop to reduce the lumbar arch and bring the lumbar region of the vertebral column parallel with the image receptor.

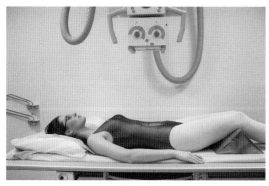

Fig. 6.21a AP patient positioning.

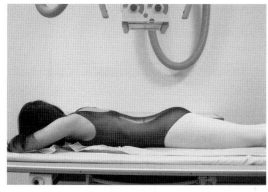

Fig. 6.21b PA patient positioning.

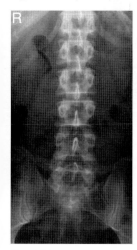

Fig. 6.21c AP projection.

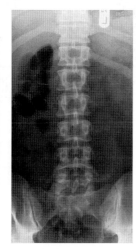

Fig. 6.21d PA projection: better visualisation of disc spaces and SI joints.

Lumbar vertebrae 6

Antero-posterior (Basic) (Figs 6.21a, 6.21b)

- If using a CR cassette this should be large enough to include the lower thoracic vertebrae and the sacro-iliac joints and is centred at the level of the lower costal margin.
- The exposure should be made on arrested expiration, as expiration will cause the diaphragm to move superiorly. The air within the lungs would otherwise cause a large difference in density and poor contrast between the upper and lower lumbar vertebrae.

Direction and location of the X-ray beam

- The collimated vertical beam is centred over the midline at the level of the lower costal margin (L3).

Essential image characteristics (Figs 6.21c, 6.21d)

- The image should include from T12 down, to include all of the sacro-iliac joints.
- Rotation can be assessed by ensuring that the sacro-iliac joints are equidistant from the spine.
- The exposure used should produce a density such that bony detail can be discerned throughout the region of interest.

Radiological considerations

The appearance of the lumbar spine on radiographs correlates poorly with symptoms and signs. Severe degenerative change on radiographs may be associated with minimal symptoms, and a prolapsed disc causing severe pain and disability be present with a normal radiograph. Since the advent of MRI, which has excellent soft-tissue resolution, the utility of plain X-ray images of the lumbar spine has reduced further still; local and national guidelines for use of lumbar spine radiography should be closely adhered to for patient safety.

Common faults and solutions

- The most common fault is to miss some or all of the sacro-iliac joint. An additional projection of the sacro-iliac joints should be performed if this is the case.

Note

- For relatively fit patients, this projection can be performed with the patient in the postero-anterior position. This allows better visualisation of the disc spaces and sacro-iliac joints, as the concavity of the lumbar lordosis faces the tube so the diverging beam passes directly through these structures. Although the magnification is increased, this does not seriously affect image quality.

6 Lumbar vertebrae

Lateral (Basic) (Figs 6.22a, 6.22b)

Position of patient and image receptor

- The patient lies on either side on the Bucky table. If there is any degree of scoliosis, then the most appropriate lateral position will be such that the concavity of the curve is towards the X-ray tube.
- The arms should be raised and resting on the pillow in front of the patient's head. The knees and hips are flexed for stability.
- The coronal plane running through the centre of the spine should coincide with, and be perpendicular to, the midline of the Bucky.
- Non-opaque pads may be placed under the waist and knees, as necessary, to bring the vertebral column parallel to the image receptor.
- The image receptor is centred at the level of the lower costal margin.
- The exposure should be made on arrested expiration.
- This projection can also be undertaken erect with the patient standing or sitting.

Direction and location of the X-ray beam

- The collimated vertical beam is centred at right-angles to the line of spinous processes and towards a point 7.5 cm anterior to the 3rd lumbar spinous process at the level of the lower costal margin.

Essential image characteristics (Fig. 6.22c)

- The image should include T12 downwards, to include the lumbar sacral junction.
- Ideally, the projection will produce adequate demonstration through the centre of the intervertebral disc space, with individual vertebral endplates superimposed.
- The cortices at the posterior and anterior margins of the vertebral body should also be superimposed.
- The imaging factors selected must produce an image density sufficient for diagnosis from T12 to L5/S1, including the spinous processes.

Radiation protection/dose

Expected DRL:
- Lateral – DAP 2.5 Gy cm^2, ESD 10 mGy.
- Antero-posterior – DAP 1.5 Gy cm^2, ESD 5.7 mGy.

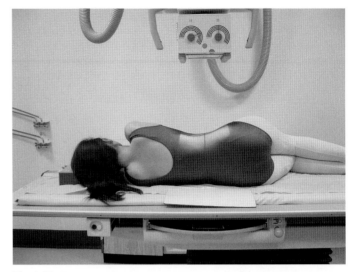

Fig. 6.22a Patient positioning.

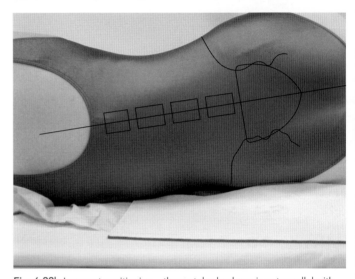

Fig. 6.22b Incorrect positioning – the vertebral column is not parallel with the table.

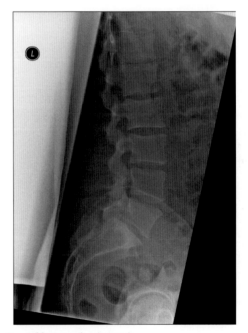

Fig. 6.22c Lateral radiograph.

Lumbar vertebrae 6

Lateral (Basic) (cont.)

Radiological considerations (Figs 6.23a, 6.23b)

- The same conditions apply as to the thoracic spine.
- Transitional vertebrae (see diagram opposite) are common at the lumbo-sacral junction and can make counting the level of an abnormality difficult. A sacralised L5 has a shape similar to S1, with large transverse processes, and is partially incorporated into the upper sacrum. The converse is lumbarisation of S1, in which the body and appendages of S1 resemble L5 and the sacro-iliac joints are often reduced in height. These anomalies may cause errors in counting the level of an abnormality, in which case the 12th rib and thoracic vertebra must be seen clearly to enable counting down from above. This is of particular importance when plain images are used to confirm the level of an abnormality detected on other imaging modalities, e.g. MRI.

Common faults and solutions (Figs 6.23c, 6.23d)

- High-contrast images will result in an insufficient or high image density over areas of high or low patient density, i.e. the spinous processes and L5/S1. A high kV or the use of other wide-latitude techniques and/or software application is recommended.
- The spinous processes can easily be excluded from the image as a result of overzealous collimation.
- Poor superimposition of the anterior and posterior margins of the vertebral bodies is an indication that the patient was rolled too far forward or backward during the initial positioning (i.e. mean sagittal plane not parallel to receptor).
- Failure to demonstrate a clear intervertebral disc space usually results as a consequence of the spine not being perfectly parallel with the receptor or is due to scoliosis or other patient pathology.

Note

- A piece of lead-rubber or other attenuator placed behind the patient will reduce scatter incident on the receptor. This will improve overall image quality as well as reduce the chance of AEC error.

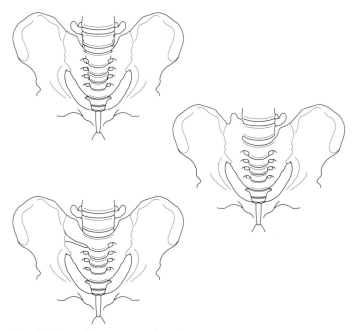

Fig. 6.23a Lumbar transitional vertebrae.

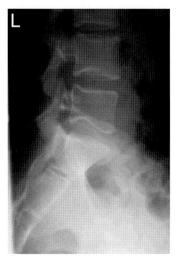

Fig. 6.23b Rudimentary disc at S1/S2.

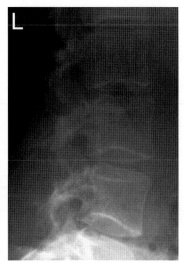

Fig. 6.23c Poor superimposition of anterior and posterior vertebral body margins due to poor positioning.

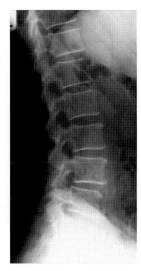

Fig. 6.23d Inappropriately high-contrast image.

6 Lumbar vertebrae

Lateral horizontal beam (Figs 6.24a, 6.24b)

A patient with a suspected fracture to the lumbar vertebrae should not be moved from the casualty trolley without medical supervision. Similarly, the patient should not be moved into the lateral decubitus position in these circumstances. This will necessitate the use of a horizontal beam technique in order to obtain the second projection required for a complete examination.

A vertical Bucky DDR system is employed or alternatively a 35 × 40 cm CR cassette is placed in landscape mode in the Bucky tray using AEC.

Position of patient and image receptor

- The trauma trolley is placed adjacent to the vertical Bucky/digital detector system.
- Adjust the position of the trolley so that the lower costal margin of the patient coincides with the vertical central line of the Bucky and the median sagittal plane is parallel to the image receptor.
- The Bucky should be raised or lowered such that the patient's mid-coronal plane is coincident with the midline of the receptor within the Bucky, along its long axis.
- If possible, the arms should be raised above the head.

Direction and location of the X-ray beam

- The collimated horizontal beam is directed parallel to a line joining the anterior superior iliac spines and centred towards a point 7.5 cm anterior to the 3rd lumbar spinous process at the level of the lower costal margin.

Essential image characteristics

- Refer to lateral lumbar spine (page 216).
- Extreme care must be taken if using the AEC. The chamber selected must be directly in line with the vertebrae, otherwise an incorrect exposure will result.
- If a manual exposure is selected, then a higher exposure will be required than with a supine lateral. This is due to the effect of gravity on the internal organs, causing them to lie either side of the spine.

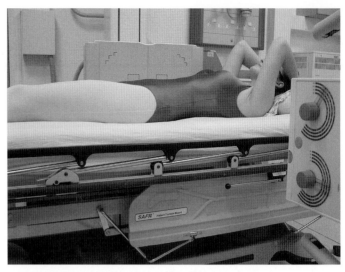

Fig. 6.24a Patient positioning seen from the side.

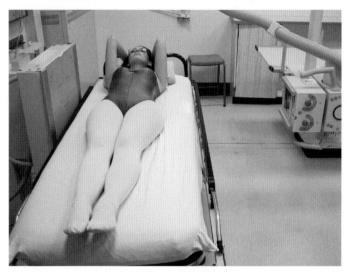

Fig. 6.24b Patient positioning seen from the feet.

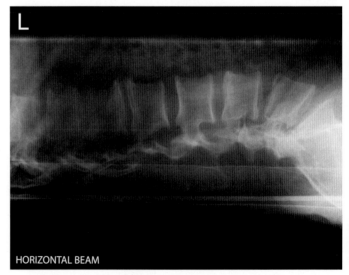

Fig. 6.24c Lateral lumbar spine image using a horizontal beam.

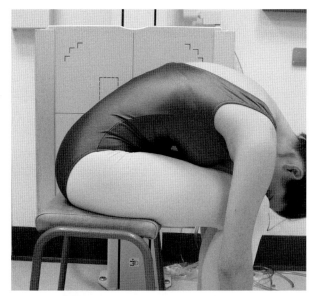

Fig. 6.25a Flexion.

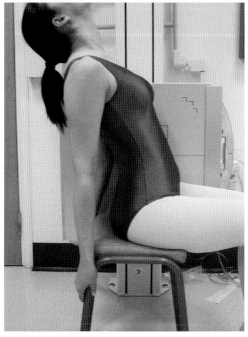

Fig. 6.25b Extension.

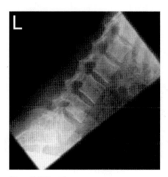

Fig. 6.25c Flexion.

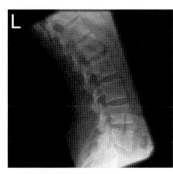

Fig. 6.25d Extension.

Lumbar vertebrae 6

Lateral flexion and extension (Figs 6.25a, 6.25b)

Lateral projections in flexion and extension may be requested to demonstrate mobility and stability of the lumbar vertebrae.

A vertical Bucky DDR system is employed or alternatively a 35 × 45 cm CR cassette is placed in portrait mode in the Bucky tray using AEC.

Position of patient and image receptor

- This projection may be performed supine, but it is most commonly performed erect with the patient seated on a stool with either side against the vertical Bucky/digital detector system.
- A seated position is preferred, since apparent flexion and extension of the lumbar region is less likely to be due to movement of the hip joints when using the erect position.
- The dorsal surface of the trunk should be at right-angles to the image receptor and the vertebral column parallel to the Bucky.
- For the first exposure the patient leans forward, flexing the lumbar region as far as possible, and grips the front of the seat to assist in maintaining the position.
- For the second exposure the patient then leans backward, extending the lumbar region as far as possible, and grips the back of the seat or another support placed behind the patient.
- The Bucky is centred at the level of the lower costal margin, and the exposure is made on arrested expiration.

Direction and location of the X-ray beam

- The collimated horizontal beam is directed at right-angles to the image receptor and centred towards a point 7.5 cm anterior to the 3rd lumbar spinous process at the level of the lower costal margin.

Essential image characteristics (Figs 6.25c, 6.25d)

- Refer to lateral lumbar spine (page 216).
- All of the area of interest must be included on both projections.

Common faults and solutions

- Extreme care must be taken if using the AEC. The AEC chamber selected must be directly in line with the vertebrae, otherwise an incorrect exposure will result.
- If a manual exposure is selected, a higher exposure will be required than with a supine lateral. This is due to the effect of gravity on the internal organs, causing them to lie either side of the spine.
- A short exposure time is desirable, as it is difficult for the patient to remain stable.

6 Lumbar vertebrae

Right or left posterior oblique (Fig. 6.26a)

These projections demonstrate the pars interarticularis and the apophyseal joints on the side nearest the image receptor. Both sides are taken for comparison.

A table Bucky DDR system is employed or alternatively a 30 × 40 cm CR cassette is placed in portrait mode in the Bucky tray using AEC.

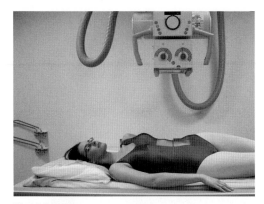

Fig. 6.26a Patient positioning.

Position of patient and image receptor

- The patient is positioned supine on the Bucky table and is then rotated 45° to the right and left sides in turn. The patient's arms are raised, with the hands resting on the pillow.
- The hips and knees are flexed and the patient is supported with a 45° foam pad placed under the trunk on the raised side.
- The image receptor is centred at the lower costal margin.

Direction and location of the X-ray beam

- The collimated vertical beam is centred towards the mid-clavicular line on the raised side at the level of the lower costal margin.

Essential image characteristics

- The degree of obliquity should be such that the posterior elements of the vertebra are aligned in such as way as to show the classic 'Scottie dog' appearance (Fig. 6.26d).

Radiological considerations (Figs 6.26b–6.26d)

The 'pars interarticularis' is part of the posterior elements of the vertebra supporting the facets that engage with the vertebra below to prevent forward slippage of one vertebra on another. A defect of pars can be unilateral or bilateral, and congenital or secondary to trauma. Abnormal mechanical stress in either case can be a cause of low back pain. If the defect is bilateral, the risk of anterior displacement of the cranial vertebra (spondylolisthesis) is increased. Spondylolisthesis can be a cause of pain, and may cause spinal stenosis resulting in symptoms due to compression of the nerve roots. The pars defect appears as a 'collar' on the 'Scottie dog', hence the importance of demonstrating the 'dog'.

Common faults and solutions

- A common error is to centre too medially, thus excluding the posterior elements of the vertebrae from the image.

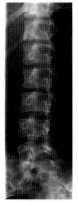
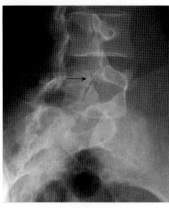

Fig. 6.26b Normal left posterior oblique.   Fig. 6.26c Defect in pars interarticularis at L5.

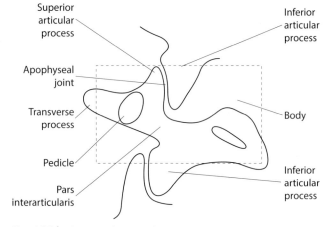

Fig. 6.26d Schematic drawing of anatomy.

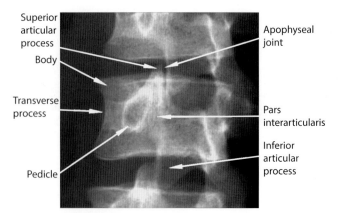

Fig. 6.26e Annotated radiograph.

Lumbar vertebrae 6

Image evaluation – 10-point plan

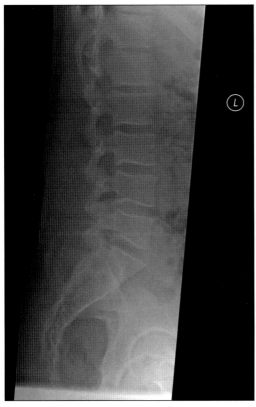

Fig. 6.27a Lateral lumber spine.

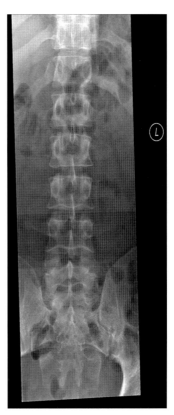

Fig. 6.27b AP lumbar spine.

IMAGE EVALUATION

Lateral lumbar spine (Fig. 6.27a)

Main points to consider:

- T12 to sacrum demonstrated.
- Centred inferiorly therefore whole sacrum visualised.
- No rotation in any plane.
- Spinous processes demonstrated.
- Good lateral collimation.
- Marker applied post processing.
- Optimal exposure with range of contrast.
- No repeat required.

Radiographer Comments/Initial report

Loss of normal lumbar lordosis with vertebral alignment intact.
No fracture or subluxation demonstrated.

IMAGE EVALUATION

AP lumbar spine (Fig. 6.27b)

Main points to consider:

- T11 to superior aspect of sacrum demonstrated.
- Cenred correctly with slightly rotated collimation.
- Posterior aspect of right sacro-iliac (SI) joint not included due to collimation.
- Optimal exposure to demonstrate bony detail of vertebral bodies.
- Marker added at post processing.
- Transverse processes of L1 and L2 not seen due to overlying bowel gas shadows.
- Further imaging required to demonstrate right SI joint.

Radiographer Comments/Initial report

Alignment of spinous processes with no loss of vertebral body height.
No fracture seen but further imaging required.

6 Lumbo-sacral junction

Lateral (Fig. 6.28a)

A table Bucky DDR system is employed or alternatively an 18 × 24 cm CR cassette is placed in portrait mode in the Bucky tray using AEC.

Position of patient and image receptor

- The patient lies on either side on the Bucky table, with the arms raised and the hands resting on the pillow. The knees and hips are flexed slightly for stability.
- The dorsal aspect of the trunk should be at right-angles to the image receptor. This can be assessed by palpating the iliac crests or the posterior superior iliac spines.
- The coronal plane running through the centre of the spine should coincide with, and be perpendicular to, the midline of the Bucky.
- The image receptor is centred at the level of the 5th lumbar spinous process.
- Non-opaque pads may be placed under the waist and knees, as necessary, to bring the vertebral column parallel to the image receptor.

Direction and location of the X-ray beam

- The collimated vertical beam is centred at right-angles to the lumbo-sacral region and towards a point 7.5 cm anterior to the 5th lumbar spinous process. This is found at the level of the tubercle of the iliac crest or midway between the level of the upper border of the iliac crest and the anterior superior iliac spine.
- If the patient has particularly large hips and the spine is not parallel with the tabletop, then a 5° caudal angulation may be required to clear the joint space.

Essential image characteristics (Fig. 6.28b)

- The area of interest should include the 5th lumbar vertebra and the first sacral segment.
- A clear joint space should be demonstrated.

Radiation protection/dose

- This projection requires a relatively large exposure so should not be undertaken as a routine projection. The lateral lumbar spine should be evaluated and a further projection for the L5/S1 junction considered if this region is not demonstrated to a diagnostic standard.

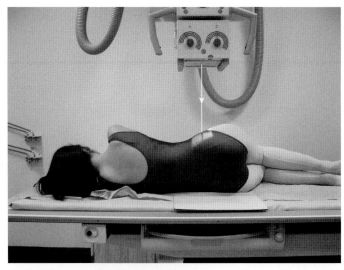

Fig. 6.28a Patient positioning.

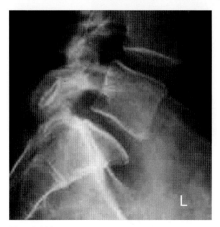

Fig. 6.28b Lateral radiograph.

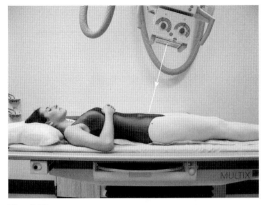

Fig. 6.29a Patient AP positioning.

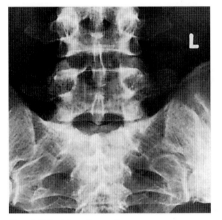

Fig. 6.29b AP radiograph.

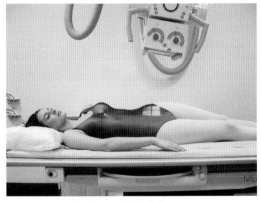

Fig. 6.29c Patient oblique positioning.

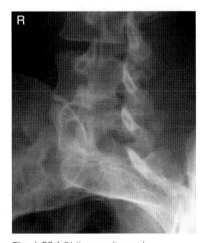

Fig. 6.29d Oblique radiograph.

Lumbo-sacral junction 6

Antero-posterior (Fig. 6.29a)

The lumbo-sacral articulation is not always demonstrated well on the antero-posterior lumbar spine, due to the oblique direction of the articulation resulting from the lumbar lordosis. This projection may be requested to specifically demonstrate this articulation.

Position of patient and image receptor

- The patient lies supine on the Bucky table, with the median sagittal plane coincident with, and perpendicular to, the midline of the Bucky.
- The anterior superior iliac spines should be equidistant from the tabletop.
- The knees can be flexed over a foam pad for comfort and to reduce the lumbar lordosis.
- The image receptor is displaced cranially so that its centre coincides with the central ray.

Direction and location of the X-ray beam

- The collimated central beam is directed 10–20° cranially from the vertical and towards the midline at the level of the anterior superior iliac spines.
- The degree of angulation of the central ray is normally greater for females than for males and will be less for a greater degree of flexion at the hips and knees.

Essential image characteristics (Fig. 6.29b)

- The image should be collimated to include the 5th lumbar and first sacral segment.

Right or left posterior oblique (Fig. 6.29c)

These projections demonstrate the pars interarticularis and the apophyseal joints on the side nearer the film.

Position of patient and image receptor

- The patient is positioned supine on the Bucky table and is then rotated to the right and left sides in turn so that the median sagittal plane is at an angle of approximately 45° to the tabletop.
- The hips and knees are flexed and the patient is supported with 45° foam pads placed under the trunk on the raised side.
- The image receptor is displaced cranially at a level to coincide with the central ray.

Essential image characteristics (Fig. 6.29d)

- The posterior elements of L5 should appear in the 'Scottie dog' configuration (see oblique lumbar spine, page 220).

Common faults and solutions

- A common error is to centre too medially, thus excluding the posterior elements of the vertebrae from the image.

6 Sacrum

Antero-posterior/postero-anterior (Figs 6.30a–6.30c)

The sacrum may be either imaged antero-posteriorly (AP) or postero-anteriorly (PA). If imaged PA, there will be various advantages, including a lower dose to the gonads and better demonstration of the sacro-iliac joints, as the joint spaces will be more parallel with the divergent central ray. The AP position may be a more realistic option when the patient is infirm or injured and therefore would find it difficult to maintain the prone position.

A table Bucky DDR system is employed or alternatively a 24 × 30 cm CR cassette is placed in portrait mode in the Bucky tray using AEC.

Position of patient and image receptor

- The patient lies supine or prone on the Bucky table, with the median sagittal plane coincident with, and at right-angles to, the midline of the Bucky.
- The anterior superior iliac spines should be equidistant from the tabletop.
- If the patient is examined supine (AP), the knees can be flexed over a foam pad for comfort. This will also reduce the pelvic tilt.
- The image receptor is displaced cranially for AP projection, or caudally for PA projections, such that its centre coincides with the angled central ray.

Direction and location of the X-ray beam

- Antero-posterior: the collimated central beam is directed 10–25° cranially from the vertical and towards a point midway between the level of the anterior superior iliac spines and the superior border of the symphysis pubis.
- The degree of angulation of the central ray is normally greater for females than for males and will be reduced for a greater degree of flexion at the hips and knees.
- Postero–anterior: palpate the position of the sacrum by locating the posterior superior iliac spine and coccyx. Centre to the middle of the sacrum in the midline.
- The degree of beam angulation will depend on the pelvic tilt. Palpate the sacrum and then simply apply a caudal angulation, such that the central ray is perpendicular to the long axis of the sacrum (see photograph opposite).

Radiological considerations

- The sacrum is a thin bone. Problems with exposure can easily lead to important pathologies such as fractures and metastases being missed.

Radiation protection/dose

Expected DRL: ESD 2.9 mGy*
* Based on a small sample size

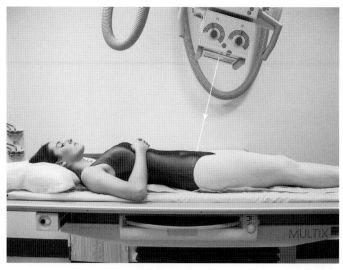
Fig. 6.30a AP patient positioning.

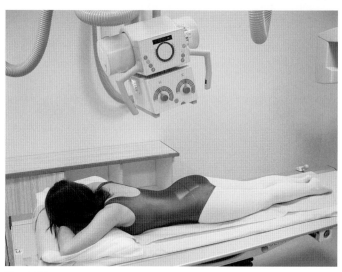
Fig. 6.30b PA patient positioning.

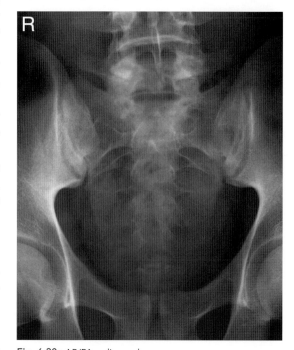
Fig. 6.30c AP/PA radiograph.

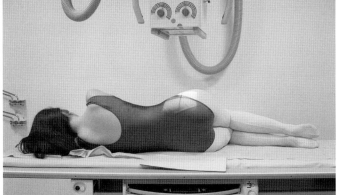

Fig. 6.31a Patient positioning.

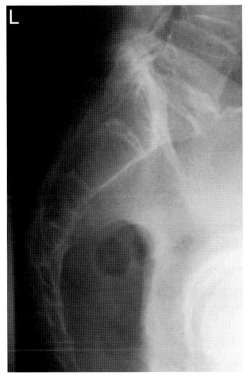

Fig. 6.31b Lateral radiograph.

Sacrum 6

Lateral (Figs 6.31a, 6.31b)

A table Bucky DDR system is employed or alternatively a 24 × 30 cm CR cassette is placed in portrait mode in the Bucky tray using AEC.

Position of patient and image receptor

- The patient lies on either side on the Bucky table with the arms raised and the hands resting on the pillow. The knees and hips are flexed slightly for stability.
- The dorsal aspect of the trunk should be at right-angles to the image receptor. This can be assessed by palpating the iliac crests or the posterior superior iliac spines. The coronal plane running through the centre of the spine should coincide with, and be perpendicular to, the midline of the Bucky.
- The image receptor is centred to coincide with the central ray at the level of the midpoint of the sacrum.

Direction and location of the X-ray beam

- The collimated vertical beam is directed at right-angles to the long axis of the sacrum and towards a point in the midline of the table at a level midway between the posterior superior iliac spines and the sacro-coccygeal junction.

Radiological considerations

- Fractures are easily missed if the exposure is poor or a degree of rotation is present.

Common faults solutions

- If using an automatic exposure control, centring too far posteriorly will result in an underexposed image.

Radiation protection/dose

Expected DRL: ESD 8.1 mGy*
* Based on a small sample size

6 Coccyx

Antero-posterior (Figs 6.32a, 6.32b)

A table Bucky DDR system is employed or alternatively an 18 × 24 cm CR cassette is placed in portrait mode in the Bucky tray using AEC.

Position of patient and image receptor

- The patient lies supine on the Bucky table, with the median sagittal plane coincident with, and at right-angles to, the midline of the Bucky.
- The anterior superior iliac spines should be equidistant from the tabletop.
- The knees can be flexed over a foam pad for comfort and to reduce the pelvic tilt.
- The image receptor is displaced caudally so that its centre coincides with the central ray.

Direction and location of the X-ray beam

- The collimated beam is directed 15° caudally towards a point in the midline 2.5 cm superior to the symphysis pubis.

Radiological considerations

- Anatomy of the coccyx is very variable (number of segments, angle of inclination, etc.).
- This is a high dose investigation with little yield unless the patient is to have a coccyxectomy, and should therefore be resisted unless requested by a specialist.

Lateral (Figs 6.32c, 6.32d)

Position of patient and image receptor

- The patient lies on either side on the Bucky table, with the palpable coccyx in the midline of the Bucky. The arms are raised, with the hands resting on the pillow. The knees and hips are flexed slightly for stability.
- The dorsal aspect of the trunk should be at right-angles to the image receptor. This can be assessed by palpating the iliac crests or the posterior superior iliac spines. The median sagittal plane should be parallel with the Bucky.
- The image receptor is centred to coincide with the central ray at the level of the coccyx.

Direction and location of the X-ray beam

- The collimated vertical beam is directed at right-angles to the long axis of the sacrum and towards the palpable coccyx.

Common faults and solutions

Care must be taken when using an AEC, as underexposure can easily result if the chamber is positioned slightly posterior to the coccyx.

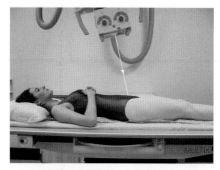
Fig. 6.32a AP patient positioning.

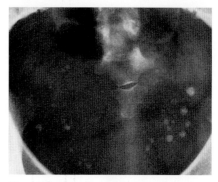
Fig. 6.32b AP radiograph.

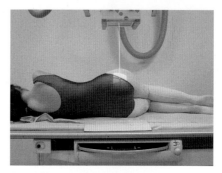
Fig. 6.32c Lateral patient positioning.

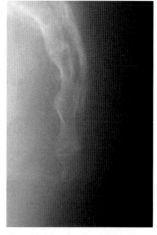
Fig. 6.32d Lateral radiograph.

Section 7

Thorax and Upper Airway

CONTENTS

THORAX: PHARYNX AND LARYNX	228
Antero-posterior	228
Lateral	229
THORAX: TRACHEA (INCLUDING THORACIC INLET)	230
Antero-posterior	230
Lateral	231
LUNGS	232
Introduction	232
Radiographic anatomy	238
General radiological considerations	239
Postero-anterior – erect	240
Antero-posterior – erect	242
Antero-posterior – supine	243
Antero-posterior – semi-erect	244
Lateral	245
Apices	246
Upper anterior region – lateral	247
Lordotic	247
Image evaluation – 10-point plan	248
HEART AND AORTA	250
Introduction	250
Postero-anterior	252
Left lateral	254
Right anterior oblique	255
BONES OF THE THORAX	256
Introduction	256
Recommended projections	257
LOWER RIBS	258
Antero-posterior (basic)	258
Right and left posterior oblique	259
UPPER RIBS	260
Right and left posterior oblique	260
First and second – antero-posterior	261
Cervical – antero-posterior	261
STERNUM	262
Anterior oblique – tube angled	262
Anterior oblique – trunk rotated	263
Lateral	264

7 Thorax: pharynx and larynx

Plain radiography is requested to investigate the presence of soft-tissue swellings and their effects on the air passages, as well as to locate the presence of foreign bodies or assess laryngeal trauma. Tomography, computed tomography (CT) magnetic resonance imaging (MRI) may be needed for full evaluation of other disease processes.

It is common practice to take two projections, an antero-posterior (AP) and a lateral. Each image is acquired using a computed radiography (CR) image receptor or alternatively within the field of view of a direct digital radiography (DDR) detector system.

For CR a 24 × 30-cm image receptor size cassette is employed.

Antero-posterior (Fig. 7.1a)

Positioning patient and image receptor

- The patient lies supine with the median sagittal plane adjusted to coincide with the central long axis of the couch.
- The chin is raised to show the soft tissues below the mandible and to bring the radiographic baseline to an angle of 20° from the vertical.
- The image receptor is centred at the level of the 4th cervical vertebra.

Direction and location of the X-ray beam

- The collimated vertical beam is directed 10° cranially and centred in the midline at the level of the 4th cervical vertebra.
- Exposure is made on forced expiration (Valsalva manoeuvre).

Essential image characteristics (Figs 7.1b, 7.1c)

- The beam should be collimated to include an area from the occipital bone to the 7th cervical vertebra.

Notes

- Image acquisition may be made either with or alternatively without a Bucky grid.
- Assessment of possible small foreign bodies may not require the AP projection, as such foreign bodies are likely to be obscured by virtue of overlying cervical spine.
- Air in the pharynx and larynx will result in an increase in subject contrast in the neck region. This may be reduced using a high kilovoltage technique.

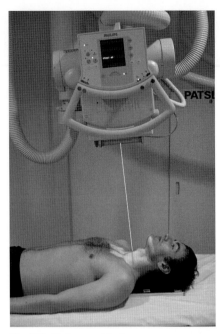

Fig. 7.1a Patient positioning.

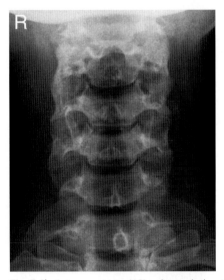

Fig. 7.1b Antero-posterior (AP) radiograph showing normal larynx.

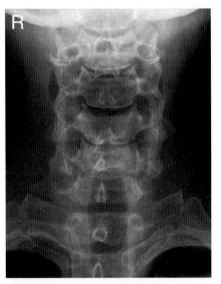

Fig. 7.1c AP radiograph of larynx showing a laryngocoele.

Thorax: pharynx and larynx 7

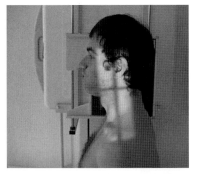

Fig. 7.2a Patient positioning.

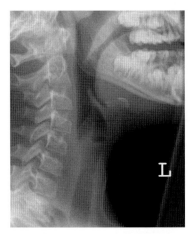

Fig. 7.2b Lateral radiograph showing normal air-filled larynx.

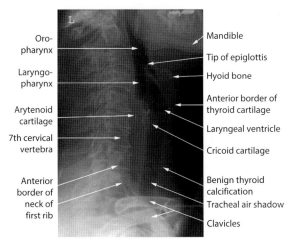

Fig. 7.2c Labelled radiograph of pharynx and larynx.

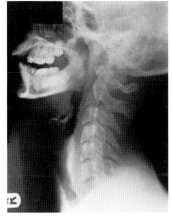

Fig. 7.2d Lateral radiograph showing fracture of the hyoid bone.

Lateral (Fig. 7.2a)

Position of patient and image receptor

- The patient stands or sits with either shoulder against the CR cassette or vertical Bucky digital detector system (a grid may be employed dependent on department protocols).
- Two 45° pads may be placed between the patient's head and the cassette to aid immobilisation.
- The median sagittal plane of the trunk and head are parallel to the image receptor.
- The jaw is slightly raised so that the angles of the mandible are separated from the bodies of the upper cervical vertebrae.
- A point 2.5 cm posterior to the angle of the mandible should be coincident with the vertical central line of the image receptor.
- The image receptor is centred at the level of the prominence of the thyroid cartilage opposite the 4th cervical vertebra.
- Immediately before exposure the patient is asked to depress the shoulders forcibly so that their structures are projected below the level of the 7th cervical vertebra.
- When carrying out this manoeuvre the head and trunk must be maintained in position.
- Exposure is made on forced expiration (Valsalva manoeuvre).

Direction and location of the X-ray beam

- The collimated horizontal central ray is centred to a point vertically below the mastoid process at the level of the prominence of the thyroid cartilage through the 4th cervical vertebra.

Essential image characteristics (Figs 7.2b–7.2d)

- The soft tissues should be demonstrated from the skull base to the root of the neck (C7).
- Exposure should allow clear visualisation of laryngeal cartilages and any possible foreign body.

Radiological considerations

- If the prevertebral soft tissues at the level of C4–C6 are wider than the corresponding vertebral body, soft-tissue swelling can be diagnosed (this may be the only sign of a lucent foreign body). This sign may be mimicked if the neck is flexed, or masked if the projection is oblique. A true lateral with adequate extension of the neck is therefore essential.
- The cartilages of the larynx typically calcify in a disparate pattern, and may mimic foreign bodies.

Radiation protection/dose

- Care should be taken when collimating to avoid including the eyes within the primary beam.

7 Thorax: trachea (including thoracic inlet)

Plain radiography is requested to investigate the presence of soft-tissue swellings in the neck and the upper thorax and to demonstrate the effects on the air passages, e.g. the presence of retrosternal goitre.

Consideration should also be given to the fact that radiography in the lateral position will involve exposure of the neck and the relatively thicker upper thorax. A high kilovoltage technique should therefore be employed to demonstrate the full length of the trachea on one image.

Two projections, an antero-posterior (AP) and a lateral are taken using a Bucky DDR detector system or CR cassette with moving grid technique. If used, a CR cassette size is selected that will include the full length of the trachea.

CT, tomography or a digital volume radiography technique of the trachea may be required for more complex problems.

Antero-posterior (Fig. 7.3a)

Position of patient and image receptor

- The patient lies supine with the median sagittal plane adjusted to coincide with the central long axis of the couch.
- The chin is raised to show the soft tissues below the mandible and to bring the radiographic baseline to an angle of 20° from the vertical.
- The image receptor is centred at the level of the sternal notch.

Direction and location of the X-ray beam

- The collimated vertical beam is directed in the midline at the level of the sternal notch.
- Exposure is made on forced expiration (Valsalva manoeuvre).

Essential image characteristics (Figs 7.3b, 7.3c)

- The beam should be collimated to include the full length of the trachea, i.e. below the level of T7.

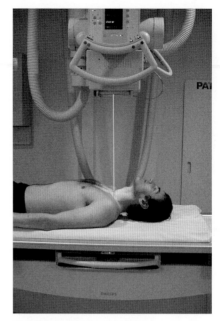

Fig. 7.3a Patient positioning.

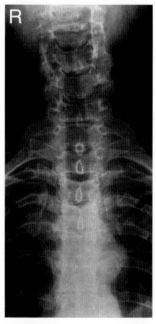

Fig. 7.3b Antero-posterior (AP) radiograph showing normal trachea.

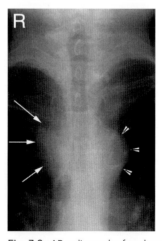

Fig. 7.3c AP radiograph of trachea showing paratracheal lymph node mass (arrows). The arrowheads indicate the aortic arch.

Thorax: trachea (including thoracic inlet) 7

Lateral (Fig. 7.4a)

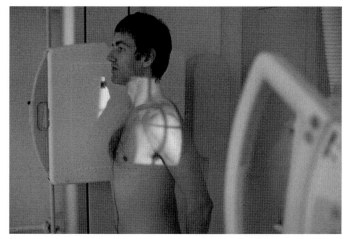

Fig. 7.4a Patient positioning.

Image acquisition is best performed with the patient erect, thus enabling the patient to position the shoulders away from the area of interest.

Position of patient and image receptor

- The patient stands or sits with either shoulder against a vertical Bucky digital detector system.
- The median sagittal plane of the trunk and head are parallel to the image receptor.
- A point 5.0 cm posterior to the sternal notch should be coincident with the vertical central line of the image receptor to ensure that the area of interest is central on the resultant image.
- If used, the CR cassette should be large enough to include from the lower pharynx to the lower end of the trachea at the level of the sternal angle.
- The shoulders are distracted posteriorly to enable the visualisation of the trachea.
- The patient clasping his hands behind the back and pulling his arms backwards aids this position.
- The image receptor is centred at the level of the sternal notch.

Direction and location of the X-ray beam

- The collimated horizontal central ray is directed to the vertical central line of the image receptor at the level of the sternal notch.
- The exposure is made on forced expiration.

Note

- The full length of the trachea can be demonstrated on a single image using a high kilovoltage technique (see page 40), which reduces the contrast between the neck and the denser upper thorax.

Radiological considerations (Figs 7.4b, 7.4c)

- This projection is sometimes helpful in confirming retrosternal extension of the thyroid gland. Most assessments of the trachea itself will be by bronchoscopy and/or CT (especially multislice CT with multiplanar reconstruction [MPR] and 3-D display).
- An anterior mediastinal mass (e.g. retrosternal thyroid) causes increased density of the anterior mediastinal window. This can also be mimicked by superimposed soft tissue if the patient's arms are not pulled backwards sufficiently away from the area of interest.

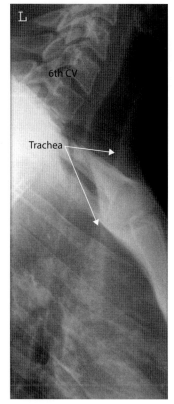

Fig. 7.4b Lateral radiograph showing normal air-filled trachea.

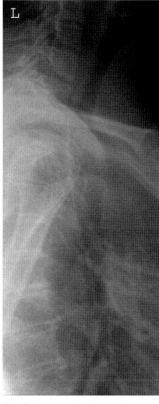

Fig. 7.4c Lateral radiograph showing compression and posterior deviation of the trachea by an enlarged thyroid. Note the shoulders are not pulled back to the ideal position and the humeral heads just overlap the trachea.

7 Lungs

Introduction (Figs 7.5a, 7.5b)

Radiographic examination of the lungs is performed for a wide variety of medical conditions, including primary lung disease and pulmonary effects of diseases in other organ systems. Such effects produce significant changes in the appearance of the lung parenchyma and may vary over time, depending on the nature and extent of the disease.

Imaging may also be performed using a variety of imaging modalities, notably CT and radionuclide imaging.

Recommended projections

Examination is performed by means of the following projections:

Basic	PA – erect
Alternative	AP – erect AP – supine AP – semi-erect
Supplementary	Lateral PA – expiration Apices Lateral – upper anterior region Decubitus with HB Tomography

AP, antero-posterior; HB, horizontal beam; PA, postero-anterior.

Positioning

The choice of erect or decubitus technique is governed primarily by the condition of the patient, with the majority of patients positioned erect. Very ill patients and patients who are immobile are X-rayed in the supine or semi-erect position (see Section 11). With the patient erect, positioning is simplified, control of respiration is more satisfactory, the gravity effect on the abdominal organs allows for the disclosure of the maximum area of lung tissue, and fluid levels are defined more easily with the use of a horizontal central ray.

The postero-anterior projection (PA) is generally adopted in preference to the antero-posterior (AP) because the arms can be arranged more easily to enable the scapulae to be projected clear of the lung fields. Heart magnification is also reduced significantly compared with the AP projection.

This projection also facilitates compression of breast tissue with an associated reduction in dose to the breast tissue. Additionally, the dose to the thyroid is reduced.

The mediastinal and heart shadows, however, obscure a considerable part of the lung fields, and a lateral radiograph may be necessary in certain situations.

Supplementary projections may be required for specific indications at the request of a clinician or radiologist (see table above).

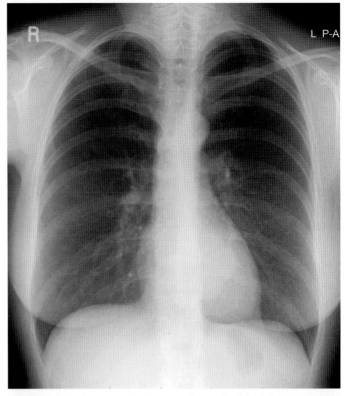

Fig. 7.5a Normal postero-anterior (PA) radiograph of chest.

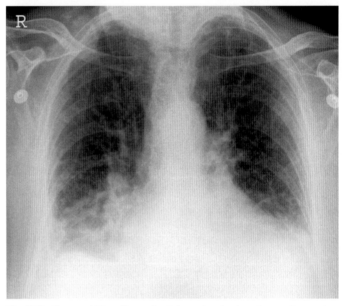

Fig. 7.5b Abnormal PA radiograph of chest showing lung bases obscured by bilateral basal pulmonary oedema.

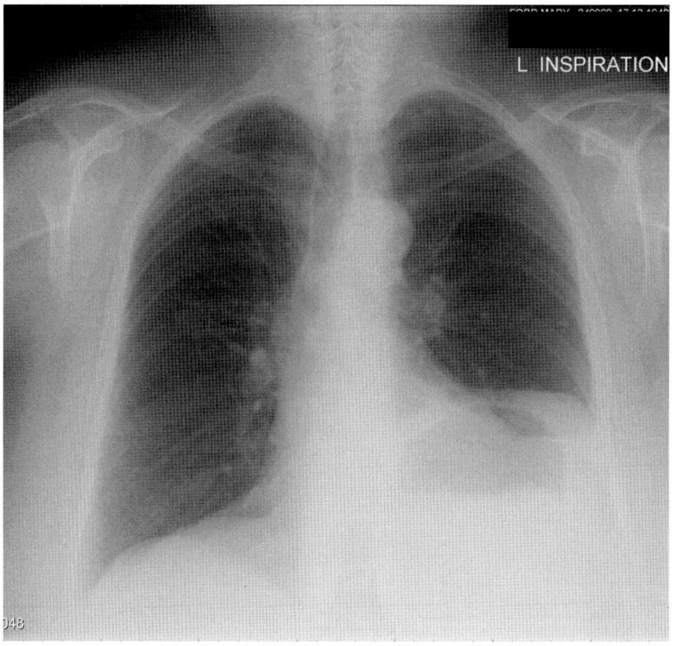

Lungs 7

Introduction (cont.) (Figs 7.6a–7.6c)

Respiration

Images are normally acquired on arrested deep inspiration, which ensures maximum visualisation of the air-filled lungs. The adequacy of inspiration of an exposed radiograph can be assessed by the position of the ribs above the diaphragm. In the correctly exposed image, it should be possible to visualise either six ribs anteriorly or ten ribs posteriorly.

A brief explanation to the patient, along with a rehearsal of the procedure, should ensure a satisfactory result. Respiratory movements should be repeated several times before the performance is considered to be satisfactory. With the patient having taken a deep breath, a few moments should be allowed to elapse to ensure stability before the exposure is made. Risk of movement is minimal by using equipment capable of using exposures in the region of 20 ms. On inspiration, there is a tendency to raise the shoulders, which should be avoided, as the shadows of the clavicles then obscure the lung apices.

A normal nipple shadow may be visible projected over the lower part of one or both lung fields on an AP radiograph, typically having a well-defined lateral border with an indistinct medial border. In cases of doubt, a simple metallic marker can be taped to the nipple and a repeat radiograph performed. If the opacity corresponds to the metal marker, then it is likely to be nipple. This may be confirmed further by an expiratory radiograph to show that both marker and opacity move together with respiration. Due to the radiation dose involved, these additional exposures should be made under the guidance of a radiologist. Soft-tissue artefacts are discussed on page 514.

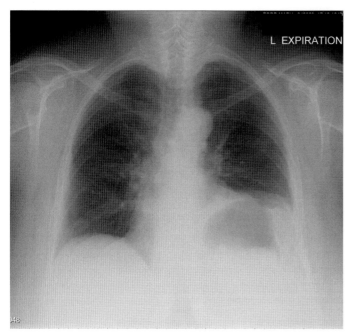

Fig. 7.6a PA radiograph on full inspiration.

Fig. 7.6b PA radiograph on expiration.

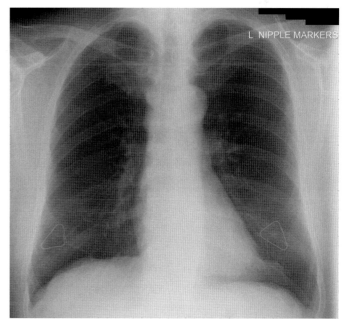

Fig. 7.6c Postero-anterior radiograph with nipple markers in situ.

7 Lungs

Introduction (*cont.*) (Figs 7.7a–7.7c)

Image acquisition

Radiography of the lung fields may be performed by a variety of imaging techniques. The following systems are available:

- Conventional screen/film with low kV.
- Conventional screen/film with high kV.
- Conventional screen/film with selective filter device.
- Digital acquisition using storage phosphor technology.
- Digital acquisition using semiconductor technology.
- Digital scanning with selenium detectors.

Selection of which imaging system is used will be dependent on the operational protocols of the imaging department. However, the overriding objective of whatever system is selected is to acquire an image of the thorax that will demonstrate all of the anatomical structures present including lung parenchyma behind the mediastinum and in the regions of the costophrenic angles (pleural reflection), where the lung fields may be obscured by abdominal structures.

The following table illustrates the optimum high and low contrast resolution criteria expected of an imaging system where the entrance surface dose (ESD) for a standard patient is 0.3 mGy using a conventional screen/film system.[1]

	High contrast	Low contrast
Small round details	0.7 mm diameter	2 mm diameter
Linear and reticular details	0.3 mm in width	2 mm in width

Imaging parameters

For adults a vertical chest stand with a stationary or moving grid is selected for patients who are able to stand unaided. Imaging without a grid is selected when a low kV technique is preferred.

The technique is modified when examining children and babies or examining adults whose medical condition is such that they require to be examined using mobile or portable X-ray equipment.

The following table illustrates the parameters necessary to provide optimum and consistent image resolution and contrast[1].

Item	Comment
Focal spot size	<1.3 mm
Total filtration	Not less than 3.0 mm Al equivalent
Anti-scatter grid	R = 10; 40/cm
Film-screen combination	Speed class 400
FFD/FRD	180 (140-200) cm
Radiographic voltage	125 kVp
Automatic exposure control	Chamber selected – right lateral
Exposure time	Less than 20 ms

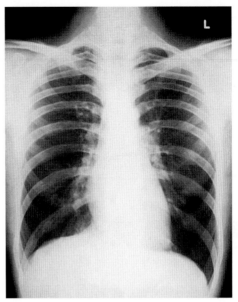

Fig. 7.7a PA chest radiograph taken using conventional screen–film combination at low kV.

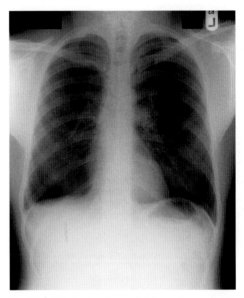

Fig. 7.7b PA chest radiograph taken using conventional screen–film combination at high kV.

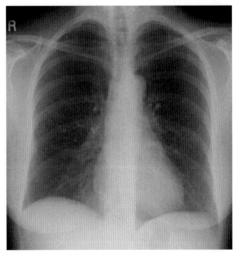

Fig. 7.7c PA chest radiograph taken using digital acquisition by storage phosphor technology.

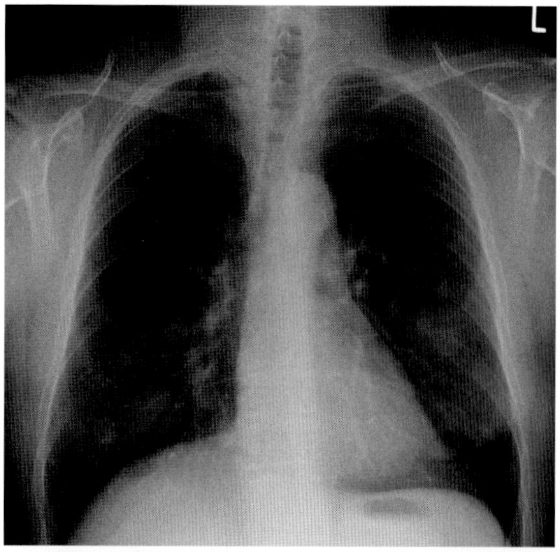

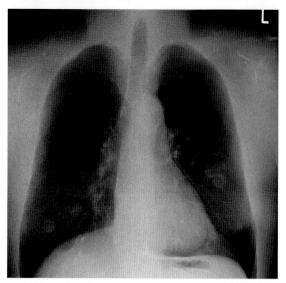

Fig. 7.8a Dual energy digital PA radiograph without subtraction.

Fig. 7.8b Dual energy digital PA radiograph with bone subtracted.

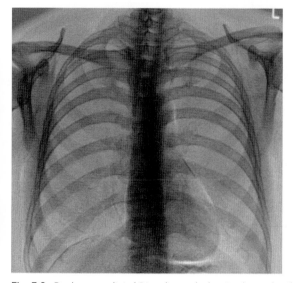

Fig. 7.8c Dual energy digital PA radiograph showing bone detail. The above example of standard, soft-tissue and bone images acquired using a dual-energy technique, with an exposure of less than 200 ms, illustrates how chest nodules can be best demonstrated on the soft-tissue image by removing overlying ribs.

Lungs 7

Introduction (cont.)

Choice of kilovoltage/dual-energy subtraction (Figs 7.8a–7.8c)

Selection of an appropriate kilovoltage should primarily provide adequate penetration from the hila to the periphery of the lung fields and should be in keeping with the patient thickness, habitus and pathology. In general, 60–70 kV provides adequate penetration for the PA projection, in which case there will be minor penetration of the mediastinum and heart. An increase in kilovoltage is necessary for penetration of the denser mediastinum and heart to show the lung behind those structures and behind the diaphragm, as well as the lung bases in a very large or heavy-breasted patient.

A high-kilovoltage technique (120–150 kV), appropriate to the film speed, reduces the dynamic range of information that needs to be recorded, thus enabling visualisation of the lung fields and mediastinum with one exposure. This technique also has the advantage of reducing radiation dose. However, with this technique there is a loss of subject contrast and therefore visualisation of small lesions of soft-tissue density becomes difficult. Additionally, rib lesions are more difficult to visualise adequately using a high-kilovoltage technique.

A range of kilovoltages (80–100 kV) midway between non-grid and high kilovoltages is used to compromise between the advantages and disadvantages of the two techniques.

Dual-energy digital subtraction can be used to overcome the problem of pathology obscured by overlying bones. In this technique, high- and low-energy images are acquired less than 200 ms apart during the same breath-hold. The low-energy image is subtracted from the standard high-kV image to produce bone and soft-tissue images. Three images are presented for viewing, similar to those shown opposite. Typically, there is up to 80 kV separating the exposures.

Maintaining general contrast/use of grid

Scattered radiation has the effect of reducing subject contrast and adding image noise. To combat these effects, especially when using a high-kV technique, selection of a grid with a grid ratio of at least 10:1 is necessary. For dedicated Bucky work, a grid designed to work at a focus-to-receptor distance (FRD) of 180 cm with a ratio of 12:1 is usually selected.

Grids with a lower grid ratio need less precise grid alignment and may be used for mobile radiography.

Air-gap technique

This technique employs the displacement of the subject from the image receptor by a distance of 15 cm. To reduce any geometric unsharpness, the FRD is increased to 300 cm. A high proportion of oblique scattered radiation from the subject will no longer fall on the image receptor because of the increased distance between subject and the receptor. A patient support, which is 15 cm in front of the image receptor, is used to steady the patient and provide the object-to-receptor distance (ORD).

7 Lungs

Introduction (cont.)

Magnification factor and focus-to-receptor distance (FRD) (Figs 7.9a, 7.9b)

To obtain minimal magnification of the intrathoracic structures, especially the heart, and structural detail at differing distances from the image receptor, FRDs in the range of 150–180 cm are selected. However, the FRD must be kept constant for any one department to allow comparison of successive images. At these distances, geometric unsharpness is greatly reduced. The selection of the focal spot size is governed by the maximum output of the generator, which enables the shortest exposure time to be selected for the examination at the kilovoltage set. Ideally, the focal spot size should be no greater than 1.3 mm for an FRD of 180 cm.

A FRD less than those recommended increases the image magnification. However, such a reduction in distance to 120 cm is a satisfactory means of obtaining a short exposure time when using low-output machines such as conventional mobile units.

Exposure time related to subject movement

Involuntary subject movement is reduced by the selection of the shortest exposure time available, preferably in the millisecond range. Ideally, exposure times should be less than 20 ms. This can be obtained with high-output units at the higher mA settings, balanced to the speed of the film and screen combination selected or speed system of the digital acquisition system and the kilovoltage selected. For conventional film technique the use of rare earth screens and fast film combinations is essential to ensure short exposure times.

With high kilovoltage, shorter exposure times are also possible, with the added advantage of selecting a smaller focal spot within the tube rating.

Uniformity

Automatic exposure control enable images to be acquired with comparable good quality over a period of time at each repeat examination. If used, automatic film processors should be monitored for constant performance. However, even without automatic exposure control (AEC), comparable good-quality images can be obtained for the same patient by the adoption of a technique that relates kV to chest thickness. This technique will also improve the possibility of greater uniformity throughout the range of patients.

If, for an average 22.5 cm thickness, for example, 67.5 kV is judged to give the required penetration and density at a selected mAs factor, then for each 1 cm difference in measured thickness, a 2–3 kV adjustment is added either as the thickness increases or as the thickness decreases.

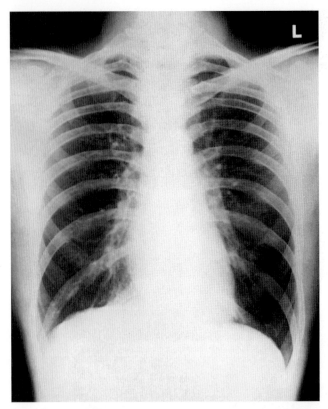

Fig. 7.9a FRD = 180 cm.

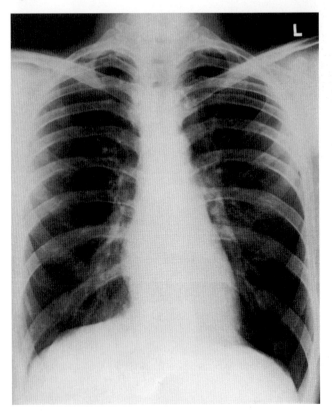

Fig. 7.9b FRD = 75 cm.

A record of exposure factors, used for each projection, should be made on either the X-ray request card or the computer records. Reference to these records will enable images of comparable good quality to be obtained over a period of time and in different sections of the same imaging department or hospital.

Lungs 7

Introduction (cont.)

Radiation protection

An adjustable rectangular diaphragm is used to collimate the radiation field to the size of the lung fields. This reduces the radiation dose to the patient. The effects of backscatter from walls can be reduced by suspending a piece of lead-rubber on the rear of the chest stand immediately behind the cassette holder or vertical Bucky.

The radiation dose to the sternum and mammary glands is minimised by employing, where possible, the PA projection of the chest in preference to the AP projection.

Film/intensifying screen combinations

Whilst digital imaging technology has mainly replaced screen/film systems various combinations of intensifying screens and film are still used in certain locations. When employed, screens are selected that enable the production of good quality radiographs that are free of movement unsharpness and quantum mottle. The radiation dose to the patient can be reduced considerably by selecting a 400 speed class screen/film combination. Faster speed systems, although reducing patient dose, have the disadvantage of introducing quantum mottle.

A major necessity in maintaining high quality radiographs is the assurance of good screen/film contact to eliminate unsharpness. Cassettes should be tested for this as well as inspecting them for damage around the hinges and corners. Intensifying screens should be cleaned regularly in accordance with the manufacturer's instructions.

Film processing equipment and processing chemicals should be subject to regular quality control to ensure high standards of image quality.

Tomosynthesis (Figs 7.10a–7.10c)

The new technique of digital tomosynthesis (DTS) can provide even greater detail and clarity of lung structure in the evaluation of equivocal abnormalities on a chest X-ray (CXR). This is described on page 526. The sensitivity of this test lies between CXR and CT, while the specificity is closer to that of CT. The time to read a DTS study is roughly twice that of a PA CXR but much less than a CT. The radiation dose is also approximately double a standard PA CXR, but 30–40 times less than CT.[2]

Identification

Accurate identification of chest radiographs is essential with information such as right or left sides, patient's name, date, hospital number and radiology identification number being clearly distinguished. Congenital transposition of the organs occurs in a small number of people and without the correct side marker the condition may be misdiagnosed. Additional information relating to orientation of the patient and tube different from the norm should also be recorded.

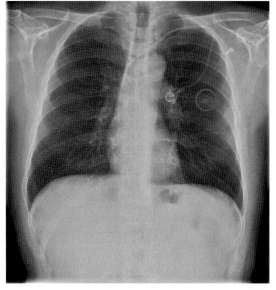

Fig. 7.10a Conventional chest PA image with suspected lesions (marked).

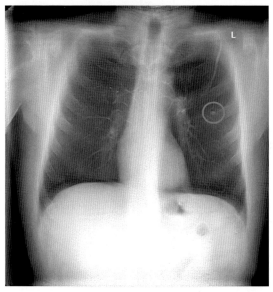

Fig. 7.10b Tomosynthesis slice image with on same patient confirming lesion.

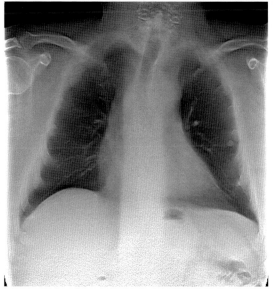

Fig. 7.10c Example of tomosynthesis slice image demonstrating a lung nodule.

7 Lungs

Radiographic anatomy (Figs 7.11a, 7.11b)

The lungs lie within the thoracic cavity on either side of the mediastinum, separated from the abdomen by the diaphragm. The right lung is larger than the left due to the inclination of the heart to the left side. In the normal radiographs of the thorax, some lung tissue is obscured by the ribs, clavicles and to a certain extent the heart, and also by the diaphragm in the PA projection.

The right lung is divided into upper, middle and lower lobes, and the left into upper and lower lobes. The fissures, which separate the lobes, can be demonstrated in various projections of the thorax, when the plane of each fissure is parallel to the beam. On a PA radiograph however, the main lobes overlap, so that for descriptive purposes the lungs are divided into three zones separated by imaginary horizontal lines. The anatomical location of pathology can sometimes be defined even on a PA view by observing the effect on visualisation of adjacent structures – for example middle lobe pneumonia obscuring the right heart border. The upper zone is above the anterior end of the 2nd ribs, the mid zone between the 2nd and 4th ribs anteriorly, and the lower zone below the level of the 4th ribs. On a lateral radiograph where horizontal and oblique fissures are visible, upper, middle and lower lobes can be defined separately. On a PA radiograph a horizontal fissure, separating upper and middle lobes, may be seen extending from the right hilum to the level of the right 6th rib laterally. An accessory lobe called the azygos lobe is sometimes seen in the right upper zone as a result of aberrant embryological migration of the azygos vein to the normal medial position. The azygos vein, surrounded by a double layer of visceral and parietal pleura, is seen as opacity at the lower end of the accessory fissure, resembling an inverted comma.

The trachea is seen centrally as a radiolucent air-filled structure in the upper thorax, which divides at the level of the 4th thoracic vertebra into the right and left main bronchi. The right main bronchus is wider, shorter and more vertical than the left, and as a result inhaled foreign bodies are more likely to pass into the right bronchial tree. The bronchi enter the hila, beyond which they divide into bronchi, bronchioles and finally alveolar air spaces, each getting progressively smaller.

As these passages are filled with air, they do not appear on a normal radiograph of the thorax, as the surrounding lung is also air filled. If the parenchyma is consolidated however, an air-filled bronchogram is shown.

The hilar regions appear as regions of increased radio-opacity and are formed mainly by the main branches of the pulmonary arteries and veins. The lung markings, which spread out from the hilar regions, are branches of these pulmonary vessels, and are seen diminishing in size as they pass distally from the hilar regions. The right dome of the diaphragm lies higher than the left mainly due to the presence of the liver on the right and the heart on the left. The costophrenic angles and lateral chest walls should be clearly defined.

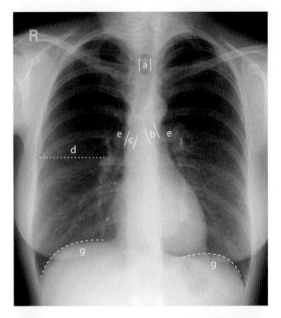

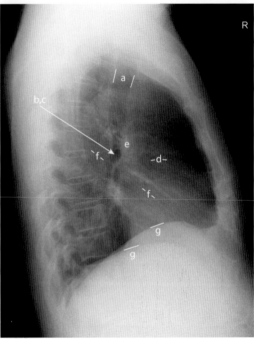

Fig. 7.11a PA radiograph of lungs. 7.11b Lateral radiograph of lungs.
(a) Trachea; (b) left main bronchus; (c) right main bronchus; (d) horizontal fissure; (e) pulmonary arteries; (f) oblique fissure; (g) diaphragm.

Special landmarks that may be seen in the PA image, although not in every image, are the subclavian vein over the apex of the left lung and the inferior vena cava appearing as a triangular shadow within the cardiophrenic angle of the right lung. Both appear as low-density shadows, as does the hair-like line of the fissure between the upper and middle lobes of the right lung.

Viewing radiographs of lung fields

Apart from AP projections all other radiographs are viewed as if the observer was looking toward the X-ray tube.

General observations

The CXR is a vital part of the investigation of many lung and cardiac conditions, often providing a differential diagnosis and thus the next appropriate examination. The CXR is complex, and not easy to interpret, but a high-technical quality examination with appropriate exposure on a digital image acquisition system or modern screen/film combination can provide a wealth of initial detail about the heart, mediastinum and thoracic cage, as well as the lung parenchyma and pulmonary vessels.

The amount of information available to the reader, and thereby the diagnostic usefulness of the examination, can be reduced by a variety of technical errors and problems. Many radiographs are initially read and acted upon by non-radiologists who may be less aware of the diagnostic limitations of a poor quality image. The aim is therefore to demonstrate the intrathoracic organs as fully as possible, though some areas (e.g. retrocardiac) will always be partially obscured.

Inspiration

Sub-maximal inspiration has several potential effects:

- The heart will swing up to a more horizontal lie and may thus appear enlarged.
- The lung bases will be less well inflated, which may simulate a variety of pathologies, or cause abnormal areas to lie hidden.
- Underinflation of the lower lobes causes diversion of blood to the upper lobe vessels, mimicking the early signs of heart failure.

Supine position

This posture is sometimes the best that can be achieved in a sick patient, but alters the appearance of some structures; these are detailed in the relevant section.

Semi-erect projection

The degree to which any patient is leaning from vertical in such a projection varies according to circumstances – age, fitness and location of patient, availability of assistance, etc. The patient may also lean to one side or the head may droop over the upper chest. It will be more difficult to ensure that the central ray is at right-angles to the image receptor. The viewer will have difficulty assessing how much allowance to make for posture and technical factors and for these reasons a supine image (being more standardised) is regarded by some radiologists as preferable to the 'semi-erect' image projection.

Antero-posterior projection

Magnification makes heart size and apical region difficult to assess as well as the mediastinum, which appears artificially widened causing difficulty in interpretation particularly when a traumatic or dissecting thoracic aortic aneurysm is suspected.

Rotation

Obliquity causes the side of the chest furthest removed from the image receptor plane to appear enlarged and hypodense, whilst the other side is partially obscured by the spine and more dense. A thoracic scoliosis may produce similar artefacts.

Lungs 7

General radiological considerations

The differing densities may simulate either abnormal density (e.g. consolidation or pleural effusion) on one side, or abnormal lucency (e.g. emphysema, air trapping) on the other.

Rotation markedly affects the appearance of the mediastinum and hila. The hilum of the raised side appears more prominent and may simulate a mass. The other hilum is overlaid by the spine, tending to obscure any mass that may be present and making other pathology such as consolidation more difficult to evaluate. Inadequate inspiration will cause the basal regions of the lungs to be obscured with similar effect.

Lordosis

An apical lordotic view is a useful view for a clearer depiction of the apices, but lordotic projection on an AP radiograph obscures more of the posterior basal part of the lung.

Exposure (see pages 234, 235)

- Overexposed images reduce visibility of lung parenchymal detail masking vascular and interstitial changes, and reducing the conspicuity of consolidation and masses. Pneumothorax becomes harder to detect.
- Underexposure can artificially enhance the visibility of normal lung markings, leading to them being wrongly interpreted as disease (e.g. pulmonary fibrosis or oedema).
- Underexposure also obscures the central areas causing failure to diagnose abnormalities of mediastinum, hila and spine.

Collimation

Good collimation is essential to optimal practice and dose reduction. Excessive collimation will exclude areas such as the costophrenic sulci (which may be the only site to indicate pleural disease). Failure to demonstrate the whole of the rib cage may lead to missed diagnosis of metastases, discrete fractures (this is especially important in patients with unexplained chest pains). Collimating off the apices can obscure early tuberculosis, apical (Pancoast) tumours and hide small pneumothoraces.

Soft-tissue artefacts

Soft-tissue artefacts are a common cause of confusion. One of the commonest of these is the normal nipple, diagnosis of which is discussed on page 233. Other rounded artefacts may be produced by benign skin lesions such as simple seborrhoeic warts or neurofibromata. Dense normal breast tissue or breast masses may also cause confusion with lung lesions. Breast implants may be obvious as a density with a thin curved line at the edge of the implant. Linear artefacts may be due to clothing or gowns, or in thin (often elderly) patients due to skin folds and creases. These are usually easy to spot but may be mistaken for the edge of the lung in a pneumothorax. Absence of soft tissue, as for example with a mastectomy, will produce hypertransradiancy of the ispilateral thorax although the lung itself is normal.

7 Lungs

Postero-anterior – erect (Fig. 7.12a)

A vertical Bucky DDR system is employed or alternatively a 35 × 43 cm or 35 × 35 cm CR cassette is selected, depending on the size of the patient. Orientation of a larger cassette will depend of the width of the thorax.

Position of patient and image receptor

- The patient is positioned facing the receptor with the chin extended and centred to the middle of the top of the receptor.
- The feet are paced slightly apart so that the patient is able to remain steady.
- The median sagittal plane is adjusted at right-angles to the middle of the receptor; the shoulders are rotated forward and pressed downward in contact with the receptor or vertical stand.
- This is achieved by placing the dorsal aspect of the hands behind and below the hips with the elbows brought forward, or by allowing the arms to encircle the vertical Bucky device.

Direction and location of the X-ray beam

- The collimated horizontal beam is directed at right-angles to the receptor and centred at the level of the 8th thoracic vertebrae (i.e. spinous process of T7) which is coincident with the lung midpoint.[3]
- The surface marking of T7 spinous process can assessed by using the inferior angle of the scapula before the shoulders are pushed forward.
- Exposure is made in full normal arrested inspiration.
- In a number of automatic chest film-changer devices the central beam is automatically centred to the middle of the receptor.

Essential image characteristics (Fig. 7.12b)

The ideal PA chest radiograph should demonstrate the following[1]:

- Full lung fields with the scapulae projected laterally away from the lung fields.
- No rotation, the anterior rib ends should be equidistant from the spine and the medial ends of the clavicles should overlap the transverse processes of the spine.
- The lungs well inflated, i.e. it should be possible to visualise either six ribs anteriorly or ten ribs posteriorly.
- Inferior to the costophrenic angles and diaphragm clearly outlined.
- The mediastinum and heart central and sharply defined.
- The fine demarcation of the lung tissues should be demonstrated from the hilum to the periphery.

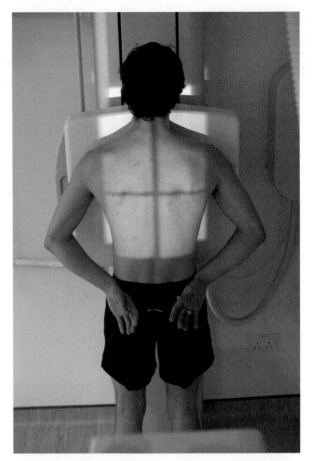

Fig. 7.12a Patient positioning.

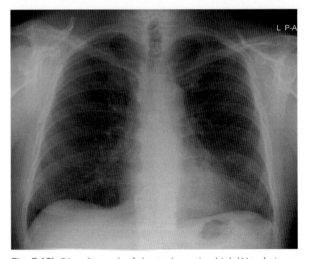

Fig. 7.12b PA radiograph of chest taken using high kV technique.

Expiration technique

A radiograph may be taken on full expiration to confirm the presence of a pneumothorax. This has the effect of increasing intrapleural pressure, which results in the compression of the lung making a pneumothorax bigger. The technique is useful in demonstrating a small pneumothorax and is also used to demonstrate the effects of air trapping associated with an inhaled foreign body obstructing the passage of air into a segment of lung, and the extent of diaphragmatic movement.

Lungs 7

Postero-anterior – erect (cont.) (Figs 7.13a, 7.13b)

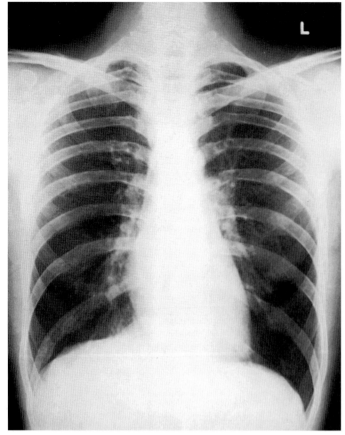

Fig. 7.13a PA radiograph of chest taken using conventional kV technique (70 kV).

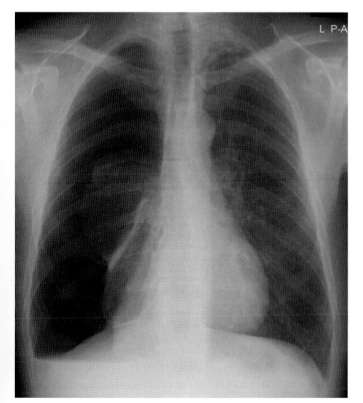

Fig. 7.13b PA radiograph of thorax showing large right pneumothorax.

Common faults and solutions

- The scapulae sometimes obscure the outer edges of the lung fields. If the patient is unable to adopt the basic arm position the arms should be allowed to encircle the vertical Bucky.
- Rotation of the patient will result in the heart not being central with assessment of heart size made impossible. Attention to how patients are made to stand is essential to ensure they are comfortable and can maintain the position. The legs should be well separated and the pelvis symmetrical in respect to the vertical Bucky.
- The lung fields sometimes are not well inflated. Explanation and rehearsal of breathing technique prior to exposure is essential.

Radiological considerations

- All comments in the general section apply.
- Soft tissues: in large patients, overlying soft tissue at the bases (obesity or large breasts) obscures detail of the lung bases and pleura as well as giving unnecessary radiation to the breast. This can be made worse by many of the factors outlined above. For diagnostic reasons and for dose reduction, female patients may hold their breasts out of the main field.
- In thin patients, skin folds can produce linear artefacts, which could mimic pleural fluid or even pneumothorax. Creasing of the skin against the Bucky or cassette should be avoided.

Notes

- Careful patient preparation is essential, with all radio-opaque objects removed before the examination.
- When an intravenous drip is in situ in the arm, care should be exercised to ensure that the drip is secured properly on a drip stand before exposure.
- Patients with underwater-seal bottles require particular care to ensure that chest tubes are not dislodged, and the bottle is not raised above the level of the chest.
- A PA side marker is normally used, and the image is identified with the identification marker set to the PA position. Care should be made not to misdiagnose a case of dextracardia.
- Long, plaited hair may cause artefacts and should be clipped out of the image field.
- Reduction in exposure is required in patients suffering from emphysema.
- For images taken in expiration, the kilovoltage is increased by five when using a conventional kilovoltage technique.

Radiation protection/dose

The radiation beam is restricted to the size of the receptor.

Expected DRL: DAP 0.1 Gy cm^2, ESD 0.15 mGy.

7 Lungs

Antero-posterior – erect (Figs 7.14a, 7.14b)

This projection is used as an alternative to the PA erect projection for elucidation of an opacity seen on a PA, or when the patient's shape (kyphosis) or medical condition makes it difficult or unsafe for the patient to stand or sit for the basic projection. For the latter, the patient is usually supported sitting erect on a trolley against a vertical Bucky direct digital radiography (DDR) system.

Position of patient and image receptor

- The patient may be standing or sitting with their back against the image receptor, which is supported vertically with the upper edge of the receptor above the lung apices.
- The median sagittal plane is adjusted at right-angles to the middle of the receptor.
- The shoulders are brought downward and forward, with the backs of the hands below the hips and the elbows well forward, which has the effect of projecting the scapulae clear of the lung fields.
- In the unwell patient, it may not be possible to perform this procedure, with the result that the scapulae may be rotated and superimposed on the lateral chest margins. This causes an increase in radiation absorption, making it difficult to observe underlying lung tissue. In this situation, it is preferable that the patient's arms are rotated laterally and supported with the palms of the hands facing forward. In this position, the scapulae are superimposed on the lungs but the effect of absorption is less, and comparison of either side of the upper lateral segments of the lung is made easier.

Direction and location of the X-ray beam

- The collimated horizontal beam is angled caudally until it is at right-angles to the sternum and centred midway between the sternal notch and the xiphisternum.
- The degree of caudal angulation for the non-kyphotic patient is dependent on the patient anatomy (5–10°). This will ensure maximum visualisation of the lung fields and that the clavicles do not obscure the lung apices).[5]
- The exposure is taken on normal full inspiration.

Notes

- The use of a lower centring point combined with a horizontal beam has the undesirable effect of projecting the clavicles above the apices of the lungs.
- The radiograph opposite is of similar appearance to that of the PA chest radiograph described on page 240. However, this projection is valuable in elucidation of relative positions of opacities seen on a PA projection.
- Small lesions, previously obscured by a rib, may also be demonstrated.

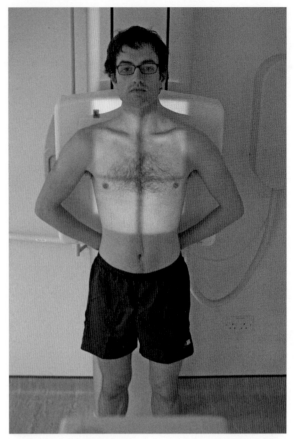

Fig. 7.14a Patient positioning.

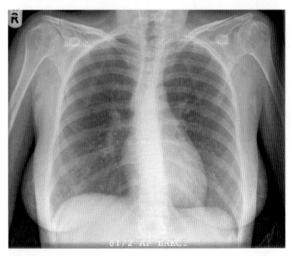

Fig. 7.14b Normal antero-posterior radiograph of the thorax – female patient.

Radiological considerations

- This projection moves the heart away from the image receptor plane, increasing magnification and reducing the accuracy of assessment of heart size (in this projection a cardio-thoracic ratio [CTR] of greater than 50% does not necessarily indicate cardiomegaly and causing apparent widening of the mediastinum).

Radiation protection/dose

Expected DRL: DAP 0.15 Gy cm², ESD 0.2 mGy.

This projection is selected when patients are unable either to stand or sit for the projections previously described. The patient is usually lying supine on a trolley or bed and a mobile DDR detector or 35 × 43 cm CR cassette is selected.

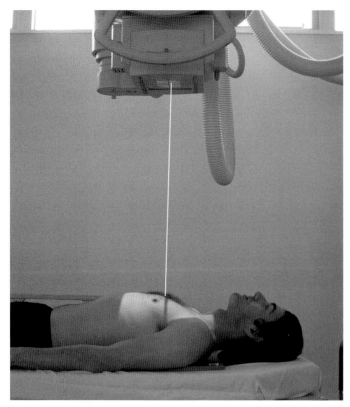

Fig. 7.15a Patient positioning.

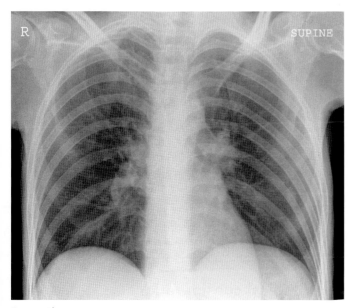

Fig. 7.15b Normal supine radiograph of thorax.

Lungs 7

Antero-posterior – supine (Figs 7.15a, 7.15b)

Position of patient and image receptor

- With assistance, the detector is carefully positioned under the patient's chest with the upper edge of the detector above the lung apices (C7 prominence). The detector is orientated to ensure that the lung fields are included on the image.
- The median sagittal plane is adjusted at right-angles to the middle of the detector, and the patient's pelvis is checked to ensure that it is not rotated.
- The arms are rotated laterally and supported by the side of the trunk. The head is supported on a pillow, with the chin slightly raised.

Direction and location of the X-ray beam

- The collimated vertical beam is angled caudally until it is at right-angles to the sternum and centred midway between the sternal notch and the xiphisternum.
- The degree of caudal angulation for the non-kyphotic patient is dependent on the patient anatomy (5–10°). This will ensure maximum visualisation of the lung fields and that the clavicles do not obscure the lung apices)[5].

Notes

- The exposure is taken on full normal inspiration.
- An FRD of at least 120 cm is essential to reduce unequal magnification of intrathoracic structures.
- In this projection maximum lung demonstration is lost due to the absence of the gravity effect of the abdominal organs, which is present in the erect position.
- Shadows caused by heavy breasts are not readily diffused.

Radiological considerations

- Compared with the PA projection, this projection moves the heart away from the image receptor plane, increasing magnification and reducing the accuracy of assessment of heart size (in this projection, a CTR of greater than 50% does not necessarily indicate cardiomegaly).
- The normal biomechanics of blood flow are different from those in the erect position, producing relative prominence of upper-lobe vessels and mimicking the signs of heart failure.
- Pleural fluid will layer against the posterior chest wall, producing an ill-defined increased attenuation of the affected hemithorax rather than the usual blunting of the costo-phrenic angle; fluid levels are not seen.
- A pneumothorax, if present, will be located at the front of the chest in the supine position. Unless it is large, it will be more difficult to detect if a lateral horizontal beam image is not employed.

7 Lungs

Antero-posterior – semi-erect (Figs 7.16a, 7.16b)

This semi-recumbent position is adopted as an alternative to the AP erect projection when the patient is too ill to stand or sit erect without support with. A mobile DDR detector or 35 × 43 cm CR cassette is selected.

Position of patient and image receptor

- The patient is supported in a semi-recumbent position facing the X-ray tube. The degree to which they can sit erect will be dependent on their medical condition.
- The image receptor is supported against the back, using pillows or a large 45° foam pad, with its upper edge above the lung fields.
- The CR cassette, if used, is orientated to ensure that the lung fields are included on the image.
- Care should be taken to ensure that the receptor is parallel to the coronal plane.
- The median sagittal plane is adjusted at right-angles to and in the midline of the image receptor.
- Rotation of the patient is prevented by the use of foam pads.
- The arms are rotated medially with the shoulders brought forward to bring the scapulae clear of the lung fields.

Direction and location of the X-ray beam

- The collimated horizontal beam is first directed at right-angles to the image receptor and then angled caudally until it is at right-angles to the sternum and centred midway between the sternal notch and the xiphisternum.
- The degree of caudal angulation for the non-kyphotic patient is dependent on the patient anatomy (5–10°). This will ensure maximum visualisation of the lung fields and that the clavicles do not obscure the lung apices.

Notes

- Difficulties sometimes arise in positioning the receptor parallel to the coronal plane, with the resultant effect that the image of the chest is foreshortened.
- The use of a horizontal central ray is essential to demonstrate fluid levels, e.g. pleural effusion. In this situation, the patient is adjusted with the chest erect as much as possible. The horizontal central ray is directed at right-angles to the middle of the image receptor. The clavicles in the resultant image will be projected above the apices.
- If the patient is unable to sit erect, fluid levels are demonstrated using a horizontal beam with the patient adopting the lateral decubitus or dorsal decubitus position.

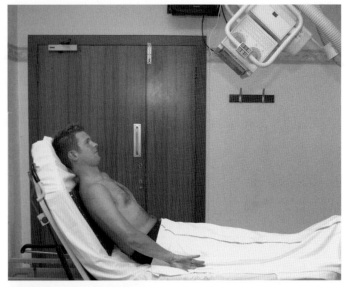

Fig. 7.16a Patient positioning.

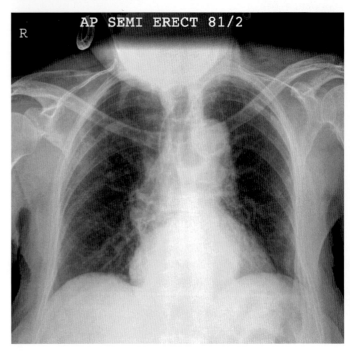

Fig. 7.16b Normal semi-erect radiograph of thorax. The chin is just superimposed on the upper thorax.

- Sick patients may be unable to support their own head in the erect position, resulting in superimposition of the chin over the upper thorax. Care should be taken to avoid or minimise this if at all possible as apical lesions will be obscured.

Radiological considerations

The use of AP semi-erect film is to look for gross pathology – lobar consolidation, big pneumothorax, position of lines. It is important that the patient is not rotated.

Lungs 7

Lateral (Figs 7.17a–7.17d)

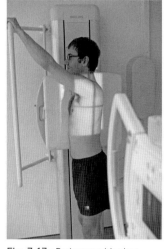
Fig. 7.17a Patient positioning.

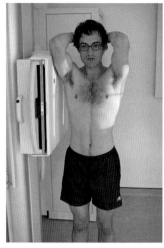
Fig. 7.17b Patient positioning.

A supplementary lateral projection may be useful in certain clinical circumstances for localising the position of a lesion and demonstrating anterior mediastinal masses not shown on the PA projection. However, it is now normal practice to undertake a CT examination if a lesion has been identified.

Lateral radiographs are not taken as part of a routine examination of the lung fields, because of the additional radiation patient dose.

A vertical Bucky DDR system is employed or alternatively a 35 × 43 cm CR cassette.

A moving or stationary grid may be used to prevent excess secondary radiation reaching the image. The FRD may be reduced to 150 cm to maintain a short exposure time.

Position of patient and image receptor

- The erect patient is turned to bring the side under investigation in contact with the image receptor.
- The median sagittal plane is adjusted parallel to the image receptor.
- The arms are folded over the head or raised above the head to rest on a horizontal bar support.
- The mid-axillary line is coincident with the middle of the Bucky, and the receptor is adjusted to include the apices and the lower lobes to the level of the 1st lumbar vertebra.

Direction and location of the X-ray beam

- The collimated horizontal beam is directed at right-angles to the middle of the image receptor coincident with the mid-axillary line.

Radiological considerations

- Insufficient elevation of the arms will cause the soft tissues of the upper arms to obscure the lung apices and thoracic inlet, and even the retrosternal window, leading to masses or other lesions in these areas being missed or incorrectly suspected.
- Rotation will also partially obscure the retrosternal window, masking anterior mediastinal masses. It will also render the sternum less distinct, which may be important in the setting of trauma when sternal fracture may be overlooked.
- For many years the lateral CXR was overused, being undertaken 'routinely' and often inappropriately for cardiac and chest clinics; this overuse has been addressed by education. The lateral CXR still has value in assessing an abnormality on the PA image and may now be underused by radiographers. If digital tomosynthesis is available however, this may replace the lateral projection for such indications.

Radiation protection/dose

- The radiation beam is restricted to the size of the receptor.

Expected DRL: ESD 0.5 mGy.

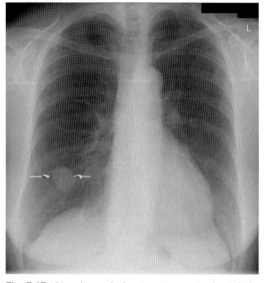
Fig. 7.17c PA radiograph showing a tumour in the right lower lobe.

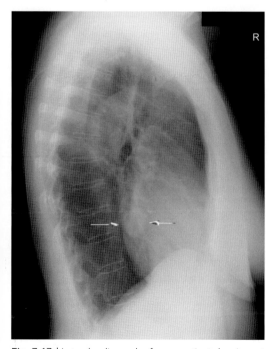
Fig. 7.17d Lateral radiograph of same patient showing a tumour in the right lower lobe.

7 Lungs

Apices (Figs 7.18a–7.18f)

Opacities obscured in the apical region by overlying ribs or clavicular shadows may be demonstrated by modification of the PA and AP projections.

Direction and location of the X-ray beam

- With the patient in the position for the PA projection, the collimated beam is angled 30° caudally and centred over the 7th cervical spinous process coincident with the sternal angle.
- With the patient in the position for the AP projection, the central ray is angled 30° cranial towards the sternal angle.
- With the patient reclining, and the coronal plane at 30° to the image receptor, to enable the nape of the neck to rest against the upper border of the CR cassette, the central ray is directed at right-angles to the receptor towards the sternal angle. Alternatively, if the patient is unable to recline 30°, the technique is adapted, with the patient reclining 15° and the tube angled 15° cranial.

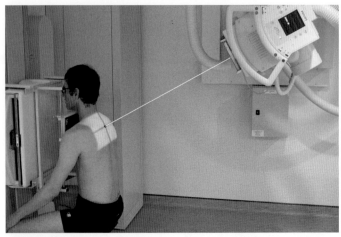

Fig. 7.18d PA 30° caudal.

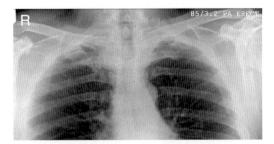

Fig. 7.18a Postero-anterior 30° caudal.

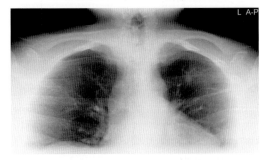

Fig. 7.18b AP 30° cranial, showing small tumour at the left apex.

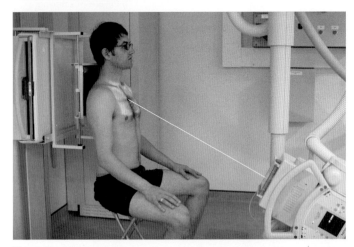

Fig. 7.18e AP 30° cranial.

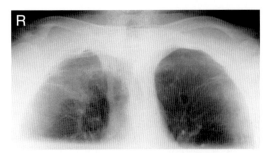

Fig. 7.18c AP coronal plane 15°, central ray 15° cranial, showing small tumour at the right apex.

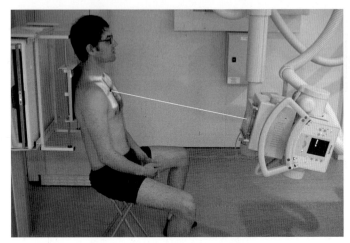

Fig. 7.18f AP coronal plane 15°, central ray 15° cranial.

Upper anterior region – lateral (Figs 7.19a, 7.19b)

This technique may be required to demonstrate an anterior lesion and the associated relationship of the trachea. A vertical Bucky DDR system is employed or alternatively a 24 × 30 cm CR cassette.

Position of patient and image receptor

- The patient is positioned with the median sagittal plane parallel to the receptor, which is centred at the level of the shoulder of the side under examination.
- Both shoulders are drawn backward and the arms extended to move the shoulders clear of the retrosternal space.
- The hands are clasped low down over the buttocks.

Direction and location of the X-ray beam

- The collimated horizontal beam is directed at right-angles to the receptor and centred over a point immediately in front of the shoulder nearest the tube.

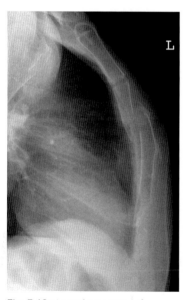

Fig. 7.19a Lateral projection of upper anterior chest in a patient with a sternal fracture.

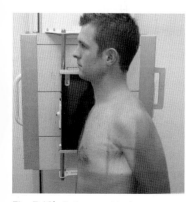

Fig. 7.19b Patient positioning.

Lungs 7

Lordotic (Figs 7.19c, 7.19d)

This technique may be used to demonstrate right middle lobe collapse or an interlobar pleural effusion. The patient is positioned to bring the middle lobe fissure horizontal.

Position of patient and image receptor

- The patient is placed for the PA projection.
- Then clasping the sides of the vertical Bucky, the patient bends backwards at the waist.
- The degree of dorsiflexion varies for each subject, but in general is about 30–40°.

Direction and location of the X-ray beam

- The collimated horizontal beam is directed at right-angles to the middle of the image receptor.

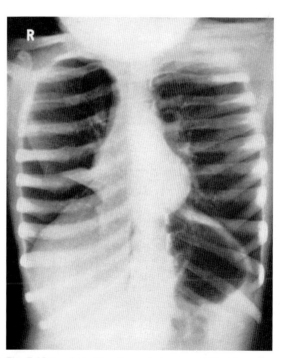

Fig. 7.19c Lordotic PA radiograph showing middle lobe collapse.

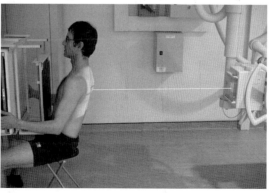

Fig. 7.19d Patient positioning.

7 Lungs

Image evaluation – 10-point plan

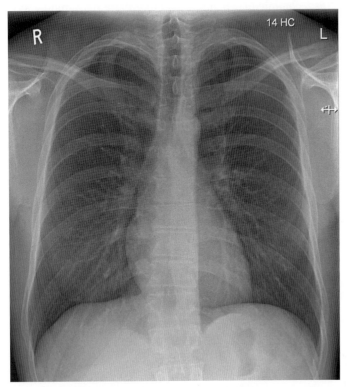

Fig. 7.20a PA chest.

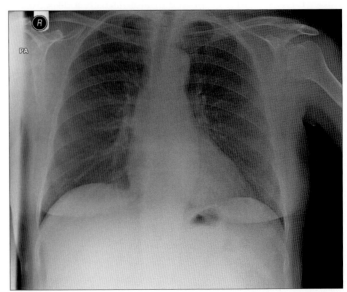

Fig. 7.20b PA chest.

IMAGE EVALUATION

PA chest (Fig. 7.20a)

Main points to consider:

- Root of neck to inferior costophrenic angles demonstrated.
- Adequate exposure with vertebral bodies demonstrated through heart shadow and lung markings well demonstrated.
- No rotation and scapulae elevated off lung fields.
- Full inspiration.

Radiographer Comments/Initial report

No repeat required.
No pathology demonstrated.

IMAGE EVALUATION

PA chest (Fig. 7.20b)

Main points to consider:

- Both apices not demonstrated.
- Rotation to the patient's left.
- Side marker applied post processing overlying original marker.
- Chest not centred to receptor/cassette.
- Inadequate inspiration.

Radiographer Comments/Initial report

Repeat required for apices.
Increased heart size (demonstrated by cardio-thoracic ratio more than 50%).
Bulky hilar markings.
No acute pathology demonstrated.

Lungs 7

Image evaluation – 10-point plan (cont.)

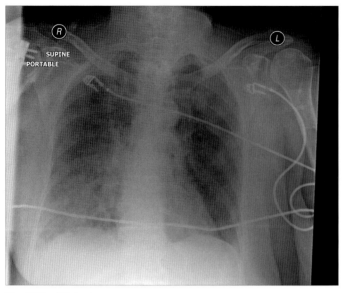

Fig. 7.21a AP chest.

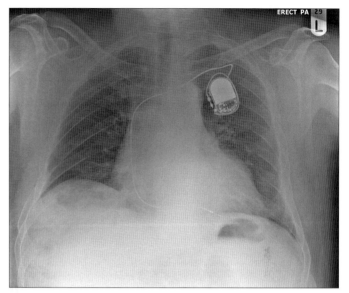

Fig. 7.21b AP chest.

IMAGE EVALUATION

AP chest – portable (Fig. 7.21a)

Main points to consider:

- AP supine – portable.
- Movement artefact (patient breathing), poor resolution.
- No radio-opaque marker was applied (markers digitally added post examination).
- Slightly rotated to the patient's left.
- Adequate inspiration.
- Scapulae overlying both lung fields.
- Chest not centred to receptor/cassette.
- Low contrast.
- Artefacts (ECG leads).

Radiographer Comments/Initial report

AP image.
Pronounced hilar markings on both sides, right lower lobe pathology and to left upper lobe, indicative of probable lung infection.

IMAGE EVALUATION

AP chest (Fig. 7.21b)

Main points to consider:

- Patient rotated – note distance of medial clavicles from spinous process.
- Inadequate inspiration, nine posterior ribs.
- Under exposed – vertebral bodies not visualised through the cardiac shadow.

Radiographer Comments/Initial report

Pacemaker in situ, heart in excess of normal CTR.

7 Heart and aorta

Introduction

Radiography of the heart and aorta is a common examination. It is performed in the routine investigation of heart disease and to assess heart size and the gross anatomy of the major blood vessels. Examination is also performed following pacemaker insertion to determine the position of the electrode leads.

The radiographic technique used is similar to that described for the lungs, and the student is referred to this section (page 240).

Imaging may also be performed using a variety of other modalities, notably echocardiography and radionuclide imaging, with angiography performed routinely to assess the heart chambers and coronary vessels. Multidetector CT and MRI are likely to be used increasingly in the future.

Examination is performed by means of the following projections:

Basic	Postero-anterior – erect
Supplementary	Left lateral
	Left anterior oblique
	Right anterior oblique

Anatomy (Fig. 7.22)

The heart is a hollow muscular organ that, together with the roots of the great vessels, is enclosed in a fibroserous sac, the pericardium. It is situated mainly to the left of the midline in the lower anterior part of the chest and attached to the central tendon of the diaphragm.

The heart has four chambers: the right and left atria and the right and left ventricles. The atria are separated by the interatrial septum and the ventricles are separated by the interventricular septum. Blood flows from the right atrium into the right ventricle through the tricuspid valve, and from the left atrium to the left ventricle through the mitral valve. The right ventricle outflow is via the pulmonary valve, and the left ventricle outflow is via the aortic valve. By rhythmic contractions, the heart

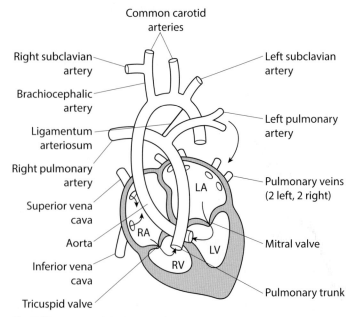

Fig. 7.22 Diagram of the heart and aorta.

serves as a pump to maintain the movement of blood throughout the circulatory system of blood vessels. At rest, there are approximately 60–80 beats per minute, with the average heart cycle occupying a time period of 0.8 s. The right side of the heart serves to perfuse the pulmonary circulation, while the left side perfuses the systemic circulation, the latter being a higher-pressure system.

The aorta, the largest of the great vessels, consists of three parts: the ascending aorta, the arch and the descending aorta, which commences at the level of the 4th thoracic vertebra.

The superior vena cava opens into the upper part of the right atrium, draining the upper limbs and head and neck. The inferior vena cava gives venous drainage from the lower limbs and abdomen, entering the inferior part of the right atrium.

Radiographically, the heart is seen as a pear-shaped structure of soft-tissue density, with its apex and inferior wall adjacent to the diaphragm and its narrower upper base overlying the spine. The size and shape of the heart vary with the build of subject, with respiration, and with the position and the clinical state of the patient.

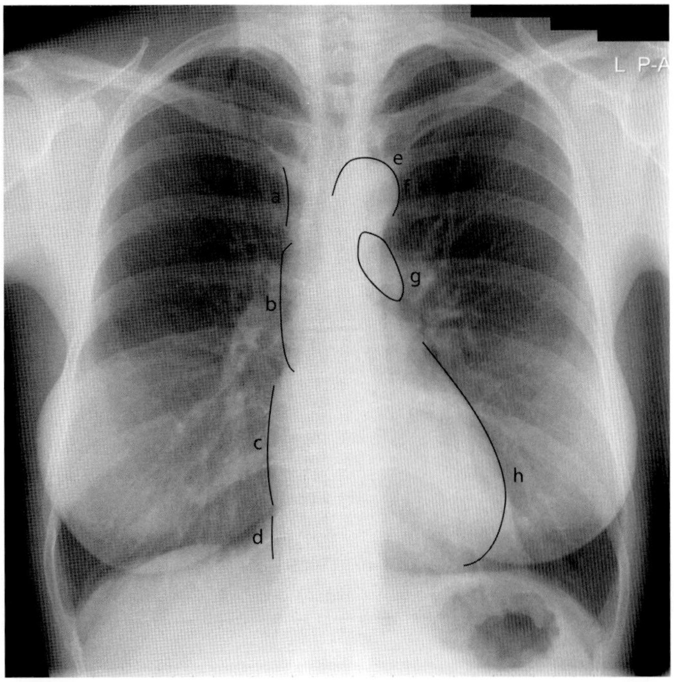

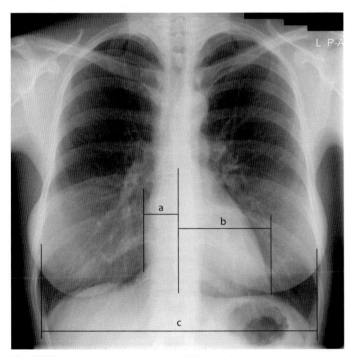

Fig. 7.23a Radiograph with labelled features of the heart and associated vessels.

Fig. 7.23b Radiograph demonstrating CTR procedure.

Heart and aorta 7

Introduction (cont.)

Radiographic anatomy (Fig. 7.23a)

In the PA radiograph of the chest seen opposite, features of the heart and associated vessels have been outlined and labelled.

The aortic knuckle is shown as a rounded protrusion slightly to the left of the vertebrae and above the heart shadow. The prominence of the aortic knuckle depends upon the degree of dilation or unfolding of the aorta and the presence (or absence) of cardiac disease. It also alters shape as a result of deformities in the thorax, intrinsic abnormalities and with old age. Calcification in the arch, when present, is demonstrated as curvilinear opacities.

a, Superior vena cava.
b, Ascending thoracic aorta.
c, Right atrium.
d, Inferior vena cava.
e, Left subclavian vein.
f, Aortic knuckle.
g, Main pulmonary artery.
h, Left ventricle.

Cardio-thoracic ratio (Fig. 7.23b)

The size of the heart is estimated from the PA radiograph of the chest by calculating the CTR. This is the ratio between the maximum transverse diameter of the heart and the maximum width of the thorax above the costo-phrenic angles, measured from the inner edges of the ribs. In adults, the normal CTR is maximally 0.5.[6,7] In children, however, the CTR is usually greater.

$$\text{Cardio-thoracic ratio (CTR)} = \frac{(a + b)}{c}$$

where a = right heart border to midline, b = left heart border to midline, and c = maximum thoracic diameter above costo-phrenic angles from inner borders of ribs.

$$\text{For example, CTR in example} = \frac{(2.5 + 10)}{29} = 0.43.$$

7 Heart and aorta

Postero-anterior (Figs 7.24a, 7.24b)

A vertical Bucky DDR system is employed or alternatively a 35 × 43 cm or 35 × 35 cm CR cassette is selected depending on the size of the patient. Orientation of a larger cassette will depend of the width of the thorax.

Position of patient and image receptor

- The patient is positioned erect, facing the receptor and with the chin extended and resting on the top of the receptor.
- The median sagittal plane is adjusted perpendicular to the middle of the receptor, with the patient's arms encircling the receptor or vertical Bucky device. Alternatively, the dorsal aspects of the hands are placed behind and below the hips to allow the shoulders to be rotated forward and pressed downward in contact with the vertical Bucky or receptor.
- The thorax must be positioned symmetrically relative to the image receptor plane.

Direction and location of the X-ray beam

- The collimated horizontal beam is directed at right-angles to the receptor and centred at the level of the 8th thoracic vertebrae (i.e. the spinous process of T7).
- The surface markings of the T7 spinous process can be assessed by using the inferior angle of the scapula before the shoulders are pushed forward.
- Exposure is made on arrested full inspiration.

Essential image characteristics

The optimal PA chest radiograph for the heart and aorta should demonstrate the following:

- The clavicles symmetrical and equidistant from the spinous processes.
- The mediastinum and heart central and defined sharply.
- The costo-phrenic angles and diaphragm outlined clearly.
- Full lung fields, with the scapula projected laterally away from the lung fields.

Notes

- A PA side marker is normally used to identify the right or left side of the patient. Care should be made to select the correct marker so as not to misdiagnose a case of dextracardia.
- The kilovoltage selected is adjusted to give adequate penetration, with the bodies of the thoracic vertebrae just visible through the heart (see page 235).
- For comparison purposes, records of exposure factors used, including FRD, should be kept for follow-up examinations.
- Care should be taken with postoperative patients with underwater seals and with intravenous drips. These should not be dislodged, and the examination time should be kept to a minimum.

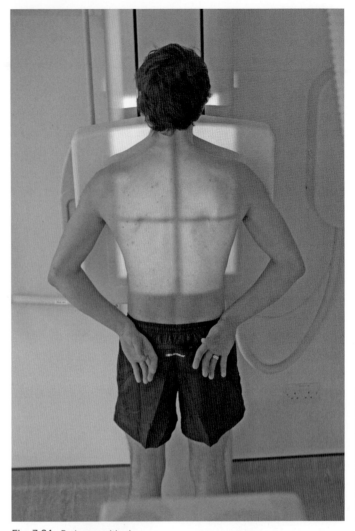

Fig. 7.24a Patient positioning.

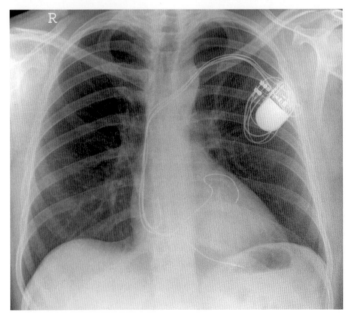

Fig. 7.24b Normal PA radiograph in a patient with a permanent pacemaker in situ.

- Underwater-seal drain bottles must be kept below the lowest point of the patient's chest at all times to prevent the contents of the bottle being siphoned back into the chest.

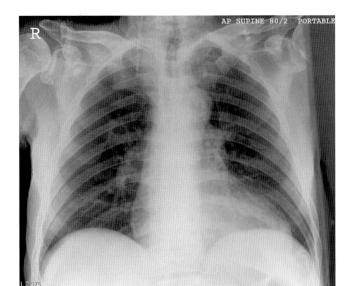

Fig. 7.25a Antero-posterior supine radiograph showing artefactual enlargement of the heart due to supine posture.

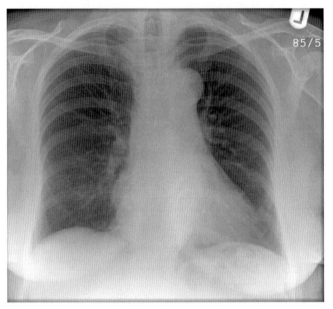

Fig. 7.25b Postero-anterior (PA) radiograph showing prosthetic aortic and mitral valves.

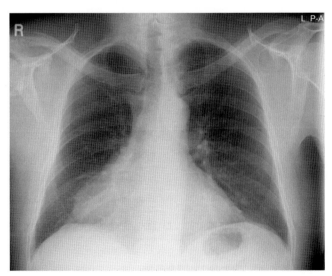

Fig. 7.25c PA radiograph in a patient with a right pericardial cyst.

Heart and aorta 7

Postero-anterior (*cont.*) (Figs 7.25a–7.25c)

Radiological considerations

- An artefactual increase in the apparent size of the heart may be produced by a number of factors, including:
  - Poor inspiration, as the heart rotates up into a more horizontal orientation.
  - Short FRD due to geometric magnification.
  - Supine posture due to a more horizontal cardiac orientation and reduced FRD.

To prevent the clinician making an erroneous diagnosis of cardiomegaly or heart failure, these factors should be avoided if possible.

- If the patient is not truly erect, there may be diversion of blood flow to the upper lobe vessels, mimicking the upper-lobe blood diversion seen in heart failure.
- Following pacemaker insertion, the clinician may wish to check that the wire is located properly and to exclude complications such as pneumothorax and pleural effusion.
- Pacemaker wires and prosthetic valves are visualised less readily on low-kV and underexposed images. A penetrated radiograph may help to demonstrate these fully. The lateral projection is also acquired to help in localisation.
- Native valve and coronary artery calcifications will be seen less well on an inadequately penetrated radiograph.

Radiation protection/dose

- The radiation beam is restricted to the size of the receptor.

Expected DRL: DAP 0.1 Gy cm^2, ESD 0.15 mGy.

7 Heart and aorta

Left lateral (Figs 7.26a, 7.26b)

A vertical Bucky DDR system is employed or alternatively a 35 × 43 cm CR cassette. A moving or stationary grid may be used to prevent excess secondary radiation reaching the image.

Position of patient and image receptor

- The patient is turned to bring the left side in contact with the image receptor.
- The median sagittal plane is adjusted parallel to the receptor.
- The arms are folded over the head or raised above the head to rest on a horizontal bar.
- The mid-axillary line is coincident with the vertical midline of the receptor, which is adjusted to include the apices and the inferior lobes to the level of the 1st lumbar vertebra.

Direction and location of the X-ray beam

- The collimated horizontal beam is directed at right-angles to the middle of the receptor in the mid-axillary line.
- Exposure is made on arrested full inspiration.

Essential image characteristics

- The thoracic vertebrae and sternum should be lateral and demonstrated clearly.
- The arms should not obscure the heart and lung fields.
- The anterior and posterior mediastinum and heart are defined sharply and the lung fields are seen clearly.
- The costo-phrenic angles and diaphragm should be outlined clearly.

Radiological considerations

- After pacemaker insertion, the lateral image confirms that the ventricular electrode lies anteriorly at the right ventricular apex.
- A lateral radiograph may help to locate cardiac or pericardial masses, e.g. left ventricular aneurysm and pericardial cyst. These are assessed better by echocardiography or CT/MRI.
- Cardiac and pericardial calcification may be confirmed and its extent assessed more fully on a lateral chest radiograph.

Notes

- An FRD of 150 or 180 cm is selected.
- Patients who have recently had a permanent pacemaker implant should not raise their arms above their head. It is sufficient to raise the arms clear of the thorax, otherwise there is a risk of damage to the recently sutured tissues and possible dislodging of the pacemaker electrodes.
- Patients on trolleys may find it difficult to remain in the vertical position. A large wedge foam pad may be required to assist the patient to remain upright.

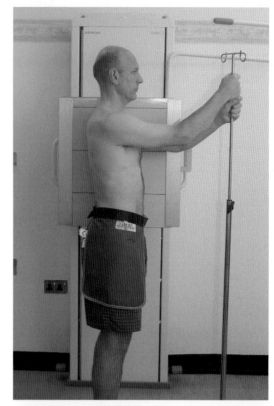

Fig. 7.26a Patient positioning following pacemaker implantation.

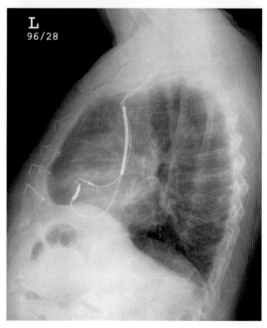

Fig. 7.26b Left lateral radiograph of heart showing position of permanent pacing system.

- Either a stationary or a moving grid may be employed. The kilovoltage selected is adjusted to give adequate penetration, with the bodies of the thoracic vertebrae, costo-phrenic and apical regions defined well.

Radiation protection/dose

- The radiation beam is restricted to the size of the receptor.

Expected DRL: ESD 0.5 mGy.

Heart and aorta

Right anterior oblique (Figs 7.27a–7.27d)

This projection is used to separate the heart, aorta and vertical column, thus enabling the path of the ascending aorta, aortic arch and descending aorta to be acquired on a large digital detector format or a 35 × 43 cm CR cassette. The projection will also demonstrate the diameter and the degree of unfolding of the aorta.

Position of patient and image receptor

- The patient is initially positioned facing the image receptor with the upper edge positioned above the lung apices.
- With the right side of the trunk kept in contact with the receptor or vertical Bucky, the patient is rotated to bring the left side away from the receptor, so that the coronal plane forms an angle of 60° to the image receptor plane.

Direction and location of the X-ray beam

- The collimated horizontal beam is directed at right-angles to the middle of the receptor at the level of the 6th thoracic vertebrae, to show the heart, aortic arch and descending aorta.

Radiological considerations

- This projection may be a useful adjunct to the lateral in cases of doubt about dilatation or tortuosity of the aorta, although CT (or MRI) will usually be requested in cases of doubt as they offer a much more accurate and complete assessment.
- This projection may be used in conjunction with a barium-swallow study to demonstrate enlargement of the heart or aorta, or abnormal vessels and vascular rings, which can produce abnormal impressions on the oesophagus and cause dysphagia. CT, MRI or angiography assess vascular rings more accurately.

Note

- The FRD may be reduced to 150 cm.

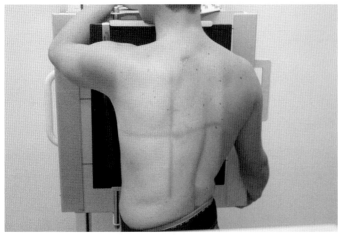

Fig. 7.27a Patient positioning.

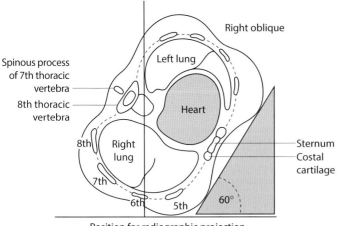

Fig. 7.27b Diagram showing gross anatomy for radiographic projection.

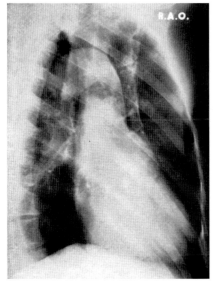

Fig. 7.27c Right anterior oblique radiograph.

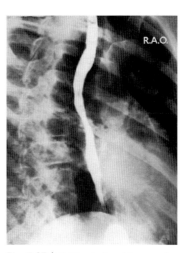

Fig. 7.27d Right anterior oblique radiograph with barium outlining the oesophagus.

7 Bones of the thorax

Introduction (Figs 7.28a, 7.28b)

The thoracic skeleton consists of the ribs and sternum, (and thoracic spine, which is covered in Section 6). The ribs and sternum may be examined radiographically in the assessment of trauma, but a good PA or AP radiograph will be more important in this setting to exclude intrathoracic complications (e.g. pneumothorax). It is no longer normal practice to perform oblique rib views for simple trauma unless a change in patient management will result (RCR guidelines), and an AP or PA projection will show much of the anterior and posterior ribs that are projected above the diaphragm.

The ribs may also be examined to detect other causes of chest wall pain, for example rib metastases when oblique rib projections are required.

In cases of severe injury to the thorax maintenance of respiratory function is of prime importance. Optimal PA or AP radiographs are required for full assessment of chest wall injury, pleural changes and pulmonary damage. In cases of major trauma, damage may occur to multiple ribs, sternum, lungs and thoracic spine, or any combination of these. Multiple rib and sternal fractures may result in a flail chest, where part of the chest collapses inwards in during inspiration, impairing or even preventing lung ventilation. In this setting a supine AP radiograph may be all that is attainable and it should be of the highest quality possible. A pneumothorax may be obscured on a supine radiograph, and in this situation a lateral radiograph is acquired using a horizontal beam.

In major trauma cases injury to the clavicle and 1st ribs may portend significant vascular injury, and these areas must be depicted clearly on any frontal projection in this situation.

Injury to the lower ribs may be associated with hepatic, splenic or renal injury, and rib projections may be requested in this situation. These could be omitted if an abdominal radiograph (Section 10) is considered necessary, though ultrasound or CT may be considered more useful, for assessment of possible internal organ damage.

Radiological considerations

- Pain impairs the ability of the patient to inspire deeply after rib trauma, reducing conspicuity of rib fractures and pulmonary contusion. Optimisation of exposure and other factors therefore becomes more critical.
- Overexposure may allow clearer depiction of rib trauma, but will tend to obscure associated pulmonary lesions, so should be avoided.
- Fluoroscopy may be useful to determine whether a peripheral chest lesion is real and whether it is related to a rib, although CT is most likely to be requested in cases of doubt.
- If available dual-energy subtraction will provide excellent visualisation of the bony aspect of the thorax.

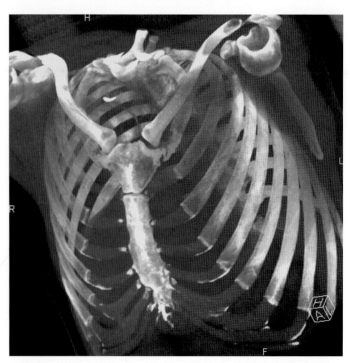

Fig. 7.28a CT reconstruction of the bony thorax created using a multislice scanner.

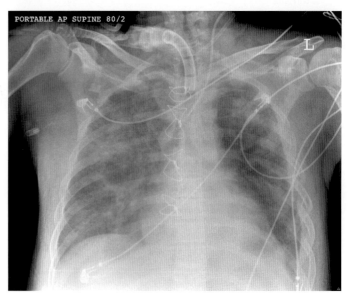

Fig. 7.28b AP supine radiograph showing multiple rib fractures and flail chest with severe pulmonary oedema.

Bones of the thorax

Recommended projections

BONES OF THORAX	Trauma – trolley patients	AP supine chest with additional lateral-horizontal beam chest if required (see this section) Other projections of chest, abdomen, ribs, sternum, thoracic vertebrae or ATLS projections on request
LOWER RIBS	Trauma – non-trolley patients	PA chest AP (basic) Posterior oblique and other projections of chest on request
	Pathology	AP (basic) Posterior oblique
UPPER RIBS	Trauma or pathology – non-trolley patients	PA chest Posterior oblique AP 1st and 2nd ribs on request
	Cervical ribs	Normally demonstrated on AP (basic) cervical vertebrae PA chest AP cervical ribs
STERNUM	Trauma – non-trolley patients	PA chest (see this section) Anterior oblique, tube angled OR Anterior oblique, trunk rotated Lateral
	Pathology	Anterior oblique, tube angled OR Anterior oblique, trunk rotated Lateral CT or tomography on request according to availability

AP, antero-posterior; ATLS, Advanced Trauma and Life Support; CT, computed tomography; PA, postero-anterior.

7 Lower ribs

Antero-posterior (basic) (Figs 7.29a–7.29e)

A table Bucky DDR system is employed or alternatively a 35 × 43 cm CR cassette to include the whole of the right and left sides from the level of the middle of the body of the sternum to the lower costal margin.

Position of patient and image receptor

- The patient lies supine on the imaging couch with the median plane coincident with the midline of the couch.
- The anterior superior iliac spines should be equidistant from the couch top.
- If selected, a cassette is placed transversely in the Bucky tray with its caudal edge positioned at a level just below the lower costal margin; otherwise the DDR detector is positioned to include the area of interest with its centre coincident with central beam.

Direction and location of the X-ray beam

- The collimated vertical beam is centred in the midline at the level of the lower costal margin and then is angled cranially to coincide with the centre of the image receptor.
- This centring assists in demonstrating the maximum number of ribs below the diaphragm.
- Exposure made on full expiration will also assist in this objective.

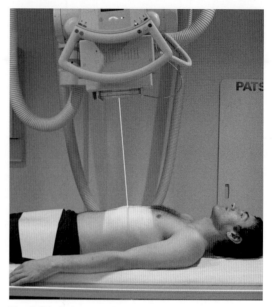

Fig. 7.29c Patient positioning.

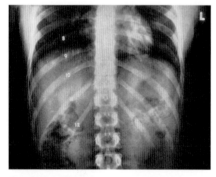

Fig. 7.29a Effect of expiration.

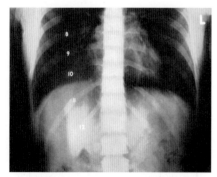

Fig. 7.29b Effect of inspiration.

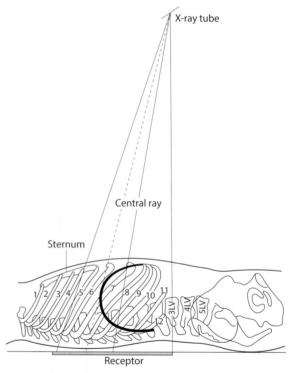

Fig. 7.29d Dotted line shows diaphragm projected upwards.

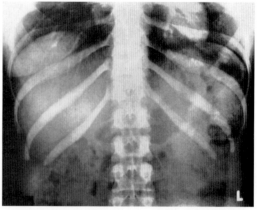

Fig. 7.29e Antero-posterior radiograph showing lower ribs on both sides.

Lower ribs 7

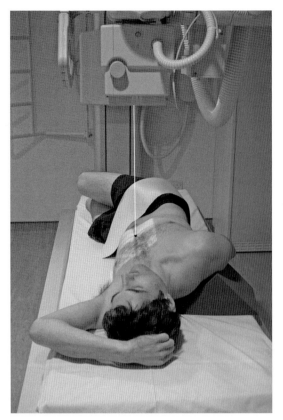

Fig. 7.30a Patient positioning – decubitus.

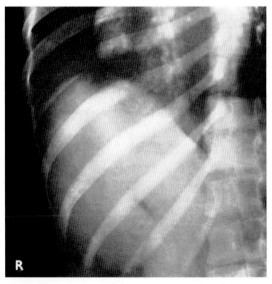

Fig. 7.30b Right posterior oblique radiograph of right lower ribs.

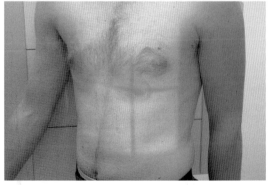

Fig. 7.30c Patient positioning – erect.

Right and left posterior oblique (Figs 7.30a–7.30c)

A table or vertical Bucky DDR system is employed or alternatively a 35 × 43cm CR cassette is selected to include either the right or left lower ribs sides. The patient may be examined erect or supine using a Bucky Grid.

Position of patient and image receptor

- The patient lies supine on the Bucky table or stands erect with the mid-clavicular line of the side under examination coincident with the midline of the Bucky grid.
- The trunk is rotated 45° onto the side being examined with the raised side supported on non-opaque pads.
- The hips and knees are flexed for comfort and to assist in maintaining patient position.
- If selected, the caudal edge of the cassette is positioned at a level just below the lower costal margin; otherwise the DDR detector is positioned to include the area of interest with its centre coincident with central beam.
- The cassette should be large enough to include the ribs on the side being examined from the level of the middle of the body of the sternum to the lower costal margin.

Direction and location of the X-ray beam

- The collimated vertical beam is centred to the midline of the anterior surface of the patient, at the level of the lower costal margin.
- From this position the central ray is then angled cranially to coincide with the centre of the image receptor.
- Exposure is made on arrested full expiration.

Notes

- The patient may find it difficult to maintain this position if they are in a great deal of pain.
- Selection of a short exposure time and rehearsal of breathing technique may be necessary to reduce the risk of movement unsharpness.

Radiation protection/dose

- The patient is provided with a waist-fitting lead-rubber apron, and the radiation beam is restricted to the size of the receptor.

7 Upper ribs

Right and left posterior oblique (Figs 7.31a–7.31e)

Radiography may be conducted with the patient erect or supine using a DDR detector or a CR cassette that is large enough to include the whole of the ribs on the side being examined from the level of the 7th cervical vertebra to the lower costal margin.

Position of patient and image receptor

- The patient sits or stands with the posterior aspect of the trunk against the vertical Bucky or lies supine on the Bucky table.
- The mid-clavicular line of the side under examination should coincide with the central line of the Bucky or table.
- The trunk is rotated 45° towards the side being examined and, if supine, is supported on non-opaque pads.
- If the condition of the patient permits, the hands should be clasped behind the head, otherwise the arms should be held clear of the trunk.
- If selected the cranial edge of the cassette should be positioned at a level just above the spinous process of the 7th cervical vertebra; otherwise the DDR detector is positioned to include the area of interest with its centre coincident with central beam.

Direction and location of the X-ray beam

- Initially direct the collimated beam perpendicular to the image receptor and towards the sternal angle.
- The beam is then angled caudally so that the central ray coincides with the centre of the receptor. This centring assists in demonstrating the maximum number of ribs above the diaphragm.
- Exposure made on arrested full inspiration will also assist in maximising the number of ribs demonstrated.

Note

- The kV should be sufficient to reduce the difference in subject contrast between the lung fields and the heart to a more uniform radiographic contrast so that the ribs are adequately visualised in both these areas.

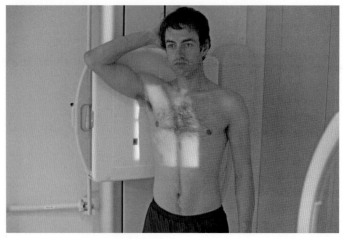

Fig. 7.31b Patient positioning – erect.

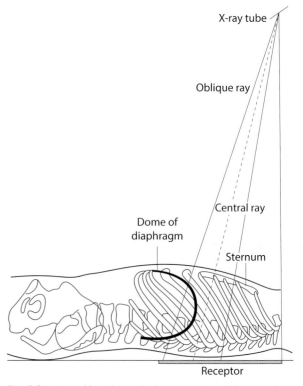

Fig. 7.31c Dotted line shows diaphragm projected downwards.

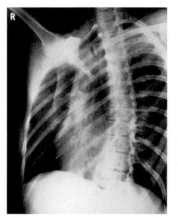 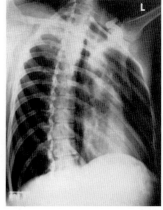

Fig. 7.31d Right posterior oblique. Fig. 7.31e Left posterior oblique.

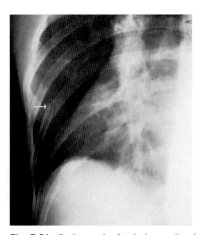

Fig. 7.31a Radiograph of right lower ribs showing acute fracture.

Upper ribs 7

First and second – antero-posterior (Figs 7.32a, 7.32b)

The 1st and 2nd ribs are often superimposed upon each other. Occasionally, a separate projection may be necessary to demonstrate them adequately. A DDR detector or 18 × 24 or 24 × 30 cm CR cassette is selected.

Position of patient and image receptor

- The patient stands with the posterior aspect of the trunk against the vertical Bucky or CR cassette. Alternatively the patient lies supine on the Bucky table.
- When the patient is erect, the cassette, if selected, is placed in a cassette holder attachment.
- The median sagittal plane is adjusted at right-angles to the image receptor.
- The image receptor is centred to the junction of the medial and middle 1/3 of the clavicle.

Direction and location of the X-ray beam

The collimated horizontal beam is directed perpendicular to the image receptor and centred over the junction of the medial and middle 1/3 of the clavicle.

Cervical – antero-posterior (Figs 7.32c, 7.32d)

Cervical ribs are normally adequately demonstrated on an AP cervical vertebrae or PA chest projection. However, occasionally a separate projection may be necessary. A DDR detector a 24 × 30 CR cassette is placed transversely on the Bucky tray.

Position of patient and image receptor

- The patient sits or stands with the posterior aspect of the trunk against a vertical Bucky or lies supine on the Bucky table.
- The median sagittal plane should be at right-angles to the image receptor and coincident with the midline of the table or Bucky.
- The CR cassette, if selected, is positioned transversely in the Bucky tray and should be large enough to include the 5th cervical to 5th thoracic vertebrae.

Direction and location of the X-ray beam

The collimated beam is angled 10° cranially from the perpendicular and centred towards the sternal notch.

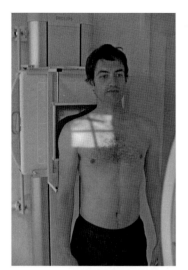

Fig. 7.32a Patient positioning.

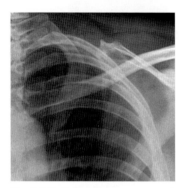

Fig. 7.32b Collimated antero-posterior radiograph of left 1st and 2nd ribs.

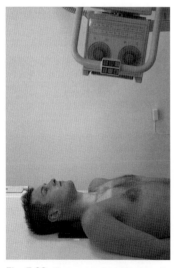

Fig. 7.32c Patient positioning – supine.

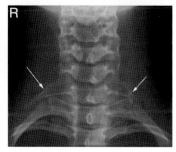

Fig. 7.32d Rudimentary bilateral cervical ribs.

7 Sternum

Anterior oblique – tube angled (Figs 7.33a–7.33d)

The projection may be performed with the patient prone or erect with the sternum at a minimal distance from the image receptor to reduce geometric unsharpness. However, if the patient has sustained a major injury to the sternum they may not be able to adopt the prone position due to pain. A 24 × 30 cm CR grid cassette is selected.

Position of patient and image receptor

- The patient lies prone on the table or stands or sits facing the vertical Bucky.
- The medial sagittal plane should be at right-angles to, and centred to, the image receptor.
- As the central ray is to be angled across the table, the cassette is placed transversely to avoid grid cut-off.
- If the DDR detector with Bucky is to be used on the table, the patient should lie on a trolley positioned at right-angles to the table, with the thorax resting on the Bucky table.
- The cassette is centred at the level of the 5th thoracic vertebra.
- Immobilisation will be assisted if it is possible to use an immobilisation band.

Direction and location of the X-ray beam

- The collimated perpendicular beam is centred initially to the axilla of either side at the level of the 5th thoracic vertebra.
- The central ray is then angled transversely so that the central ray is directed to a point 7.5 cm lateral to the midline on the same side.

Notes

- The patient is allowed to breathe gently during an exposure time of several seconds using a low mA.
- This technique diffuses the lung and rib shadows that otherwise tend to obscure the sternum.

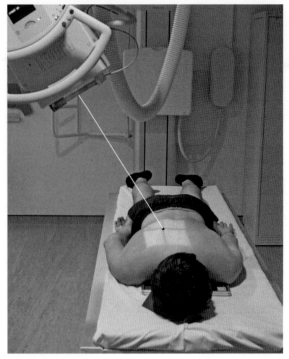

Fig. 7.33a Left anterior oblique – prone.

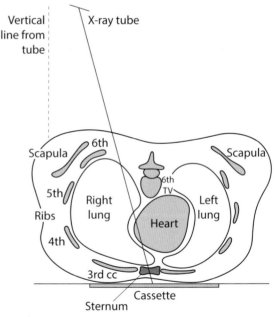

Fig. 7.33b Cassette to image receptor.

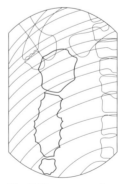

Fig. 7.33c Diagram showing sternum in anterior oblique position.

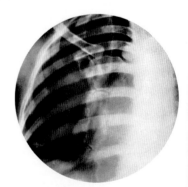

Fig. 7.33d Postero-anterior oblique radiograph of sternum taken during gentle respiration.

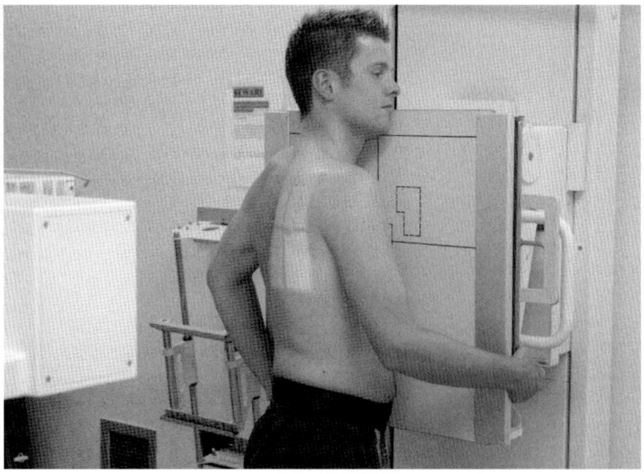

Sternum 7

Anterior oblique – trunk rotated (Figs 7.34a–7.34d)

A vertical Bucky DDR system is employed or a 24 × 30 cm CR cassette is selected for use in the Bucky mechanism. Alternatively a grid cassette may be used in the vertical cassette holder. The patient may also be examined prone on the DDR Bucky table.

Position of patient and image receptor

- The patient initially sits or stands facing the vertical Bucky or lies prone on the Bucky table with the median sagittal plane at right-angles to, and centred to, the image receptor.
- The patient is then rotated approximately 20–30° with the right side raised to adopt the left anterior oblique position, which will ensure that less heart shadow obscures the sternum.
- The patient is supported in position with non-opaque pads and an immobilisation band where possible.
- The image receptor is centred at the level of the 5th thoracic vertebra.

Direction and location of the X-ray beam

- The collimated perpendicular beam is directed towards a point 7.5 cm lateral to the 5th thoracic vertebra on the side nearest the X-ray tube.

Note

- The patient is allowed to breathe gently during an exposure time of several seconds using a low mA, providing immobilisation is adequate.

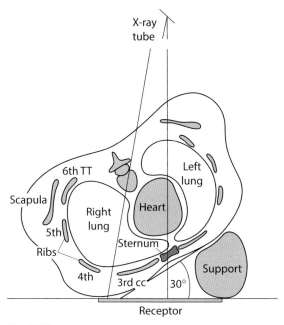

Fig. 7.34a Right anterior oblique – erect.

Fig. 7.34b Diagram of the cross-section of the thorax.

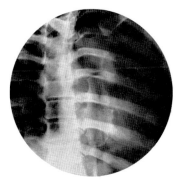

Fig. 7.34c Postero-anterior oblique radiograph of sternum taken during gentle respiration.

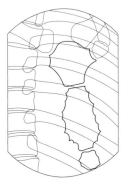

Fig. 7.34d Diagram of the sternum in anterior oblique projection.

7 Sternum

Lateral (Figs 7.35a–7.35c)

A vertical Bucky DDR system is employed or a 24 × 30 cm CR cassette is selected for use in the Bucky mechanism. Alternatively a grid cassette may be used in the vertical cassette holder.

Position of patient and image receptor

- The patient sits or stands, with either shoulder against a vertical Bucky or cassette stand.
- The median sagittal plane of the trunk is adjusted parallel to the image receptor.
- The sternum is centred to the image receptor or Bucky.
- The patient's hands are clasped behind the back and the shoulders are pulled well back.
- The receptor/cassette is centred at a level 2.5 cm below the sternal angle.

Direction and location of the X-ray beam

- The collimated horizontal beam is centred towards a point 2.5 cm below the sternal angle.
- Exposure is made on arrested full inspiration.

Notes

- Immediately before exposure, the patient is asked to pull back the shoulders.
- If the patient is standing, the feet should be separated to aid stability.
- An FRD of 120 or 150 cm is selected.

Radiological considerations

- The lateral sternal projection can be confusing to read, especially in elderly patients, who often have heavily calcified costal cartilages.
- Interpretation of the lateral projection is much easier when the sternum is truly lateral and at right-angles to the image receptor, with corresponding superimposition of ribs and cartilage.
- It is important to remember that the initial interpretation is often done in the emergency department by inexperienced observers; therefore, care should be exercised to ensure that the sternum is projected in the true lateral position.
- Sternal fracture, especially when there is overlap of the bone ends, may be associated with compression (wedge) fracture of the 4th to 6th thoracic vertebrae. It is appropriate to image the thoracic spine if this is suspected.

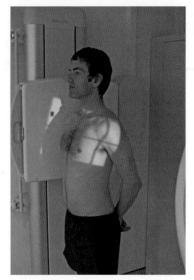

Fig. 7.35a Patient positioning.

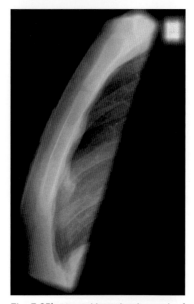

Fig. 7.35b Normal lateral radiograph of sternum.

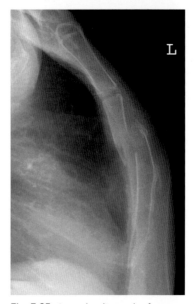

Fig. 7.35c Lateral radiograph of sternum showing fracture of the body with overlap of bone ends.

Section 8
Skull, Facial Bones and Sinuses

CONTENTS

SKULL	266
Introduction	266
Anatomical terminology	266
Radiographic anatomy	267
Positioning terminology	270
Patient preparation	272
Radiological considerations	273
CRANIUM	274
Radiographic technique	274
Lateral – supine with horizontal beam	274
Lateral erect	275
Occipito-frontal	276
Fronto-occipital	278
Half axial, fronto-occipital 30° caudal (Towne's projection)	279
Occipito-frontal 30° cranial angulation (reverse Towne's projection)	281
Submento-vertical	282
Sella turcica – lateral	283
Optic foramina and jugular foramina	**284**
Optic foramina – postero-anterior oblique	284
Jugular foramina – submento-vertical 20° caudal	285
Temporal bones	**286**
Frontal-occipital 35° caudal	286
Submento-vertical	287
Mastoid – lateral oblique 25° caudal	288
Mastoid – profile	289
Petrous – anterior oblique (Stenver's)	290
FACIAL BONES AND SINUSES	291
Introduction	291
Equipment	291
Radiographic anatomy	292
Radiological considerations	293
Recommended projections	293
Facial bones	**294**
Occipito-mental	294
Modified mento-occipital	295
Occipito-mental 30° caudal	296
Modified reverse occipito-mental 30° for the severely injured patient	297
Lateral	298
Zygomatic arches – infero superior	299
Orbits – occipito-mental (modified)	300
Nasal bones – lateral	301
Mandible – lateral 30° cranial	302
Mandible – postero-anterior	303
Mandible – postero-anterior oblique	304
Temporo-mandibular joints – lateral 25° caudal	305
PARANASAL SINUSES	306
Occipito-mental	306
Occipito-frontal 15° caudal	307
Lateral	308
SKULL	309
Image evaluation – 10-point plan	309
FACIAL BONES AND SINUSES	310
Image evaluation – 10-point plan	310

8 Skull

Introduction

The importance of plain radiography of the skull has diminished in recent years due to the widespread availability of other imaging modalities, i.e. computed tomography (CT) and magnetic resonance imaging (MRI). The specificity of both modalities does allow for a faster and more definitive diagnosis than plain radiography. Skull radiography can play a significant role in the management of patients with certain skeletal conditions and, to a limited extent in trauma, e.g. when a depressed or penetrating injury is suspected or if the patient is difficult to assess. Also the ability to refer patients for multiplanar skull/head imaging may be dependent upon local availability. Consequently, a significant number of referrals are still received from the accident and emergency department.

In order to produce high-quality diagnostic images of the cranium and minimise risk, i.e. radiation dose for the patient, the radiographer must have a good understanding of the relevant anatomy, positioning landmarks and equipment used for imaging.

This chapter will enable the radiographer to balance the technical factors with individual patient needs in order to maximise diagnostic outcome.

Interpretation of skull images

Skull images are recognised to be amongst the most difficult to interpret due to the complexity of the bony construction with numerous irregular bones forming a sphere joined by sutures. The arterial and venous markings in the inner skull table may add confusion and can mimic fractures. Anteriorly, the complex facial skeleton is superimposed over the lower part of the skull vault; the dense petrous temporal bone also obscures detail in specific radiographic projections. Fractures of the skull base are important because of the risk of cerebrospinal fluid (CSF) leak and spread of infection to the intracranial contents, but they are difficult to demonstrate due to the thin, flat nature of the bones and superimposition of the aforementioned facial skeleton and petrous bone.

Superimposition of other unnecessary radio-opaque structures, including hair extensions, clips and hair matted with blood, can cause some confusion at interpretation. Surgical clips used for wound closure should not cause confusion, and they may help by marking the site of injury.

The initial interpretation of a skull series will often be done by a clinician who is relatively inexperienced in trauma radiology. Therefore the images must be of diagnostic quality.

Anatomical terminology (Figs 8.1a–8.1d)

All radiography of the skull is undertaken with reference to a series of palpable/visible landmarks and recognised lines or planes of the skull and face. It is vital that the radiographer possesses a good understanding of these before undertaking any radiographic positioning.

Landmarks

Outer canthus of the eye: the lateral point where the upper and lower eyelids meet.
Infraorbital margin/point: the lowest point of the inferior rim of the orbit
Nasion: the articulation between the nasal and frontal bones.
Glabella: a bony prominence found on the frontal bone immediately superior to the nasion.
Vertex: the highest point of the skull in the median sagittal plane.
External occipital protuberance (inion): a bony prominence found on the occipital bone, usually coincident with the median sagittal plane.
External auditory meatus (EAM): the opening within the ear that leads into the external auditory canal.

Lines

Interpupillary (interorbital) line: joins the centre of the two orbits or the centre of the two pupils when the eyes are looking straight forward.
Infraorbital line: joins the two inferior infraorbital points.
Anthropological baseline: passes from the infraorbital point to the upper border of the EAM (also known as the Frankforter line).
Orbito-meatal baseline (radiographic baseline): extends from the outer canthus of the eye to the centre of the EAM. This is angled approximately 10° to the anthropological baseline.

Planes

Median sagittal plane: divides the skull into right and left halves. Landmarks on this plane are the nasion anteriorly and the external occipital protuberance (inion) posteriorly.
Coronal planes: are at right-angles to the median sagittal plane and divide the head into anterior and posterior parts.
Anthropological plane: a horizontal plane containing the two anthropological baselines and the infraorbital line. It is an example of an axial plane.
Auricular plane: perpendicular to the anthropological plane and passes through the centre of the two EAMs. It is an example of a coronal plane.

The median sagittal, anthropological and coronal planes are mutually at right-angles.

Skull 8

Radiographic anatomy

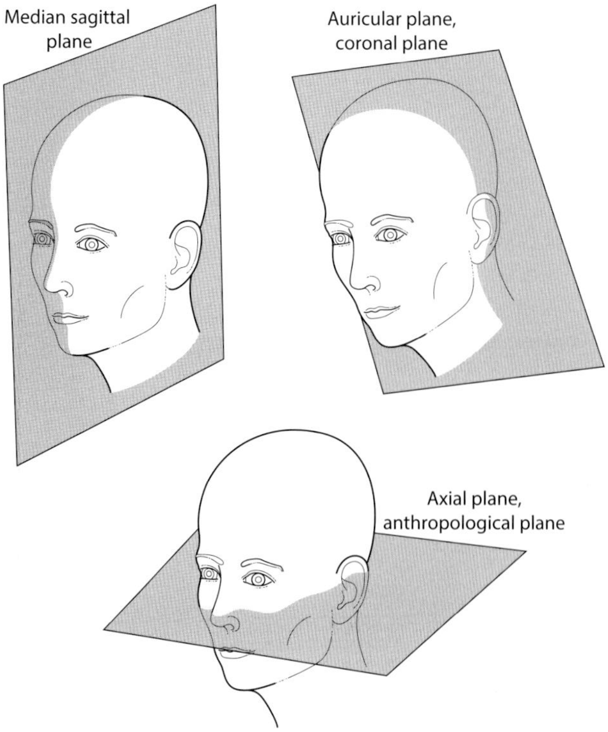

Fig. 8.1a Diagram of planes.

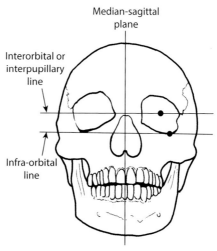

Fig. 8.1d Frontal line diagram of skull showing primary positioning lines.

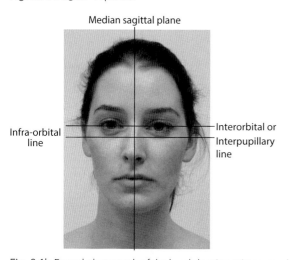

Fig. 8.1b Frontal photograph of the head showing primary positioning lines.

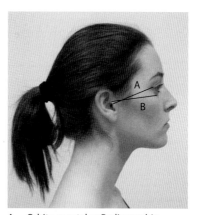

A = Orbito-meatal or Radiographic baseline (RBL)
B = Anthropological baseline

Fig. 8.1e Lateral photograph of the head showing primary positioning lines.

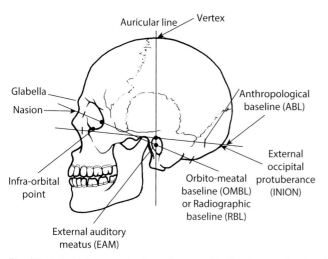

Fig. 8.1c Lateral diagram showing primary positioning lines and landmarks.

8 Skull

Radiographic anatomy (cont.)

In order to evaluate radiographs successfully it is important to be aware of a range of anatomical features demonstrated on the standard skull projections. This will enable a judgement to be made in relation to the quality of the radiograph with respect to positioning.

The radiographs (Figs 8.2a–8.2c) show a range of features that are used in image evaluation and will be regularly referred to in the remainder of this chapter.

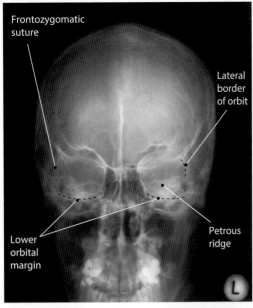

Fig. 8.2a OF radiograph showing anatomical features.

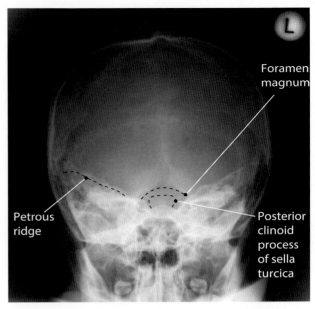

Fig. 8.2b FO 30° radiograph showing anatomical features.

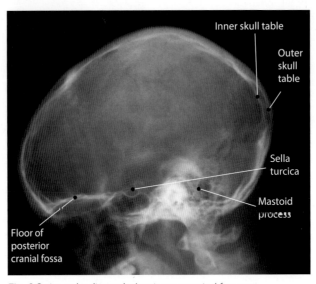

Fig. 8.2c Lateral radiograph showing anatomical features.

Skull 8

Radiography of the skull can be carried out using an ordinary erect Bucky with direct digital radiography (DDR) or computed radiography (CR) cassettes, or simply a fine stationary grid and X-ray tube with CR imaging. A specialised skull unit may also be used but in the majority of hospitals in the UK they have been superseded by other imaging systems.

Each method has specific advantages and disadvantages in any given situation and these will be considered later. Problems arise for the radiographer as the different methods use slightly different imaging techniques, which in turn utilise different planes and beam angulations to achieve the same projection. It is important for the radiographer to be fully aware of each technique in order to maximise the diagnostic outcome for their patients.

Skull units (Figs 8.3a, 8.3b)

Images taken on skull units yield the highest quality skull images. All aspects of tube and receptor/cassette support design have been optimised for skull radiography. Their use is to be recommended where possible when undertaking skull radiography, providing the patient's condition will allow this.

Advantages include:

- Reduction in distortion.
- High-resolution images resulting from a grid with a large number of gridlines per unit length (grid lattice) and very fine focal spot on the tube anode (typically 0.3–0.4 mm^2).
- Projections accurate and consistent as the patient is placed in one or a limited number of positions and the tube is then positioned at differing angulations around the patients head.
- Can be more comfortable for the patient as usually only one position has to be achieved and maintained.
- Purpose designed circular collimators allow close collimation to the head, reducing the dose produced by scatter and minimising secondary radiation.

Radiographic anatomy (*cont.*)

Disadvantages include:

- With some skull units the patient is required to lie on a narrow table. This may not make it suitable for some patients who are unable to co-operate.
- Most units are accompanied by their own technique manual, requiring the radiographer to acquire a set of skills unique to one piece of equipment.
- Equipment may be expensive to purchase and maintain.
- Can be lacking in versatility for sick patients or those with conditions such a thoracic lordosis.

Types of skull unit

Isocentric: this is the most widely available unit and will produce the highest quality images. This is achieved by the design of the equipment, which ensures the image receptor/cassette and collimated X-ray beam are always perpendicular to each other, thus eliminating distortion and grid cut-off. Note that the point around which the tube pivots is always adjusted so that it is at the centre of the object of interest.

The technique used by each manufacturer will vary slightly but all use the anthropological baseline rather than the radiographic baseline (RBL) when describing projections.

Lysholm: this differs from the isocentric type because the point around which the tube pivots is always in the same plane as the receptor. This has the potential to produce distorted images if large angulations are used. The techniques used to operate these units are very similar to skull radiography carried out with a simple tube and Bucky and utilise the RBL when describing techniques. This type of skull unit is not widely used in modern imaging departments.

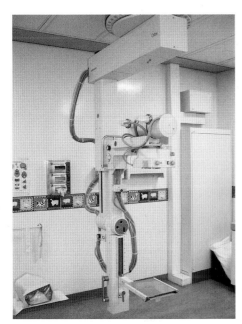

Fig. 8.3a Isocentric skull unit.

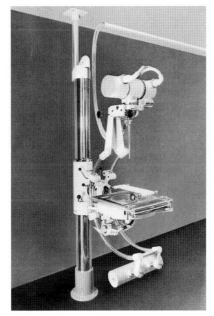

Fig. 8.3b Lysholm skull unit.

8 Skull

Positioning terminology

To describe a skull projection it is necessary to state the relative positions of: the skull planes to the image receptor, the central ray relative to skull planes/image receptor and give a centring point or area to be included within the collimated X-ray beam.

Traditionally a centring point has always been given but this may not always be appropriate with skull radiography. This is because some centring points will lead to the irradiation of a large number of radiosensitive structures that are of no diagnostic interest. Rather than focussing entirely on centring points, it is often better for the radiographer to be mindful of the anatomy that needs to be demonstrated for a diagnosis to be made and ensure that this is included within the collimated primary beam, whilst ensuring it is not obscured by other anatomical structures.

Occipto-frontal projection

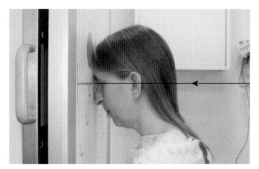

Fig. 8.4a Head position for OF projection.

Projections in which the collimated X-ray beam is parallel to the sagittal plane are named according to the direction of the central ray. In the photograph above the central ray enters the skull trough the occipital bone and exits through the frontal bone. This is therefore an occipto-frontal (OF) projection (Fig. 8.4a).

Fronto-occipital projection

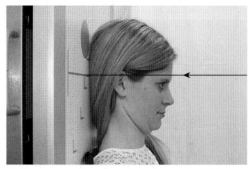

Fig. 8.4b Head position for FO projection.

Again the central ray is parallel to the sagittal plane except now the central ray enters the skull through the frontal bone and exits through the occipital bone. This is a fronto-occipital (FO) projection (Fig. 8.4b).

Beam angulation

Many OF or FO projections will require the central ray to pass along the sagittal plane at some angle to the orbital-meatal plane. In these cases the degree of angulation is stated after the name of the projection. The direction of angulation is also given. Cranial angulation involves the beam directed up the body towards the head (written in short form as ↑). If the central ray is angled toward the feet, the beam is then said to be angled caudally (written in short form as ↓).

The photograph below shows a FO 30° caudal projection (FO30°↓) (Fig. 8.4c).

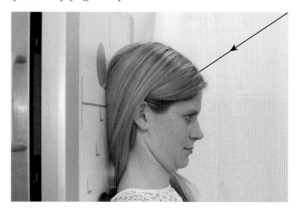

Fig. 8.4c Head position for FO30°↓ projection.

Lateral

For the lateral projection, the collimated central ray passes along a coronal plane at right-angles to the median sagittal plane. It is named according to the side of the head closest to the image receptor/cassette. In the example below the beam enters the skull on the left side, passes along a coronal plane and exits the head on the right side where the image receptor is located. This is therefore a right lateral (Fig. 8.4d).

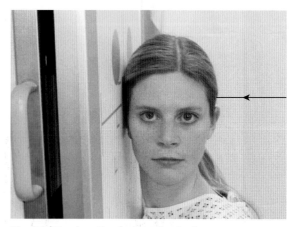

Fig. 8.4d Head position for lateral projection.

Warning

When undertaking oblique skull radiography always ensure the beam is angled in the same direction as the grid lattice, i.e. parallel to the grid lines. If any angulation is applied such that beam is angled across the grid lines, i.e. perpendicular to their direction of travel, then a grid cut-off artefact will result and the image will need to be repeated.

Lateral with angulation

If the collimated central ray passes along a coronal plane at some angle to the median sagittal plane then the degree of angulation is stated. The photograph below shows a right lateral with 30° caudal angulation (R Lat 30°↓) (Fig. 8.5a).

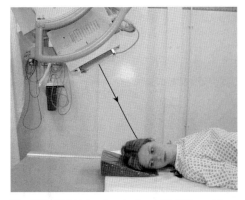

Fig. 8.5a Right lateral projection with 30° caudal angulation.

Oblique projections

An oblique projection is obtained when the central ray is at some angle to the median sagittal plane and the coronal plane. The naming of the projection will depend on two factors: firstly, whether the anterior or posterior portion of the head is in contact with the receptor/cassette; and secondly, whether the left or right side of the head is in contact with the receptor/cassette.

Forty degree left anterior oblique (40°LAO)

In this example the head is rotated to the left such that the median sagittal plane is 40° to the image receptor and the left side of the head is in contact with the image receptor (Fig. 8.5b).

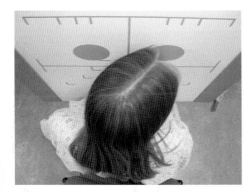

Fig. 8.5b 40° LAO from a superior aspect.

Complex oblique projections

Oblique projections may become more complex when a caudal or cranial angulation is added in relation to a specified baseline. This additional angle is usually achieved by raising or lowering the chin such that the relevant baseline makes the required angle to the image receptor. Alternatively the X-ray tube can be angled or a combination of both approaches may be useful if the patient has limited mobility. The photograph on the top right is an example of one such projection used for plain imaging of the optic foramina (Fig. 8.5c).

Skull 8

Positioning terminology (cont.)

Fifty five degree left anterior oblique with 35° caudal angulation (55°LAO35°↓)

The head has been rotated such that the right side of the face is in contact with the receptor/cassette and the median sagittal plane makes an angle of 55° with the image receptor. In the example below the central ray has a 35° caudal angulation. Alternatively this angulation may be achieved by raising the orbito-meatal plane by 35° whilst using a horizontal beam (Figs 8.5c, 8.5d).

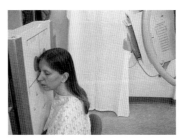

Fig. 8.5c 55° right anterior oblique with 35° caudal angulation (lateral aspect).

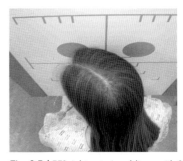

Fig. 8.5d 55° right anterior oblique with 35° caudal angulation (superior aspect).

The photograph below shows how the same projection has been achieved with a combination of tube and orbital-meatal plane angulation. In this case the plane has been raised 20° and the tube has been given a 15° caudal angulation, in effect producing a total beam angulation of 35° to the orbital-meatal plane (Fig. 8.5e).

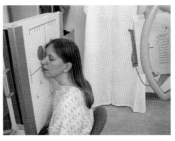

Fig. 8.5e 55° right anterior oblique with 35° caudal angulation (lateral aspect). RBL raised 20° with 15° caudal angle on the tube.

8 Skull

Patient preparation

Before undertaking skull radiography the following specific considerations should be made.

- Ensure all metal/radio-opaque objects are removed from the patient, e.g. hair clips or pins.
- Ponytails/bunches of hair often produce artefacts and thus should be loosened.
- If the area of interest includes the mouth then false teeth containing metal or metal dental bridges should be removed unless the patient has facial injuries as they may be assisting retention of the airway.
- The patient should be provided with a clear explanation of any movements and image receptor positions associated with the normal operation of the skull unit (if being used).

Useful accessories

- Foam pads can be useful as an aid to patient immobilisation. The photograph opposite shows a specially designed pad for skull radiography. It is available in a range of sizes to accommodate different age groups/head sizes (Fig. 8.6a).
- 45° triangular pads are also extremely useful for immobilising children. They can be held by the parent and enable immobilisation without the parent placing their hands in the primary beam (Fig. 8.6b).
- Individual side markers are essential for skull radiography.

General image quality guidelines and radiation protection considerations

The European Guidelines on Quality Criteria for Diagnostic Images describe various criteria by which images should be assessed. Many of these criteria are included with the specific projection descriptions and in the introduction to the chapter, but some more general points and other considerations are included below.

- Images should have high resolution of all the skull structures such as outer and inner lamina of the cranial vault, the trabecular structure of the cranium, the various sinuses and

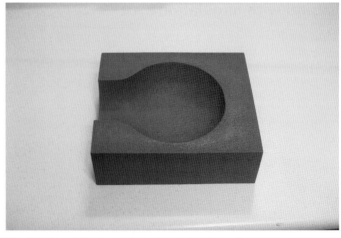

Fig. 8.6a Immobilisation pads used in skull radiography.

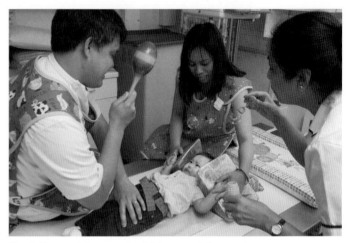

Fig. 8.6b Immobilisation of a child using 45° foam pads.

sutures where visible, vascular channels, petrous part of the temporal bone and the pituitary fossa.
- Important image details in the 0.3–0.5 mm range achieved by using fine focus and 70–85 kV tube voltage.
- Whenever possible, use an OF (PA) rather than an FO (AP) technique as this greatly reduces the dose to the orbits.
- 24 × 30 cm CR cassettes are generally utilised for plain skull radiography or appropriate collimation when using DDR.
- A grid, moving or stationary, should be used for skull radiography to ensure high resolution and definition of fine detail in the bony anatomy of the skull.

Skull 8

Radiological considerations (Figs 8.7a–8.7c)

As mentioned in the introduction skull imaging using plain DDR or CR systems is relatively rare in the UK. Any patient who has suffered a head injury or any severe trauma affecting the skull is referred for a CT scan using the National Institute for Health and Care Excellence (NICE) guidelines.

NICE guidelines are used for several NHS protocols across Trusts and have been updated in Jan 2014 (to replace NICE Clinical guideline 56).

Research shows that head injury in the under 40s is the commonest cause of death. These latest guidelines state that 1/5 of the 200,000 people seen annually in accident and emergency (A&E) departments in the UK, have features suggesting a skull fracture or brain injury. Therefore, early detection and treatment is crucial to preserving life.[1]

The previous guidelines, which were updated in 2007, resulted in CT imaging replacing plain imaging of the skull for trauma-referred patients. CT is now a quick and relatively simple examination that is protocol driven and has a high sensitivity to identifying brain injury.

The NICE CT referral guidelines[2] for head injury patients rely upon the understanding and application of the Glasgow Coma Scale (GCS). The GCS is used to assess the level of a patient's coma: their ability to open their eyes, move and speak. The total score is calculated by the adding up of the scores for each section, seen in the table opposite, and ranges from a minimum of 3 to a maximum of 15.[3]

The criteria for performing a head CT scan is dependent upon the patient age, i.e. adult or child, and their presentation, symptoms and thus GCS score. The severity of their presentation is dependent on the injury sustained and thus their risk factors. In the image opposite the criteria for an adult referral is indicated.[4]

The key change to the NICE guidelines in 2014 was the recommendation of a provisional radiological report on all CT scans for trauma within 1 hour of the scan having been performed. This forced change in some radiology departments from their previous reporting framework to ensure compliance with these national guidelines.[5]

This relatively new modification to referral criteria has ensured that patients referred via A&E suffering a suspected brain injury gain access to the optimum imaging modality to allow rapid diagnosis and treatment. If CT is to be performed according to these guidelines, skull radiography will very rarely be justifiable.

Glasgow Coma Scale - Best motor response	
6	Obeying commands
5	Movement localised to stimulus
4	Withdraws
3	Abnormal muscle bending and flexing
2	Involuntary muscle straightening and extending
1	None

Glasgow Coma Scale - Verbal responses	
5	Orientated response
4	Confused conversation
3	Inappropriate words
2	Incomprehensible sounds
1	None

Glasgow Coma Scale - Eye opening	
4	Spantaneous
3	To speech
2	To pain
1	None

Fig. 8.7a Glasgow Coma Scale[2] table used throughout the medical world.

Criteria for performing a CT head scan

- For adults who have sustained a head injury and have any of the following risk factors, perform a CT head scan within 1 hour of the risk factor being identified:
  - GCS less than 13 on initial assessment in the emergency department.
  - GCS less than 15 at 2 hours after the injury on assessment in the emergency department.
  - Suspected open or depressed skull fracture.
  - Any sign of basal skull fracture (haemotympanum. 'panda' eyes, cerebrospinal fluid leakage from the ear or nose, Battle's sign).
  - Post-traumatic seizure.
  - Focal neurological deficit.
  - More than 1 episode of vomiting.

A provisional written radiology report should be made available within 1 hour of the scan being performed. [new 2014]

Fig. 8.7b NICE criteria[3] for adult CT scan following head injury.

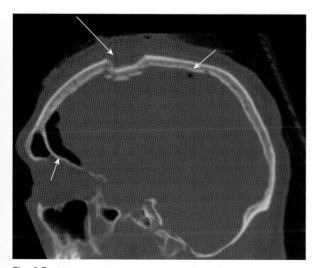

Fig. 8.7c CT image showing comminuted skull fractures with intracranial air.[6]

8 Cranium

Radiographic technique

Basic skull technique should be undertaken for specific conditions and referrals and only when the patients' condition allows. The technique below is for a patient who is supine, on a trolley and thus restricted due to health from sitting erect. Stationary grids are used when it is not possible to use the Bucky grid system.

Lateral – supine with horizontal beam (Figs 8.8a, 8.8b)

Position of patient and image receptor

- The patient lies supine with the head raised and immobilised on a non-opaque skull pad. This will ensure the occipital region is included on the image.
- The head is adjusted such that the median sagittal plane is perpendicular to the table/trolley and the interpupillary line is perpendicular to the image receptor.
- The image receptor is supported vertically against the lateral aspect of the head parallel to the median sagittal plane with its edge 5 cm above the vertex of the skull.

Direction and location of the X-ray beam

- The collimated horizontal beam is directed parallel to the interpupillary line such that it is at right-angles to the median sagittal plane.
- The centring point is midway between the glabella and the external occipital protuberance to a point approximately 5 cm superior and posterior to the EAM.
- The long axis of the image receptor should be coincident with the long axis of the skull.

Essential image characteristics

- The image should contain all of the cranial bones and the 1st cervical vertebrae.
- A true lateral will result in superimposition of the lateral portions of the floors of the anterior and the posterior cranial fossa. The clinoid processes of the sella turcica should also be superimposed.

Radiological considerations

- Skull imaging as previously mentioned is used to identify brain injury that cannot be assessed by skull radiography, so the prime modality currently used is a CT scan.
- Basal skull fractures are potentially life threatening due to the risk of intracranial infection, and are often very difficult to detect. Lateral skull projections taken supine with a collimated horizontal beam may reveal (sphenoid) sinus fluid levels, which may be a discrete indicator of skull base injury. They may also help to confirm the presence of free intracranial air, which is another sign of a discrete fracture to the cranium.
- Fracture of the very thin squamous temporal bone may be associated with bleeding from the middle meningeal artery and can cause rapid death due to extradural haematoma. Good optimisation of imaging this region is therefore essential.

Common faults and solutions

- Failure to include the occipital region as a result of not using a pad or similar to ensure the head is elevated adequately from the trolley surface.
- Poor superimposition of the lateral floors of the cranial fossa. Always ensure the interobital line is perpendicular to the cassette/receptor and the median sagittal plane is perpendicular to the trolley surface.

Notes

- The choice of lateral will depend on the site of the suspected pathology.
- If the suspected pathology is to the left side of the head then a left lateral should be undertaken with the image receptor supported on the left side of the patient and vice versa. This will ensure the pathology is shown at the maximum resolution possible due to the minimisation of geometric unsharpness.
- This is the projection of choice for the majority of trauma cases on a trolley if CT is not been undertaken.

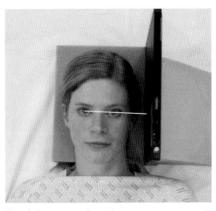

Fig. 8.8a Position from the anterior aspect with the line showing the interorbital line relation to image receptor; the patient is supported in the correct position.

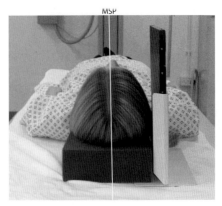

Fig. 8.8b Patient positioning from the superior aspect showing MSP, CR cassette position and pad.

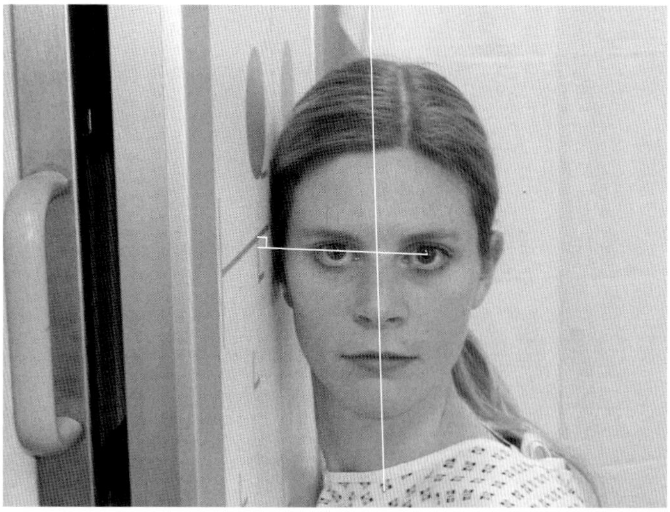

Cranium 8

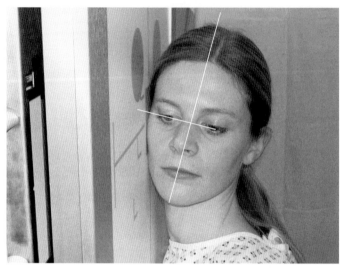

Fig. 8.9a Correct positioning for erect lateral skull.

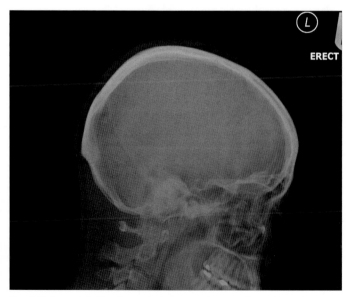

Fig. 8.9b Incorrect positioning for erect lateral skull.

Fig. 8.9c Lateral skull radiograph demonstrating superimposition of sphenoid wings.

Lateral erect (Figs 8.9a–8.9c)

This position may be used for a co-operative patient. Variations from the supine horizontal beam technique are noted below but all other imaging criteria remain the same.

Position of patient and image receptor

- The patient sits facing the erect Bucky/receptor and the head is then rotated such that the median sagittal plane is parallel to the Bucky/receptor and the interpupillary line is perpendicular to the Bucky/ receptor.
- The shoulders may be rotated slightly to allow the correct position to be attained and the patient may grip the Bucky inferiorly for stability.
- Position the image receptor transversely such that its upper border is 5 cm above the vertex of the skull.
- A radiolucent pad may be placed under the chin/lower half of the face, for support.

Direction and location of the X-ray beam

- The X-ray tube should be centred to the Bucky/image receptor and the 'tracking' facility utilised if available.
- Adjust the height of the Bucky/tube so that the patient is comfortable (NB: do not decentre the tube from the Bucky at this point).
- Centre with a collimated horizontal beam midway between the glabella and the external occipital protuberance to a point approximately 5 cm superior and posterior to the EAM.

Common faults and solutions

- This is not an easy position for the patient to maintain. Check the position of all planes immediately prior to the exposure; the patient may have moved.

Notes

- This projection can also be performed with the patient prone on a floating-top table with a collimated vertical beam.
- The projection may usefully be performed on babies in the supine position with the head rotated to either side.
- An air/fluid level in the sphenoid sinus (an indicator for a base of skull fracture) will not be visible if the patient is imaged with a collimated vertical central ray. This is not relevant in young babies, as the sinus is not fully developed.

Expected DRL: ESD 1.1 mGy

8 Cranium

Occipito-frontal (Figs 8.10a–8.10e)

Occipito-frontal (OF) projections can be employed with different degrees of beam angulation. The choice of projection will depend upon departmental protocol and the anatomy that needs to be demonstrated.

Position of patient and image receptor

- This projection may be undertaken erect or in the prone position. The erect projection will be described, as the prone projection may be uncomfortable for the patient and will usually only be undertaken in the absence of a vertical Bucky/image receptor.
- The patient is seated facing the erect Bucky/receptor so that the median sagittal plane is coincident with the midline of the image receptor and is also perpendicular to it.
- The neck is flexed so that orbito-meatal baseline is perpendicular to the image receptor. This can usually be achieved by ensuring the nose and forehead are in contact with the Bucky/receptor.
- Ensure the mid part of the frontal bone is positioned in the centre of the Bucky/receptor.
- The patient may place the palms of each hand either side of the head (out of the primary beam) for stability.

Direction and location of the X-ray beam

OF:
- The collimated horizontal beam is directed perpendicular to the Bucky/receptor along the median sagittal plane.
- The beam collimation should include the vertex of the skull superiorly, the region immediately below the base of the occipital bone inferiorly and the lateral skin margins. It is important to ensure the tube is centred to the centre of the Bucky receptor.

OF10°↓, OF15°↓, OF20°↓:
- The technique used for these three projections is similar to that employed for the OF except a caudal angulation is applied. The degree of angulation will depend upon the technique, i.e. for an OF20↓ projection a 20° caudal angulation will be employed.
- Ensure the collimated horizontal beam is always centred to the centre of the Bucky/image receptor after the tube angulation has been applied and not before.

Essential image characteristics

- All the cranial bones should be included within the image including the skin margins.
- It is important to ensure the skull is not rotated. This can be assessed by measuring the distance from a point in the midline of the skull to the lateral margin. If this is the equidistant from both sides of the skull then it is not rotated.

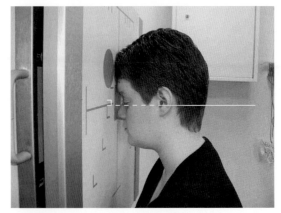

Fig. 8.10a Positioning for OF skull projection.

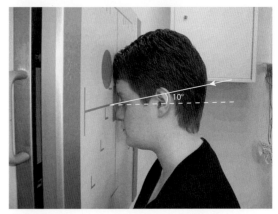

Fig. 8.10b Positioning for OF10°↓ skull projection.

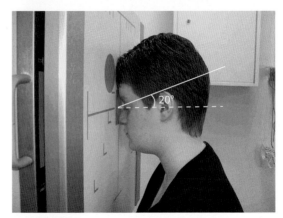

Fig. 8.10c Positioning for OF20°↓ skull projection.

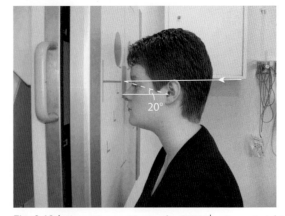

Fig. 8.10d Alternative positioning for OF20°↓ using a straight tube with the orbito-meatal baseline raised 20°.

Cranium 8

Occipito-frontal (cont.)

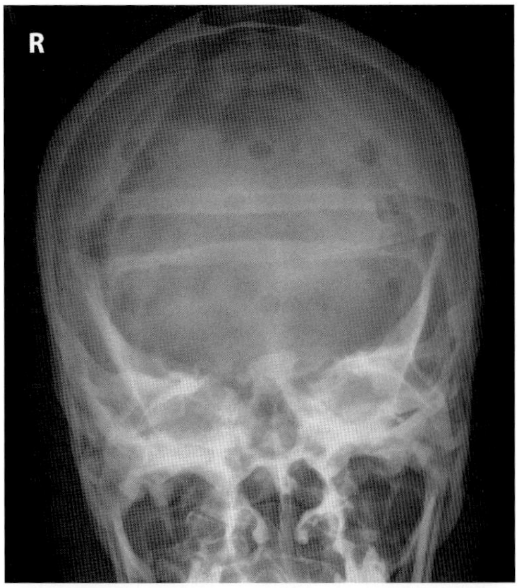

Essential image characteristics (cont.) (Figs 8.11a–8.11c)

- The degree of beam angulation can be evaluated from an assessment of the position of the petrous ridges within the orbits:
- OF: the petrous ridges should be completely superimposed within the orbit with their upper borders coincident with the upper 1/3 of the orbit.
- OF10°↓: the petrous ridges appear in the middle 1/3 of the orbit.
- OF15°↓: the petrous ridges appear in the lower 1/3 of the orbit.
- OF20°↓: the petrous ridges appear just below the inferior orbital margin.

Radiological considerations

- Asymmetry of projection of the squamo-parietal suture due to rotation increases the risk of it being mistaken for a fracture.
- As the beam angle increases, more of the orbital region is demonstrated. Thus the site of the suspected pathology should be considered when selecting the beam angle, e.g. an injury to the superior orbital region can be best evaluated with an OF20°↓ projection.

Common faults and solutions

- Rotation: ensure the patient has maintained their position immediately before the exposure is made.
- Incorrect beam angulation: NB: increased beam angulations will result in the petrous ridges appearing more inferiorly in the orbit. If an OF20°↓ is undertaken and the petrous bones appear in the middle 1/3 of the orbit, then a greater angle should have been applied, in this case a further 10°.

Notes: alternative technique

Patients often find it difficult to maintain their orbito-meatal baseline perpendicular to the image receptor as this is an uncomfortable position. Instead of angling the X-ray beam to achieve the desired position of the petrous ridge within the orbits, a collimated vertical central ray, i.e. perpendicular to the image receptor may be used. The desired angulation for the projection can then be achieved by raising the orbito-meatal baseline by the desired angle, e.g. for an OF20°↓ the chin can be raised such that the orbito-meatal baseline will be at an angle of 20° to the horizontal (see Fig. 8.10d). Similarly for an OF10°↓ the orbito-meatal line will be raised by 10°.

Expected DRL: ESD 1.8 mGy

Fig. 8.11a OF (all images are taken using a phantom).

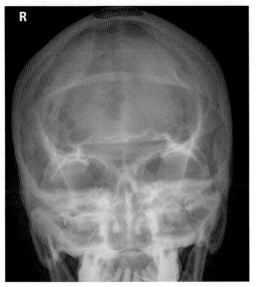

Fig. 8.11b OF 15°.

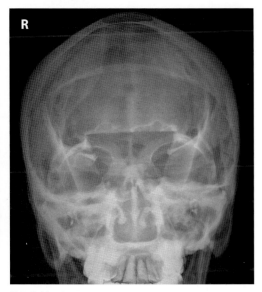

Fig. 8.11c OF 20°.

8 Cranium

Fronto-occipital (Figs 8.12a–8.12c)

Fronto-occipital (FO) projections of the skull will demonstrate the same anatomy as OF projections. The orbits and frontal bone however, will be magnified as they are positioned further from the image receptor.

Such projections should only be undertaken when the patient cannot be moved and must be imaged supine. These projections result in an increased radiation dose to the orbits and some loss of resolution of the anterior skull structures due to increased object-to-receptor distance.

Position of patient and image receptor

- The patient lies supine on the trolley (or X-ray table) with the posterior aspect of the skull resting on the image receptor/ gridded CR cassette.
- The head is adjusted to bring the median sagittal plane at right-angles to the image receptor and coincident with its midline. In this position the EAMs are equidistant from the image receptor to ensure no rotation.
- The orbito-meatal baseline should be perpendicular to the image receptor.

Direction and location of the X-ray beam

- All angulations for FO projections are made cranially.
- The collimated vertical X-ray beam is directed perpendicular to the image receptor along the median sagittal plane.
- The collimated field should be set to include the vertex of the skull superiorly, the base of the occipital bone inferiorly and the lateral skin margins. It is important to ensure that the tube is centred to the image receptor and 'tracking' applied if available.

FO10°↑, FO15°↑, FO20°↑:

- The technique used for these three projections is similar to that employed for the OF except cranial angulations are applied. The degree of angulation will depend upon the projection required.
- Remember that the image receptor must be displaced superiorly to allow for the tube angulation, otherwise the area of interest will be projected off the image.

Essential image characteristics, radiological considerations and DRL

See OF projections.

Common faults and solutions

- See OF projections.
- Remember increasing the degree of cranial angulation will project the petrous ridges more inferior in the orbits.

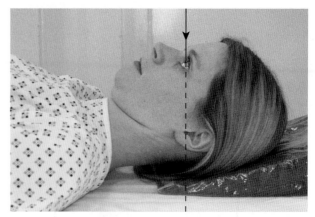

Fig. 8.12a FO projection.

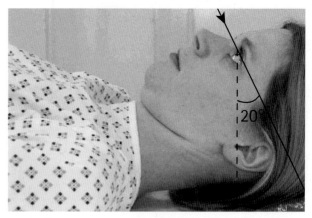

Fig. 8.12b FO 20° projection.

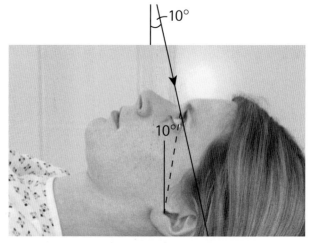

Fig. 8.12c FO 20° projection achieved with 10° tube angle and RBL raised 10°.

Notes: alternative technique

- As for the OF projections.
- In the example given below, an FO20°↑ projection is required but the patient can only maintain their orbito-meatal baseline in a position 10° back from perpendicular (i.e. with the chin raised slightly). In order to achieve an overall 20° angle, a 10° cranial angulation will need to be applied to the tube.
- Similarly if the patients chin was raised such that the baseline was 20° to the perpendicular, an FO20°↑ projection can be achieved by using a straight tube perpendicular to the image receptor.

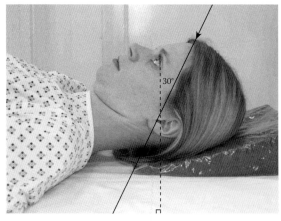

Fig. 8.13a FO 30' Towne's projection.

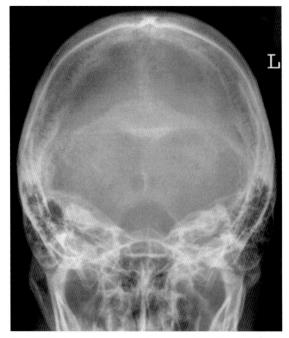

Fig. 8.13b Correctly positioned townes with sella turcica seen within the foramen magnum.

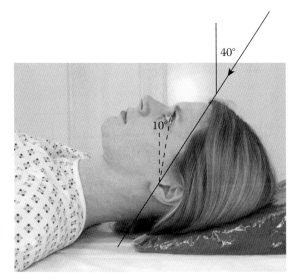

Fig. 8.13c The chin is raised such that the baseline makes an angle of 10° to the perpendicular, therefore a 40° tube angle must employed to ensure a 30° angle to the orbito-meatal plane.

Cranium 8

Half axial, fronto-occipital 30° caudal (Towne's projection) (Figs 8.13a, 8.13c)

Position of patient and image receptor

- The patient lies supine on a trolley (or X-ray table) with the posterior aspect of the skull resting on an image receptor/gridded CR cassette.
- The head is adjusted to bring the median sagittal plane at right-angles to the image receptor and so that it is coincident with its midline.
- The orbito-meatal baseline should be perpendicular to the image receptor.

Direction and location of the X-ray beam

- The collimated vertical beam is angled caudally so it makes an angle of 30° to the orbito-meatal plane.
- To avoid irradiating the eyes the collimation is set to ensure the lower border is coincident with the superior-orbital margin and the upper border includes the skull vertex. Laterally the skin margins should also be included within the field.[7]
- The top of the receptor should be positioned adjacent to the vertex of the skull to ensure the beam angulation does not project the area of interest off the bottom of the image.

Essential image characteristics (Fig. 8.13b)

- The sella turcica of the sphenoid bone is projected to appear within the foramen magnum.
- The image must include all of the occipital bone and the posterior parts of the parietal bone and the lambdoidal suture should be clearly visualised.
- The skull should not be rotated. This can also be assessed by ensuring the sella turcica appears centrally in the foramen magnum.

Radiological considerations

- The foramen magnum should be clearly seen on this projection. The margins may be obscured by incorrect angulation, thus hiding serious fractures.
- The zygoma is well demonstrated on this projection and if fractured gives a clue to the presence of associated facial injury.

8 Cranium

Half axial, fronto-occipital 30° caudal (Towne's projection) (cont.) (Figs 8.14a–8.14c)

Common faults and solutions

- Under angulation: the foramen magnum is not clearly demonstrated above the petrous ridges. This is probably the most common fault as the patient may find it difficult to maintain their radiographic baseline perpendicular to the image receptor.
- If the patient's chin cannot be sufficiently depressed to bring the orbito-meatal baseline perpendicular to the image receptor then it will be necessary to increase the angulation of the tube to more than 30° to the vertical. A 30° angle to the orbito-meatal plane must be maintained (see picture).
- Over angulation: the posterior arch of the atlas bone (C1) is visible within the foramen magnum.
- The large tube angle introduces a significant degree of distortion in the resultant image.
- Some patients, particularly those with an increased thoracic kyphosis may have difficulty in positioning their back against the image receptor. This can be somewhat overcome by angling the Bucky/image receptor as shown in the photograph.

Notes

- Some of the 30° angle required for this projection can be applied by using a skull board. If a 30° board is used and the patient's orbito-meatal baseline is perpendicular to the top of the board, then a vertical central ray should be employed. If a 15° board is used a 15° caudal angulation must be applied.
- If a skull board with a 20° angle is used then a 10° caudal angulation will be required to give the correct overall beam angulation.

Modified half axial (Fig. 8.14d)

Denton (1998) has suggested an alternative projection that avoids irradiating the eyes and thyroid.

- The central ray is angled caudally so it makes an angle of 25° to the orbito-meatal plane.
- Instead of using a centring point, a collimation field is set. The lower border of this field should be limited immediately above the supraorbital ridges at their highest point. The upper border of the light beam should just include the vertex of the skull at its highest point. Collimate laterally to include the skin margins within the field.[9]

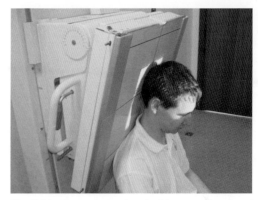

Fig. 8.14a The Bucky can be tilted for ease of imaging kyphotic patients.

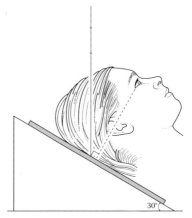

Fig. 8.14b FO30° Towne's projection using a 30° skull board.

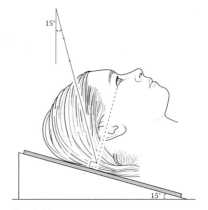

Fig. 8.14c FO30° Towne's projection using a 15° skull board.

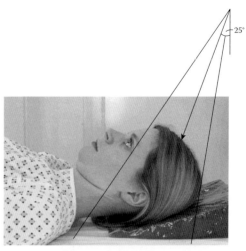

Fig. 8.14d Modified half axial.

Position of patient and image receptor

- This projection is usually undertaken with the patient in the erect position facing the erect Bucky/image receptor, although it may be performed with the patient prone.
- Initially the patient is asked to place their nose and forehead against the image receptor.

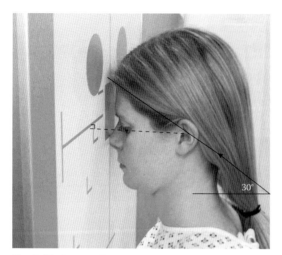

Fig. 8.15a Reverse Towne's.

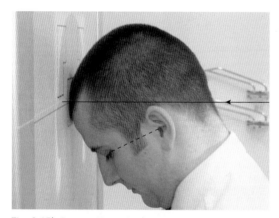

Fig. 8.15b Reverse Towne's, alternative positioning.

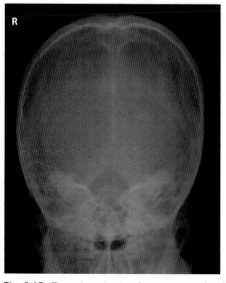

Fig. 8.15c Towne's projection demonstrating the clivus centred within the sella turcica.

Cranium 8

Occipito-frontal 30° cranial angulation (reverse Towne's projection) (Figs 8.15a, 8.15b)

- The head is adjusted to bring the median sagittal plane at right-angles to the image receptor so it is coincident with its midline.
- The orbito-meatal baseline should be perpendicular to the image receptor.
- The patient may place their hands on the Bucky/receptor for stability.

Direction and location of the X-ray beam

- The central ray is angled cranially so it makes an angle of 30° to the orbito-meatal plane.
- Adjust the collimation field such the whole of the whole of the occipital bone and the parietal bones up to the vertex are included within the field. Avoid including the eyes in the primary beam.
- Laterally the skin margins should also be included within the field.

Essential image characteristics

- The sella turcica of the sphenoid bone is projected within the foramen magnum.
- The image must include all of the occipital bone and the posterior parts of the parietal bone and the lambdoidal suture should be clearly visualised.
- The skull should not be rotated. This can also be assessed by ensuring the sella turcica appears centrally in the foramen magnum.

Radiological considerations (Fig. 8.15c)

- The foramen magnum should be clearly visualised on this projection. The margins may be obscured by incorrect angulation, thus hiding important fractures.
- The zygoma may be well seen on this projection and if fractured gives a clue to the presence of associated facial injury.

Common faults and solutions

- As per FO30°↓ projection (page 280).

Notes

- This projection will carry a lower radiation dose to sensitive structures than the equivalent fronto–occipital 30° caudal projection.
- Positioning may be easier for patients who find it difficult to achieve the position required for the equivalent AP half axial projections.

8 Cranium

Submento-vertical (Figs 8.16a, 8.16c)

Position of patient and image receptor

The patient may be imaged erect or supine. If the patient is unsteady then a supine technique is advisable as this is a difficult position to maintain.

Supine:
- The patient's shoulders are raised and neck hyperextended to bring the vertex of the skull in contact with the image receptor/gridded CR cassette (or X-ray table).
- The head is adjusted to bring the EAMs equidistant from the image receptor.
- The median sagittal plane should be at right-angles to the image receptor along its midline.
- The orbito-meatal plane should be as near as possible parallel to the image receptor.

Erect:
- The patient sits facing the X-ray tube a short distance away from the vertical Bucky/ receptor.
- The neck is hyperextended to allow the head to fall back until the vertex of the skull makes contact with the centre of the vertical image receptor.
- The remainder of the positioning is as described for the supine technique.

Direction and location of the X-ray beam

- The collimated perpendicular beam is directed at right-angles to the orbito-meatal plane and centred midway between them.

Essential image characteristics (Fig. 8.16b)

- An optimum projection will demonstrate the mandibular angles clear of the petrous portions of the temporal bone.
- The foramina of the middle cranial fossa should be seen symmetrically either side of the midline.

Radiological considerations

- Erosion of the bony margins of the skull base foramina is an important indicator of destruction by tumour. Under/overtilting or any rotation, reduces the visibility of these foramina.
- This is now an uncommon projection as CT imaging demonstrates fine bone detail of the skull base with the ability to produce 3D reconstructions. However, this may be used as an alternative projection to demonstrate the zygomatic arches in profile for facial injury. MRI offers multiplanar imaging with detail of the soft tissues as well as the skull base.

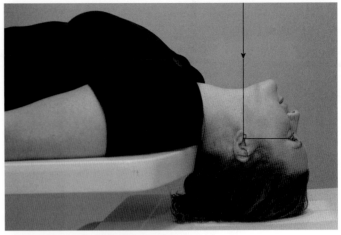

Fig. 8.16a SMV using supine technique.

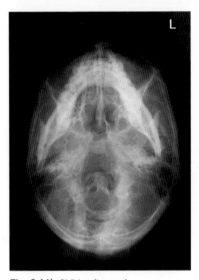

Fig. 8.16b SMV radiograph.

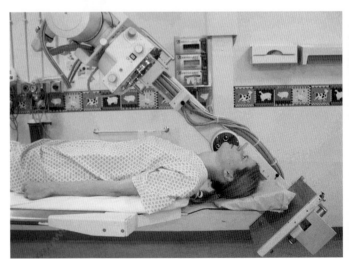

Fig. 8.16c SMV using skull unit.

Common faults and solutions

- This projection involves positioning that can be very uncomfortable for the patient. It is important to ensure the equipment is fully prepared before commencing the examination so the patient need only maintain the position for a minimum period.

Cranium 8

Sella turcica – lateral (Fig. 8.17a)

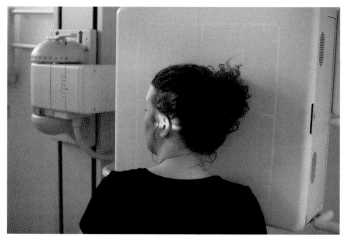

Fig. 8.17a Patient positioning.

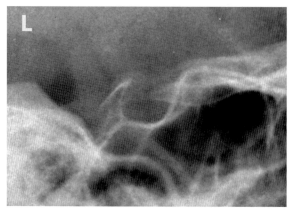

Fig. 8.17b Example of a collimated lateral sella turcica image.

Position of patient and image receptor

- The patient sits facing the erect Bucky/image receptor and the head is then rotated such that the median sagittal plane is parallel to the image receptor and the interpupillary line is perpendicular to it.
- The shoulders may be rotated slightly to allow the correct position to be attained and the patient may grip the image receptor for stability.
- The head and image receptor heights are adjusted to enable centring as indicated below.
- A radiolucent pad may be placed under the chin and lower face for support.

Direction and location of the X-ray beam

- A collimated horizontal beam is centred to a point 2.5 cm vertically above a point 2.5 cm along the baseline from the auditory meatus nearest the X-ray tube.

Radiological considerations (Fig. 8.17b)

This examination is increasingly uncommon, as in the presence of good clinical or biochemical evidence of a pituitary tumour, MRI or CT examinations along with other diagnostic tests will be undertaken. If these modalities are unavailable, evidence of sella expansion by a large lesion may be demonstrated by this projection. A double floor to the sella turcica may be a sign of smaller intrapituitary tumour, but can also be a normal variant due to a slope of the sella floor or suboptimal positioning; this may be confirmed by use of a well-collimated OF20°↓ projection.

8 Cranium

Optic foramina and jugular foramina (Figs 8.18a–8.18c)

The main indication for imaging these foramina is detection of tumour (e.g. glomus jugulare hypervascular tumour, optic nerve glioma), which currently is best demonstrated by CT and/or MRI. These modalities demonstrate optimal specificity for these complex pathologies.

Optic foramina – postero-anterior oblique

The optic canal opens posteriorly within the bony orbit at the optic foramen. The canal passes forwards and laterally at approximately 35° to the median sagittal plane and downwards at approximately 35° to the orbito-meatal plane, and therefore this is the path the central ray must take to demonstrate the foramen for imaging.

Both sides are usually imaged separately for comparison.

Position of patient and image receptor

- The patient sits erect with the nose cheek and chin of the side being examined in contact with Bucky/image receptor.
- The centre of the orbit of the side under examination should coincide with the centre of the image receptor.
- The median sagittal plane is adjusted to make an angle of 35° to the vertical (55° to the receptor).
- The orbito-meatal baseline is raised 35° from the horizontal.

Direction and location of the X-ray beam

- The collimated horizontal central ray should be centred to the middle of the image receptor. This is to a point 7.5 cm superior and 7.5 cm posterior to the uppermost EAM, so that the central ray emerges from the centre of the orbit in contact with the image receptor.
- A side marker may be placed above the superior orbital margin.

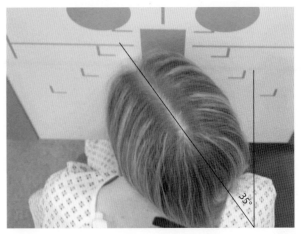

Fig. 8.18a Superior view of optic foramina projection showing MSP angle with film.

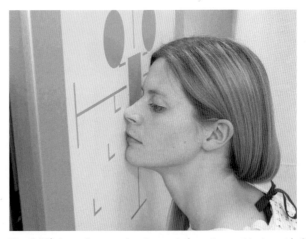

Fig. 8.18b Lateral aspect showing optic foramina positioning with OM base line superimposed.

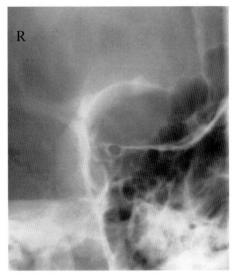

Fig. 8.18c Radiograph of correct positioning for optic foramina.

Cranium 8

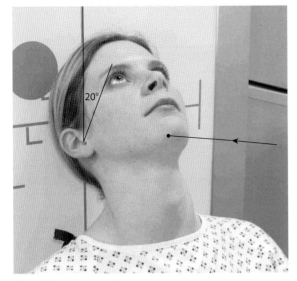

Fig. 8.19a Patient positioning.

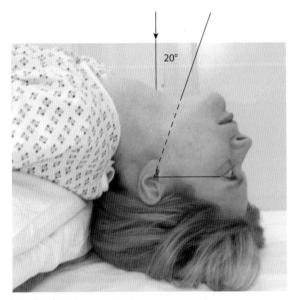

Fig. 8.19b Patient positioning.

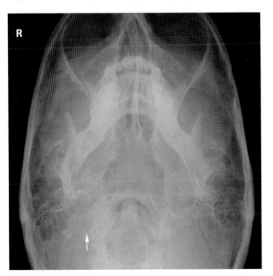

Fig. 8.19c SMV 20° with the jugular foramen arrowed.

Jugular foramina – submento-vertical 20° caudal (Figs 8.19a–8.19c)

The jugular foramina lie in the posterior cranial fossa between the petrous temporal and occipital bones on each side of the foramen magnum. Both sides are imaged simultaneously on a single image by undertaking a submento-vertical (SMV) 20° caudal projection.

Position of patient and image receptor

- As per the SMV projection described previously in this chapter.

Direction and location of the X-ray beam

- Using a collimated horizontal beam, the central ray is angled caudally so that it makes an angle of 70° to the orbito-meatal plane and is centred in the midline to pass midway between the EAMs.

Notes: alternative technique

- With the patient's neck less extended the head can be positioned with the orbito-meatal plane at an angle of 20° to the Bucky/image receptor, in which case a horizontal central ray will make the required angle of 70° to the base plane (see photograph).

8 Cranium

Temporal bones

These projections are traditionally difficult to perform, and are also difficult to interpret, especially if the examination is not of the highest quality. CT imaging with the software for 3D reconstruction affords exquisite demonstration of the temporal bone detail and has thus eradicated the need for these projections.

Frontal-occipital 35° caudal (Figs 8.20a–8.20c)

Position of patient and image receptor

- The patient may be erect with their back to the erect Bucky/receptor or supine in the midline of the X-ray table
- The head is adjusted to bring the EAMs equidistant from the Bucky/receptor so that the median sagittal plane is at right-angles to and in the midline.
- The chin is depressed so that the orbito-meatal line is at right-angles to the Bucky/receptor.
- If used a (24 × 30 cm) CR cassette is placed transversely in the Bucky tray and is centred to coincide with the angled collimated central ray.

Direction and location of the X-ray beam

- A caudal angulation is employed such that it makes an angle of 35° to the orbito-meatal plane.
- The collimated X-ray beam is centred midway between the EAMs.
- Collimate laterally to include the lateral margins of the skull and supero-inferiorly to include the mastoid and petrous parts of the temporal bone. The mastoid process can be easily be palpated behind the pinna of the ear.

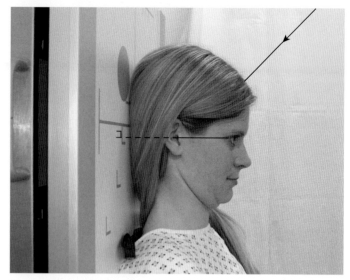

Fig. 8.20a Patient positioning.

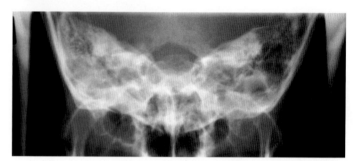

Fig. 8.20b Radiograph of collimated FO 35°.

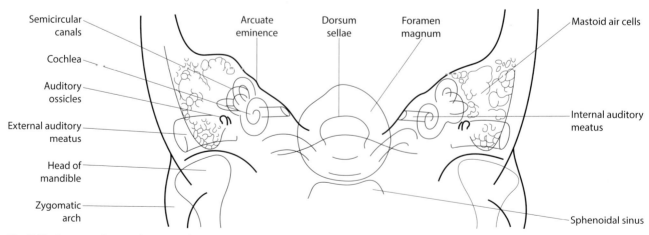

Fig. 8.20c Diagram of required anatomy demonstrated by FO 35°.

Cranium 8

Frontal-occipital 35° caudal (cont.)

Essential image characteristics

- The sella turcica of the sphenoid bone should be projected within the foramen magnum.
- The skull should not be rotated. This can also be assessed by ensuring the sella turcica appears in the middle of the foramen magnum.
- All the anatomy included on the radiograph and line diagrams opposite should be included (Fig. 8.21c).

Common faults and solutions

- Underangulation: the foramen magnum is not clearly demonstrated above the petrous ridges. This is probably the most common fault as the patient may find it difficult to maintain the baseline perpendicular to the receptor.
- If the patient's chin cannot be sufficiently depressed to bring the orbito-meatal baseline perpendicular to the receptor then it will be necessary to increase the angle of the tube more than 35° to the vertical. A 35° angle to the orbito-meatal plane must be maintained.

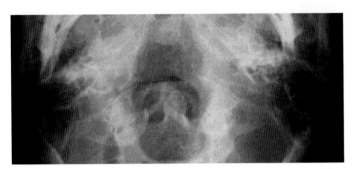

Fig. 8.21a Example of patient positioned for SMV projection using an isocentric skull unit.

Fig. 8.21b SMV radiograph.

Submento-vertical (Figs 8.21a–8.21c)

As an alternative a SMV projection (see earlier in chapter for details) collimated to include only the petrous and mastoid parts of the temporal bone is a further projection that has been employed to demonstrate this specific region of bony anatomy.

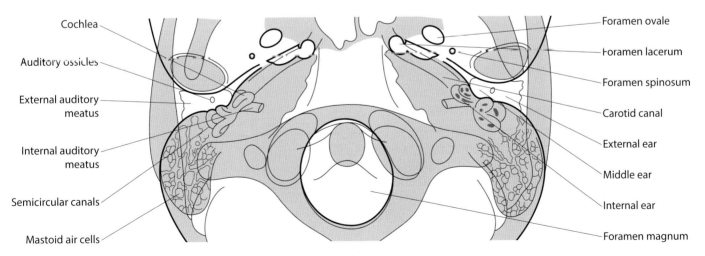

Fig. 8.21c Diagram of required anatomy demonstrated by SMV.

287

8 Cranium

Mastoid – lateral oblique 25° caudal (Fig. 8.22a)

Position of patient and receptor

- The patient sits facing the erect Bucky/receptor and the head is then rotated so that the median sagittal plane is parallel to the Bucky/receptor and the interpupillary line is perpendicular to the Bucky/receptor.
- The shoulders may be rotated slightly to allow the correct position to be maintained and the patient may grip the Bucky/receptor for stability.
- The auricle of the ear adjacent to the table is folded forward to ensure its soft-tissue outline is not superimposed over the region of interest.
- Position the mastoid process in the centre of the Bucky/receptor.
- If used, a 18 × 24 cm CR cassette is positioned longitudinally in the Bucky tray and is centred to coincide with the collimated horizontal beam and mastoid process.

Direction and location of the X-ray beam

- A 25° caudal angulation is applied to the collimated horizontal beam and is centred 5 cm above and 2.5 cm behind the EAM remote from the receptor/cassette.
- Limit the collimation to the mastoid area under examination.

Essential image characteristics (Figs 8.22b, 8.22c)

- Ensure all of the mastoid air cells have been included within the image. The size of these structures can vary greatly from individual to individual.

Common faults and solutions

- Failure to centre far enough posteriorly might exclude part of the mastoid air cells from the image if these structures are very well-developed.
- Failure to ensure the auricle of the ear is folded forward will result in a soft-tissue artefact. Check the ear is in the correct position just before the exposure is undertaken.

Note

- Examine both sides for comparison.

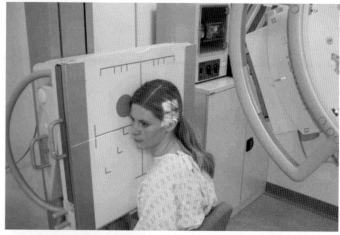

Fig. 8.22a Patient positioning.

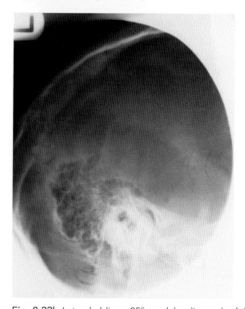

Fig. 8.22b Lateral oblique 25° caudal radiograph of the left mastoid.

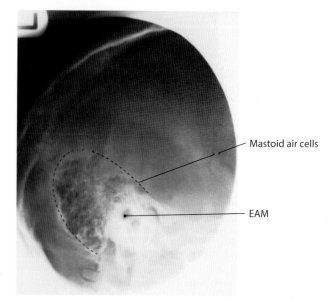

Fig. 8.22c Labelled radiograph.

Cranium 8

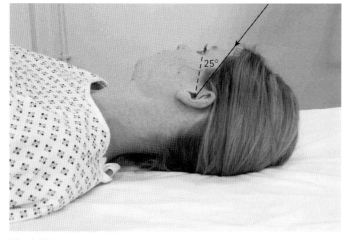

Fig. 8.23a Patient positioning.

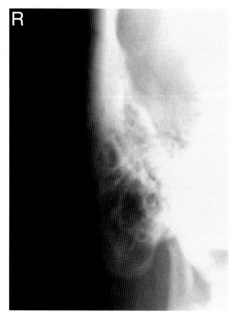

Fig. 8.23b Radiograph of mastoid – profile.

Mastoid – profile (Figs 8.23a, 8.23b)

Position of patient and image receptor

- The patient sits erect with their back to the erect Bucky/receptor or lies supine on the X-ray table with the orbito-meatal baseline perpendicular to the receptor/Bucky.
- From a position with the median sagittal plane perpendicular to the table/receptor, the head is rotated through an angle of 35° away from the side under examination such that the median sagittal plane now makes an angle of 55° to the table/Bucky.
- The vertical tangent to the skull should now be at the level of the middle of the mastoid process under examination so that the mastoid process is in profile.
- Finally the head is moved transversely across the Bucky/table so that the mastoid process being examined is in the midline of the CR cassette/receptor.

Direction and location of the X-ray beam

- The collimated beam is angled caudally so that it makes an angle of 25° to the orbito-meatal plane and is centred to the middle of the mastoid process on the side under examination.
- Collimate to the margins of the mastoid process.

Notes

- Both sides are often imaged for comparison.
- A small side marker may be included within the collimated field.

8 Cranium

Petrous – anterior oblique (Stenver's) (Figs 8.24a–8.24d)

Position of patient and image receptor

- The patient may be prone but may be more comfortable examined erect facing a vertical Bucky/receptor.
- The middle of the supra-orbital margin on the side being examined is centred to the middle of the Bucky/receptor.
- The neck is flexed so that the nose and forehead are in contact with the Bucky/receptor and the orbito-meatal line is perpendicular to it.
- From a position where the median sagittal plane is perpendicular to the table/receptor, the head is rotated toward the side under examination such that the median sagittal plane is now at an angle of 45° to the Bucky/receptor. This brings the petrous part of the temporal bone parallel to the receptor.
- The neck is extended so that the orbito-meatal line is raised 5° from horizontal.
- If used, an 18 × 24 cm CR cassette is placed transversely in the Bucky tray and is centred at a level to coincide with the collimated X-ray beam.

Direction and location of the X-ray beam

- A 12° cranial beam angulation is used, i.e. at an angle of 7° to the orbito-meatal plane, to separate the occiput from the petrous bone.
- Centre midway between the external occipital protuberance and the EAM furthest from the Bucky/receptor.
- Collimate to the mastoid and petrous parts of the temporal bone under examination.

Note

- This projection is almost completely redundant due to the superior diagnostic capabilities of CT imaging.

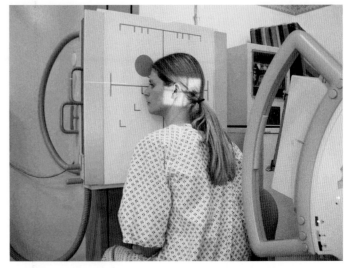

Fig. 8.24b Patient positioning.

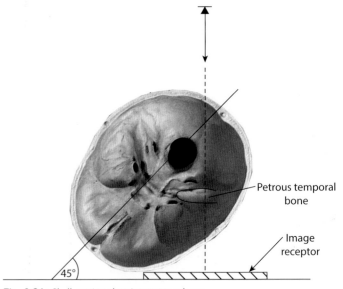

Fig. 8.24c Skull section showing petrous bone.

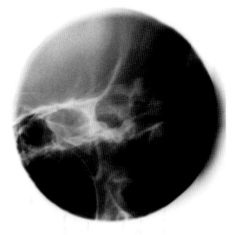

Fig. 8.24d Radiograph of petrous bone.

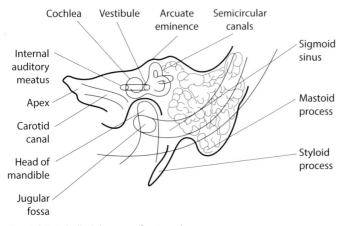

Fig. 8.24a Labelled diagram of petrous bone.

Facial bones and sinuses 8

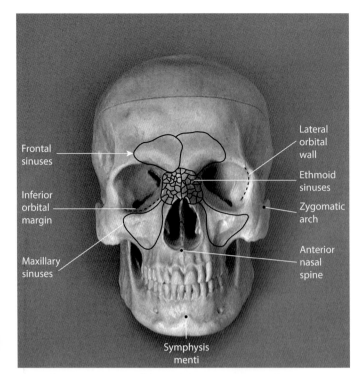

Fig. 8.25a Anterior aspect of the skull showing important structures.

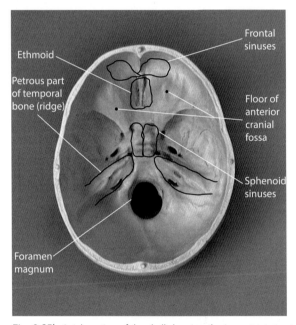

Fig. 8.25b Axial section of the skull showing the important structures.

Introduction (Figs 8.25a, 8.25b, 8.26a–8.26c)

The facial skeleton is complex and the series of images produced are difficult to assess radiologically for diagnosis; optimal projections are therefore extremely important. The facial bones are a series of 14 irregular bones that collectively are attached to the antero-inferior aspect of the skull. Within these bones, and some of the bones forming the cranial base, are a series of air-filled cavities known as the paranasal air sinuses. These communicate with the nasal cavity and the margins of them appear of higher radiographic density than surrounding bones, as the air within them offers little attenuation to the X-ray beam. If the sinuses become filled with fluid due to pathology, e.g. blood in trauma or chronic infection, this results in a decrease in radiographic density and increase in radio-opacity. The sinuses are therefore best imaged by using a horizontal beam, with the patient in the erect position thus demonstrating fluid levels.

The following comprise the paranasal air sinuses:

- Maxillary sinuses (maxillary antra): paired, pyramidal-shaped structures located within the maxillary bone either side of the nasal cavity. These are the largest of the sinuses.
- Frontal sinuses: these are paired structures located within the frontal bone adjacent to the fronto-nasal junction (acanthion). They are very variable in size and shape and in some individuals they may be absent.
- Sphenoid sinus: this structure lies immediately beneath the sella turcica and posterior to the ethmoid sinuses.
- Ethmoid sinuses: a labyrinth of small air spaces that collectively form part of the medial wall of the orbit and the supero-lateral walls of the nasal cavity.

Radiological considerations

The facial bones and sinuses are complicated structures and the radiographer must be aware of their anatomical position and radiographic appearances in order to assess the diagnostic suitability of an image. The accompanying diagrams and radiographs outline the position of the major structures and landmarks used for image assessment. If serious facial injury is suspected clinically, CT will give more detailed information, with the ability to perform 3D reconstructions.

Equipment

Given the subtle pathologies often encountered in this region, resolution is an important consideration. The optimum quality images will be obtained using a moving grid in the vertical tilting Bucky/detector. Alternatively stationary grids may be used, preferably with a high grid lattice with more than 40 grid lines/cm will give far superior results in terms of resolution.

The use of a skull unit if still available, offers considerable advantages for positioning, patient comfort and immobilisation.

8 Facial bones and sinuses

Radiographic anatomy

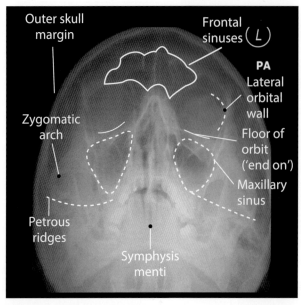

Fig. 8.26a Labelled radiograph showing important structures.

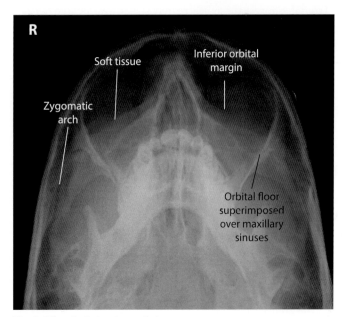

Fig. 8.26b Labelled radiograph showing important structures.

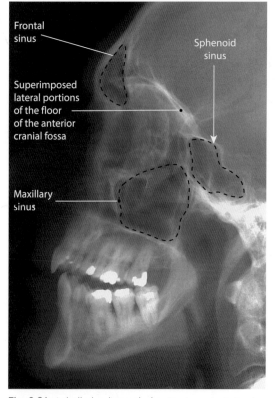

Fig. 8.26c Labelled radiograph showing important structures.

Facial injuries may be complex and difficult to demonstrate on plain imaging as the facial skeleton is a 3D structure. Therefore, once a fracture is demonstrated involving the facial bones then further multiplanar imaging such as CT is usually undertaken, to demonstrate the full extent of the facial injury and fracture pattern.

Positive CT facial examinations generally include 3D reconstruction to allow maxillary-facial specialists a clear aid to facilitate surgery planning.[6]

Due to the complexity of facial fracture patterns there are some well-known fracture classifications and assessment models to allow radiographers and clinicians viewing/reporting upon plain facial images to demonstrate the severity and involvement of the facial skeleton.

Assessment tools

McGrigors' lines are lines on the facial skeleton that can be followed to exclude or confirm any breach in continuity and thus a facial fracture.

The lines are visible on any OM image.[6]

Follow all 3 lines:

- Line 1: fronto-zygomatic suture across the superior orbital margin, nasion and opposing side.
- Line 2: superior aspect of zygomatic arch, frontal process of zygoma, inferior orbital margin, nasal bones and opposing side.
- Line 3: inferior aspect zygomatic arch, base of maxillary sinuses, maxilla at base of upper teeth and opposing side.[6]

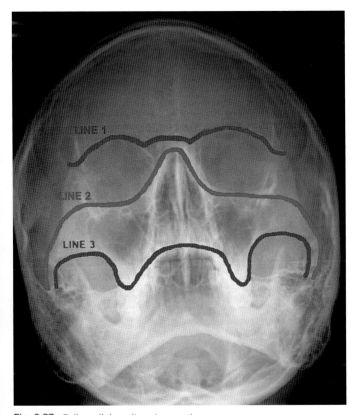

Fig. 8.27a Follow all three lines (see text).

Facial bones and sinuses 8

Radiological considerations (Figs 8.27a, 8.27b)

Facial fracture classifications

Le Fort classifications are a well-known method of classifying mid-face injuries and have three different grades:

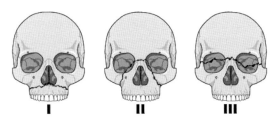

Fig. 8.27b Le Fort classifications.

These are complex bilateral fractures associated with a large unstable fragment ('floating face') and invariably involve the pterygoid plates. This indicates three planes of weakness, with a Le Fort III the most serious and possibly involving severe brain injury.[8]

Facial projections must clearly demonstrate the commonly predicted sites of facial fracture, especially in the mid-facial area. These include the orbital floor, lateral orbital wall and fronto-zygomatic suture, lateral maxillary antral wall, and zygomatic arch. Facial fractures although often localised may be bilateral and symmetrical.[9,10]

Recommended projections

Trauma & pathology	Occipito-mental Occipito-mental 30°↓ (basic series)
Gross trauma	Basic series & usually CT
Suspected depressed zygoma fracture	Basic series & consider modified infero-superior/SplitTownes/SMV for zygomatic arches
Nasal injury	Usually clinical diagnosis; collimated occipito-mental may be indicated
Foreign body in eye	Modified occipito-mental for orbits
Mandible trauma	PA mandible + either tomography (OPG [DPT]) or lateral obliques Anterior oblique for symphysis menti injury
TMJ pathology	Tomography & consideration of lateral 25°↓
TMJ trauma	Tomography & lateral 25° caudal + OPG

CT, computed tomography; DPT, dental panoramic tomography; OPG, orthopantomography; PA, postero-anterior; SMV, submento-vertical; TMJ, temporo-mandibular joint.

8 Facial bones and sinuses

Facial bones

Occipito-mental (Fig. 8.28a)

The occipito-mental (OM) projection shows the floor of the orbits in profile, nasal region, the maxillae, inferior parts of the frontal bone and the zygomatic bone. The zygomatic arches can be seen but they are visualised 'end-on' and thus appear foreshortened. The OM projection is designed to project the petrous parts of the temporal bone (which overlies the region and would cause unwanted 'noise' on a facial bone image) below the inferior part of the maxilla.

Position of patient and image receptor

- The projection is best performed with the patient erect, seated facing the Bucky/receptor.
- The patient's nose and chin are placed in contact with the midline of the Bucky/receptor and then the head is adjusted to bring the orbito-meatal baseline to a 45° angle to the Bucky/receptor.
- The horizontal central line of the Bucky/receptor should be at the level of the lower orbital margins.
- Ensure the median sagittal plane is at right-angles to the Bucky/receptor by checking the outer canthus of the eyes and the EAMs are equidistant.

Direction and location of the X-ray beam

- The collimated horizontal beam is centred to the Bucky/receptor before positioning is undertaken.
- To check the beam is centered properly, the crosslines on the Bucky/receptor should coincide with the patient's anterior nasal spine.

Essential image characteristics (Figs 8.28b, 8.28c)

- The petrous ridges should be demonstrated inferior to the floors of the maxillary sinuses.
- There should be no rotation. This can be checked by ensuring the distance from the lateral orbital wall to the outer skull margins is equidistant on both sides.

Common faults and solutions

- Petrous ridges superimposed over the inferior part of the maxillary sinuses. In this case several faults may have occurred. The orbito-meatal baseline may not have been positioned at 45° to the cassette/receptor; a 5–10° caudal angulation could be applied to the tube to compensate for this.
- As this is an uncomfortable position to maintain, always check the baseline angle immediately before exposure.

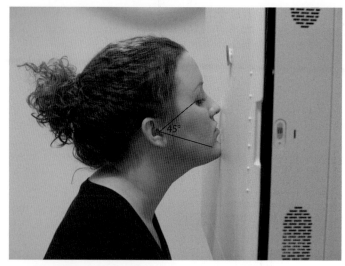

Fig. 8.28a Patient positioning.

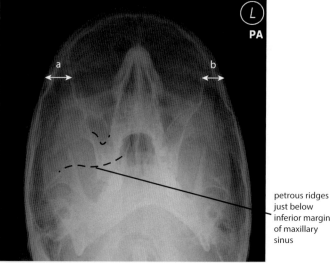

Fig. 8.28b Labelled OM radiograph showing petrous ridges just below inferior margin of maxillary sinus.

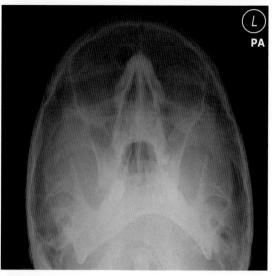

Fig. 8.28c OM radiograph with right zygomatic arch fracture.

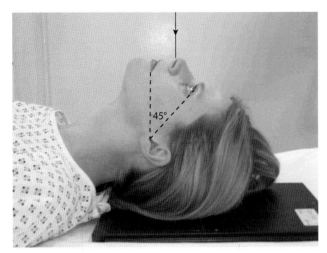

Fig. 8.29a Patient imaged supine with 45° baseline.

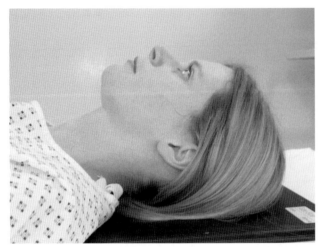

Fig. 8.29b Patient imaged supine with 20° baseline and 25° cranial angulation.

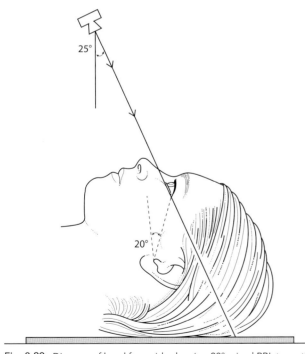

Fig. 8.29c Diagram of head from side showing 20° raised RBL to vertical and 25° cranial angulation.

Facial bones and sinuses 8

Modified mento-occipital (Figs 8.29a–8.29c)

Patients who have sustained trauma will often present supine on a trolley, in a hard collar, with the radiographic baseline in a fixed position. Modifications in technique will therefore be required by imaging the patient in the antero-posterior position and adjusting the beam angle to ensure the petrous bones are projected away from the facial bones.

The optimum solution for this presentation is to avoid facial imaging until the cervical spine is cleared and thus erect OM facial views can be taken. Otherwise, if a serious head injury or obvious facial injury is evident CT imaging with 3D reconstructions would be the optimum procedure.

Modified mento-occipital (MO) projections are recommended only in specific cases where CT imaging may not be available.

Position of patient and image receptor

- The patient will be supine on the trolley and should not be moved. The gridded CR cassette/receptor is placed either in the cassette tray in the trolley or under the patient.
- The top of the CR cassette/receptor should be at least 5 cm above the top of the head to allow for any cranial beam angulation.

Direction and location of the X-ray beam

- The patient should be assessed for position (angle) of the orbito-meatal line in relation to the receptor and obviously any modifications must be made to the tube angulation and the patient not moved.
- If the baseline makes an angle of 45° back from vertical (chin raised), then a perpendicular beam can be employed centred to the midline at the level of the lower orbital margins.
- If the orbito-meatal baseline makes an angle of less than 45° with the cassette/receptor because of the cervical hard collar then the difference between the measured angle and 45° should be added to the beam in the form of a cranial angulation. The centring point remains the same.
- For example, if the orbito-meatal baseline was estimated to be 20° from vertical as the chin was raised, then a 25° cranial angulation would need to be applied to the tube to maintain the required angle (see image).
- The beam is collimated to the area of interest.

Notes

- As the cranial angulation increases, the top of the CR cassette/receptor should be displaced further from the top of the head.
- The image quality is greatly affected by poor resolution resulting from magnification and distortion from the cranial angulation. As mentioned above, if possible consider postponing the examination until any spinal injury can be ruled out and the patient can be examined without the cervical hard collar or moved onto a skull unit if other injuries will allow.

8 Facial bones and sinuses

Occipito-mental 30° caudal (Figs 8.30a–8.30c)

This projection demonstrates the lower orbital margins and the orbital floors 'en face'. The zygomatic arches are more visible compared with the OM but are still somewhat foreshortened.

Position of patient and image receptor

- The projection is best performed with the patient seated facing the vertical Bucky/receptor.
- The patient's nose and chin are placed in contact with the midline of the Bucky/receptor and then the head is adjusted to bring the orbito-meatal base line to a 45° angle to the Bucky/receptor.
- The horizontal central line of the Bucky/receptor should be at the level of the symphysis menti.
- Ensure the median sagittal plane is at right-angles to the Bucky/receptor by checking that the outer canthus of the eyes and the EAMs are equidistant.

Direction and location of the X-ray beam

- The tube is angled 30° caudally from the horizontal and centred along the midline such that the central ray exits at the level of the lower orbital margins.
- To ensure the collimated beam is centered properly, the crosslines on the Bucky/cassette holder should coincide approximately with the upper aspect of the symphysis menti region (this will vary with anatomical differences between patients).

Essential image characteristics

- The orbital floors will be clearly visible through the maxillary sinuses and the lower orbital margin should be clearly demonstrated.
- There should be no rotation. This can be checked by ensuring the distance from the lateral orbital wall to the outer skull margins is equidistant on both sides.

Common faults and solutions

- Failure to demonstrate the whole of the orbital floor due to under angulation and failure to maintain the orbito-meatal baseline at 45°. This may be compensated by increasing the caudal tube angle.

Note

- If using a skull unit, the tube and cassette holder are permanently fixed, such that the tube is perpendicular to the cassette. This presents a problem for this projection, as the baseline should be 45° to the cassette. This would not be feasible when the 30° tube angle is applied. The patient

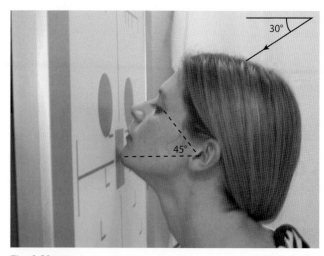

Fig. 8.30a Patient positioning.

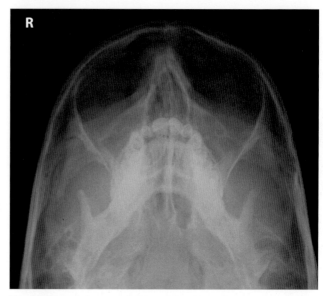

Fig. 8.30b Occipito-mental 30° caudal radiograph.

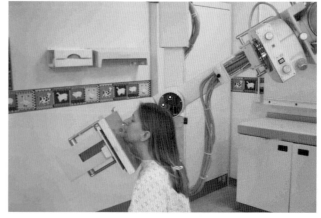

Fig. 8.30c Patient positioning with skull unit.

must therefore be positioned with their orbito-meatal line positioned at 45° to an imaginary vertical line from the floor (see Fig. 8.30c). Although such an arrangement makes positioning and immobilisation more difficult, it does have the advantage of producing an image free from distortion.

Facial bones and sinuses 8

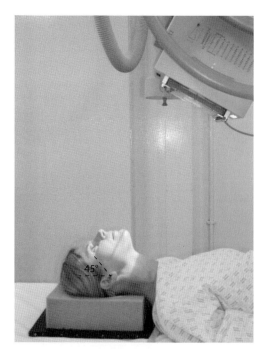

Fig. 8.31a Positioning for reverse OM30°. This will result in image distortion.

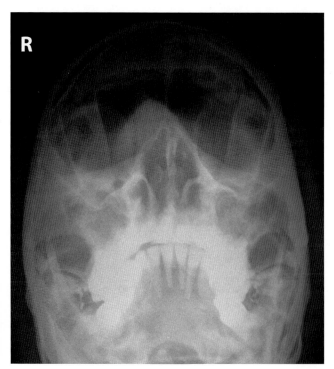

Fig. 8.31b Distorted modified OM30°. (Phantom used for radiograph to demonstrate loss of image quality.)

Modified reverse occipito-mental 30° for the severely injured patient (Fig. 8.31a)

Any modified facial projection has certain limitations to its diagnostic quality and this projection is only recommended for specific referrals. It is possible to undertake a reverse OM30°↓ (i.e. an MO30°↑) with the patient supine on a trolley provided the patient can elevate their orbito-meatal baseline to 45°. Problems arise when the baseline is less than 45° as additional cranial angulation causes severe distortion in the resultant image. This results from the additional cranial angulation that must be applied to the X-ray tube. Clements & Ponsford (1991)[1] have proposed an effective solution to this problem, which is described below.

Position of patient and image receptor

- The patient is supine on the trolley with head adjusted such that the median sagittal plane and orbito-meatal baseline are perpendicular to the trolley top.
- A gridded CR cassette is positioned vertically against the vertex of the skull and supported with foam pads and sandbags such that it is perpendicular to the median sagittal plane.

Direction and location of the X-ray beam

- The tube is angled 20° cranially and centred to the symphysis menti in the midline.
- A 100 cm FRD is used but it may be necessary to increase this for obese or large patients, as the tube will be positioned close to the chest. Remember to increase the exposure if the FRD is increased.

Essential image characteristics (Fig. 8.31b)

- The floors of the orbits will be clearly visible through the maxillary sinuses and the lower orbital margin should be clearly demonstrated.
- There should be no rotation. This can be checked by ensuring the distance from the lateral orbital wall to the outer skull margins is equidistant on both sides.

Notes

- If the orbito-meatal baseline is raised by any degree, there will have to be a corresponding correction of the tube angle to compensate. This may be required if the patient is in a hard collar when the neck must not be moved.
- The main radiological indicator for mid-face fractures is a fluid level in the maxillary sinuses and this would not be indicated on a supine projection. Thus this projection has limited use.
- If the patient has other injuries and is unable to be in the erect position, then CT may be the optimal modality if a facial fracture is strongly suspected.

8 Facial bones and sinuses

Lateral (Figs 8.32a, 8.32b)

This examination is rarely undertaken as an erect OM and OM30° are the optimum and standard projections in the UK. Complex facial injuries will undergo CT imaging with 3D reconstruction.

In cases of injury this projection should be specifically requested and taken using a horizontal beam, in order to demonstrate any fluid levels in the paranasal sinuses. The patient may be positioned erect or supine.

Position of patient and image receptor

Erect
- The patient sits facing the vertical Bucky/receptor. The head is rotated such that the side under examination is in contact with the Bucky/receptor.
- The arm on the same side is extended comfortably by the trunk whilst the other arm may be used to grip the Bucky/receptor for stability. The Bucky/receptor height is altered such that its centre is 2.5 cm inferior to the outer canthus of the eye.

Supine
- The patient lies on the trolley with their arms extended by the sides and the median sagittal plane vertical to the trolley top.
- A gridded CR cassette is supported vertically against the side under examination so that the centre of the receptor is 2.5 cm inferior to the outer canthus of the eye.

In either case the median sagittal plane is brought parallel to the Bucky/receptor by ensuring that the interorbital line is at right-angles to the Bucky/receptor and the nasion and external occipital protuberance are equidistant from it.

Direction and location of the X-ray beam

- The collimated horizontal beam is centred to a point 2.5 cm inferior to the outer canthus of the eye.

Essential image characteristics (Fig. 8.32c)

- The image should contain all of the facial bones sinuses, including the frontal sinus and posteriorly to the anterior border of the cervical spine.
- A true lateral will have been obtained if the lateral portions of the floor of the anterior cranial fossa are superimposed.

Notes

- This projection is often reserved for gross trauma as the facial structures are superimposed.
- For foreign body imaging see Miscellaneous, Chapter 14.

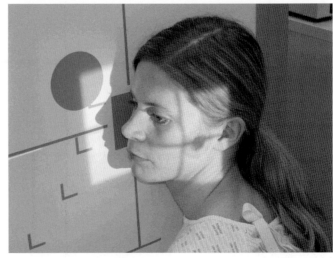

Fig. 8.32a Patient positioning, erect.

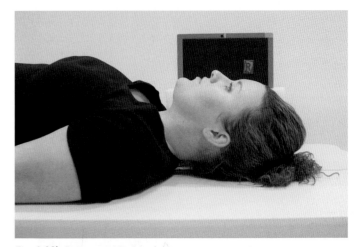

Fig. 8.32b Patient positioning, supine.

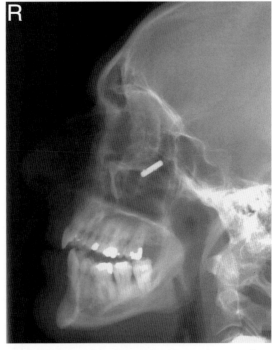

Fig. 8.32c Radiograph of lateral facial bones showing a foreign body.

Facial bones and sinuses 8

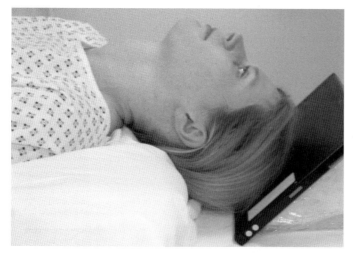

Fig. 8.33a Supine positioning for infero-superior zygomatic arch.

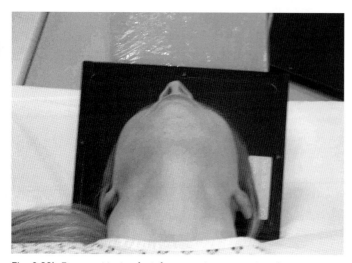

Fig. 8.33b Erect positioning for infero-superior zygomatic arch.

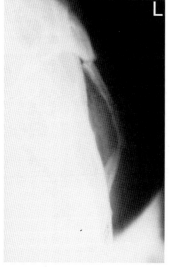

Fig. 8.33c Zygomatic arch demonstrating double fracture.

Zygomatic arches – infero superior (Figs 8.33a, 8.33b)

This projection is essentially a modified SMV projection. It is often referred to as the 'jug handle' projection as the whole length of the zygomatic arch is demonstrated in profile against the side of the skull and facial bones.

Position of patient and image receptor

- The patient lies supine with one or two pillows under the shoulders to allow the neck to be fully extended.
- An 18 × 24 cm CR cassette is placed against the vertex of the skull such that its long axis is parallel with the axial plane of the body. It should be supported in this position with foam pads and sandbags.
- The flexion of the neck is now adjusted to bring the long axis of the zygomatic arch parallel to the CR cassette.
- The head in now tilted 5–10° away from the side under examination. This allows the zygomatic arch under examination to be projected onto the image without superimposition of the skull vault or facial bones.

Direction and location of the X-ray beam

- The central ray should be perpendicular to the CR cassette and long axis of the zygomatic arch.
- A centring point should be located such that the central ray passes through the space between the midpoint of the zygomatic arch and the lateral border of the facial bones.
- Close collimation should be applied to reduce scatter and to avoid irradiating the eyes.

Essential image characteristics (Fig. 8.33c)

- The whole length of the zygomatic arch should be demonstrated clear of the cranium.
- If this has not been achieved it may be necessary to repeat the examination and alter the degree of head tilt to try and bring the zygomatic arch clear of the skull.

Radiological considerations

- Depressed fracture of the zygoma can be missed clinically due to soft-tissue swelling making the bony defect less obvious radiologically. Radiography has an important role in ensuring that potentially disfiguring depression of the cheekbones is not overlooked.

Note

- It is important for the radiographer to have a good understanding of facial anatomy to locate the position of the zygomatic arch correctly and thus allow for accurate positioning and collimation. In some individuals variations in anatomy may not allow the arch to be projected clear of the skull.

8 Facial bones and sinuses

Orbits – occipito-mental (modified) (Fig. 8.34a)

This is a frequently undertaken projection used to assess injuries to the orbital region (e.g. blow-out fracture of the orbital floor) and to exclude the presence of metallic foreign bodies in the eyes prior to MRI investigations. The projection is essentially an 'undertilted' OM with the orbito-meatal baseline raised 10° less than standard OM projection.

Position of patient and image receptor

- The projection is best performed with the patient seated facing the skull unit cassette holder or vertical Bucky.
- The patient's nose and chin are placed in contact with the midline of the cassette holder and then the head is adjusted to bring the orbito-meatal baseline to a 35° angle to the image receptor.
- The horizontal central line of the vertical Bucky/receptor should be at the level of the midpoint of the orbits.
- Ensure the median sagittal plane is at right-angles to the Bucky/receptor by checking the outer canthi of the eyes and the EAMs are equidistant from the image receptor.

Direction and location of the X-ray beam

- If using a skull unit the central ray will be perpendicular to the cassette holder and by design will thus be centered.
- If using an erect Bucky the tube should be centered to the Bucky using a collimated horizontal beam before positioning is undertaken. Again, if the above positioning is accurately performed and the Bucky height is not altered, the beam will already be centered.
- To check the beam is centered properly the crosslines on the Bucky/receptor should coincide with the midline at the level of the mid-orbital region.

Essential image characteristics (Figs 8.34b, 8.34c)

- The orbits should be roughly circular in appearance (they will be more oval in the OM projection).
- The petrous ridges should appear in the lower 1/3 of the maxillary sinuses.
- There should be no rotation. This can be checked by ensuring the distance from the lateral orbital wall to the outer skull margins is equidistant on both sides to the Bucky/receptor.

Notes

- If the examination is purely to exclude foreign bodies in the eye tight 'letter box' collimation to the orbital region should be applied.

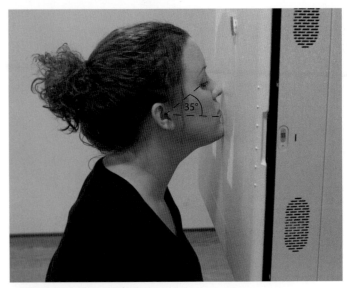

Fig. 8.34a Patient positioning.

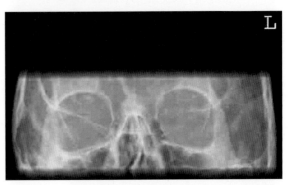

Fig. 8.34b Collimation used for foreign body projection.

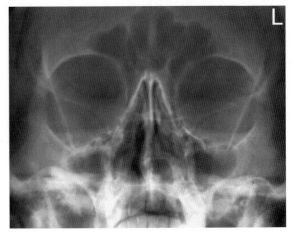

Fig. 8.34c Radiograph of orbits.

- A dedicated CR cassette should be used for foreign bodies, which should be regularly cleaned to avoid small artefacts on the screens being confused with foreign bodies.
- If a foreign body is suspected, a second projection may be undertaken with the eyes in a different position to differentiate this from an image artefact. The initial exposure could be taken with the eyes pointing up and the second with the eyes pointing down.

Facial bones and sinuses 8

Nasal bones – lateral
(Figs 8.35a, 8.35b)

Position of patient and image receptor

- The patient sits facing an 18 × 24 cm CR cassette supported in the cassette stand of a vertical Bucky or within the field of view of a vertical DDR unit with the grid removed.
- The head turned so the median sagittal plane is parallel with the image receptor and the interpupillary line is perpendicular to the image receptor.
- The nose should be roughly coincident with the centre of the image receptor.

Direction and location of the X-ray beam

- A horizontal central ray is directed through the centre of the nasal bones and collimated to include the nose.

Radiological considerations

- Nasal fracture can usually be detected clinically and is rarely treated actively. If a fracture causes nasal deformity or breathing difficulty it may be straightened, but lateral projections will not help in this.
- Due to the dose of radiation to the eye, this projection should be avoided in most instances.

Notes

- This projection may also be used to demonstrate foreign bodies in the nose. In this case a soft-tissue exposure should be employed.
- In the majority of cases severe nasal injuries will only require an OM projection to assess the nasal septum and surrounding structures.
- The projection can also be undertaken with the patient supine with a CR cassette supported against the side of the face.

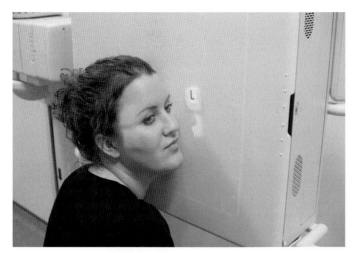

Fig. 8.35a Patient positioning.

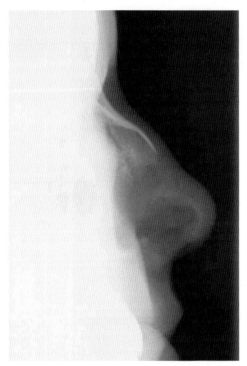

Fig. 8.35b Lateral radiograph of the nose.

8 Facial bones and sinuses

Mandible – lateral 30° cranial (Figs 8.36a, 8.36b)

Dependent on patient presentation this can be undertaken using either of the two different techniques described below.

Position of patient and image receptor

Position 1

- The patient lies in the supine position and the trunk is rotated slightly and then supported with pads to allow the side of the face being examined to come in to contact with CR cassette, which is supported by the use of a thin wedge foam pad.
- The median sagittal plane should be parallel with the CR cassette and the interpupillary line perpendicular to one another.
- The neck may be flexed slightly to clear the mandible from the spine.
- The CR cassette and head can now be adjusted and supported so the above positioned is maintained but is comfortable for the patient.
- The long axis of the CR cassette should be parallel with the long axis of the mandible and the lower border positioned 2 cm below the lower border of the mandible.

Position 2

- The projection may also be performed with a horizontal beam in trauma cases when the patient cannot be moved.
- In this case the patient will be supine with the median sagittal plane at right-angles to the tabletop. The CR cassette is supported vertically against the side under examination.

Direction and location of the X-ray beam

- The central ray is angled 30° cranially at an angle of 60° to the receptor and is centred 5 cm inferior to the angle of the mandible remote from the receptor.
- Collimate to include the whole of the mandible and temporo-mandibular joint (TMJ) (include the EAM at the edge of the collimation field).

Essential image characteristics (Fig. 8.36c)

- The body and ramus of each side of the mandible should not be superimposed.
- The image should include the whole of mandible from the TMJ to the symphysis menti.

Radiological considerations

- Do not mistake the mandibular canal, which transmits the inferior alveolar nerve, for a fracture.

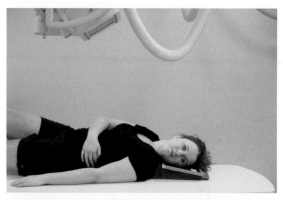

Fig. 8.36a Positioning with the patient's head on the side.

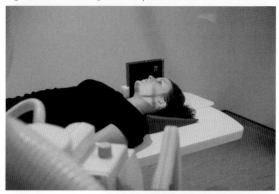

Fig. 8.36b Positioning with the patient supine.

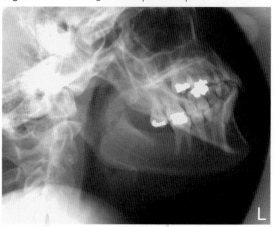

Fig. 8.36c Radiograph of 30° oblique mandible.

Common faults and solutions

- Superimposition of the mandibular bodies will result if the angle applied to the tube is less than 30° or the centring point is too high.
- If the shoulder is obscuring the region of interest in the horizontal beam projection, a slight angulation toward the floor may have to be applied or, if the patient's condition will allow, tilt the head toward the side under examination.

Notes

- In cases of injury both sides should be examined to demonstrate a possible contre-coup fracture.
- If the patient is mobile this may be done erect using similar technique as described for the supine examination above.

Facial bones and sinuses

Mandible – postero-anterior (Figs 8.37a, 8.37b)

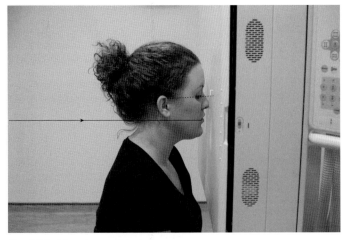

Fig. 8.37a PA patient positioning – erect.

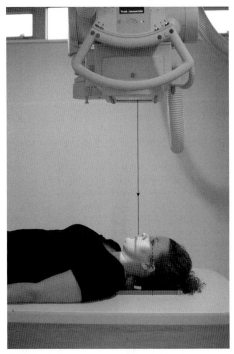

Fig. 8.37b AP patient positioning – supine.

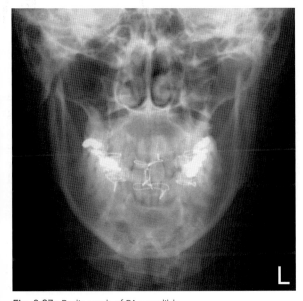

Fig. 8.37c Radiograph of PA mandible.

Position of patient and image receptor

- The patient sits erect facing the vertical Bucky/receptor (in the case of trauma the projection may be taken antero-posterior).
- The patient's median sagittal plane should be coincident with the midline of the Bucky/receptor and the head is then adjusted to bring the orbito-meatal baseline perpendicular to the Bucky/receptor.
- The median sagittal plane should be perpendicular to the receptor. Check the EAMs are equidistant from the Bucky/receptor.
- An 18 × 24 cm CR cassette, if used, should be positioned such that when placed longitudinally in the Bucky, it is centred at the level of the angles of the mandible.

Direction and location of the X-ray beam

- The collimated central ray is directed perpendicular to the receptor and centred in the midline at the levels of the angles of the mandible.

Essential image characteristics

- The whole of the mandible from the lower portions of the TMJs to the symphysis menti should be included in the image.
- There should be no rotation evident.

Radiological considerations (Fig. 8.37c)

- This projection demonstrates the body and rami of the mandible and may show transverse or oblique fractures not evident on other projections or a OPG (DPT).
- The region of the symphysis menti is superimposed over the cervical vertebra and will be more clearly seen using the anterior oblique projection.

Common faults and solutions

- Superimposition of the upper parts of the mandible over the temporal bone will result if the orbito-meatal baseline is not perpendicular to the receptor.

Note

- A 10° cranial angulation of the beam may be required to demonstrate the mandibular condyles and TMJs.

8 Facial bones and sinuses

Mandible – postero-anterior oblique (Figs 8.38a, 8.38b)

This projection demonstrates the region of the symphysis menti and body of the mandible.

Position of patient and image receptor

- The patient sits facing the vertical Bucky/receptor or, in the case of trauma the projection may be supine on a trolley giving an antero-posterior projection.
- The patient's median sagittal plane should be coincident with the midline of the Bucky/receptor and the head is then adjusted to bring the orbito-meatal baseline perpendicular to the receptor.
- From a position with the median sagittal plane perpendicular to the receptor, the head is rotated 20° to either side so the cervical vertebra will be projected clear of the symphysis menti.
- The head is now repositioned so the region of the symphysis menti is coincident with the middle of the receptor.
- An 18 × 24 cm CR cassette, if used, should be positioned such that the middle of an 18 × 24cm CR cassette, when placed longitudinally in the Bucky/cassette holder, is centred at the level of the angles of the mandible.

Direction and location of the X-ray beam

- The collimated central ray is directed perpendicular to the receptor and centred 5 cm from the midline, away from the side being examined at the level of the angle of the mandible.

Essential image characteristics (Fig. 8.38c)

- The symphysis menti should be demonstrated without any superimposition of the cervical vertebra.

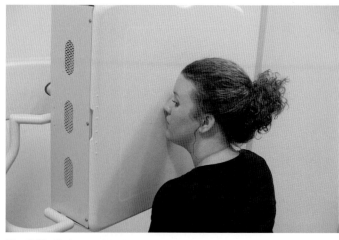

Fig. 8.38a Patient positioning.

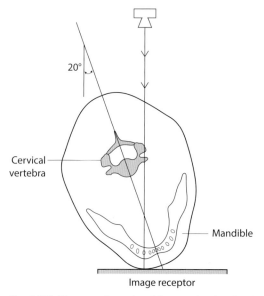

Fig. 8.38b Diagram of anterior oblique projection showing rational for projection.

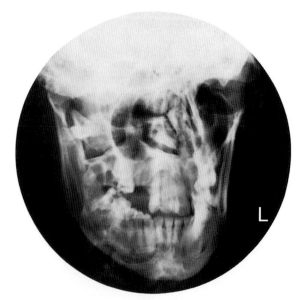

Fig. 8.38c Radiograph of anterior oblique mandible.

Facial bones and sinuses 8

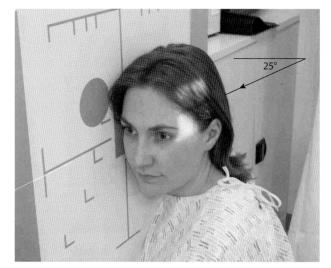

Fig. 8.39a Patient positioning.

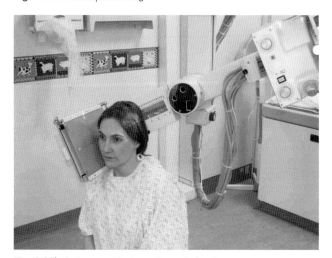

Fig. 8.39b Patient positioning using a skull unit.

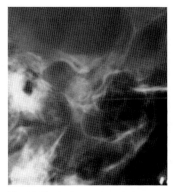

Fig. 8.39c Radiograph with the mouth open.

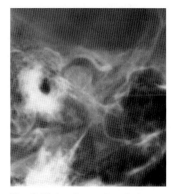

Fig. 8.39d Radiograph with the mouth closed.

Temporo-mandibular joints – lateral 25° caudal (Figs 8.39a, 8.39b)

It is usual to examine both TMJs. For each side, a projection is obtained with the mouth open as far as possible and then another projection with the mouth closed. An additional projection may be required with the teeth clenched.

Position of patient and image receptor

- The patient sits facing the vertical Bucky/skull unit/cassette holder or lies prone on the Bucky table. In either case the head is rotated to bring the side of the head under examination in contact with the table/Bucky face. The shoulders may also be rotated slightly to help the patient achieve this position.
- The head and Bucky/CR cassette holder level is adjusted so the centre crosslines are positioned to coincide with a point 1 cm along the orbito-meatal baseline anterior to the EAM.
- The median sagittal plane is brought parallel to the receptor by ensuring the interpupillary line is at right-angles to the tabletop and the nasion and external occipital protuberance are equidistant from it.
- A CR cassette, if used, is placed longitudinally in the cassette holder such that two exposures can be made without superimposition of the images.

Direction and location of the X-ray beam

- Using a well-collimated beam or an extension cone, the central ray is angled 25° caudally and will be centred to a point 5 cm superior to the joint remote from the receptor, so the central ray passes through the joint nearest to it.

Radiological considerations (Figs 8.39c, 8.39d)

- TMJ projections are useful in assessing joint dysfunction, by demonstrating erosive and degenerative changes.
- Open and closed mouth projections can be very helpful in assessing whether normal anterior gliding movement of the mandibular condyle occurs on jaw opening. MRI promises greater accuracy as it also demonstrates the articular cartilages and fibrocartilage discs, and how they behave during joint movement.

Notes

- The image should include the correct side marker and labelled to indicate the position of the mouth when the exposure was taken (open, closed).
- If using a skull unit, in which the tube cannot be angled independently of the cassette holder, the interpupillary line is at right-angles to an imaginary vertical line drawn from the floor.
- This projection may supplement OPG (DPT) images of the TMJs. PA projections may be undertaken by modifying the technique described for PA mandible on page 304.

8 Paranasal sinuses

Plain imaging of the sinuses are unreliable for diagnosis of inflammatory sinus disease, since many asymptomatic people will have sinus opacification, and sinus symptoms may be present in the absence of gross sinus opacification. Acute sinusitis (especially infective) may manifest radiologically as fluid levels in the maxillary antrum, but it is questionable whether this alters clinical management. Malignant sinus disease requires more comprehensive imaging by CT and/or MRI. Some radiology departments will no longer perform plain sinus radiographs.

Occipito-mental (Figs 8.40a, 8.40b)

This projection is designed to project the petrous part of the temporal bone below the floor of the maxillary sinuses so that fluid levels or pathological changes in the lower part of the sinuses can be clearly visualised.

Position of patient and image receptor

- The projection is best performed with the patient seated facing the vertical Bucky/receptor.
- The patient's nose and chin are placed in contact with the midline of the receptor and then the head is adjusted to bring the orbito-meatal baseline to a 45° angle to the Bucky/receptor.
- The horizontal central line of the Bucky/receptor should be at the level of the lower orbital margins.
- The median sagittal plane is at right-angles to the Bucky/receptor by checking the outer canthi of the eyes and the EAMs are equidistant.
- The patient should open their mouth as wide as possible prior to exposure. This will allow the posterior part of the sphenoid sinuses to be projected through the mouth.

Direction and location of the X-ray beam

- The collimated horizontal beam should be centered to the Bucky/receptor before positioning is undertaken.
- To check the beam is centered properly the crosslines on the Bucky/receptor should coincide with the patient's anterior nasal spine.
- Collimate to include all of the sinuses.
- If using a skull unit the central ray should be perpendicular to the cassette holder and will automatically be centered to the middle of the image receptor.

Essential image characteristics (Fig. 8.40c)

- The petrous ridges must appear below the floors of the maxillary sinuses.
- There should be no rotation. This can be checked by ensuring the distance from the lateral orbital wall to the outer skull margins is equidistant on both sides.

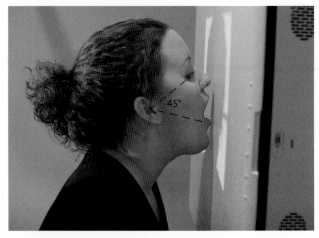

Fig. 8.40a Patient positioning.

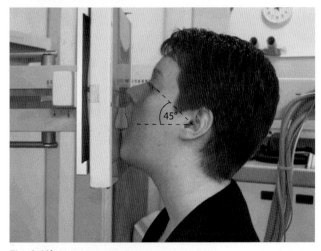

Fig. 8.40b Patient positioning.

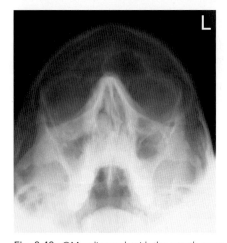

Fig. 8.40c OM radiograph with the mouth open.

Common faults and solutions

- Petrous ridges appearing over the inferior part of the maxillary sinuses. In this case several things may have occurred: the orbito-meatal baseline was not positioned at 45° to the film; a 5–10° caudal angulation may be applied to the tube to compensate. As this is an uncomfortable position to maintain, patients often let the angle of the baseline reduce between positioning and exposure.
- Always check the baseline angle immediately before exposure.

Paranasal sinuses 8

Occipito-frontal 15° caudal (Fig. 8.41a)

This projection is used to demonstrate the frontal and ethmoid sinuses.

Position of patient and image receptor

- The patient is seated facing the vertical Bucky/skull unit cassette holder so the median sagittal plane is coincident with the midline of the Bucky and is also perpendicular to it.
- The head is positioned so that orbito-meatal baseline is raised 15° to the horizontal.
- Ensure the nasion is positioned in the centre of the Bucky.
- The patient may place the palms of each hand either side of the head (out of the primary beam) for stability.
- An 18 × 24 cm cassette, if used, is placed longitudinally in the Bucky tray, with the image receptor (DDR detector/CR cassette) height adjusted so that its centre coincides with the nasion.

Direction and location of the X-ray beam

- The central ray is directed perpendicular to the vertical Bucky along the median sagittal plane so the beam exits at the nasion.
- A collimation field or extension cone should be set to include the ethmoidal and frontal sinuses. The size of the frontal sinuses can vary drastically from one individual to another.

Essential image characteristics (Fig. 8.41b)

- All the relevant sinuses should be included within the image.
- The petrous ridges should be projected just above the lower orbital margins.
- It is important to ensure the skull is not rotated. This can be assessed by measuring the distance from a point in the midline of the skull to the lateral orbital margins. If this is the same on both sides of the skull then it is not rotated.

Notes

- The degree of angulation may vary according to local preferences. The baseline is then raised to the angle required by the projection, e.g. a 10° angulation will be employed if an OF10°↓ projection is required.
- To distinguish a fluid level from mucosal thickening, an additional projection may be undertaken with the head tilted such that a transverse plane makes an angle of about 20° to the floor.

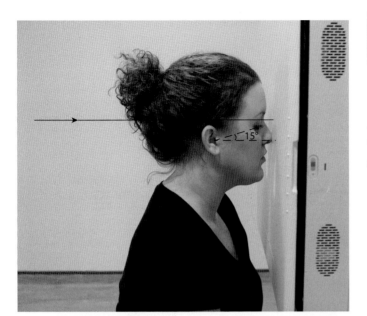

Fig. 8.41a Patient positioning.

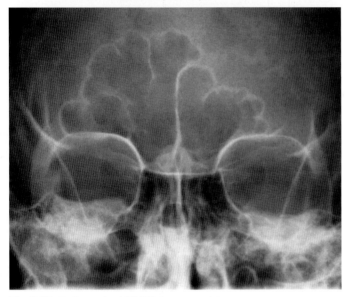

Fig. 8.41b Radiograph of OF 15° sinuses caudal.

8 Paranasal sinuses

Lateral (Figs 8.42a, 8.42c)

Position of patient and image receptor

- The patient sits facing the vertical Bucky/receptor and the head is then rotated such that the median sagittal plane is parallel to the Bucky/receptor and the interpupillary line is perpendicular to it.
- The shoulders may be rotated slightly to allow the correct position to be attained and the patient may grip the Bucky for stability.
- The head and Bucky heights are adjusted so that the centre of the Bucky/receptor is 2.5 cm along the orbito-meatal line from the outer canthus of the eye.
- If used, an 18 × 24 cm CR cassette is positioned longitudinally in the erect Bucky such that its lower border is 2.5 cm below the level of the upper teeth.
- A radiolucent pad may be placed under the chin for support.

Direction and location of the X-ray beam

- A collimated horizontal central ray should be employed to demonstrate fluid levels.
- The X-ray tube should have previously been centred to the Bucky/receptor such that the central ray will now be centred to a point 2.5 cm posterior to the outer canthus of the eye.

Common faults and solutions

- This is not an easy position for the patient to maintain. Check the position of all planes immediately prior to the exposure; the patient will have probably moved.

Essential image characteristics (Fig. 8.42b)

- A true lateral will have been achieved if the lateral portions of the floors of the anterior cranial fossa are superimposed.

Radiological considerations

- Plain X-ray projections of the paranasal sinuses for inflammatory disease are rarely used today as CT is a quick and very accurate way of obtaining all the information required by the surgeon, as well as providing the surgeon with a 'road map' to assist surgical orientation.
- MRI is also being used in many places to provide the same information without any use of ionising radiation.

Note

- This projection may also be undertaken with the patient supine with a gridded CR cassette supported vertically against the side of the face. Again a horizontal beam is used to demonstrate fluid levels.

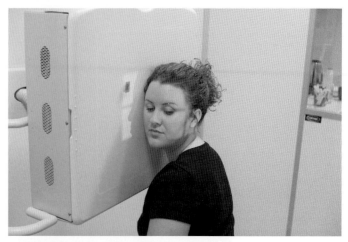

Fig. 8.42a Patient positioning.

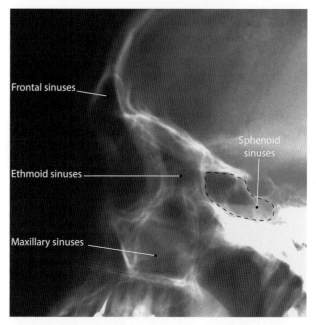

Fig. 8.42b Radiograph of lateral sinuses.

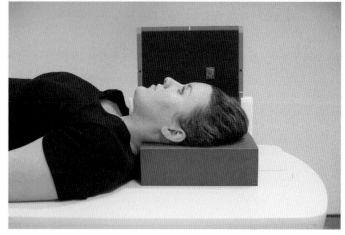

Fig. 8.42c Patient positioning, lateral.

Skull 8

Image evaluation – 10-point plan

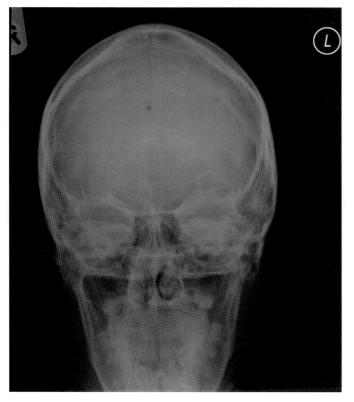

Fig. 8.43a Radiograph.

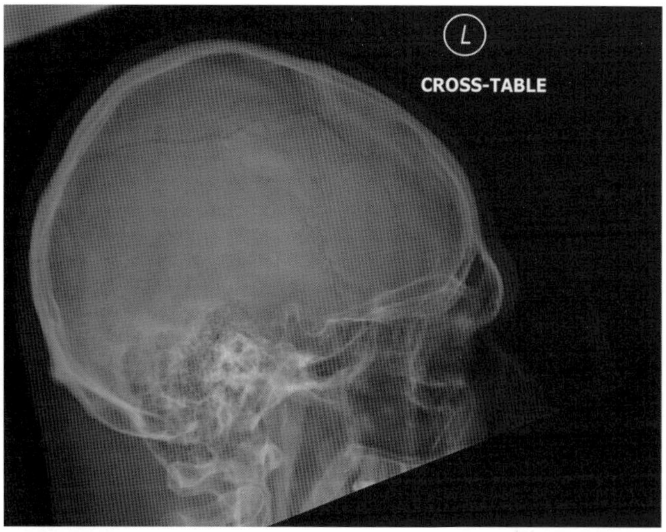

Fig. 8.43b Radiograph.

IMAGE EVALUATION

Occipito-frontal skull (cranium) (Fig. 8.43a)

The main points to consider are:
- Marker applied at time of imaging and post processing.
- No rotation.
- Petrous ridges in the mid-orbital region, therefore chin could be minimally elevated or caudal angulation reduced.
- No repeat needed.

Radiographer Comments/Initial report

Diagnostic image with a well-demarcated lucent line demonstrated in the right temporal region, indicating need for further imaging, CT.

IMAGE EVALUATION

Lateral skull (cranium) (Fig. 8.43b)

The main points to consider are:
- Marker applied post processing.
- Minimal rotation in the facial region but with the sella floor in true lateral position.
- Adequate elevation of chin.
- No repeat needed.

Radiographer Comments/Initial report

Comminuted complex skull fracture extending through the left parietal and temporal bones with a depressed segment centrally.
Further imaging required to assess for brain injury; CT.

8 Facial bones and sinuses

Image evaluation – 10-point plan

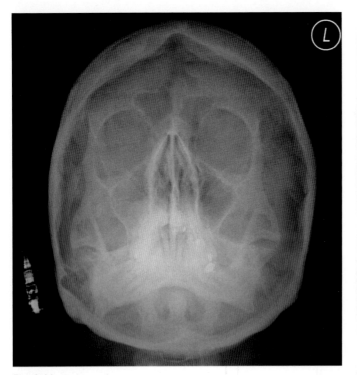

Fig. 8.44a Radiograph.

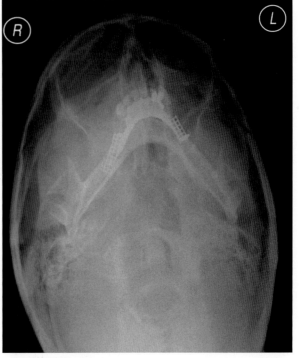

Fig. 8.44b Radiograph.

IMAGE EVALUATION

Occipito-mental facial bones (Fig. 8.44a)

The main points to consider are:
- Marker applied post processing.
- Hearing aid artefact.
- Minimal rotation to the patient's right.
- Adequate elevation of chin to demonstrate maxillary sinuses.
- No repeat needed.

Radiographer Comments/Initial report

Fluid level and opacity right maxillary sinus.
? right orbital floor and lateral maxillary wall fracture.

IMAGE EVALUATION

Occipito-mental – 30° caudal facial bones (Fig. 8.44b)

The main points to consider are:
- Marker applied post processing.
- Right lateral tilt with minimal rotation to the patient's left.
- Denture artefact.
- Adequate elevation demonstrating inferior orbital margin.
- No repeat needed.

Radiographer Comments/Initial report

Opacity right maxillary sinus.
? fracture right lateral maxillary wall and right zygomatic arch.

Section 9
Dental Radiography

CONTENTS

INTRODUCTION	312
Intraoral radiography	312
Extraoral radiography	312
The dentition	312
Dental formula	314
Terminology	316
Occlusal planes	316
X-ray equipment features	317
Image receptors	318
Image acquisition	320
Film mounting and identification of intraoral films	321
Radiation protection	322
Cross-infection control	322
Principles for optimal image geometry	323
BITEWING RADIOGRAPHY	324
Quality standards for bitewing radiography	326
PERIAPICAL RADIOGRAPHY	327
Bisecting angle technique	327
Paralleling technique	332
Third molar region	336
Complete mouth survey or full mouth survey	337
OCCLUSAL RADIOGRAPHY	338
Terminology	338
Recommended projections	338
Radiological considerations	338
Vertex occlusal of the maxilla	339
True occlusal of the mandible	340
Oblique occlusal of the maxilla	342
Oblique occlusal of the mandible	344
LATERAL OBLIQUE OF THE MANDIBLE AND MAXILLA	346
General imaging principles	346
Lateral oblique of the body of the mandible and maxilla	346
Lateral oblique of the ramus of the mandible	348
DENTAL PANORAMIC TOMOGRAPHY	350
Principles of panoramic image formation	350
Image acquisition considerations	351
Problems with panoramic radiography	356
CEPHALOMETRY	357
X-ray equipment features	357
Lateral projection	358
Postero-anterior projection	359
CONE BEAM COMPUTED TOMOGRAPHY	360

9 Introduction

In 2002 it was estimated that 41.5 million medical and dental X-ray examinations were undertaken in the UK, which represented 0.70 examinations per head of the population. Dental radiography has been recognised as the most common radiographic examination constituting 33% of all radiological examinations. By 2008, published numbers of dental radiographs provided within and external to the NHS was 46 million, which included intraoral, panoramic and cephalometric images. The majority of dental radiographs are taken in the primary care dental setting by general dental practitioners, hygienists and dental practice nurses, who have obtained qualifications to allow them to conduct a dental X-ray examination. Many dental practices now employ digital technology to provide both intraoral and extraoral radiographs. Cone beam computed tomography (CBCT) is now being used increasingly in both hospitals and in practices that specialise in endodontic and surgical treatments. The use of CBCT allows clinicians to acquire accurate bone depth measurements for implant planning at a much reduced dose to that which was previously required for multislice computed tomography (MSCT).

Radiographs are used in dentistry for many reasons, summarised below:

- Detection of pathology associated with the teeth and their supporting structures such as caries, periodontal disease and periapical pathology.
- Detection of anomalies/injury associated with the teeth, their supporting structures, the maxilla and the mandible.
- Determination of the presence/absence of teeth and the localisation of any unerupted teeth.
- Root length determination of teeth prior to endodontic therapy.
- Detection of the presence/absence of radio-opaque salivary calculi and foreign bodies.
- Detection of anomalies/injury/pathology of adjacent facial structures.
- Evaluation of skeletal and /or soft tissues prior to orthodontic treatment.
- Monitoring the progress of orthodontic treatment and dental disease.
- The preoperative assessment of skeletal and soft-tissue patterns prior to orthognathic surgery.
- Assessment of bone levels prior to implant placement.
- Monitoring the healing and effectiveness of surgical treatment of the patient postoperatively.

Dental radiography involves techniques in which the image receptor is placed either inside the mouth (intraoral radiography) or outside the mouth (extraoral radiography).

Intraoral radiography

The most frequently requested intraoral projections are bitewing radiography, periapical radiography and occlusal radiography.

Bitewing radiography is a lateral projection of the posterior regions of the jaws. The view demonstrates the crowns of the teeth and the alveolar crestal bone of the premolar and molar regions of both the maxilla and mandible.

Periapical radiography is a lateral projection displaying both the crown and root of the tooth and the surrounding bone.

Occlusal radiography comprises a number of projections in which the image receptor is positioned in the occlusal plane.

Extraoral radiography

The most frequently requested extraoral projections are dental panoramic radiography, oblique lateral radiography and cephalometry.

Dental panoramic radiography is a projection that produces an image of both jaws and their respective dentitions on a single extraoral image receptor.

Oblique lateral radiography demonstrates large areas of the maxilla and mandible with the region imaged dependent on the technique chosen.

Cephalometry employs techniques that produce standardised and reproducible images of the facial bones for use in orthodontic, orthognathic and implant treatment.

CBCT has become an accepted radiographic technique in clinical dentistry during the last decade. The technique differs from conventional intraoral and extraoral radiography in that it produces a cone shaped X-ray beam covering the maxilla and mandible, which offers the clinician the ability to review the area of interest as a 3D image. The accuracy of the technique enables the clinician to quantify the extent of pathosis prior to surgery and also allows an accurate assessment of bone depth prior to implant placement.

The dentition

The primary or deciduous dentition comprises 20 teeth, with five in each quadrant of the jaws. These are replaced from 6 years onwards by a permanent dentition of 32 teeth. With eruption of all 32 permanent teeth, there will be eight permanent teeth in each quadrant. Some teeth may fail to develop or erupt, a complication most commonly affecting the 3rd permanent molars (the wisdom teeth).

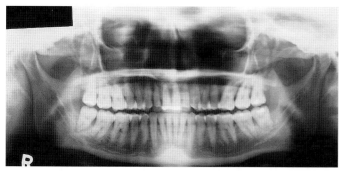

Fig. 9.1a A dental panoramic tomograph of an adult dentate patient.

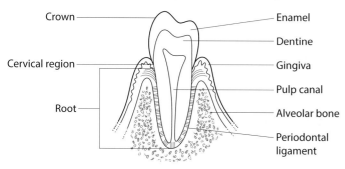

Fig. 9.1b A schematic view of the basic components of the tooth and its supporting tissue.

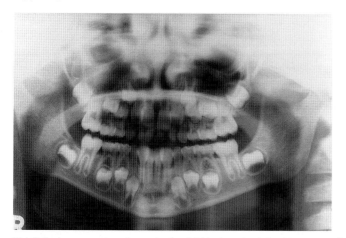

Fig. 9.1c A panoramic radiograph of a child in the mixed dentition stage of tooth development.

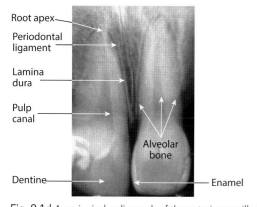

Fig. 9.1d A periapical radiograph of the anterior maxilla illustrating normal radiographic anatomy of the tooth and supporting structures.

Introduction 9

The dentition (*cont.*)

The teeth (Figs 9.1a–9.1d)

From the midline moving posteriorly, the teeth in the anterior part of the jaws comprise the central incisor, the lateral incisor and the canine (cuspid). This terminology is used in both deciduous and permanent dentitions. In the permanent dentition posterior to the canine, there are a 1st and a 2nd premolar (bicuspid) followed by a 1st, a 2nd and, if they develop, a 3rd permanent molar. The deciduous dentition differs in that there are only two teeth posterior to the deciduous canine, a 1st and a 2nd deciduous molar.

Each tooth consists of a variety of hard mineralised tissues with a central area, the pulp chamber and canal, consisting of blood vessels and nerves supported by loose connective tissue. The part of the tooth that projects above the dental gingiva and is evident in the mouth, is the crown, and the portion embedded within the jaw is known as the root. The constriction between the crown and the root is known as the cervical region.

The outer surface of the crown of the tooth consists of enamel and a less mineralised tissue, dentine, below it. The enamel, containing 96% by weight of inorganic material, is radiographically distinguishable from the dentine that is 70% mineralised with hydroxyapatite. Enamel is limited to the crown of the tooth whereas dentine encircles the pulp chamber in the crown of the tooth and extends into the root of the tooth enveloping the pulp canal. Cementum is a thin layer of bone-like material (50% mineralised with hydroxyapatite) covering the dentine of the root and forming the periphery of the root surface. It is not possible to distinguish radiographically between cementum and dentine. Nerves and nutrient vessels enter the pulp through the root apex.

The tooth, depending on its position in the mouth, may have one or more roots. In the anterior region of the jaws, in both dentitions, the incisor and canine teeth are single rooted. The molar teeth, in both dentitions, have several roots. As a generality, in the upper jaw the molar teeth have three roots, whilst in the lower jaw two-rooted molars are the norm. The roots associated with the 3rd permanent molar in both jaws may vary in their number and complexity.

The tooth is supported in its alveolar socket by a periodontal ligament, the fibres of which are embedded in the cementum of the root surface and the surrounding alveolar bone. A thin layer of dense bone encircles the tooth socket. Radiographically, this appears as a linear radio-opacity and is referred to as the lamina dura. The periodontal ligament appears as a uniform (0.4–1.9 mm) linear radiolucency around the root. In the absence of periodontal disease, the alveolar bone should extend to a point 1.5 mm below the cemento-enamel junction.

9 Introduction

Dental formula

There are several internationally recognised methods of identifying the teeth that require radiography. In those cases in which a patient is edentulous (i.e. no teeth visible within the dental arches), a clinician will continue to use the dental formula to denote the part of the oral cavity requiring radiography.

The two most commonly used methods of notation are:

- Palmer notation.
- Federation Dentaire International (FDI) notation.

Palmer notation

This technique is known by other names, Zsigmondy–Palmer, Chevron and the Set Square system.

Each dental quadrant extends from the midline of the oral cavity posteriorly and, individually, corresponds to the upper left and right quadrants in the maxilla and the lower left and right quadrants in the mandible.

The Palmer notation is depicted schematically with a vertical line between the central maxillary and mandibular incisors and a horizontal line between the maxilla and mandible, dividing the oral cavity into quadrants.

The clinician requesting intraoral radiography uses these vertical and horizontal lines to denote the appropriate quadrant in which the tooth/teeth to be radiographed are sited.

To avoid confusion between the permanent and deciduous dentition, the following convention is observed:

- **For the deciduous dentition:** five teeth in each quadrant are assigned the letters 'A' to 'E' from the central deciduous incisor to the second deciduous molar, respectively (Fig. 9.2a).
- **For the permanent dentition:** eight teeth in each quadrant are assigned the number 1–8 from the central incisor to the 3rd permanent molar respectively (Fig. 9.2b).

The number or letter of the tooth to be radiographed is then added to complete the notation.

Examples using this system are:

- C⌋: upper right deciduous canine.
- ⌈78: lower left 2nd and 3rd molars.

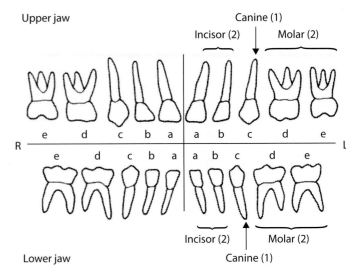

Fig. 9.2a Deciduous teeth.

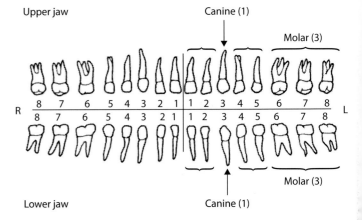

Fig. 9.2b Permanent teeth.

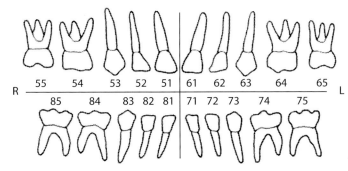

5 Upper jaw									6
R	55	54	53	52	51	61 62 63 64 65			L
	85	84	83	82	81	71 72 73 74 75			
8 Lower jaw									7

Deciduous teeth

Fig. 9.3a Deciduous teeth.

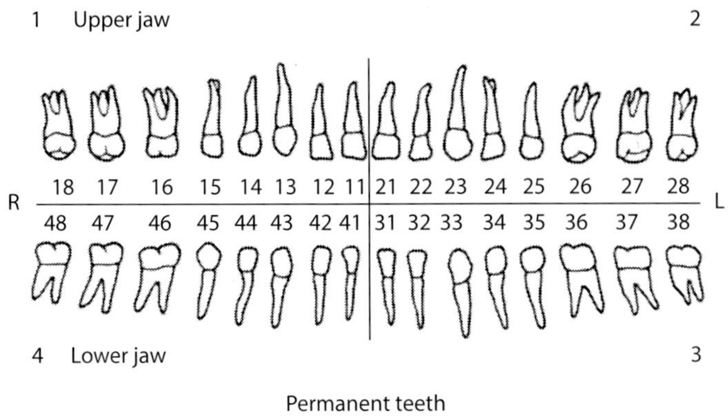

1 Upper jaw	2
R 18 17 16 15 14 13 12 11	21 22 23 24 25 26 27 28 L
48 47 46 45 44 43 42 41	31 32 33 34 35 36 37 38
4 Lower jaw	3

Permanent teeth

Fig. 9.3b Permanent teeth.

Introduction

Dental formula (*cont.*)

Federation Dentaire International notation (Figs 9.3a, 9.3b)

The formula devised by the FDI identifies each tooth using two digits. This method of notation is preferred by some clinicians to avoid typographical errors that can sometimes affect the Palmer system.

The dentition is again divided into four quadrants. These are assigned the numbers 1–4 for the permanent teeth and 5–8 for the deciduous dentition. In both dentitions, the quadrants follow on numerically starting from the upper right, to upper left to lower left and, finally, the lower right. The number of the quadrant precedes the number of the tooth to be radiographed.

The convention is for individual teeth in either dentition to be numbered sequentially from 1 (for the central incisor) to the most distal molar, i.e. 1–8 in each quadrant in the permanent dentition and 1–5 for the deciduous dentition.

Examples using this system are:

- 53: upper right deciduous canine.
- 37, 38: lower left 2nd and 3rd molars.

9 Introduction

Terminology (Figs 9.4a, 9.4b)

Dentists use the following terms to describe the tooth surfaces:

- Mesial represents that surface of the tooth adjacent to the median plane following the curvature of the dental arch.
- Distal represents that surface of the tooth furthest away from the median plane following the curvature of the dental arch.
- Lingual or palatal refers to the inner aspect of the teeth or dental arches adjacent to the tongue or palate respectively.
- Buccal or labial refers to the outer aspect of the teeth or dental arches adjacent to the cheeks or lips respectively.
- Occlusal refers to the biting surface of both premolar and molar teeth.
- Incisal refers to the horizontal flat surface of the incisor teeth.

Occlusal planes (Figs 9.4c, 9.4d)

The occlusal plane is that which passes through the opposing biting surfaces of the teeth. The terms upper and lower occlusal planes are used in radiographic positioning when carrying out intraoral radiography.

It is necessary to adjust the position of the patient's head prior to intraoral radiography to ensure that the appropriate occlusal plane is horizontal and the median plane is vertical. Common radiographic centring points are used to achieve these aims with the patient seated and the head adequately supported.

With the mouth open, the upper occlusal plane lies 4 cm below and parallel to a line joining the tragus of the ear to the ala of the nose.

The lower occlusal plane lies 2 cm below and parallel to a line joining the tragus of the ear to the angle of the mouth with the mouth open.

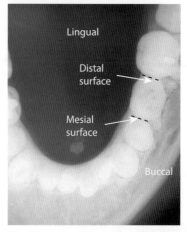

Fig. 9.4a True occlusal radiograph of the mandible.

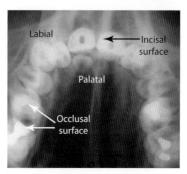

Fig. 9.4b Vertex occlusal radiograph.

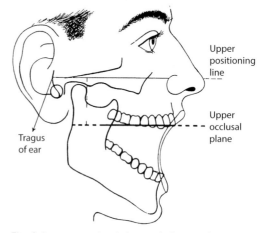

Fig. 9.4c Upper occlusal plane with the mouth open.

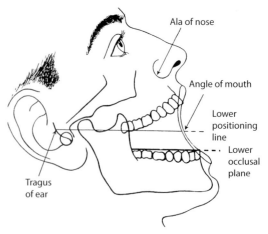

Fig. 9.4d Lower occlusal plane with the mouth open.

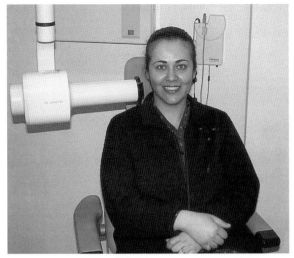

Fig. 9.5a Patient sitting in dental chair with adjacent intraoral X-ray. X-ray equipment is fitted with a long open-ended spacer cone (beam-indicating device).

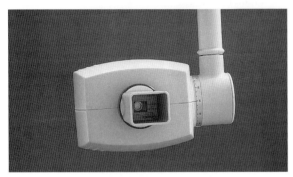

Fig. 9.5b Intraoral X-ray equipment fitted with metallic rectangular spacer cone.

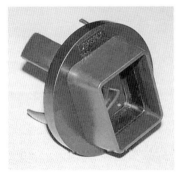

Fig. 9.5c An example of a removable collimator (Dentsply Rinn® Universal collimator).

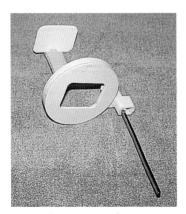

Fig. 9.5d Dentsply Rinn® stainless steel collimator attached by tabs to a Densply Rinn XCP® film holder.

Introduction

X-ray equipment features

Dental equipment for intraoral radiography is designed in order to comply with radiation protection legislation and to ensure that the patient dose is minimised. Equipment features include:

- X-ray tube potential:
  - Nominal tube potential not lower than 50 kV.
  - Recommended operating range of 60–70 kV.
- X-ray tube filtration:
  - 1.5 mm aluminum equivalent for dental units up to 70 kV.
  - 2.5 mm aluminum equivalent (of which 1.5 mm should be permanent) for dental units over 70 kV.
- X-ray beam dimensions:
  - Beam diameter at the patients' skin not greater than 60 mm.
  - Rectangular collimation to be provided on new equipment and retrofitted to existing equipment.
- Minimum focus-to-skin distance:
  - 200 mm: dental units of 60 kV or greater.
  - 100 mm: dental units less than 60 kV.

Recommended kV operating range

The use of a higher kilovoltage (60–70 kV) in dental radiography represents a prudent compromise between minimising surface dose to the patient and obtaining sufficient contrast to allow effective radiological diagnosis of dental and bony tissue.

Rectangular collimation

The use of rectangular collimation for intraoral dental has been shown to reduce patient dose by up to 50% compared with a 6 cm round beam and should be routinely installed on every intraoral X-ray unit, either as an integral component of the X-ray unit or as a retrofitted accessory (Fig. 9.5a).

Rectangular collimation is available as:

- Manufactured component of the X-ray tube head (Fig. 9.5b).
- 'Removable' universal fitting to open-ended cylinder type of equipment (Fig. 9.5c).
- Additional component of some types of image receptor holders (Fig. 9.5d).

Proprietary devices to stabilise the image receptor

The use of a proprietary holder is necessary to stabilise the image receptor of choice. An ideal device should be robust and incorporate an extraoral aiming device to ensure accurate alignment of the X-ray tube relative to the intraoral image receptor. These devices when used correctly ensure that there is no evidence of cone cutting on the resultant image (Fig. 9.5a).

The use of rectangular collimation and a longer focus-to-image receptor distance (FRD) has been shown to improve image quality by a reduction in the amount of scattered radiation and by reducing the penumbra effect.

9 Introduction

Image receptors

The following types of image receptors are used in dental radiography:

- **Intraoral:**
  - Direct or non-screen image receptor.
  - Digital receptors:
    - Solid state.
    - Storage phosphor.
- **Extraoral:**
  - Image receptor -screen (usually rare-earth).
  - Digital receptor:
    - Solid state.
    - Storage phosphor.

Direct or non-screen image receptor

Dental radiography uses a direct image receptor. For the dental clinician, the direct (or packet) image receptor has the advantage of producing a high-resolution image that provides the fine detail needed to assess pathological changes (Fig. 9.6a).

The contents of a conventional film packet consists of:

- An outer plastic wrapper to prevent moisture contamination. The reverse side of which has a two-toned appearance to differentiate it as the 'non-imaging' side of the image receptor.
- Black paper that is wrapped around the image receptor to protect it from light ingress and damage during handling.
- Lead foil with an embossed pattern is positioned at the back of the image receptor to reduce the possibility of fogging from scattered radiation. If the packet is inadvertently positioned back to front, the foil pattern is evident on the processed image receptor identifying the cause of underexposure.
- The image receptor itself comprises an emulsion which is adherent to each side of a plastic base. It is possible to purchase film packets containing two emulsions. This enables the practitioner to retain one for the patient's records whilst the other can be used for referral purposes (Fig. 9.6b).

Intraoral image receptor sizes (Fig. 9.6c)

Several image sizes are available:

- Size 0: 22 mm × 35 mm. Used for small children and anterior periapicals when using the paralleling technique.
- Size 1: 24 mm × 40 mm. Used for bitewings in young children and also for anterior projections in adults.
- Size 2: 31 mm × 41 mm. Used for bitewings in adults and older (generally 6 years plus) children and periapical projections. It can be used for occlusal views in young children.
- Size 3: 27 mm × 54 mm. Listed for use as a bitewing film by the manufacturer.
- Size 4: 57 mm × 76 mm. Used for occlusal projections of the maxilla and mandible.

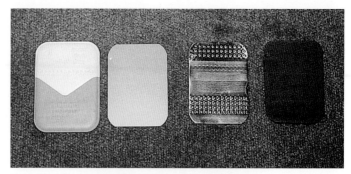

Fig. 9.6a The contents of a film packet from left to right: the outer plastic wrapper, the film, the sheet of lead foil and the black paper.

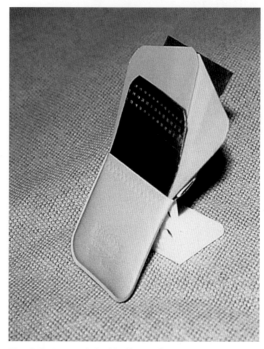

Fig. 9.6b Intraoral double film packet.

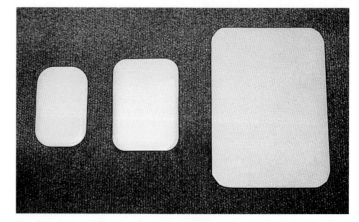

Fig. 9.6c Intraoral film sizes from left to right: small periapical/bitewing film (size 0), large periapical/bitewing film (size 2) and an occlusal film (size 4).

Note

Intraoral film is available, in some sizes, as double film packets. This enables the practitioner to forward one to, for instance, the insurer funding the treatment whilst retaining the other within the patient's records.

Digital receptors

Many manufacturers are now producing digital imaging systems specifically for dental radiography.

The two methods of image capture used are:

- Solid state.
- Storage phosphor.

Solid state (SS): manufacturers employ a range of electronic sensor technology within digital imaging systems. These include the charge-coupled device (CCD), the charge-injection device

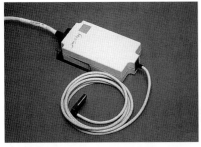

Fig. 9.7a An intraoral CCD/CMOS sensor of the Regam Medical Sens-A-Ray® system.

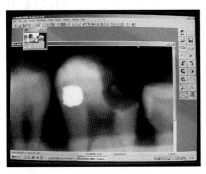

Fig. 9.7b Monitor display of Dentsply's Visualix^USB system.

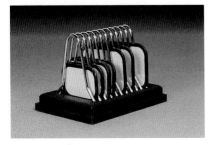

Fig. 9.7c The imaging plates of the Soredex Digora® photostimulable phosphor digital imaging system.

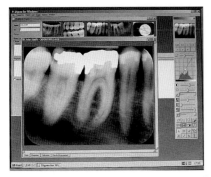

Fig. 9.7d Monitor display of Soredex Digora® system.

Introduction 9

Image receptors (*cont.*)

(CID) and the complementary metal oxide semiconductor (CMOS) based sensors. The sensor is linked directly to the computer via a cable. There is an instantaneous image display with these systems (Figs 9.7a, 9.7b).

Storage phosphor (SP): these systems are commonly found in general radiography departments and may be referred to as computed radiography (CR). Other terminologies variously used to describe the technique are: photostimulable phosphor radiography (PPR), storage phosphor radiography (SPR) and photostimulable phosphor (PSP). The PSP imaging plates consist of europium-activated barium fluorohalide. When exposed to X-rays, the energy of the incident X-ray beam is stored in valency traps in the phosphor. This 'latent image' of stored energy is released as light following scanning of the exposed plate by a laser beam. The pattern of light released is received and then amplified by a CCD and photomultiplier respectively. The image is displayed on a monitor (Figs 9.7c, 9.7d).

The advantages of SS and SP are:

- Instant image in the case of SS systems.
- Almost instant images with SPs. There is a negligible delay of 20 seconds as the plate is 'read' by the laser.
- Image manipulation.

The advantages of SP are:

- Very wide exposure latitude.
- Sensors identical in size and thickness to conventional intraoral image receptors and these are tolerated well by patients.

Disadvantages of SS and SP systems are:

- Cost.
- In some SS systems, the sensor may have a smaller sensitive area than the outer dimensions of the actual image receptor, thereby requiring more exposures to cover areas of interest.
- A number of SS sensors are bulky and some have an attached cable.
- Some imaging systems provide insubstantial intraoral positioning devices.

Both of these techniques require the sensor to be securely located within a sealed water-proof disposable plastic envelope when placed in the oral cavity to prevent moisture contamination. This is a one-use technique with the outer covering being discarded in clinical waste following the exposure. Designated holders are also available to support both SS and SP systems. These devices should be used routinely to ensure optimal geometry.

Before purchasing a digital system, careful consideration should be given to the robustness of the recommended receptor holder. It is important to ensure that the digital receptor is not too bulky as this will often compromise their acceptance by patients, resulting in possible repeat exposures thereby negating the dose benefit for the patient.

9 Introduction

Image acquisition

Alignment devices for use in intraoral radiography (Figs 9.8a, 9.8b)

These devices have been developed in order to simplify intraoral (bitewing and periapical) radiography for both the operator and the patient. Although bitewing and periapical radiography may be carried out without these devices, research has shown that alignment devices noticeably reduce technical errors.

Types available include:

- **Simple devices:** localise the image receptor intraorally (Fig. 9.8a).
- **Beam alignment and image receptor locating instruments:** localise the image receptor intraorally and align the X-ray tube relative to the image receptor (Fig. 9.8b).

An ideal device must incorporate the following features:

- A bite block to stabilise and locate the device correctly.
- A rigid backing to prevent bending if using conventional packet film or some types of phosphor plate digital systems with thin image receptors.
- An extraoral arm (or extension) to ensure correct angulation.

The image receptor/beam alignment types of film holders are, in most cases, designed with an aiming ring attached to an external indicator rod. This type of device has the advantage of accurate localisation. The ring must be positioned in contact with the skin surface to achieve the correct focal spot-to-skin distance.

Specialised image receptor holders (Figs 9.8c–9.8g)

Specialised holders are available for use when conducting endodontic treatment, periodontal assessment and when clinicians are using digital sensors such as SS or SP systems.

During endodontic treatment, the image receptor/beam aiming instrument allows a working length calculation or enables length determination of a master cone. This is achieved by replacing the conventional rigid bite block with an open 'basket' design.

The specialised periodontal image receptor-holding beam alignment instrument allows assessment of bone loss in advanced periodontal disease by stabilising the intraoral image receptor with its long axis vertically.

Alignment devices have also been developed to accommodate intraoral digital sensors. Before purchasing a digital system, the clinicians should confirm that the film holder supplied for digital sensors does also incorporates the ideal factors listed above to ensure that the resultant image is of optimal quality.

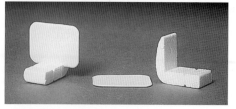

Fig. 9.8a The Rinn Greene Stabe® intraoral film holder with and without film in position.

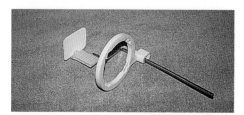

Fig. 9.8b The Rinn XCP® posterior film holder.

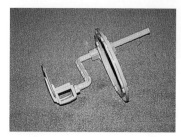

Fig. 9.8c Lateral view of the Rinn Endoray®.

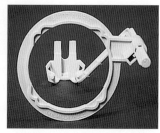

Fig. 9.8d Anterior-posterior view of the Rinn Endoray® showing open 'basket' arrangement to accommodate endodontic instruments.

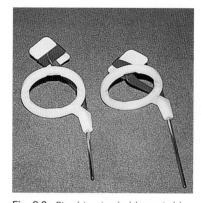

Fig. 9.8e Rinn bitewing holders suitable for (from left to right) a horizontal bitewing and a vertical bitewing. The latter is appropriate in patients with advanced periodontal disease.

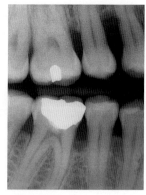

Fig. 9.8f An adult right vertical bitewing of the right premolar/molar region.

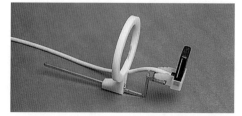

Fig. 9.8g An intraoral CCD/CMOS sensor of the Regam Medical Sens-A-Ray® system positioned in a specially designed Rinn XCP anterior film holder. Note modification to bite block to accommodate bulky sensor. The sensor is always covered by a moisture-proof barrier envelope prior to being placed in the oral cavity.

Film mounting and identification of intraoral films (Fig. 9.9)

If a conventional image receptor is used then the image receptor is mounted with the (embossed) dot towards the radiographer and as though the operator was looking at the patient. This ensures that the mounted images exactly match the dental charting.

- Arrange all images to be mounted on the viewing box.
- Arrange each image as to whether it was taken in the maxilla or the mandible followed by the region, i.e. anterior and posterior. Use anatomical landmarks for guidance as well as root formation.
- Arrange the images of the maxillary teeth by placing the crowns of the teeth towards the bottom of the viewer.
- Arrange the images of the mandibular teeth with the crowns of the teeth towards the top of the viewer.
- When maxillary and mandibular teeth have been identified, radiographs are then arranged as belonging to either the right or left side of the patient.

Radiographs of the central incisors are placed in the centre of the mount and the radiographs of the lateral and canine teeth (correctly positioned according to side) are placed adjacent to them. This is repeated successively for premolars and molar to complete mounting in both dental arches.

General comments

- Most dental projections examinations require the patient to be seated with the head supported and usually with the occlusal plane horizontally positioned and parallel to the floor.
- Prior to the examination, any spectacles, orthodontic appliances, partial/full dentures should be removed, as should jewellery such as earrings, necklaces, tongue bar, nose ring and a nose stud may also be necessary for certain views.

Dental radiographic examinations of the mouth may be complicated by a variety of factors. These include:

- The patient's medical and dental condition.
- The degree of patient co-operation.
- Anatomical factors, i.e. large tongue, shallow palate and narrow dental arches.

Other factors such as a careful explanation of the procedure including information on the placement of the image receptor will reassure the patient, thereby reducing the need for repeat radiographs.

Small children often find the equipment very intimidating and need careful reassurance. Elderly patients may find difficulty in maintaining the position for dental radiography and movement during the exposure may be a problem. Both these groups of individuals can often benefit from a clear explanation of the procedure and the use of short exposure times.

The X-ray request form should be checked to ensure the examination has been justified and that the appropriate X-ray equipment is available. Exposure factors should be set prior to the examination.

Processing of analogue films

Processing of analogue films may employ either manual or automatic techniques. The operator should pay particular attention to careful handling of the image receptor and should ensure that the processing and darkroom techniques employed will not result in:

- Pressure marks on image receptor.
- Emulsion scratches.
- Roller marks (automatic processing only).
- Evidence of film fogging.
- Chemical streaks/splashes/contamination.
- Evidence of inadequate fixation/washing.

Introduction 9

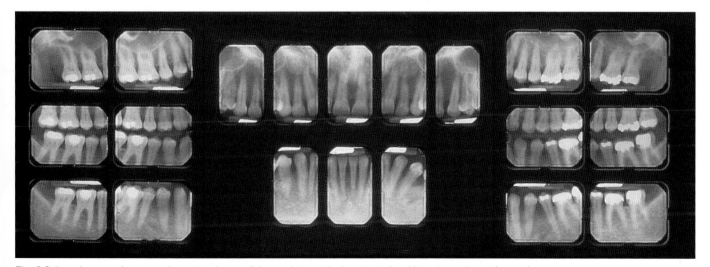

Fig. 9.9 Complete mouth survey taken using the paralleling technique. Both periapical and bitewing radiographs are shown.

9 Introduction

Radiation protection

Dental radiography is a low-dose but high-volume technique. The following comprise the basic requirements of radiation protection legislation as it relates to dental radiography, which has been adopted for dental practice within the UK:

- Each request for dental radiography must be justified.
- Radiographers must never position themselves in the direction of the primary beam.
- Controlled areas are determined in consultation with the Radiation Protection Adviser (RPA).
- The radiographer must never physically support an image receptor inside the patient's mouth.
- Image receptor film holders should be used routinely for intraoral radiography.
- Quality assurance procedures must be adopted when employing conventional radiography.
- The use of a higher kilovoltage (60–70 kV) X-ray in dental radiography represents a prudent compromise between minimising surface dose to the patient and obtaining sufficient contrast to allow radiological diagnosis of dental and bony tissue.
- The use of rectangular collimation for intraoral dental radiography has been shown to reduce patient dose by up to 50% compared with a 6 cm round beam.
- The use of an image receptor holder, incorporating an extraoral aiming arm to ensure accurate alignment of the X-ray tube relative to the intraoral image receptor. The latter not only ensures optimal geometry and is essential when using rectangular collimation in order to prevent 'cone-cut'.
- Image quality is improved when employing rectangular collimation and longer FRD by reducing the amount of scattered radiation and reducing the penumbra effect respectively.

There is no indication for the routine use of lead aprons in dental radiography as it is well recognised that lead protection for the patient has no demonstrable effect against internal scatter and only provides a practicable degree of protection in the case of the very infrequently used vertex occlusal projection. The document 'Selection criteria for Dental Radiography' states that within the field of dental radiography it is unusual for an X-ray beam to be pointed at the abdomen and the only projection in which this occurs is the vertex occlusal radiograph which is a rarely requested dental radiographic technique.

The publication *Guidance Notes for Dental Practitioners on the Safe Use of X-Ray Equipment* highlights Regulation 6 (1)(e) of the IR(ME)R 2000 regulations, which prohibits the carrying out of a medical exposure of a female of child-bearing age without an enquiry as to whether she is pregnant, if this is relevant. Section 2.40 of the Guidance Notes details the possible courses of action open to the clinician if the patient is pregnant.

Cross-infection control

Dental radiography is not an invasive procedure and is generally considered low risk for the operator except when blood is present, i.e. after dental extraction/dental trauma. Saliva and/or blood can contaminate the image receptor, the work surfaces and also the radiographic equipment. As such meticulous cross-infection control is required and this is provided by the use of barrier techniques. It is important that written procedures are in place in the X-ray department to eliminate the possibility of cross infection occurring.

To ensure compliance the following procedures must be observed:

- All surfaces to be disinfected using recommended proprietary disinfectants.
- Disinfected work surfaces must be covered by an appropriate barrier.
- Surface barrier techniques must be used to isolate X-ray equipment from direct contact by the clinician with regard to difficult-to-clean areas on the radiographic equipment, such as the tube head and the control panels of the equipment. Materials used for achieving this are usually plastic sheets and must be changed between patients.
- Other surfaces that must be disinfected are the dental chair, head rest, lead apron and thyroid collar.
- Effective cleaning of work surfaces and disinfection between patients must be ensured.
- The radiographer should wash his/her hands before and after each examination. When multiple patients are seen, an alcohol based hand wash is also recommended
- If the operator has any open wounds on their hands, these areas should be covered with an appropriate dressing.
- Disposable gloves must be worn for all radiographic examinations. Powder-free gloves are preferred as the powder component can cause artifacts on the dental film.
- The radiographer should employ eye protection if there is a possibility of exposure to body fluids.

All staff members involved in dental X-ray examinations should be aware of and be following written policies relating to cross-infection control when conducting either an intraoral or an extraoral dental examination of a patient. These are:

- The use of autoclavable X-ray accessories such as film holders or disposable devices.
- The use of high-level disinfectants for heat sensitive items.
- The use of surface covers and intermediate-level chemical disinfectants for clinical surfaces.
- Clinicians should routinely use barrier envelopes for conventional intraoral image receptors and intraoral digital sensors. The routine use of these barrier techniques has been found to reduce significantly the risk of microbial contamination by saliva and/or blood.
- If barrier envelopes are not available, exposed film packets should be disinfected before they are handled and processed.

Cross-infection control (cont.)

The use of a disposable tray system containing the image receptor and the film holder reduces the possibility of contamination of the clinical work surface.

Following completion of the intraoral radiographic examination, the operator must ensure that empty conventional intraoral film packets, barrier envelopes, gloves, cotton wool rolls and the disposable tray should be discarded as clinical waste.

Intraoral image film-holding devices should be sterilised according to manufacturer's guidelines. Most manufacturers recommend rinsing and steam autoclaving of these devices after use. Some manufacturers produce film-holding devices that are disposable.

Surface disinfectants should be used on all work surfaces, the dental chair, film cassettes, the control panel, X-ray tube head and the exposure switch after each patient.

Manufacturers of panoramic equipment provide individual autoclavable bite blocks. During radiography, panoramic bite blocks are used once and then autoclaved. Lateral restraints are wiped using a recommended proprietary antibacterial wipe and are then covered with a new disposable plastic cover for the next patient. Following the panoramic examination, the removable biteblock should be sterilised, and the plastic cover discarded as clinical waste. Chin rests and head positioning guides must be routinely cleaned by a recommended antiseptant between patients using the manufacturer's recommended cleansing regime.

Most manufacturers of dental imaging equipment provide both medical grade key boards and a medical grade mouse. These are fully sealed items and require to be covered with a sterilised disposable barrier envelope.

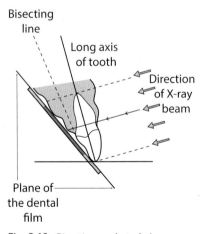

Fig. 9.10a Bisecting angle technique.

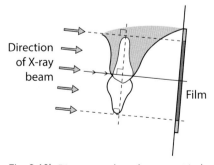

Fig. 9.10b Diagram to show the geometrical relationship between X-ray beam, tooth and film in the paralleling technique.

Introduction 9

Principles for optimal image geometry

In order to minimise distortional effects and achieve optimal image geometry, the following principles have been advocated for intraoral radiography:

- The focal spot should be as small as possible.
- The focal spot-to-object distance (FOD) should be as great as possible.
- The object-to-image receptor distance (ORD) should be as small as possible.
- The image receptor should be parallel to the plane of the object.
- The central ray should be perpendicular to both the object and the image receptor.

Both bitewing and periapical radiography benefit from an accurate and stable position of the image receptor. Bitewing radiography requires that the beam, in the horizontal plane, meets the teeth and the image receptor at right-angles and passes through all the contact areas. For periapical radiography, the ideal principles for optimal image geometry cannot be satisfied in all patients due to a variety of factors. To overcome these problems, two techniques have been developed:

- The bisecting angle technique: the technique is based upon the geometric theorem of isometry. It requires the central ray of the X-ray beam to pass through the root of the tooth at right-angles to a plane, which is the bisector of the angle formed by the long axis of the tooth and the plane of the image receptor (Fig. 9.10a).
- The paralleling technique: the technique requires that the X-ray image receptor is positioned parallel with the long axes of the teeth or tooth to be imaged. This enables the central ray of the X-ray beam to pass at right-angles, i.e. perpendicular to the beam to the long axes of the teeth and the plane of the image receptor (Fig. 9.10b).

9 Bitewing radiography

Bitewing radiography (Fig. 9.11a) is used for:

- The detection of dental caries in the upper and lower pre-molar and molar teeth.
- Monitoring the progression of dental caries.
- The assessment of existing restorations.
- The assessment of the periodontal condition.

The methods available to position the image receptor intraorally include:

- **Bitewing tab:** a heavy-duty paper tab attached to an intraoral image receptor. The attachment can be either by an adhesive backing to the tab or by a bitewing loop with an attached tab for the patient to bite on (Fig. 9.11b).
- **Film-holding instrument:** this is a simple device to localise the image receptor comprising a biteblock and image receptor-positioning slot (Fig. 9.11c).
- **Film-holding beam alignment instrument:** a device with a biteblock, rigid backing and an extraoral arm to position correctly the tube relative to the image receptor. These are available for both analogue films and digital sensors (Fig. 9.11d).

Irrespective of the method used to position the image receptor intraorally, the imaging surface of the image receptor must be positioned facing the X-ray tube.

Radiological considerations

It is important to use the correct sized image receptor/digital sensor for the patient:

- In an adult, a size 2 image receptor (31 mm × 41 mm) is usual.
- An adult with erupted 3rd molars and in those patients with larger jaws, two size 2 image receptors may be needed to cover the dental arch adequately.
- For younger children, the convention is to use a size 0 image receptor (22 mm × 35 mm) or a digital sensor.
- In the older child, a common sense approach will determine when to upgrade from a size 0 to a size 2 image receptor to obtain adequate coverage.
- It is important to recognise that some digital sensors may have a smaller sensor area compared with the identical conventional image receptor. This will obviously negate the obvious dose benefit of using digital radiography.

When using bitewing tabs: correct position and angulation of the X-ray tube is needed to ensure adequate image receptor coverage without evidence of coning off (Fig. 9.11e).

Incorrect vertical angulation of the X-ray tube causes distortion of the image. Incorrect horizontal placement of the X-ray tube results in horizontal overlap of the contact points of the teeth reducing the diagnostic yield for the clinician (Fig. 9.11f).

When using a bitewing film-holding beam alignment instrument: young children often find these devices uncomfortable. If the patient clinically exhibits periodontal bone loss of >6 mm, two vertically positioned image receptors (i.e. with the narrower length positioned parallel to the floor of the mouth) are required to enable the bone of the periodontium to be imaged.

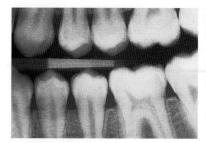

Fig. 9.11a A left horizontal adult bitewing radiograph.

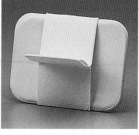

Fig. 9.11b An intraoral film packet with tab attached.

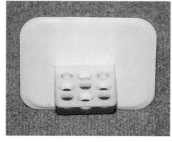

Fig. 9.11c Twix® film holder and with intraoral film packet positioned in localising slot.

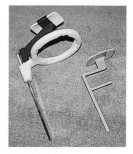

Fig. 9.11d Horizontal bitewing film holders. From left to right: Rinn bitewing holder and Hawe-Neos Kwikbite with beam-aiming rod.

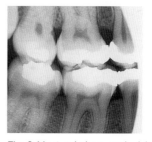

Fig. 9.11e A right horizontal adult bitewing radiograph showing coning off or cone cutting.

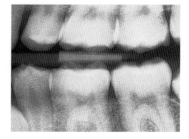

Fig. 9.11f A left horizontal adult bitewing radiograph showing incorrect horizontal angulation of the X-ray tube head.

Notes

- Access to previous radiographs may reveal the need for vertical bitewings.
- The correct image receptor size is chosen and placed in an ideal film holder.
- The film holder is introduced into the mouth, rotated over the tongue and positioned in the lingual sulcus.
- The anterior edge of the image receptor should be located opposite to the distal edge of the lower canine (see Fig. 9.12a).
- The biteblock rests on the occlusal surface of the lower teeth (see Fig. 9.13a).
- The patient is told to bite gently on the biteblock and, at the same time, the operator ensures that there is good contact between the image receptor and the teeth.
- Inform patient to continue biting on the biteblock to position the image receptor holder securely.
- See section on specialised film holders and the importance of their use when using digital sensors.

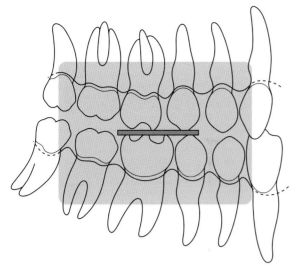

Fig. 9.12a Diagram to show the correct position of the adult horizontal bitewing.

Bitewing radiography 9

Position of patient and image receptor using a bitewing tab attached to the image receptor packet

- The correct image receptor size is chosen and the bitewing tab attached.
- The patient's head must be adequately supported with the medial plane vertical and the occlusal plane horizontal.
- Hold the tab between thumb and forefinger.
- Place the image receptor in the lingual sulcus.
- The anterior edge of the image receptor should be located opposite to the distal aspect of the lower canine (Fig. 9.12a).
- The tab rests on the occlusal surface of the lower teeth (Fig. 9.12b).
- The patient is told to bite gently on the tab and, when the teeth are almost in contact, the operator pulls the tab laterally to ensure that there is good contact between the image receptor and the teeth.
- The operator releases their hold on the tab and concomitantly informs the patient to continue biting on the tab.

Direction and location of the X-ray beam

The tube is angled 5–8° downward (caudal) with the central ray at the level of the occlusal plane and perpendicular to the contact points of the teeth (Fig. 9.12c).

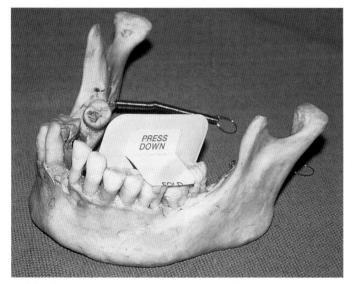

Fig. 9.12b The ideal position for a left adult horizontal bitewing using a bitewing tab.

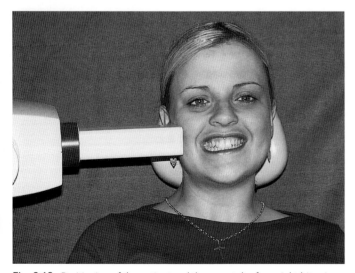

Fig. 9.12c Positioning of the patient and the x-ray tube for a right bitewing radiograph using a bitewing tab.

9 Bitewing radiography

Position of patient and image receptor when using a bitewing image receptor-holding/beam alignment instrument

- The correct image receptor size is chosen and placed in the film holder. For digital sensors, most manufactures will provide appropriate holders.
- The film holder is introduced into the mouth, rotated over the tongue and positioned in the lingual sulcus.
- The anterior edge of the image receptor should be located opposite to the distal edge of the lower canine (see Fig. 9.12a).
- The biteblock rests on the occlusal surface of the lower teeth (Fig. 9.13a).
- The patient is told to bite gently on the biteblock and, at the same time, the operator ensures that there is good contact between the image receptor and the teeth.
- Inform patient to continue biting on the biteblock to position the holder securely.

Direction and location of the X-ray beam

- As directed by the extraoral aiming device of the holder (Fig. 9.13b).

Quality standards for bitewing radiography

Evidence of optimal image geometry

- There should be no evidence of bending of the teeth on the image.
- There should be no foreshortening or elongation of the teeth.
- Ideally, there should be no horizontal overlap.

If overlap is present, it should not obscure more than 1/2 of the enamel thickness. This may be unavoidable due to anatomical factors (i.e. overcrowding, shape of dental arch) necessitating an additional bitewing or periapical radiograph.

Correct coverage

- The image receptor should cover the distal surfaces of the canine teeth and the mesial surfaces of the most posterior erupted teeth.
- The periodontal bone level should be visible and equally imaged in the maxilla/mandible confirming ideal centring.

Good density and contrast

- There should be good density and adequate contrast between the enamel and the dentine.

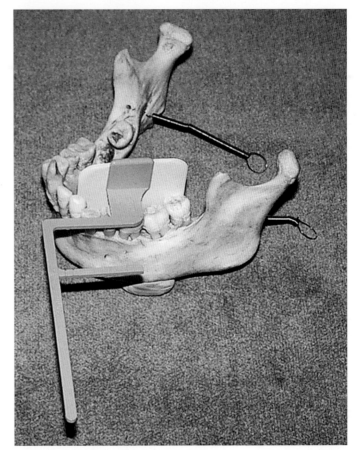

Fig. 9.13a Lateral view of a Hawe-Neos Kwikbite film holder positioned for a left bitewing radiograph on a dried mandible.

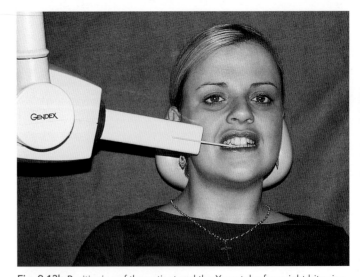

Fig. 9.13b Positioning of the patient and the X-ray tube for a right bitewing radiograph using a Hawe-Neos Kwikbite film holder and rectangular collimation of the X-ray tube.

Adequate number of images

- When the 3rd molars are erupted or partially erupted and impacted and all the other teeth are present, two image receptors may be needed on each side to evaluate the dentition.

Periapical radiography 9

Periapical radiography provides an image of the teeth, the surrounding periodontal tissues and the alveolar bone (Fig. 9.14a). There are many clinical indications for periapical radiography:

- Assessment of the periodontium, encompassing the periapical and the periodontal status.
- Assessment of apical pathology and other lesions situated within alveolar bone.
- Pre- and postoperative assessment of alveolar surgery.
- Following trauma to teeth and alveolar bone.
- Localisation of teeth, presence/absence of teeth.
- Prior to extraction to assess root morphology and the relationship of roots to vital structures, i.e. the inferior dental canal, the maxillary antrum.
- During endodontic therapy.
- Pre- and postoperative assessment of implants.

The two available techniques are:

- The bisecting angle technique (Fig. 9.14b).
- The paralleling technique (Fig. 9.14c).

Irrespective of the technique used, the imaging surface of the image receptor must be positioned facing the X-ray tube.

Bisecting angle technique

The technique is based upon the geometric theorem of isometry. It requires the central ray of the X-ray beam to pass through the root of the tooth at right-angles to a plane, which is the bisector of the angle formed by the long axis of the tooth and the plane of the image receptor (Fig. 9.14b).

- Advantages: positioning is relatively simple.
- Disadvantages: too many variables in the technique often resulting in poor image quality.

Two methods are employed to stabilise the image receptor intraorally:

- A film holder.
- The patient's finger.

The use of an image receptor-holding instrument is preferred as it reduces distortion within the image and stabilises the image receptor, ensuring better patient co-operation. However, the resulting X-ray image may exhibit image shape distortion as a result of incorrect vertical angulation of the tube (Fig. 9.14d).

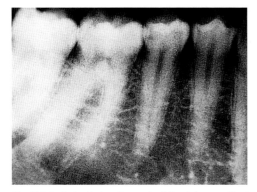

Fig. 9.14a Periapical radiograph of the right mandibular molar region.

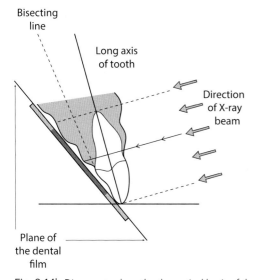

Fig. 9.14b Diagram to show the theoretical basis of the bisecting angle technique.

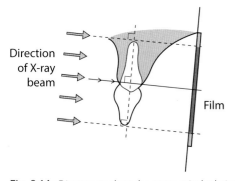

Fig. 9.14c Diagram to show the geometrical relationship between X-ray beam, tooth and film in the paralleling technique.

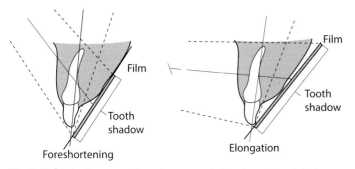

Fig. 9.14d Left: diagram to show the geometric foreshortening of the image by using too steep a vertical angulation of the X-ray tube. Right: diagram to show the geometric elongation of the image by using a too shallow vertical angulation of the X-ray tube.

327

9 Periapical radiography

Bisecting angle technique (*cont.*)

The convention for intraoral image receptor placement is as follows:

- Anterior teeth (incisors and canines): the long axis of image receptor is vertical.
- Posterior teeth (premolars and molars): the long axis of image receptor is horizontal.

Position of patient and image receptor

- The patient's head must be adequately supported with the medial plane vertical and the occlusal plane horizontal (i.e. upper occlusal plane and lower occlusal plane for maxillary and mandibular radiography, respectively).

If an image receptor holder is used:

- The correct film/sensor size is chosen and placed in the receptor holder (Fig. 9.15a).
- Position the holder intraorally adjacent to the lingual/palatal aspects of the tooth/teeth to be imaged.
- Insert a cotton wool roll between the opposing teeth and the biteblock.
- Ask the patient to close together slowly, to allow gradual accommodation of the film holder intraorally.
- Inform patient to continue biting on the biteblock to position the film holder securely (Fig. 9.15b).

If the patient's finger is used:

- The correct conventional film/sensor size is chosen and positioned intraorally.
- Ensure that the tooth/teeth being examined are in the middle of the image receptor.
- 2 mm of the film packet should extend beyond the incisal or occlusal margin to ensure that the entire tooth is imaged.
- Patient is instructed to support the film packet gently using either their index finger or thumb (Fig. 9.15c).
- Apply the patient's finger/thumb solely to the area of film that overlies the crown and gingival tissues of the teeth. This reduces the possibility of distortion by bending of the film covering the root and periapical tissues.

Direction and location of the X-ray beam

- The X-ray beam should be centred vertically on the midpoint of the tooth to be examined.
- Look at the tooth; look at the image receptor; and the bisecting the angle between the two. This achieves the correct vertical angulation of the tube.
- It is important to remember that proclined teeth will require more angulation, whilst retroclined teeth will need less.
- The x-ray tube must be positioned so that the beam is at right-angles to the labial or buccal surfaces of the teeth to prevent horizontal overlap.

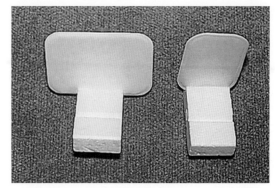

Fig. 9.15a Rinn Greene Stabe® film holder with (from left to right) horizontal film placement for the premolars and molars and vertical film placement for the incisors and canines.

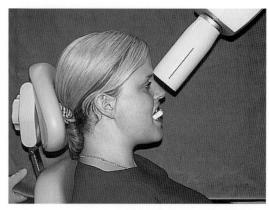

Fig. 9.15b Positioning of the patient and the X-ray tube for a periapical radiograph of the maxillary incisors using the Rinn Greene Stabe® film holder.

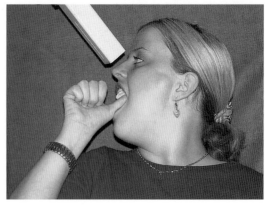

Fig. 9.15c Positioning of the patient and the X-ray tube for a periapical radiograph of the maxillary incisors using the thumb for support.

Periapical radiography 9

Bisecting angle technique (cont.)

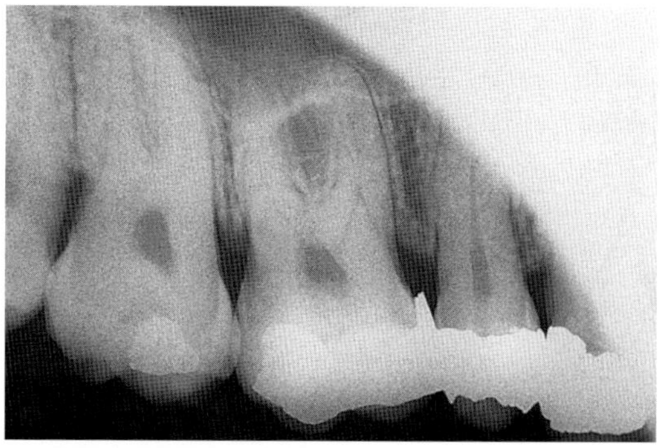

Notes

- Correct position and angulation of the X-ray tube is needed to ensure adequate image coverage without evidence of coning off (Fig. 9.16a).
- Incorrect vertical angulation of the X-ray tube causes distortion of the image and may result in inaccuracies in diagnosis (Fig. 9.16b).
- The image can be distorted due to incorrect placement of image receptor and/or the patient's finger (Fig. 9.16c).
- Inaccurate vertical angulation of the X-ray tube results in misrepresentation of the alveolar bone levels (Fig. 9.16d).
- Incorrect horizontal placement of the X-ray tube results in horizontal overlap of the contact point of the teeth (Fig. 9.16e).
- The image of the zygomatic bone frequently overlies the roots of upper molars (Fig. 9.16f).

Radiological considerations

- Conventionally, the technique uses a short tube-to-image receptor distance and the object distance is reduced by close approximation of the image receptor to the palatal or lingual aspect of the alveolar ridge.
- With the occlusal plane horizontal, the X-ray tube is positioned vertically by an assessment of the bisected plane for each individual patient. This technique is preferred to the use of the standardised vertical tube angulations (see tables) as it allows for anatomical variations.

Fig. 9.16a Coning off or cone cutting occurs when the X-ray tube is incorrectly poisoned. The X-ray tubehead was positioned too far posteriorly so the anterior region of the periapical radiograph was not exposed.

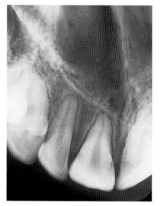

Fig. 9.16b Foreshortened image due to the vertical angle being too steep.

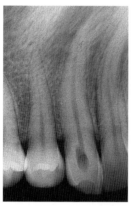

Fig. 9.16c Excessive pressure when stabilising the film or incorrect placement of the film in the mouth results in bending of the film packet during exposure.

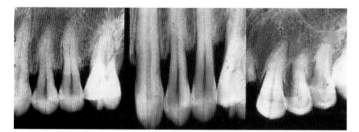

Fig. 9.16d The effect of beam angulation on periodontal bone levels. A steep vertical angle (extreme right) masks bone loss, whilst too shallow an angle (centre) amplifies the extent of bone loss. The image on the extreme left of this dried skull series represents the correct geometry and accurate bone levels.

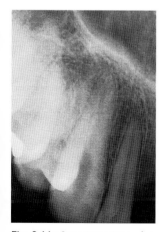

Fig. 9.16e Superimposition of structures due to incorrect horizontal angulation of the tube.

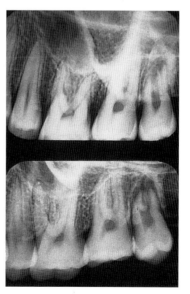

Fig. 9.16f The upper periapical was taken using the bisecting angle technique resulting in the dense radio-opacity of the zygomatic buttress overlying and obscuring the apices of the upper molar teeth. In the lower image, taken using the paralleling technique, the shadow of the buttress is well above the apices as it is a true lateral image.

329

9 Periapical radiography

Bisecting angle technique (cont.)

Table 9.1 Angulations and centring points for the bisecting angle technique in the maxilla

Region	Centring point	Vertical angulation (degrees)
Incisor: central Incisor: lateral	Midline through tip of nose Ala of nose, 1 cm from midline	50–60° (average 50°)
Canine	Ala of nose	45–50°
Premolar	On the cheek: at the point of intersection of a line down from mid-point of inner and outer canthus of the eye and the ala–tragus line	35–40
Molar	On the cheek: at point of intersection of a line down from a point 1 cm posterior to outer canthus of the eye and the ala–tragus line	20–30

Table 9.2 Angulations and centring points for the bisecting angle technique in the mandible (negative angle indicates upward [cranial] angulation of the tube)

Region	Centring point	Vertical angulation (degrees)
Incisors	Midline, 1 cm above the lower border of the mandible	−20 to −30
Canine	Vertical line down from the outer aspect of the ala of nose, centring 1 cm above the lower border of the mandible	−20 to −30
Premolars	Vertical line down from the midpoint between inner and outer canthus of eye, centring 1 cm above the lower border of the mandible	−10 to −15
Molars	Vertical line down from a point 1 cm posterior to outer canthus of eye centring 1 cm above the lower border of the mandible	0 to −10

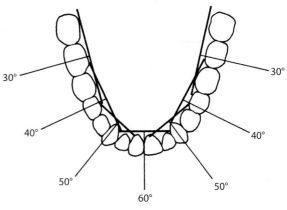

Fig. 9.17a Diagram of upper teeth showing caudal angulations.

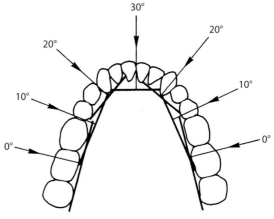

Fig. 9.17b Diagram of lower teeth showing cranial angulations.

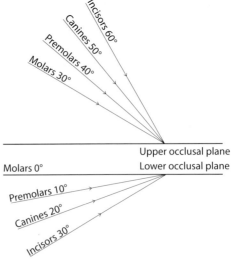

Fig. 9.17c Schematic of angulations to upper and lower occlusal planes.

Periapical radiography 9

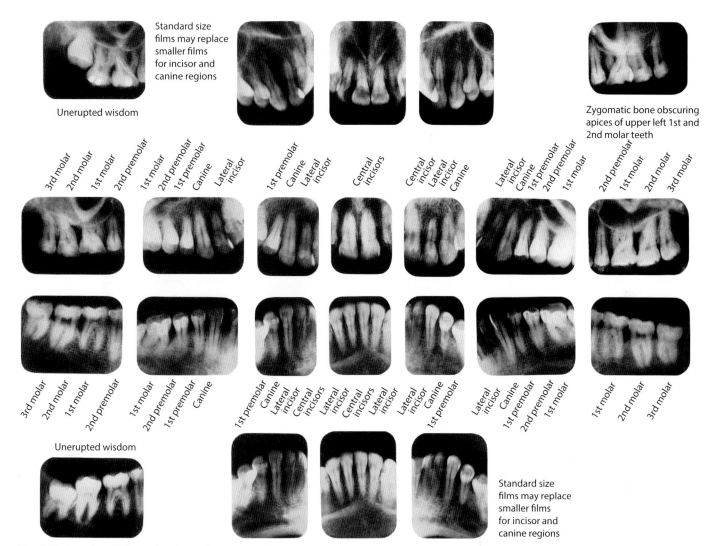

Fig. 9.18 Examples of full mouth radiography (upper and lower jaw).

9 Periapical radiography

Paralleling technique

The paralleling technique requires that the x-ray image receptor is positioned parallel with the long axes of the teeth. The central ray of the X-ray beam passes at right-angles, i.e. perpendicular, to the tooth (Fig. 9.19a).

In order to minimise magnification of the image and subsequent loss of image sharpness, the technique uses an increased focal spot-to-object distance (FOD) ensuring a more parallel X-ray beam is incident to the object and image receptor (Figs 9.19b, 9.19c).

Advantages of the paralleling technique include:

- Minimal elongation/foreshortening/distortion.
- An increased focus-to-skin distance (FSD) reduces surface dose.
- An increased FSD improves image quality by reducing the penumbra effect.
- Reduction in distortional effects due to bending of the image receptor /image receptor.

Disadvantages of the paralleling technique:

- The paralleling technique can be used when using X-ray equipment with a short FRD (i.e. <20 cm) providing the operator accepts increased magnification.
- Anatomical limitations, such as a shallow palate, principally in the maxillary molar and anterior regions preclude true parallel placement of the image receptor relative to the tooth.

Radiological considerations

- The use of the paralleling technique along with film-holding beam alignment instruments allows the operator to obtain images that have reproducibility and standardisation. This allows the clinician to study longitudinal disease progression and to assess accurately treatment outcomes.
- Provided the image receptor position does not diverge from the long axis (or axes) of the tooth by more than 20°, the image will demonstrate no evidence of longitudinal distortion.
- In endodontic treatment, it may be necessary to separate superimposed root canals using two radiographs at different horizontal angles. Obtain one 'normal' image and one with a 20° oblique horizontal beam angle for all molars and maxillary 1st premolars.
- Assessment of some horizontally impacted mandibular 3rd molars may require two image receptors to image the apex. Obtain one 'normal' image and one with a more posterior 20° oblique horizontal beam angle.

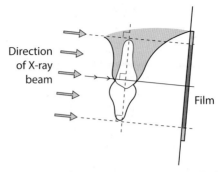

Fig. 9.19a Diagram to show the geometrical relationship between X-ray beam, tooth and film in the paralleling technique.

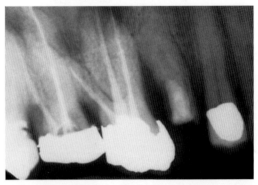

Fig. 9.19b Paralleling periapical radiograph of upper right molar region. Endodontic treatment has been carried out on each of the molar teeth.

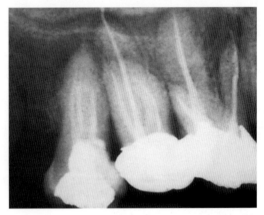

Fig. 9.19c Second paralleling periapical radiograph of the same region as the figure above, but using a 20° posterior horizontal tube shift. This has the effect of identifying and separating the root canals of the upper right 1st molar.

Periapical radiography 9

Paralleling technique (cont.)

Film-holding beam alignment instruments (Figs 9.20a, 9.20b)

Most devices require the use of different sized image receptors in the anterior and posterior regions of the oral cavity. The usual convention for image receptor use is:

- Anterior teeth (incisors and canines): size 0 or size 1 film with long axis of image receptor vertical. The alternative use of a size 1 image receptor is governed solely by operator preference.
- Posterior teeth (premolars and molars): size 2 (31 mm × 41 mm) film with the long axis of image receptor horizontal.
- Some operators use size 0 or size 1 for premolars.
- Adopting these techniques limits longitudinal distortion and ensures patient comfort (Fig. 9.20c).

Digital sensors follow the same convention as conventional radiography for imaging anterior and posterior teeth. Most digital systems either supply or recommend commercially available digital sensor-holding devices to ensure accurate geometry for the resultant image.

Essential image characteristics

- There should be no evidence of bending within the imaging of the teeth and the periapical region of interest on the image.
- There should be no foreshortening or elongation of the teeth.
- Ideally, there should be no horizontal overlap. If overlap is present, it must not obscure pulp/root canals.
- The image receptor should demonstrate all the tooth/teeth of interest (i.e. crown and root[s]).
- There should be 3 mm of periapical bone visible to enable an assessment of apical anatomy.
- No pressure marks on the image receptor.
- For conventional processing there should be:
  - No pressure marks on the image receptor, no emulsion scratches.
  - No roller marks (automatic processing only).
  - No evidence of image receptor fog.
  - No chemical streaks/splashes/contamination.
  - No evidence of inadequate fixation/washing.

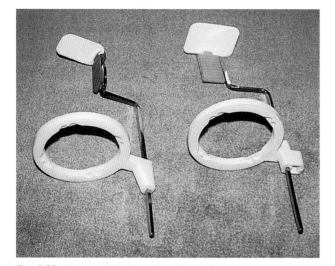

Fig. 9.20a The Rinn XCP film holder: from left to right the anterior and posterior devices with size 0 and size 2 films respectively.

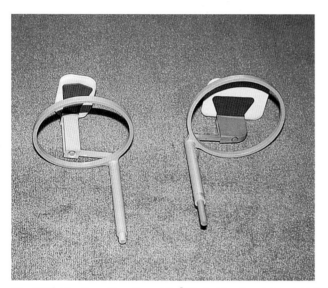

Fig. 9.20b The Hawe-Neos Super Bite® film holder: from left to right the anterior and posterior devices with size 0 and size 2 films respectively.

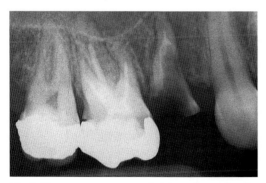

Fig. 9.20c A posterior periapical of the right maxilla taken using the paralleling technique.

9 Periapical radiography

Paralleling technique (*cont.*) (Figs 9.21a, 9.21b)

Position of patient and image receptor

- The patient's head must be adequately supported with the median plane vertical and the occlusal plane horizontal.
- The appropriate film/sensor holder and periapical image receptor are selected and assembled.
- Place the biteblock in contact with the edge of the tooth to be imaged and ensure that the image receptor covers the particular tooth/teeth to be examined.
- **Maxilla:** (Figs 9.21c, 9.21d)
  - For the incisor, canine, premolar and molar regions, the film/sensor holder must be positioned palatally some distance from the tooth to achieve parallelism. This requires using the entire horizontal length of the biteblock with the image receptor occupying the highest part of the palate.
- **Mandible:**
  - For the lower incisor teeth, the image receptor is positioned lingually to the tooth/ teeth selected for imaging.
  - For the mandibular premolars and molars, the film holder is positioned in the lingual sulcus adjacent to the teeth selected for imaging.
- Insert a cotton wool roll between the opposing teeth and the biteblock.
- Ask the patient to close together slowly to allow gradual accommodation of the image receptor holder intraorally.
- As the patient closes together rotate biteblock in an upward/downward direction (as appropriate).
- Instruct the patient to close firmly on the biteblock and to continue biting until the examination is completed.
- Slide the aiming ring down the indicator rod to approximate the skin surface.

Direction and location of the X-ray beam

- Correctly align the X-ray tube adjacent to the indicator rod and aiming ring in both vertical and horizontal planes.

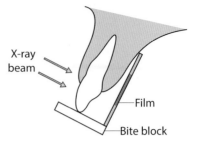

Fig. 9.21a Diagram showing the correct position of the film in the film-holder biteblock relative to an anterior tooth in the maxilla.

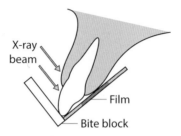

Fig. 9.21b Diagram showing the incorrect position of the film in the film-holder biteblock. When the holder is positioned adjacent to the tooth (mimicking the set up for the bisecting technique), true parallelism cannot be achieved and the holder is extremely uncomfortable for the patient.

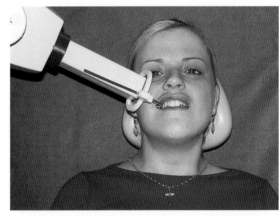

Fig. 9.21c Positioning of the patient and the X-ray tube for a periapical radiograph of the maxillary molar region using the Rinn XCP posterior film holder.

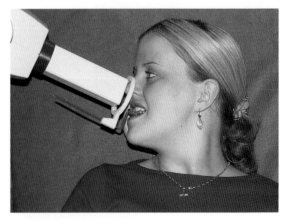

Fig. 9.21d Positioning of the patient and the X-ray tube for a periapical radiograph of the maxillary central incisors using the Rinn XCP anterior film holder.

Periapical radiography 9

Paralleling technique (*cont.*)

Common faults and solutions

- Care must be taken in the partially dentate patient as edentulous areas can displace the holder and 'prop' open the bite (Fig. 9.22a).
- To overcome this problem cotton wool rolls can be used to support the image receptor in the edentulous area (Fig. 9.22b).
- In edentulous patients, the effect of tooth loss is to alter the height of the palate and the depth of the lingual sulcus. To overcome these anatomical factors, the placement of a cotton wool roll on the maxillary and mandibular alveolar ridge with the biteblock between will stabilise the image receptor/film holder.
- Ensure that the patient understands that they must continue to bite on the biteblock. Failure to do this results in loss of apices from the resultant image (Fig. 9.22c).

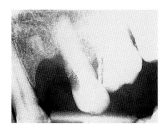

Fig. 9.22a Radiograph of the upper left maxilla shows the biteblock being trapped against the upper left canine due to the adjacent edentulous region. This has the effect of 'propping' open the bite.

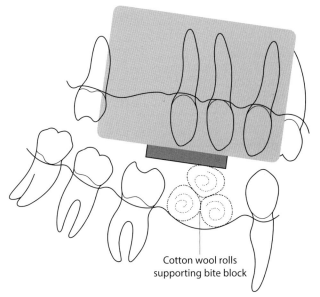

Fig. 9.22b Use of cotton wool rolls to stabilise the biteblock in an edentulous area.

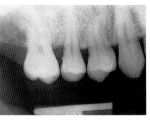

Fig. 9.22c Loss of apices due to lack of continuous biting pressure.

9 Periapical radiography

Third molar region

Positioning of the image receptor using a conventional image receptor/ holder can be uncomfortable for the patient in the 3rd molar region. To overcome these problems, the following techniques should be adopted.

Imaging mandibular 3rd molars

Surgical haemostats or needle holders can be used to stabilise the image receptor. One beak of the device is modified into a biteblock by soldering a semi-circular stainless wire onto the needle holder and covering it with heavy-duty autoclavable plastic. This simple addition significantly reduces the problem of the patient inadvertently moving the holder (Fig. 9.23a).

Position of patient and image receptor (Fig. 9.23b)

- The upper leading anterior edge of a size 2 image receptor is securely attached to the beaks of the needle holder ensuring that the front aspect (or imaging surface) will face the X-ray tube when positioned intraorally.
- The image receptor is positioned in the lingual sulcus as far posterior as possible.
- The patient is instructed to bring their teeth together slowly. This has the effect of lowering the floor of the mouth and, thereby, providing more space to accommodate the image receptor. Simultaneously, the operator positions the image receptor holder so that the leading edge of the image receptor lies adjacent to the mesial aspect of the mandibular 1st molar. It is important to do this gradually to reduce discomfort for the patient.
- The patient is instructed to hold the handles of the needle holder.
- Problems may be encountered with patient acceptance if a solid state digital sensor is the only available image receptor, irrespective of the presence of an appropriate film holder.

Direction and location of the X-ray beam

The tube is centred and angulated as outlined in the table on page 330 for the mandibular molar region (Fig. 9.23c). The X-ray tube must be positioned so that the beam is at right-angles to the labial or buccal surfaces of the teeth to prevent horizontal overlap and the image receptor exposed.

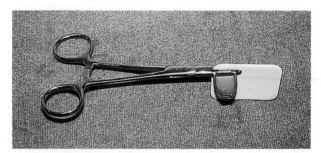

Fig. 9.23a Modified surgical haemostats with soldered biteblock.

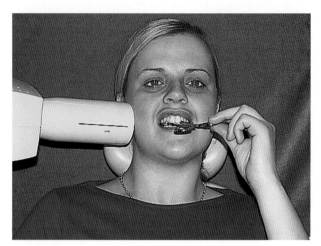

Fig. 9.23b Positioning of the patient and the X-ray tube for a periapical radiograph of the mandibular 3rd molar. The holder is stabilised by the patient's hand.

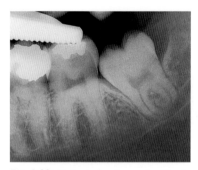

Fig. 9.23c Periapical radiograph of the lower left 3rd molar showing a complex root form and close approximation of root apices to the mandibular canal.

Periapical radiography 9

Third molar region (cont.)

Imaging maxillary 3rd molars (Figs 9.24a, 9.24b)

The use of a film holder in this region is dependent on the patient's ability to tolerate the device. If the use of a film holder is impossible, then the bisecting angle technique is adopted. Problems may be encountered with patient acceptance if a solid state digital sensor is the only available image receptor irrespective of the presence of an appropriate film holder.

Position of patient and image receptor

- The patient's head must be adequately supported with the medial plane vertical and the maxillary occlusal plane horizontal.
- Position the image receptor intraorally so that the front aspect (or imaging surface) will face the X-ray tube.
- The image receptor is positioned far enough posteriorly to cover the 3rd molar region with the anterior border just covering the 2nd premolar.
- The image receptor is supported by the patient's index finger or thumb. It is positioned with 2 mm of image receptor packet extending beyond the occlusal plane to ensure that the entire tooth is imaged. The image plane must be flat to reduce the distortional effects of bending.

Direction and location of the X-ray beam

- The X-ray tube is centred and angulated as outlined in the table on page 330 for the maxillary molar region.
- The X-ray tube must be positioned so that the beam is at right-angles to the labial or buccal surfaces of the teeth to prevent horizontal overlap and the image receptor exposed.

Complete mouth survey or full mouth survey

The complete mouth survey or full mouth survey is composed of a series of individual periapical image receptors covering all the teeth and tooth-bearing alveolar bone of the dental arches. Most patients require 14 periapical image receptors to fulfil these requirements. Careful technique is essential to reduce the need for repeat examinations (see Fig. 9.9).

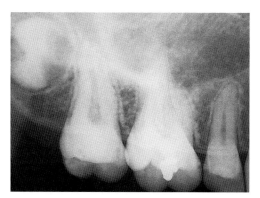

Fig. 9.24a Periapical of the right molar region showing a developing 3rd maxillary molar.

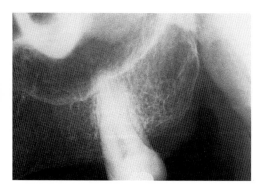

Fig. 9.24b Periapical of the left molar region showing normal anatomy of the tuberosity, the antral floor and the inferior aspect of the zygoma.

9 Occlusal radiography

Occlusal projections are used to image relatively large areas of the dental arches. Their main uses are:

- To localise accurately unerupted teeth, supernumeraries, retained roots, odontomes, foreign bodies, radio-opaque salivary calculi, etc in regions of the oral cavity where the occlusal view provides a 'plan' view of the jaw.
- To localise accurately unerupted teeth, supernumeraries, retained roots, odontomes, foreign bodies using parallax when combined with another image receptor of the region taken using a different vertical angulation.
- To evaluate a patient with severe trismus or who cannot tolerate periapical radiography.
- To evaluate a patient in cases of trauma, when information is required on the extent and location of fractures to teeth and to the maxillary and mandibular bones.
- To evaluate the medial–lateral extent of pathology, i.e. cysts, tumours, malignancy, osteodystrophies and other anomalies.

Terminology

There is a diversity of terminology used to describe the various types of occlusal projections, which reflects the beam angulation or the anatomical region in which the tube is positioned.

In this section alternative, but synonymous, nomenclature appears in parentheses to ensure a common understanding amongst the wider readership of this text.

Recommended projections

The occlusal projections that are necessary for full examination of the dental arches can be seen in the diagram. These are presented as true and oblique projections.

Radiological considerations

The clinician should ensure that their request for certain occlusal projections (i.e. true occlusal) should indicate the tooth over which the beam is centred.

Occlusal radiography – The family tree
(Italics designate a soft tissue exposure)

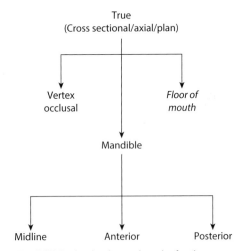
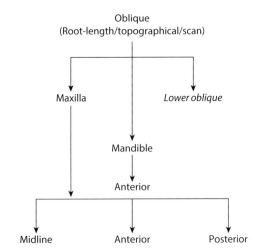

Fig. 9.25 Occlusal radiography – the family tree

Occlusal radiography 9

Vertex occlusal of the maxilla

This projection demonstrates a 'plan' view of the maxillary teeth and is used to demonstrate the bucco-palatal relationship of unerupted teeth in the maxilla (Fig. 9.26a).

The conventional radiographic examination requires the use of an intraoral cassette with rare-earth intensifying screens to reduce dose to the patient. The loaded cassette, prelabeled with a lead letter to designate side, is placed inside a small plastic disposable bag to prevent saliva contamination. Statutory requirements require the use of a lead apron for this projection. (See section on Radiation Protection.)

Position of patient and image receptor

- The patient should be seated comfortably with the head supported with the median plane vertical and occlusal plane horizontal.
- The occlusal cassette is positioned with its long axis antero-posteriorly (i.e. parallel to the median plane) within the oral cavity.
- The cassette should be placed flat in the patient's mouth adjacent to the occlusal surface of the lower teeth.
- Position the cassette as far posteriorly as possible, at least to the level of the 1st permanent molars.
- The patient should bite together gently to stabilise the cassette intraorally.

Direction and location of the X-ray beam

- The tube is positioned over the vertex of the skull and the central ray is directed along the median plane downward (caudal) through the long axis of the upper central incisor teeth (Figs 9.26b, 9.26c).

Notes

- It is important to remember that the beam is NOT at right-angles to the occlusal plane.
- The phosphor plate digital system provides an appropriate size sensor with which to undertake occlusal examinations.
- At the time of writing, occlusal size DDR detectors such as CCD/CMOS systems are not available for this examination.

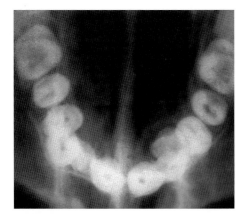

Fig. 9.26a A vertex occlusal radiograph.

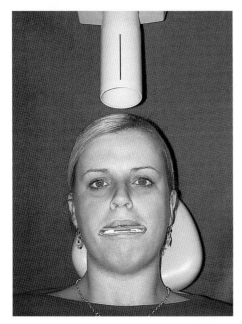

Fig. 9.26b Positioning of the patient and the X-ray tube for a vertex occlusal.

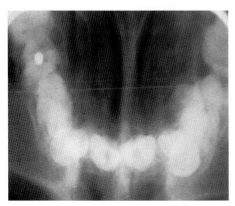

Fig. 9.26c A vertex occlusal radiograph showing buccally positioned left canine and palatally positioned left 2nd premolar.

9 Occlusal radiography

True occlusal of the mandible

(Synonyms: submental occlusal; lower true occlusal; occlusal plan view of the lower jaw; cross sectional mandibular occlusal projection)

Midline

This projection shows a 'plan' view of the mandible with the teeth and the lingual and buccal cortices seen in cross section (Fig. 9.27a).

Position of patient and image receptor

- The image receptor should be placed as far posteriorly in the mouth as the patient will tolerate with the image receptor resting on the occlusal surfaces of the lower teeth. The tube side of the image receptor faces the floor of the mouth with the long axis of image receptor extending across the oral cavity (i.e. perpendicular to the sagittal plane).
- The anterior leading edge of the image receptor should extend 1 cm beyond the labial aspects of the mandible incisor teeth.
- The patient is instructed to extend their head backwards so that the ala–tragus line is almost perpendicular to the floor. The head is then adequately supported in this position.
- The patient should bite together gently to avoid pressure marks on the image receptor.

Direction and location of the X-ray beam

- The tube is placed well down below the patient's chin and directed vertically at 90° to the occlusal plane and the image receptor (Fig. 9.27b).
- Centre the tube in the midline at 90° to an imaginary line joining the 1st permanent molars (i.e. approximately 3 cm distal to the midline of the chin).

Anterior

- This projection is designed to image the anterior regions of the mandible (Fig. 9.27c).
- The only modification to the technique described for the midline true occlusal is that the tube is centered on the symphysis menti, with the beam positioned so that the central ray passes through the root canals of the lower central incisors.

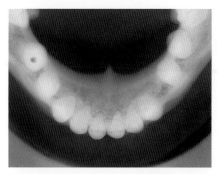

Fig. 9.27a A true occlusal radiograph of the mandible.

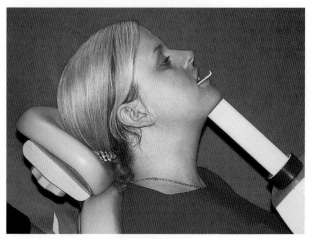

Fig. 9.27b Positioning of the patient and the X-ray tube for a true occlusal radiograph of the mandible.

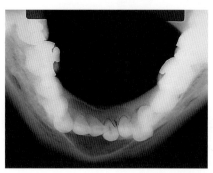

Fig. 9.27c A true occlusal radiograph of the mandible showing a cystic lesion in the anterior region of the jaw.

Occlusal radiography 9

True occlusal of the mandible (cont.)

Posterior

If pathology is related only to one side of the mandible, the posterior view is used (Figs 9.28a, 9.28b). To achieve this projection, some modifications of the technique outlined for the midline true occlusal are needed.

These modifications are as follows:

- The image receptor is positioned with its long axis anteroposterior (i.e. parallel with the sagittal plane) on the side of interest.
- The lateral aspect of the image receptor extends approximately 1 cm buccally to the dental arch but remains parallel to the buccal surfaces of the posterior teeth.
- The tube is centred below the body of the mandible on the side of interest (approximately 3 cm distal to the antero-lateral aspect of the chin) at 90° to the image receptor.

Digital sensors are available for this radiographic examination. However, the receptor must be protected by a sealed barrier technique.

Floor of mouth

This projection is performed to image radio-opaque calculi in the anterior aspect of the floor of the mouth and to identify effectively fragments of fractured tooth and radio-opaque foreign bodies embedded within the lower lip (Fig. 9.28c). Positioning of the patient, along with the image receptor and tube placement are identical to those previously described for the midline true occlusal. Exposure is reduced by a factor of approximately 50% to that used to produce an image of the teeth and mandible.

Radiological considerations

More than 1/3 of submandibular calculi (35%) are found at the hilum of the gland. Whilst the true occlusal of the mandible (see previous section) adequately images the anterior aspects of the submandibular duct, the posterior portion is obscured by the image of the lingual cortex of the mandible. The posterior oblique occlusal (see later) overcomes the problem.

Notes

Other radiographic projections are available to image calculi in this region, they include: (i) true lateral with floor of mouth depressed and (ii) panoramic view.

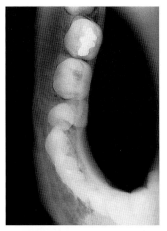

Fig. 9.28a Posterior true occlusal radiograph of right mandible.

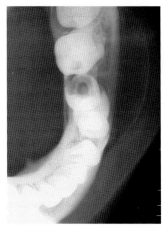

Fig. 9.28b Posterior true occlusal radiograph of the left mandible. A cystic lesion is apparent in the premolar region.

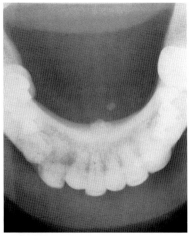

Fig. 9.28c True occlusal showing a discrete salivary calculus in the midline, adjacent to the left submandibular duct orifice.

9 Occlusal radiography

Oblique occlusal of the maxilla

Midline occlusal

(Synonyms: upper standard occlusal, standard occlusal, 70° maxillary occlusal)

The projection is used to show the anterior maxilla (Fig. 9.29a).

Position of patient and image receptor

- The patient should be seated comfortably with the head supported and the median plane vertical and occlusal plane horizontal.
- An occlusal image receptor is placed flat in the patient's mouth, resting on the occlusal surfaces of the lower teeth, with the tube side of the image receptor facing the vault of the palate.
- The convention for positioning the image receptor in the mouth is:
  - Adults: long axis of image receptor extending across the oral cavity (i.e. perpendicular to the sagittal plane).
  - Children: long axis of image receptor positioned antero-posteriorly in the oral cavity (i.e. parallel to the sagittal plane). NB: in younger children with small mouths, a periapical image receptor can be effectively substituted.
- The anterior leading edge of the image receptor should extend 1 cm beyond the labial aspects of the maxillary incisor teeth.
- The image receptor should be placed as far back as the patient will tolerate.
- Patient should bite together gently to avoid pressure marks on the image receptor.

Direction and location of the X-ray beam

- The tube is positioned above the patient in the midline and angled downwards (caudal) at 65–70°, the central ray passing through the bridge of the nose towards the centre of the image receptor (Fig. 9.29b).

Modifications of the technique

Using a soft-tissue exposure, this projection is effective in identifying fragments of tooth and/or radio-opaque foreign bodies within the upper lip following trauma (Fig. 9.29c).

Another useful projection to identify radio-opaque structures embedded within the lips is the **true lateral** (Fig. 9.29d). The patient holds the occlusal image receptor parallel to the sagittal plane using the thumb to support the lower edge and the fingers to stabilise the image receptor against the cheek. This projection is taken using soft-tissue settings. Unless the object is confirmed clinically to be solitary and situated in the midline, the true lateral must be supplemented by other projections (i.e. at right-angles to it) to enable accurate localisation.

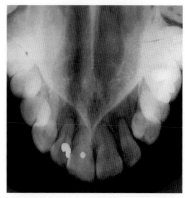

Fig. 9.29a Upper standard oblique occlusal radiograph.

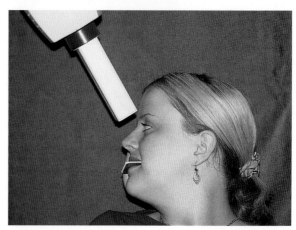

Fig. 9.29b Positioning of the patient and the X-ray tube (from the side) for an upper standard oblique occlusal radiograph.

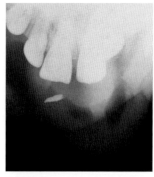

Fig. 9.29c Upper standard oblique occlusal radiograph (with soft-tissue exposure) showing fractured tooth fragment localised to soft tissues of upper lip.

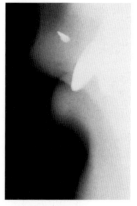

Fig. 9.29d True lateral projection of the case illustrated above. Embedded tooth fragment is clearly seen.

Anterior oblique occlusal

This projection is used to image the anterior region of maxilla and is used commonly combined with a periapical image receptor of this region to assist in localisation of supernumerary teeth, unerupted canines, etc. (Fig. 9.30a).

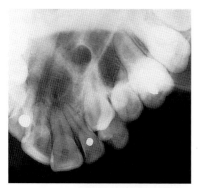

Fig. 9.30a Anterior oblique occlusal of the left maxilla showing an unerupted left canine.

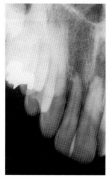

Fig. 9.30b Anterior oblique occlusal of the right maxilla. The region has sustained trauma. The upper right central and lateral incisors are partially extruded.

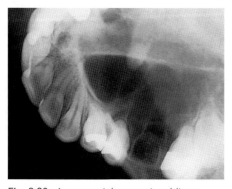

Fig. 9.30c An upper right posterior oblique occlusal. During the extraction of the 1st permanent molar, the palatal root has been displaced into the maxillary antrum. It is clearly seen overlying the floor of the nasal fossa.

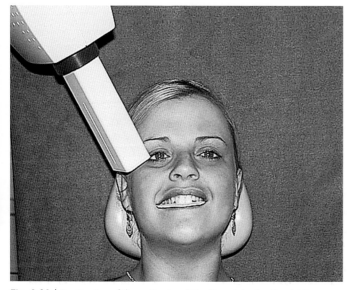

Fig. 9.30d Positioning of the patient and the X-ray tube for the right upper posterior oblique occlusal.

Occlusal radiography 9

Oblique occlusal of the maxilla (cont.)

Position of patient and image receptor

Positioning is identical to the midline occlusal except image receptor coverage is restricted to anterior region of interest.

Direction and location of the X-ray beam

The X-ray tube is centred over the lateral/canine region with downward (caudal) angulation of 60° (Figs 9.30a, 9.30b).

Posterior oblique occlusal

(Synonyms: upper oblique occlusal, oblique maxillary occlusal, oblique occlusal of the upper jaw, lateral maxillary occlusal projection)

This projection demonstrates the posterior quadrant of the maxillary arch, the teeth, the alveolar bone, part of the maxillary antrum, the floor of the antrum and the zygomatic process of the maxilla superimposed over the roots of the molar teeth (Fig. 9.30c).

Position of patient and image receptor

- The patient should be seated comfortably with the head supported and the median plane vertical and occlusal plane horizontal.
- An occlusal image receptor is placed flat in the patient's mouth on the side of interest.
- The image receptor lies on the occlusal surfaces of the lower teeth, with the tube side of the image receptor facing the vault of the palate. The convention for positioning the image receptor is that the long axis of the image receptor lies anteroposteriorly in the oral cavity (i.e. parallel to the median plane).
- The edge of the image receptor adjacent to the cheek should extend 1 cm lateral to the buccal surfaces of the posterior teeth to be imaged.
- The image receptor should be positioned as far back as the patient will tolerate.
- The patient should bite together gently to avoid pressure marks on the image receptor.

Direction and location of the X-ray beam

- The X-ray tube is positioned towards the side of the face where pathology is suspected and angled downwards (caudal) at 65–70° through the cheek (Fig. 9.30d).
- The centring point is medial to the outer canthus of the eye but level with the pupil. It is important to ensure that the central ray is at right-angles to the dental arch.

Notes

It is important not to position the tube more laterally than the centring point outlined above or the body of the zygoma will obscure important detail in the area of interest.

9 Occlusal radiography

Oblique occlusal of the mandible

Anterior oblique occlusal

(Synonyms: lower anterior occlusal, lower midline oblique occlusal, oblique mandibular occlusal, anterior mandibular occlusal projection)

This projection shows the anterior teeth and the inferior cortical border (Figs 9.31a, 9.31c).

Position of patient and image receptor

- The patient should be seated comfortably with the head supported and the median plane vertical.
- An occlusal image receptor is placed flat in the patient's mouth, resting on the occlusal surfaces of the lower teeth. The image receptor should be placed with the tube side of the image receptor facing the floor of the mouth.
- The long axis of image receptor is positioned so that it extends across the oral cavity (i.e. perpendicular to the sagittal plane).
- The anterior leading edge of the image receptor should extend 1 cm beyond the labial aspects of the mandibular incisor teeth.
- The patient should bite together gently to avoid pressure marks on the image receptor.
- The patient is instructed to extend their head backwards so that the occlusal plane is 35° to the horizontal. This allows the tube to be more easily positioned adjacent to the chin. The head is adequately supported in this position.

Direction and location of the X-ray beam

The X-ray tube is positioned in the midline achieving an upward angle of 10° (i.e. overall upward angulation of 45°) to the plane of the image receptor, centring through the midpoint of the chin (Fig. 9.31b).

Radiological considerations

More than 1/3 of submandibular calculi (35%) are found at the hilum. Whilst the true occlusal of the mandible (see previous section) adequately images the anterior aspects of the submandibular duct, the posterior portion is obscured by the image of the lingual cortex of the mandible.

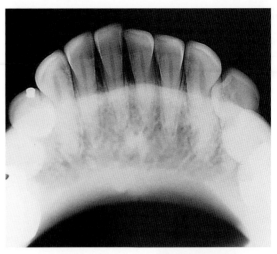

Fig. 9.31a Anterior oblique occlusal image of the mandible.

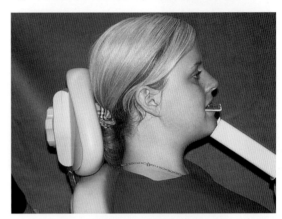

Fig. 9.31b Positioning of the patient and the X-ray tube for an anterior oblique occlusal of the mandible.

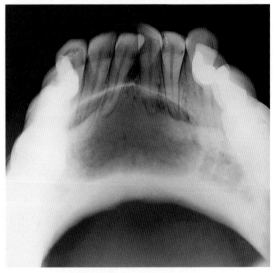

Fig. 9.31c An anterior oblique occlusal image showing a large unilocular radiolucency in the midline region.

Lower oblique occlusal

(Synonym: oblique occlusal)

This projection demonstrates the soft tissues of the middle and posterior aspects of the floor of the mouth (Fig. 9.32a).

Position of patient and image receptor

- The patient should be seated comfortably with the head supported and the median plane vertical and occlusal plane horizontal.
- An occlusal image receptor is placed flat in the patient's mouth on the side of interest.
- The image receptor lies on the occlusal surfaces of the lower teeth, with the tube side of the image receptor facing the floor of the mouth. The convention for positioning the image receptor is that the long axis of image receptor lies antero-posteriorly in oral cavity (i.e. parallel with the sagittal plane).
- The edge of the image receptor adjacent to the cheek should extend 1 cm lateral to the buccal surfaces of the posterior teeth to be imaged.
- The image receptor must be positioned as far back as the patient will tolerate and the patient should bite together gently to avoid pressure marks on the image receptor.
- The operator then supports the patient's head and rotates it away from the side of interest and simultaneously elevates the chin.
- This rotation and elevation allows the X-ray tube to be positioned below the angle of the mandible.

Direction and location of the X-ray beam

- The X-ray tube is positioned 2 cm below and behind the angle of the mandible.

Occlusal radiography 9

Oblique occlusal of the mandible (cont.)

- The centring point is the angle of the mandible with an upward angle (cranial) to the plane of the image receptor of 115° (Fig. 9.32b).
- It is important to ensure that the beam is parallel to the lingual plate of the mandible.

Alternative technique

- Elderly or short-necked patients can be difficult to image with this technique but an effective modification has been devised (Fig. 9.32c).
- The patient is seated adjacent to a flat surface (i.e. table or work surface). With the image receptor positioned intraorally, the head is tipped over so that the forehead and nose are in contact with the table and the head rotated with the affected side 20° away from the table.
- The X-ray tube is positioned above and behind the patient's shoulder. Use identical centring points as detailed above with the tube position 25° from the vertical.

Modifications of the technique

Using a soft-tissue exposure this projection is employed primarily to detect radio-opaque calculi in the proximal regions of the submandibular duct as it crosses the free edge of the mylohyoid muscle. This modification is also referred to as the posterior oblique occlusal and postero-anterior lower occlusal.

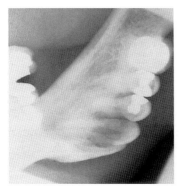

Fig. 9.32a Lower oblique occlusal image of the mandible.

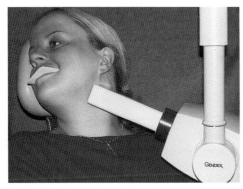

Fig. 9.32b Positioning of the patient and the X-ray tube for a lower oblique occlusal of the mandible.

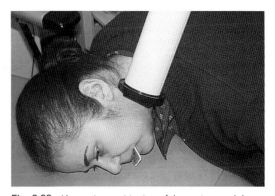

Fig. 9.32c Alternative positioning of the patient and the X-ray tube for a lower oblique occlusal of the mandible.

9 Lateral oblique of the mandible and maxilla

The lateral oblique radiograph is an extraoral projection produced using conventional intraoral X-ray equipment that reveals a larger area of the jaws than intraoral radiography. It can also be produced using a skull unit or conventional radiography equipment. Despite the growth of panoramic radiography, lateral oblique radiography remains a valid technique.

Although intraoral radiography remains the obvious imaging modality for the majority of dental patients, there will be a relatively small number of dental/oral conditions that because of their size and/or location cannot be imaged adequately using intraoral techniques. These are outlined as follows:

- Assessment of the presence/absence of teeth and also the position of unerupted teeth (especially 3rd molars).
- Detection and assessment of fractures of the mandible.
- Assessment of large pathological lesions (i.e. cysts, tumours, osteodystrophies, etc).
- When intraoral radiography is impossible (i.e. trismus, severe gagging).
- Patients with physical and/or medical conditions in which large coverage and a rapid imaging technique is needed.

As a variety of different lateral oblique projections are carried out, the exact positioning of each of these projections depends on the area or region of the jaws under examination. This section will confine itself to describing the two most commonly requested lateral oblique projections:

- A lateral oblique projection imaging the body of the mandible and the maxilla.
- A lateral oblique projection imaging the ascending ramus of the mandible.

Radiographers requiring a fuller description of the range of oblique lateral projections should refer to the specialist textbooks on dental radiography listed at the end of this chapter.

General imaging principles

- The head is rotated to ensure that the area under examination is parallel to the image receptor.
- The image receptor and the median plane are not parallel.
- To avoid superimposition of the opposite side of the jaws, the combined angulation of the angle between the median plane and the image receptor plus the angulation of the X-ray beam must not be less than 20°.
- The central ray is perpendicular to the image receptor but oblique to the median plane.

Lateral oblique of the body of the mandible and maxilla

This projection shows the dentition in the premolar/molar region of the maxilla and mandible, the inferior cortex of the mandible and the angle and ascending ramus of the mandible (see Fig. 9.33c).

Position of patient and image receptor

- The patient should be seated comfortably with the head supported and the median plane vertical.
- A 13 cm × 18 cm cassette is used with removable image receptor marker attached to designate the side of the mandible to be imaged.
- The cassette is positioned against the patient's cheek overlying the region of the mandible under investigation, with the lower border parallel to the inferior border of the mandible but lying at least 2 cm below it.
- The positioning achieves a 10° angle of separation between the median sagittal plane and the image receptor.
- The patient is instructed to stabilise the cassette in this position.
- The patient's head is then rotated to the side of interest. This positions the contralateral ascending ramus forwards and increases the area between the neck and the shoulder to provide space for the X-ray tube.
- The chin is raised slightly to increase the space between the posterior aspect of the mandible and the cervical spine.
- The patient is asked to protrude the mandible.

Direction and location of the X-ray beam

- Direct the central ray at a point 2 cm below and behind the angle of the contralateral side of the mandible (see Fig. 9.33b).
- Positioning of the X-ray tube is dependent upon the area of clinical interest (see Fig. 9.33a), which can be:
  - 3rd molar region for assessment of the position of 3rd molars and possible pathology in this region.
  - Premolar region for assessment of the developing dentition.
  - Lower canine region if there is evidence of mandibular fracture (see section on modification of the projection).
- The choice of beam angulation varies between 10° upward and 10° downward (see section on modification of the projection).
- The central ray is perpendicular to the plane of the image receptor.

Lateral oblique of the mandible and maxilla 9

Lateral oblique of the body of the mandible and maxilla (*cont.*)

Modification of the projection

- The choice of a downward beam angulation is related to the (clinical) need to avoid superimposition of the hyoid bone on the body of the mandible.
- To image the maxillary and mandibular canine/incisor region requires further rotation of the head to a point where the patient's nose is flattened against the cassette.
- It is important to ensure that the area of interest is parallel to the image receptor. This technique reduces the angle of separation between the median sagittal plane and the image receptor to 5°.

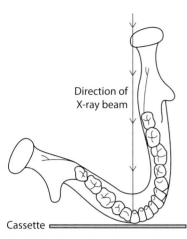

Fig. 9.33a Schematic to illustrate the direction of the beam for a lateral oblique radiograph of the body of the mandible and maxilla.

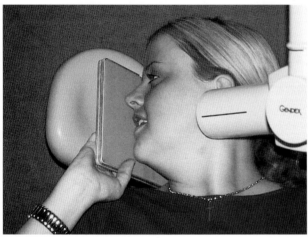

Fig. 9.33b Cassette and the X-ray tube positions for a right lateral oblique radiograph of the body of the mandible and maxilla. Note the rotation of the head with flattening of the nose against the cassette.

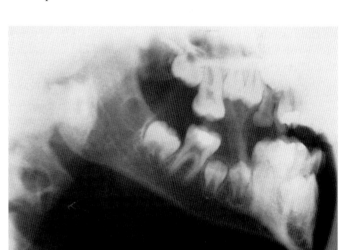

Fig. 9.33c Lateral oblique radiograph of the body of the mandible and maxilla of a child in the mixed dentition.

9 Lateral oblique of the mandible and maxilla

Lateral oblique of the ramus of the mandible

This projection gives an image of the ramus from the angle of the mandible to the condyle (Figs 9.34a, 9.34b).

Position of patient and image receptor

- The patient should be seated comfortably with the head supported and the median plane vertical.
- A 13 cm × 18 cm cassette is used with removable image receptor marker attached to designate the side of the mandible to be imaged.
- The cassette is positioned against the patient's cheek overlying the ascending ramus and the posterior aspect of the condyle of the mandible under investigation.
- The cassette is positioned so that its lower border is parallel with the inferior border of the mandible but lies at least 2 cm below it.
- The positioning achieves a 10° angle of separation between the median sagittal plane and the image receptor.
- The patient is instructed to support the cassette in this position.
- The mandible is extended as far as possible.
- Limit rotation of the head (approximately 10°) towards the cassette.

Direction and location of the X-ray beam

- The central ray is directed posteriorly with upward angulation (cranial) of 10° towards the centre of the ramus of the mandible on the side of interest.
- The centering position of the X-ray tube is the contralateral side of the mandible at a point 2 cm below the inferior border in the region of the 1st/2nd permanent molar (Fig. 9.34c).

Notes

- Some operators prefer a slight (10°) downward (caudal) angulation of the tube to prevent the image of the hyoid bone being superimposed on the body of the mandible.

Essential image characteristics

- No removable metallic foreign bodies.
- No motion artifacts.
- No antero-posterior positioning errors.
- No evidence of excessive elongation.
- No evidence of incorrect horizontal angulation.

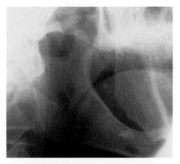

Fig. 9.34a Lateral oblique radiograph of the ramus of the mandible.

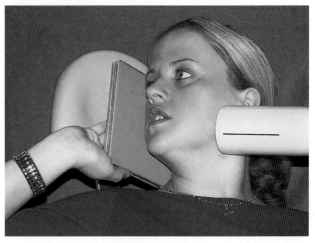

Fig. 9.34b Cassette and the X-ray tube positions for a right lateral oblique radiograph of the ramus of the mandible.

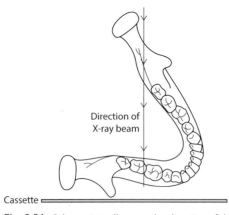

Fig. 9.34c Schematic to illustrate the direction of the beam for a lateral oblique radiograph of the ramus of the mandible.

- Minimal superimposition of the hyoid bone on the region of (clinical) interest.
- There should be good density and adequate contrast between the enamel and the dentine.
- No pressure marks on image receptor, no emulsion scratches.
- No roller marks (automatic processing only).
- No evidence of image receptor fog.
- No chemical streaks/splashes/contamination.
- No evidence of inadequate fixation/washing.
- Name/date/left or right marker all legible.

Modification of the projection – with the patient supine

In a general department, the most convenient method of achieving the lateral oblique view is with the patient supine on the X-ray couch.

Position of patient and image receptor

- Use a 10° foam wedge-shaped pad to achieve separation of one side of the mandible from the other.

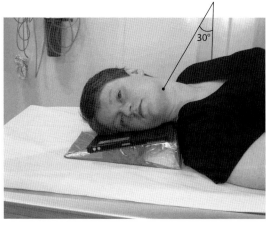

Fig. 9.35a Patient lying supine on the X-ray couch and positioned for a right lateral oblique.

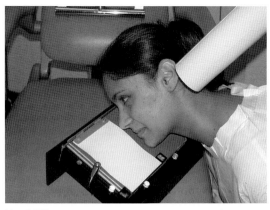

Fig. 9.35b Patient positioned on an angle board for a right lateral oblique.

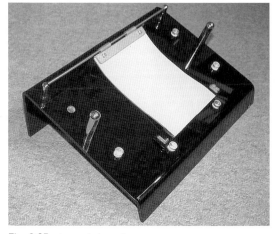

Fig. 9.35c An angle board.

Lateral oblique of the mandible and maxilla

Lateral oblique of the ramus of the mandible (cont.)

- Attach a removable image receptor marker to the cassette to designate the side of the mandible to be imaged.
- With the cassette on the pad, the patient's head is rotated so the side of the jaw to be examined is parallel to the image receptor with the median sagittal plane parallel to the cassette.
- The head is tilted back on the spine to achieve further extension of the contralateral mandible away from the region of interest.

Direction and location of the X-ray beam

- Centre 5 cm below the angle of the mandible remote from the image receptor with the X-ray tube angled 10° to the head (cranial) (Fig. 9.35a).

Modification of the projection using an angle board

An angle board is a device incorporating an incline to help separate the sides of the mandible (Fig. 9.35c).

Position of patient and image receptor

- The head is positioned parallel to the angle board and cassette but with the sagittal plane inclined to the vertical by the degree of angulation set by the device.
- Some angle boards incorporate ear-rods to ensure accurate localisation of the patient.
- A small forward tilt of the chin avoids superimposition of the cervical vertebrae on the ramus.

Direction and location of the X-ray beam

- The X-ray tube is positioned below the angle of the mandible remote from the image receptor and the central ray is directed towards the vertex.
- To avoid superimposition of the opposite side of the face, there must be an effective separation of 20° (Fig. 9.35b).
- For example with a sagittal plane angled at 15° by the angle board, the central ray must be angled 5° to the vertex to achieve the required separation of 20°.

Bimolar projection

This technique is used in orthodontic practice. It shows both left and right oblique lateral views on one image receptor. The technique incorporates a hinged lead shield to prevent exposure of the other side of the image receptor.

9 Dental panoramic tomography

(Synonyms: rotational panoramic radiography, orthopantomography [OPG], dental panoramic tomography [DPT], panoral)

Dental panoramic radiography is an extraoral radiographic technique that produces an image of both jaws and their respective dentitions on a single image receptor, either using conventional film screen technology or a direct digital detector (DDR) (Fig. 9.36a).

Panoramic radiography has supplanted lateral oblique radiography in that it is most useful in those patients who require an imaging modality providing a wide coverage of the jaws, such as:

- Orthodontic assessment of the presence/absence of teeth.
- The detection and assessment of fractures of the mandible.
- An assessment of large pathological lesions (i.e. cysts, tumours, osteodystrophies, etc).
- When intraoral radiography is impossible (i.e. trismus, severe gagging).
- An assessment of 3rd molars prior to surgical removal.

Principles of panoramic image formation (Fig. 9.36b)

Panoramic equipment is based upon a simultaneous rotational movement of the tubehead and image receptor cassette/carriage in equal but opposite directions around the patient's head, which remains stationary. The technique employs a slit collimated vertical X-ray beam, with an 8° upward inclination, in association with a similar collimation slit in front of the image receptor cassette/carriage to receive the image.

Improvements in image production have centred upon refining the rotational movement and determining the 'correct' form of the image layer. Obviously, manufacturers vary in the methods employed to produce the panoramic image. However, irrespective of the type of rotational movement involved, the result is the production of an elliptical image layer with 3D form (i.e. height and width) in the shape of the dental arch. This image layer is referred to as the focal trough.

Within the different types of panoramic equipment, there are noticeable variations in the width of this image layer. This variability is much more apparent in equipment employing a continuous moving rotational centre, resulting in a narrow anterior layer compared to the lateral aspects of the focal trough.

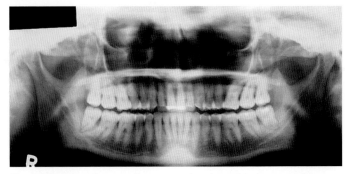

Fig. 9.36a A dental panoramic tomography of an adult dentate patient.

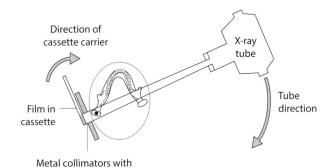

Fig. 9.36b The schematic illustrates the relative positions and movement of the X-ray tubehead, cassette carrier and film during three stages of the exposure cycle of a continuous mode panoramic unit. The stages shown are: A, start of the exposure; B, intermediate stage of panoramic exposure; C, end of exposure. Throughout the exposure, a different part of the receptor is exposed as illustrated.

Dental panoramic tomography 9

Image acquisition considerations

There are a number of factors inherent to panoramic radiography that reduce the diagnostic quality of the final image. These factors are:

- Magnification variation.
- Tomographic blur.
- The overlap of adjacent teeth.
- The superimposition of soft tissue and secondary shadows.
- The limitations of resolution imposed by the image receptor, exposure parameters and processing conditions.

Magnification variation

While all types of radiographic projections exhibit a degree of magnification, the type associated with panoramic radiography is more complex. The individualised movement patterns, variations in the width of the beam, differing focus/object/image receptor relationships and the chosen position/shape of the image layer chosen by the manufacturer can produce variations in magnification of 10–30% between units.

Horizontal and vertical magnifications are only equal for structures at the centre of the focal plane. The degree of horizontal magnification in panoramic images varies considerably depending upon the relationship of the structure to the image layer. Objects lying closer to the X-ray source (i.e. situated inside the focal trough; Fig. 9.37a) will display a greater degree of horizontal magnification. This situation is reversed for objects lying closer to the cassette (i.e. placed outside the focal trough) as they will be imaged with a relatively diminished horizontal magnification whilst the vertical shape remains virtually the same. This variability in horizontal shape is apparent by examining the appearance of anatomical structures within the focal trough (tongue, hyoid bone) and those outside it (zygomatic arch).

Minor inaccuracies in the antero-posterior positioning of the patient can easily lead to discrepancies between the vertical and horizontal magnification of teeth, with consequent distortions of tooth shape. These errors are most marked in the anterior region of the jaws where the focal plane is narrower (Fig. 9.37b).

Correct patient positioning is therefore essential for good image production. To achieve this, panoramic equipment employs various positioning aids to assist the operator. These include a system of light alignment beams to position the patient correctly along with combinations of some or all of the following: a chin rest, a biteblock and two or more head supports (Fig. 9.37c).

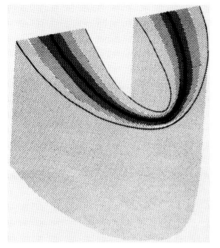

Fig. 9.37a The focal trough.

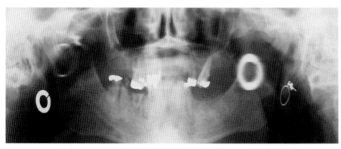

Fig. 9.37b Patient position to close to the receptor with very obvious reduction in the width of the anterior teeth. The patient is also wearing earrings (of different design) and their ghost shadow appears at a higher level on the contralateral side of the image.

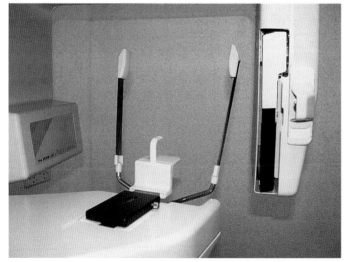

Fig. 9.37c Patient-positioning devices on the Planmeca PM2002 panoramic unit: bite-peg, chin and temporal supports.

9 Dental panoramic tomography

Image acquisition considerations (*cont.*)

Tomographic blur

Panoramic radiography is known as a modified form of tomography but only when tomography is described in the most general terms as a 'layer-forming imaging system'. The majority of panoramic systems have only one predesignated rotational movement, resulting in one fixed form of image layer. The parameters of that image layer have been chosen to enable radiography of the 'average' jaw. Therefore, accurate patient positioning is always necessary to accommodate consistently the tooth-bearing regions of the maxilla and diagnostic quality. If a patient presents with a gross skeletal abnormality of one jaw relative to another, two panoramic image receptors may be required. If there are gross discrepancies within a single jaw, the limitation of the imaging modality is obvious and has to be accepted (Fig. 9.38a).

The overlap of adjacent teeth

Although different movement patterns of the beam are adopted in different units, the aim of the manufacturer is to produce a beam of radiation that is perpendicular to the average arch. The maximum deviation from the ideal orthoradial (i.e. 90°) projection occurs in the canine/premolar region, resulting in a variable amount of overlap of contact points, reducing caries diagnosis in these areas (Fig. 9.38b).

The superimposition of soft tissue and secondary shadows (Figs 9.38c–9.38e)

Panoramic images are further degraded, to a variable degree, by shadows of soft tissues and surrounding air. Whilst many of these shadows are on the periphery of the image, the presence of air between the dorsum of the tongue and the hard palate leads to a band of relative overexposure of the roots of the maxillary teeth and associated alveolar bone. Elimination of this shadow is easily accomplished by positioning the tongue against the palate during radiography.

Secondary images of the spine and mandible further reduce diagnostic quality. In some panoramic equipment, compensation is made for the density of the cervical spine by stepping up the kV or mA as the anterior structures are imaged. Whilst this technique is successful, it cannot compensate for incorrect positioning of the patient that can result in the spine being imaged as a dense radio-opacity in the midline of the image. The same principles apply to the secondary imaging of the mandible, with these images becoming apparent and intrusive when careful patient positioning is not achieved.

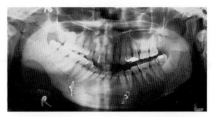

Fig. 9.38a Patient suffers from hemifacial hypoplasia affecting the right side of the face. This has resulted in a marked reduction in the size of the bones on this side, affecting correct positioning the patient in the focal trough.

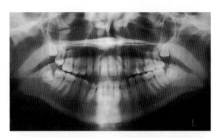

Fig. 9.38b The problems of overlap in the premolar/molar region.

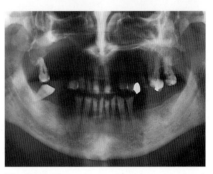

Fig. 9.38c The presence of air between the dorsum of the tongue and the hard palate. This produces a band of relative overexposure of the roots of the maxillary teeth and the alveolar bone.

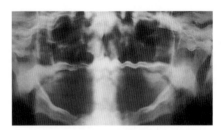

Fig. 9.38d Incorrect positioning of the patient resulting in the presence of the dense radio-opacity of the spine in the midline of the panoramic image. The patient has moved throughout the exposure in a vertical direction. This is evidenced by the undulating outline of the lower border of the mandible and that of the hard and soft palate.

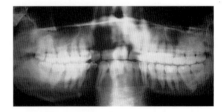

Fig. 9.38e Patient positioned too far from the film resulting in the horizontal magnification of the anterior teeth and also blurring of the teeth. Incorrect positioning has also resulted in the production of secondary images of the mandible. These are seen as dense radio-opacities overlying the posterior maxillary and mandibular teeth.

Limitations of resolution imposed by the image receptor, exposure parameters and processing conditions

- There is an inevitable reduction in resolution when using screen film as the image receptor. In addition, the exposure factors and processing conditions profoundly influence the perception of detail.
- The quality of the panoramic image is heavily dependent upon careful attention to technique and processing. Failure to observe these principles have been reported in a study that found 1/3 of all panoramic images were diagnostically unacceptable.

Dose reduction in panoramic radiography

Newer panoramic equipment incorporates improved methods of X-ray generation, such as direct current generators. It also employs field limitation that enables the operator to image selected areas of interest, thereby reducing dose to the patient. Further dose reduction is achieved by the provision of a variable mA and kV facility, allowing the equipment to be used with faster image receptor/screen combinations. The adoption of digital sensors has now become commonplace as the method of acquiring the panoramic image.

Recent advances in panoramic imaging

Newer panoramic equipment, combined with linear tomography, offers greater versatility for the clinician than conventional equipment. Most manufacturers provide field size limitation as standard (Fig. 9.39). The programmes provided by the

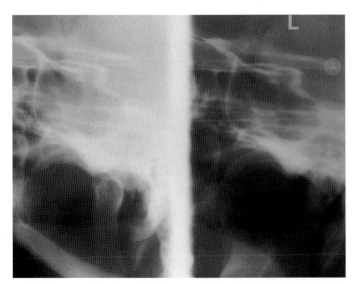

Fig. 9.39 Sectional image of the left temporomandibular joint region

Dental panoramic tomography 9

Image acquisition considerations (cont.)

manufacturer may include some or all of the following: the jaws, the maxillary sinuses, a temporo-mandibular joint (TMJ) programme, a child programme. A wide range of projections can be achieved that include; frontal and lateral images of the TMJ, tomographic images of the paranasal sinuses, as well as cross sectional images of the maxilla and mandible using pre-programmed detector movements.

Most equipment has a facility for a cephalometric attachment and also a facility for an automated exposure control (AEC). Newer panoramic units are supported by digital technology and include an optional cephalometric facility that allows standardised skull projections to be obtained. This type of newer equipment has the ability to adjust to the wide range of the size of patients who require panoramic imaging.

Reported benefits of digital panoramic radiography

- Digital technology reduces clinical time as the resultant image is not reliant on chemical processing.
- Shadows of the spinal column can be reduced by modulation of the kV.
- All images are of consistently high quality that are produced rapidly.
- The equipment provides a wide range of imaging programmes that can optimise patient dose. These include:
  - A facility for AEC.
  - Frontal and lateral images of the TMJ.
  - Tomographic views of the paranasal sinuses.
  - Cross sectional imaging of designated areas of the maxilla and mandible.
  - Facility for a cephalometric device.
  - Easily achieved post processing.
  - The technique removes the need for chemical processing thereby eliminating the need for chemicals that are toxic.
  - Both digital panoramic and cephalometric images can be acquired.
  - The equipment provides a 3D stitching programme.
  - The panoramic computer-controlled multimodality equipment facilitates the speed and the movement of the tube head and the image receptor.

9 Dental panoramic tomography

Image acquisition considerations (*cont.*)

Patient preparation

- If the patient is wearing a bulky coat, it should be taken off as it can interfere with the rotational movement of the panoramic equipment.
- The patient should remove all radio-opaque objects from the head and neck areas. These include spectacles, metallic hair clips at the neckline on the back or side of head, hearing aids, earrings, tongue-studs, nose jewellery and necklaces (Fig. 9.40a). This instruction also includes intraoral devices such as complete/partial dentures and removable orthodontic appliances. High-necked sweaters with metal zippers/fasteners should also be removed. Chewing gum appears as a radio-opaque mass on the image and should be disposed of prior to imaging.
- If the patient is unable to remove their earrings from the lobule of the ear, the lobule and attached earring should be folded inwardly on the antitragus and taped to the helix/antihelix of the external ear. The use of this technique ensures that the ghost images of the earrings will not appear on the final image.

General comments

- The unit should be readied in the start position and raised sufficiently to allow the patient to walk into the equipment.
- Depending on the type of equipment used, the examination can be carried out with the patient either standing or seated.
- Careful explanation of the procedure must be given to the patient as the exposure times vary from 12 seconds for newer equipment and up to 20 seconds for older panoramic units.
- In view of the exposure time involved, this technique should not be used to image the following patients:
  - Children unable to remain motionless for the duration of the 10–20 second exposure.
  - Patients suffering from medical conditions resulting in uncontrollable involuntary movement and lack of coordination.

Position of patient and image receptor

- If used a 15 cm × 30 cm cassette should be inserted in the cassette carrier, otherwise the digital unit is placed in the start position (Fig. 9.40b).
- Position a biteblock on the machine (or chin rest if this is all that is available).
- Ask the patient to walk straight into the machine, gripping the handles if available, and ask them to adopt the 'ski position'. Often patients are afraid of the equipment and hence only tentatively enter with their neck 'craning' forward.

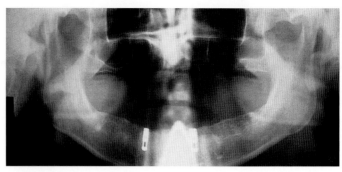

Fig. 9.40a Ghost shadow of radio-opaque necklace obscuring the mandible.

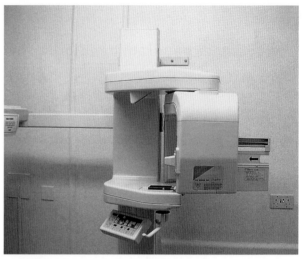

Fig. 9.40b Panoramic unit in start position.

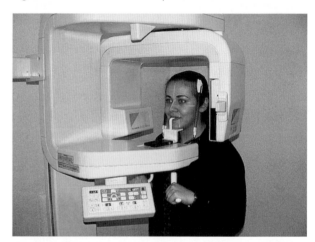

Fig. 9.40c Patient positioned in Planmeca PM2002. The biteblock, chin rest and temporal supports and the light beam marker lines ensure correct positioning.

- The patient's head should be tilted down towards the floor so that the Frankfort plane is parallel to floor. In this position ala–tragus line is 5° caudal.
- Turn on positioning lights (Fig. 9.40c):
  - Sagittal plane light should be down the middle of the face.
  - Frankfort plane should be 5° down from ala–tragus line.
  - Antero-posterior light should be centred distal to the upper lateral incisor (i.e. the lateral/canine interproximal space).

- Adjust the height of the machine to the patient, not vice versa.
- Ask the patient to bite into the biteblock groove. Check that the upper and lower incisors are both in the groove. In patients with a prominent mandible relative to the maxilla (i.e. Class III patients), at least ensure that the upper incisors are in the groove.
- Position the patient chin on the chin rest. If the chin is not on the support, or if the cassette is too far below the mandible, adjust to prevent the image being positioned too high with consequent loss of the upper portion of the image.
- Stand behind the patient and check the symmetry of position; adjust if needed by holding shoulders.
- Close head restraints.
- Make any fine adjustments at this point.
- Ask the patient to close their lips and press their tongue to the roof of their mouth. The latter instruction is particularly important as if it is not done a dark radiolucent shadow of the air space above the tongue will obscure the apices of the maxillary teeth. Closing the lips around the biteblock reduces the air shadow that can be mistaken for caries where it overlies the dentition in the premolar region.
- Explain again that he/she must stay absolutely still for about 20 seconds.
- Make the exposure.

Dental panoramic tomography 9

Image acquisition considerations (*cont.*)

Essential image characteristics (Fig. 9.41)

- Edge to edge incisors.
- No removable metallic foreign bodies.
- No motion artefacts.
- The tongue should be against the roof of the mouth.
- Minimisation of spine shadow.
- No antero-posterior positioning errors.
- No mid sagittal plane positioning errors.
- No occlusal plane positioning errors.
- Correct positioning of spinal column.
- There should be good density and adequate contrast between the enamel and the dentine.
- Conventional image acquisition benefits from the use of a wide latitude image film.
- Name/date/left/right markers are legible.

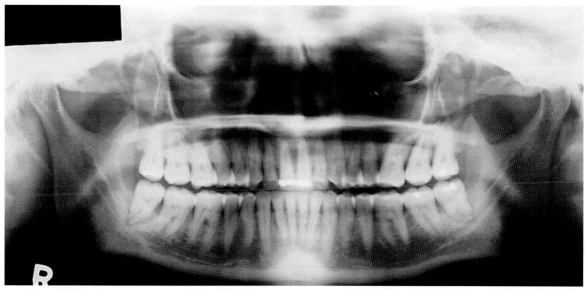

Fig. 9.41 A dental panoramic tomograph of an adult dentate patient.

9 Dental panoramic tomography

Problems with panoramic radiography (Figs 9.42a, 9.42b)

The technique is plagued with problems relating to positioning errors. The more common positioning errors and those related to movement are outlined in Table 9.3 below.

Table 9.3 Common panoramic image receptor faults and how to correct them

Panoramic Image Receptor Fault	Appearance of Fault	Remedy
Anterior teeth positioning errors: a) Head too far forward i.e. dental arch positioned anterior to focal trough	Narrow unsharp image of anterior teeth present. Spine overlaps the rami.	Ensure occlusal plane slightly tilted downward and teeth biting in grooves on bite-block as outlined in the procedures for this examination.
b) Head too far back i.e. dental arch positioned posterior to focal trough).	Wide unsharp image of anterior teeth present. TMJ region not evident.	
Mid saggital plane positioning errors Head off-centre. Tilting of the head.	Mid-saggital plane off centre, rami and posterior teeth unequally magnified.	Ensure correct saggital position of the patient.
b) Twisted position of patient.	Side tilted towards x-ray tube enlarged, side closer towards the image receptor looks smaller.	
Occlusal plane positioning errors: a) Excessive downward angulation	Severe curvature of the occlusal plane. Lack of definition of the lower incisors	Ensure correct position of the occlusal plane
b) Upward over-angulation	Flattening of occlusal plane, superimposition of apices of maxillary teeth on hard palate	Ensure correct position of the occlusal plane
Spinal column positioning error	Underexposed region in the midline of the image due to excessive attenuation of energy of beam by the spinal column	Ensure patients adopt 'ski position'. Operator must correct position, before exposure, if patient position is 'slumped' forward
Patient's shoulder interfering with movement of cassette	Slows cassette and resulting in dark band, due to prolonged exposure, in region where obstructed occurred.	Patient usually has short neck. Elevate chin until ala-tragus line parallel to floor. Positioning cassette 1cm higher may also help.

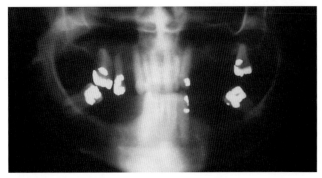

Fig. 9.42a Panoramic radiograph with the patient's chin too far down.

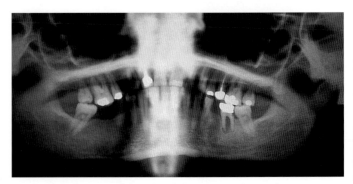

Fig. 9.42b Panoramic radiograph with the patient's chin too far up.

Cephalometry 9

Cephalometric radiography ensures standardisation and reproducibility of the images taken. Lateral and postero-anterior projections are used as part of the initial evaluation of patients who are being considered for orthodontic treatment and/or orthognathic surgery. The technique is also use in the assessment of dento-facial abnormalities (Figs 9.43b, 9.43c).

X-ray equipment features (Fig. 9.43a)

The equipment can be 'stand-alone' (i.e. existing X-equipment employed with a separate cephalostat). More commonly, the equipment is an integral component of a panoramic unit. The cephalostat (or craniostat) provides the mechanism by which the projection is standardised. It consists of two Perspex arms with attached ear pieces/rods to position the patient accurately within the unit.

The stand-alone equipment uses a fixed FRD of 200 cm, whilst that employed in combined panoramic/cephalometric equipment is less (150 cm). Whichever method is used, the longer FRD ensures that the beam is parallel thereby minimising magnification in the image. It is important that the X-ray equipment employed has sufficient output to produce a final image exhibiting adequate penetration.

A filter attenuates the beam in the anterior regions so that the soft tissues of the face can also be demonstrated on a single image receptor. Prepatient image enhancement is obtained when the filter is attached to the tube head covering the anterior part of the emerging beam. Postpatient image enhancement can be achieved by placing a filter between the patient and the anterior part of the cassette. The former technique is preferable, as, in this position, the filter leaves no line of demarcation on the image receptor and also provides dose reduction. A beam collimator must be incorporated at the tube head to limit the beam to those areas containing the main cephalometric points. Unfortunately, the method of manufacture of the newer cephalometric units precludes adoption of this technique as the tube head is covered by the outer casing of the X-ray unit.

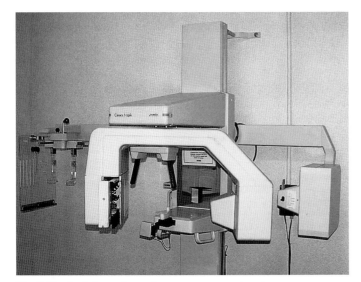

Fig. 9.43a Cephalometric attachment to a panoramic unit.

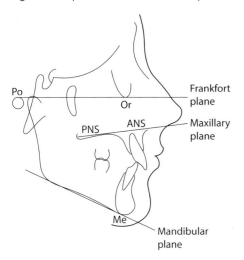

Fig. 9.43b A diagram showing the main cephalometric planes.

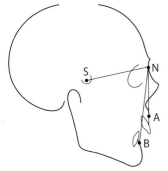

Fig. 9.43c A diagram illustrating the SNA and SNB lines. SNA: relates the antero-posterior (AP) position of the maxilla, represented by the A point, to the cranial base; SNB: relates the AP position of the mandible, represented by the B point, to the cranial base.

357

9 Cephalometry

Lateral projection

The projection is a standardised true lateral projection of the skull (Figs 9.44a, 9.44d).

Position of patient and image receptor

- The patient sits or stands inside the cephalometric unit with the sagittal plane vertical and parallel to the cassette.
- The Frankfort plane should be horizontal.
- The head is immobilised by guiding the earpieces carefully into the external auditory meati (EAMs). Metal circular markers within the earpieces allow the operator to recognise 'off-centring' of the cephalostat (Figs 9.44b, 9.44c).
- The nose support is positioned against the nasion.
- A wedge-shaped filter is positioned so that it will be superimposed on the face with its thick edge placed anteriorly.
- The patient is instructed to close the mouth and to bite together on their back teeth (i.e. in centric occlusion). Some children find this difficult to do so it is worth checking prior to exposing the radiograph.
- The lips should be relaxed.

Direction and location of the X-ray beam

- The direction and centring of the x-ray beam will normally be fixed and the horizontal beam is centred on the EAMs (Fig. 9.44d).

Essential image characteristics

- No removable metallic foreign bodies.
- No distortion due to movement.
- Frankfort plane perpendicular to image receptor.
- No sagittal plane positioning errors.
- No occlusal plane positioning errors.
- Teeth in centric occlusion.
- Lips relaxed.
- Name/date/left or right marker all legible.

Radiological considerations

The use of beam collimation has dramatically reduced the dose to patients whilst adequately imaging the patient without loss of that information which is necessary for orthodontic or orthognathic diagnosis. The edge collimation limits the dose to the superior aspects of the calvarium above the orbits and to the lower aspects of the cervical spine. Unfortunately, when using modern panoramic equipment, it is impossible with some models to access the tube head to add the additional wedge collimation.

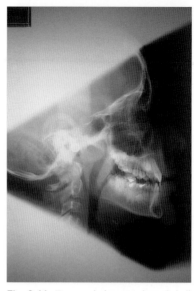

Fig. 9.44a True cephalometric lateral skull radiograph. Images of metal ear rods are superimposed over one another and image displays optimal collimation.

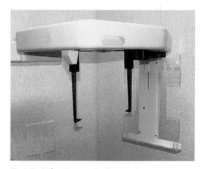

Fig. 9.44b The cephalostat.

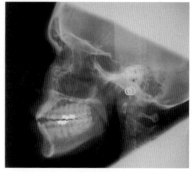

Fig. 9.44c True cephalometric lateral skull radiograph with images of metal ear rods separated indicating 'off centring'.

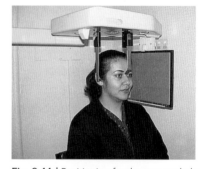

Fig. 9.44d Positioning for the true cephalometric lateral skull radiograph.

Cephalometry 9

Postero-anterior projection

Most cephalometric equipment has the facility to allow this projection to be taken. It is an important view in assessing patients with facial asymmetry (Figs 9.45a, 9.45b).

Position of patient and image receptor

- The equipment is rotated through 90°.
- The patient is set up as for posterior-anterior (PA) projection of the mandible.
- The orbitomeatal base line is parallel to floor.
- The head is immobilised using earpieces inserted into the EAMs.

Direction and location of the X-ray beam

- The horizontal X-ray beam is fixed.
- The central beam is centred through the cervical spine at the level of the rami.

Essential image characteristics

- No removable metallic foreign bodies.
- No distortion due to movement.
- Median sagittal plane and radiographic baseline are at right-angles to the image receptor.
- No sagittal plane positioning errors.
- No radiographic baseline positioning errors.
- Teeth in centric occlusion.
- Lips relaxed.
- Name/date/left or right marker all legible.

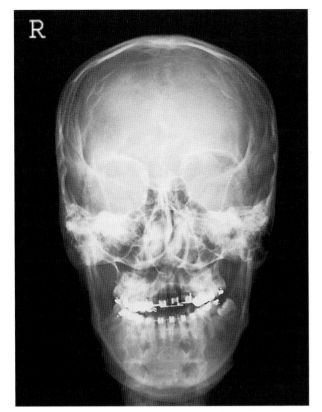

Fig 9.45a A cephalometric postero-anterior skull.

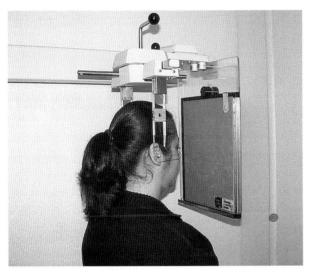

Fig. 9.45b Positioning for the cephalometric postero-anterior skull projection.

9 Cone beam computed tomography

(Synonyms: dental volumetric tomography; dental computed tomography; cone beam volumetric tomography; cone beam imaging.

Cone beam computed tomography (CBCT) has been in existence in medical radiography for the last 20 years and in the last decade has become an accepted and proven radiographic technique in clinical dentistry. The technique differs from conventional intraoral and extraoral radiography as it provides the clinician with a 3D dataset and the possibility of multiplanar reformatting.

The imaging technique uses a rotating gantry comprising an X-ray source at one end and an image detector at the other. Both the X-ray source and the detector rotate about the area of interest under consideration within the dento-maxillofacial region of the jaws. The acquisition of the image requires the collection of multiple 2D 'basis' images that are subsequently reformatted by a Feldkamp back-projection algorithm. Between around 150 and 600 basis images are acquired, varying according to the manufacturer. CBCT scanners employ a well-collimated cone-shaped X-ray beam and the image data are acquired by a 2D detector. The type of detector employed may differ amongst manufacturers; however, in most cases this is an amorphous silicon flat panel. A few manufacturers use an image intensifier/CCD detector, but this is likely to be superseded in the future. CBCT equipment also varies in that patients may be standing, seated or supine. The chairs may have a weight limit and this must be considered when imaging patients. There are head immobilisation devices to ensure correct positioning and stabilisation of the patient's head during imaging. In recent years, there has been an increasing manufacture of integrated panoramic/cephalometric/CBCT machines; these 'hybrid' units may be more cost-effective for hospital departments and dental practices.

The 3D dataset in CBCT is almost always cylindrical, with a defined height and diameter, and CBCT equipment may be classified by the field-of-view (FoV) capabilities. Some equipment designs have a single, fixed, FoV, while others have several FoV options. The largest FoVs may cover the whole head, or at least the facial bones. The smallest FoVs are appropriate for imaging single teeth or small regions of the jaws and may be as small as 4 cm height × 4 cm diameter. Particularly with these small FoVs, scout views (lateral and antero-posterior [AP]) are taken on the machine as a preliminary stage of CBCT imaging.

On average, radiation dose increases with larger FoV selection, so it is important to use the smallest FoV consistent with the diagnostic task.

Voxels on CBCT are isotropic and may be as small as <0.1 mm, giving the possibility of very fine detail. Soft-tissue contrast is extremely limited, however, so dental CBCT should be seen as a hard tissue imaging modality only. Image resolution often defaults to lower resolution with larger FoVs on equipment with options of FoV.

Image display is usually provided as four windows on the monitor: axial, coronal, sagittal and a 'volume-rendered' or 'pseudo-3D' image, with mouse-driven navigation through the dataset. Secondary multiplanar reconstruction (MPR) is almost always used to produce ideally-orientated images. The most commonly used MPR technique is to produce panoramic sections, analogous to panoramic radiographs, with cross-sectional images perpendicular to this for dental implant planning purposes. It is unacceptable, however, to perform a CBCT examination purely for the purpose of making a panoramic radiographic image, as this would be at a higher radiation dose than achievable with panoramic X-ray equipment.

Advantages

- 3D dental imaging.
- High-resolution capabilities.
- Lower radiation dose than conventional multislice CT.
- Rapid scan times.
- Dimensionally accurate, allowing measurements to be used for dental implant planning.

Disadvantages

- Very limited soft-tissue contrast, meaning that it can only be used for hard-tissue imaging.
- Inflexible FoV options on some systems.
- Metal-related artefact from dental restorations may obscure areas of interest.

Clinical concerns

Concerns have been raised as this type of radiographic equipment has been found to be used inappropriately in some clinical situations as a replacement for conventional dental imaging, rather than as a supplement for selected cases. A recent systematic review of the literature on CBCT has reviewed all the relevant publications in the field of CBCT and has produced guidelines on the use of CBCT in clinical practice.

Cone beam computed tomography 9

Imaging procedure (Figs 9.46a–9.46c)

The imaging procedure is very much equipment dependent and will be subject to the type of equipment selected. Whilst there are similarities in the positioning technique associated with hybrid units as described for panoramic tomography, users are directed to the manufacturer's literature for detailed use of equipment.

Image analysis

From the acquired volume image set various 3D modelling software tools are available to provide a comprehensive visualisation of the jaw anatomy on a supporting workstation. With the aid of multi-planar reconstruction, images can readily be viewed in the orthogonal and oblique planes including volume rendering of the face and jaw. With the application of appropriate software, cephalometric analysis is undertaken as well as precise dental implant planning, i.e. accurate bone depth, width and density and the location of anatomical structures such as nerve canals and sinuses. The following pages illustrates the capabilities of the equipment.

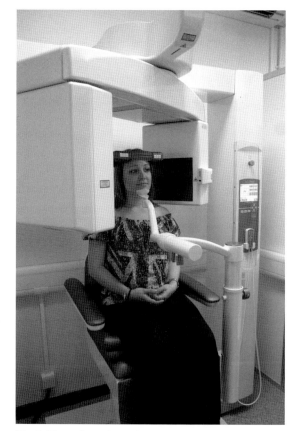

Fig. 9.46a Dedicated cone beam computed tomography (CBCT) equipment.

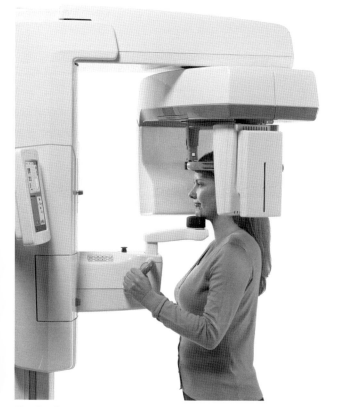

Fig. 9.46b Hybrid OPG/ CBCT equipment.

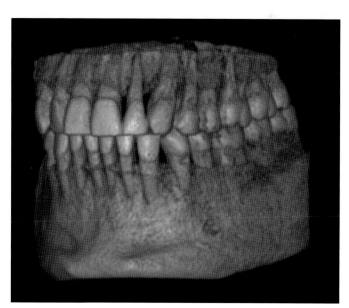

Fig. 9.46c Volume-rendered image from a OPG/CBCT unit.

9 Cone beam computed tomography

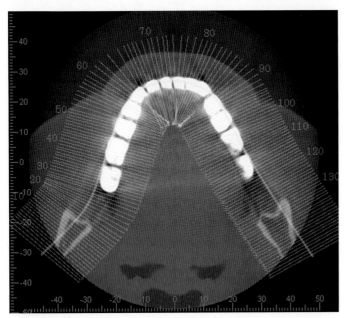

Fig. 9.47a Typical cross-sectional axial image of the lower jaw. A line has been positioned along the line of the dental arch, as represented by a radio-opaque radiographic guide. Multiple lines are automatically produced perpendicular to this at preset intervals, to produce cross-sectional images.

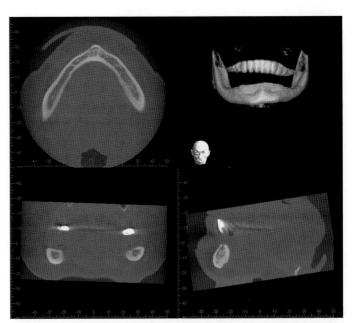

Fig. 9.47b Typical image set of an edentulous patient showing three orthogonal planes including a volume-rendered image of the upper and lower jaw. A radio-opaque radiographic guide is in the patient's mouth to aid the dentist to relate the images to the clinical situation.

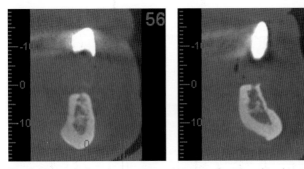

Fig. 9.47c Examples of cross-sectional images of proposed implant sites.

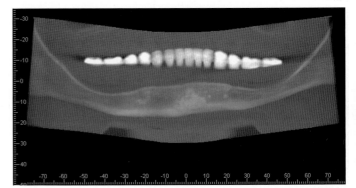

Fig. 9.47d Panoramic image reformatted from the CBCT dataset.

Cone beam computed tomography 9

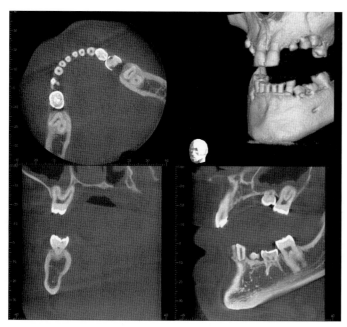
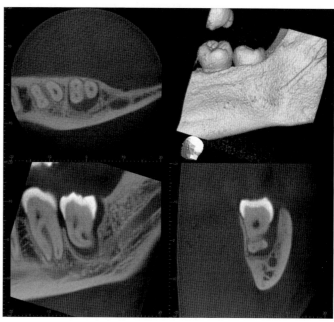

Fig. 9.48a and 48b Example of image sets demonstrating the difference in appearance of a large field of view (FoV) (left image) and the application of a smaller FoV (right image). The image on the left is of a patient with retained deciduous teeth due to hypodontia of the permanent teeth.

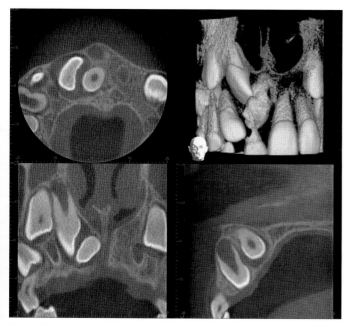

Fig. 9.48c Image set showing unerupted and supernumerary teeth.

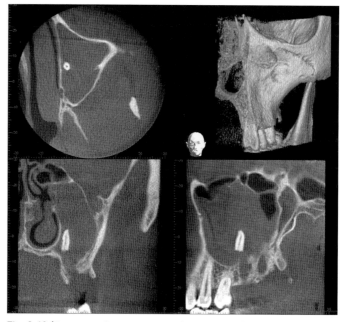

Fig. 9.48d Image set showing a retained root in the left maxillary antrum, displaced during attempted extraction.

9 Cone beam computed tomography

Acknowledgements

The author is indebted to Dr. Michael Rushton, PhD BDS for the diagrams and photography that accompany the text.

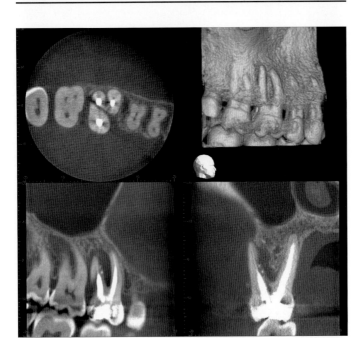

Fig. 9.49 Image set showing a fractured 1st maxillary molar.

Section 10

Abdomen and Pelvic Cavity

CONTENTS

INTRODUCTION	366	AP cross-kidney (upper abdomen)	377
Planes and regions	366	Right posterior oblique	378
Most common referral criteria	368	Left posterior oblique	378
Typical imaging protocols	368		
Recommended projections	368	URINARY BLADDER	379
Image parameters	369	Antero-posterior 15° caudal	379
Radiological considerations	370	Right or left posterior oblique	379
ABDOMEN AND PELVIC CAVITY	372	BILIARY SYSTEM	380
Antero-posterior – supine	372	Left anterior oblique	380
Antero-posterior – erect (standing or sitting)	374	Right posterior oblique	381
Antero-posterior – left lateral decubitus	375	ABDOMEN AND PELVIC CAVITY	382
Lateral – dorsal decubitus (supine)	375	Image evaluation – 10-point plan	382
URINARY TRACT – KIDNEYS–URETERS–BLADDER	376		
Antero-posterior	376		
Urinary tract	377		

10 Introduction

This section deals only with plain radiography of the abdomen and pelvic contents; examinations including the introduction of contrast media will be in the companion volume *Clark's Procedures in Diagnostic Imaging*.

Planes and regions (Figs 10.1a, 10.1b)

The abdominal cavity extends from the inferior surface of the diaphragm to the pelvic inlet inferiorly and is contained by the muscles of the abdominal walls.

To mark the surface anatomy of the viscera, the abdomen is divided into nine regions by two transverse planes and two parasagittal (or vertical) planes.

The upper transverse plane, called the transpyloric plane, is midway between the suprasternal notch and the symphysis pubis – approximately midway between the upper border of the xiphisternum and the umbilicus. Posteriorly it passes through the body of the 1st lumbar vertebra near its lower border and anteriorly passes through the tips of the right and left 9th costal cartilages; also in most cases the plane also cuts through the level of the pylorus of the stomach.

The lower transverse plane, called the transtubercular plane is at the level of the tubercles of the iliac crest anteriorly and near the upper border of the 5th lumbar vertebra posteriorly.

The two parasagittal planes are at right-angles to the two transverse planes. They run vertically passing through a point midway between the anterior superior iliac spine and the symphysis pubis on each side, in the mid-clavicular line.

These planes divide the abdomen into nine regions centrally from above to below epigastric, umbilical and hypogastric regions and laterally from above to below right and left hypochondriac, lumbar and iliac regions.

The pelvic cavity is continuous with the abdominal cavity at the pelvic inlet, extends inferiorly to the muscles of the pelvic floor and is contained within the bony pelvis.

Although viscera are said to occupy certain regions of the abdomen, and surface markings can be stated, it must be remembered that surface markings of viscera are variable, particularly those organs that are suspended by a mesentery. The main factors affecting the position and surface markings of organs are: (a) body build, (b) phase of respiration, (c) posture (erect or recumbent), (d) loss of tone of abdominal muscles that may occur with age, (e) change of organ size due to pathology, (f) quantity of contents of hollow viscera, (g) the presence of an abnormal mass and normal variants within the population.[1]

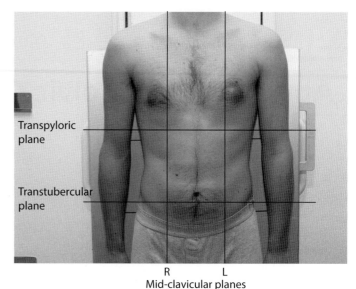

Fig. 10.1a Planes and regions.

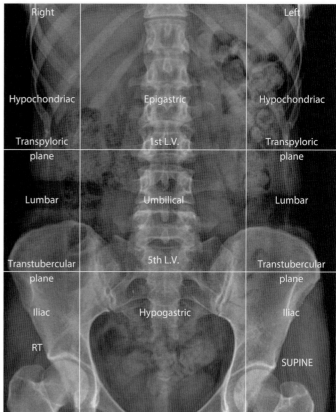

Fig. 10.1b Radiographic image of planes and regions.

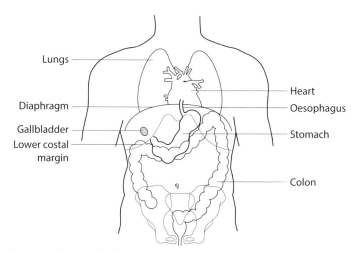

Fig. 10.2a Hypersthenic.

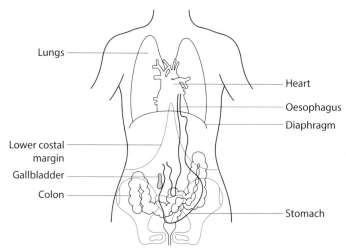

Fig. 10.2b Asthenic.

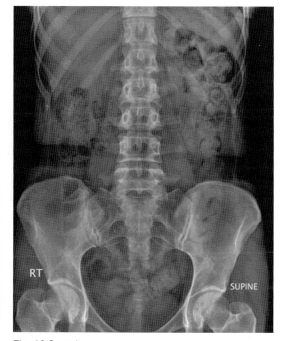

Fig. 10.2c Asthenic.

Introduction 10

Planes and regions (*cont.*) (Figs 10.2a–10.2d)

Individuals have been classified according to body build, into four types – hypersthenic, sthenic, hyposthenic and asthenic. The shape and position of organs tend to follow a particular pattern typifying each type.

Hypersthenic – massively built. The dome of the diaphragm is high and the lower costal margin is at a high level with a wide angle, resulting in the widest part of the abdomen being its upper part. The stomach and transverse colon are in the upper part of the abdomen. The fundus of the gall bladder is pushed upwards so that the gall bladder lies horizontally in the abdomen well away from the midline.

Asthenic – thin and slender. The elongated narrow thorax with a narrow costal angle is associated with a low position of the dome of the diaphragm. The abdominal cavity is shallow being widest in its lowest region. The pylorus of the stomach is low and the long stomach may reach well below the iliac crests, while the transverse colon can loop down into the pelvic cavity. The gall bladder lies vertically close to the midline with the fundus below the level of the iliac crests.

Between these two extremes of body build are the sthenic (tending towards hypersthenic, but not as broad in proportion to height) and the hyposthenic (tending towards asthenic, but bariatric – these are obese patients defined as weighing in excess of 159 kg (25 stone).

Increasingly, radiographers are asked to image morbidly obese patients. The challenges facing radiology departments include difficulties in transporting patients to the department, inability to accommodate large patients on currently designed imaging equipment and difficulties in acquiring desired images of diagnostic quality (see page 494).[1]

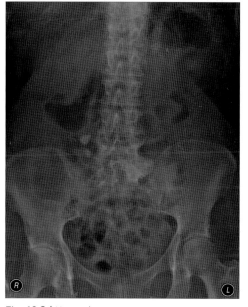

Fig. 10.2d Hypersthenic.

10 Introduction

Most common referral criteria

Radiographic examination of the abdomen and pelvic cavity is performed for a variety of reasons. These include:

- Obstruction of the bowel.
- Perforation.
- Renal pathology.
- Acute abdomen (with no clear clinical diagnosis).
- Foreign body localisation (see also Paediatric Radiography, Section 13, and Miscellaneous, Section 14).
- Toxic mega colon.
- Aortic aneurysm.
- Prior to the introduction of a contrast medium, e.g. intravenous urography (IVU) to demonstrate the presence of radio-opaque renal or gall stones and to assess the adequacy of bowel preparation, if used.
- To detect calcification or abnormal gas collections, e.g. abscess.
- Alimentary studies using barium preparations.

Typical imaging protocols

The following table illustrates projections used to diagnose common clinical conditions (see also iRefer RCR guidelines 2014[2]).

Recommended projections

Examination is performed by means of the following:

Basic	• Antero-superior - supine
Alternative	• Postero –anterior – prone
Supplementary	• Antero-posterior – erect • Antero-posterior or Postero-anterior – left lateral decubitus • Lateral – dorsal decubitus • Posterior obliques

Condition	Supine abdomen	Additional projections
Obstruction	Yes	
Perforation	Yes	• Erect PA or AP chest • AP or PA left lateral decubitus • Lateral dorsal decubitus
Renal pathology	Yes	• Supine on inspiration • Right or left posterior oblique
Acute abdomen	Yes	• Erect PA or AP chest
Foreign body • Swallowed • Inhaled • Penetrating • Other	 Not indicated unless FB is potentially poisonous/sharp No Yes Yes	• Lateral soft-tissue neck • Erect PA or AP chest • Erect PA or AP chest to include soft-tissue neck • Lateral • Lateral rectum or lateral bladder
Toxic megacolon	Yes	• Erect abdomen
Aortic aneurysm	Yes	• Lateral • Erect PA or AP chest

AP, antero-posterior; FB, foreign body; PA, postero-anterior.

Introduction 10

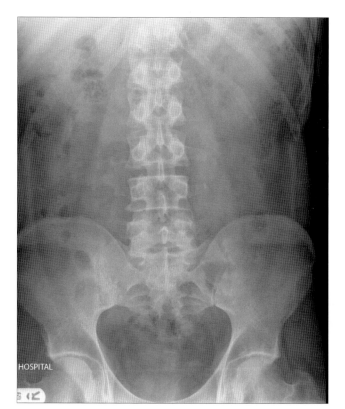

Fig. 10.3a Plain abdomen demonstrating optimal contrast.

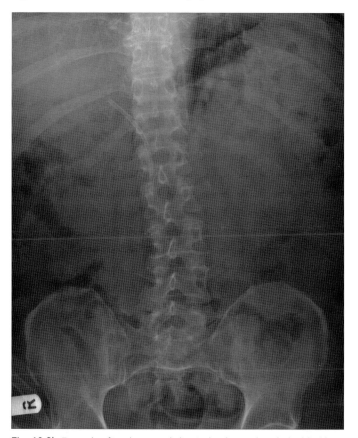

Fig. 10.3b Example of inadequate abdominal radiograph with the bladder region not included.

Image parameters (Figs 10.3a, 10.3b)

Although the radiographic technique used will depend on the condition of the patient, there are a number of requirements common to any plain radiography of the abdomen and pelvic cavity. Maximum image sharpness and contrast must be obtained so that adjacent soft tissues can be differentiated.

Radiography is normally performed using a standard imaging table with a moving grid. However, depending on the condition of the patient imaging may be performed on a trauma trolley with computed radiography (CR) cassettes or a mobile direct digital radiography (DDR) detector using a stationary grid.

The patient should be immobilised and exposure is made on arrested respiration, usually after full expiration.

The following table illustrates the parameters necessary to provide optimum and consistent image resolution and contrast for the antero-posterior (AP) supine abdomen projection with screen/film technology.[3]

Item	Comment
Focal spot size	≤1.3 mm
Total filtration	1.3 mm Al equivalent
Antiscatter grid	R=10; 40/cm
Screen/film combination	Speed class 400
FRD	115 (100–150) cm
Radiographic voltage	75–90 kV
Automatic exposure control	Chamber(s) selected – central or central and right upper lateral
Exposure time	<200 ms

FRD, focus-to-receptor distance.

Note

By choosing all three chambers on the automatic exposure control (AEC) this avoids the risk of underexposure due to the beam passing through regions containing mainly bowel gas.

Essential image characteristics

- Coverage of the whole abdomen to include diaphragm to inferior to the symphysis pubis and lateral properitoneal fat stripe.
- Reproduction of the whole of the urinary tract (kidneys–ureters–bladder [KUB]).
- Demonstration of the kidney outlines.
- High resolution of the bones and the adequate contrast to demonstrate the interface between air-filled bowel and surrounding soft tissues.

Radiation protection

- The exclusion of pregnancy via the 28/10 day rules should be observed unless it has been decided to ignore it in the case of an emergency.
- Gonad shielding can be used for males.

10 Introduction

Radiological considerations

General observations

The abdominal radiograph is a vital first-line investigation in a range of acute abdominal pathologies. Interpretation can be very difficult and is often initially performed by a relatively inexperienced doctor. High-quality imaging is important, but may be difficult to achieve as these patients are often in pain, unable to fully co-operate and may be distended with bowel gas.

Selection of the appropriate strategy for imaging the acute abdomen depends largely upon the clinical indication for the investigation. The following is a discussion of possible indications for this investigation, some of the radiological signs that may be demonstrated, and the role of other modalities.[4]

Renal calculi

Acute renal colic is a severe sharp intermittent pain on one side of the abdomen, often radiating to the groin or testicle. Frequently the patient has some degree of haematuria. Calculi may be visible on plain radiographs, depending on their chemical composition, in up to 90% of cases. Visible calculi appear as foci of increased attenuation, often tiny, and more often oval than round. Some chemical types are relatively low density, and even when calcified are hard to see if very small, especially when obscured by overlying gas, faeces, or bone. Larger calculi appear more round, and very large calculi may assume the shape of the calyceal system (staghorn calculi).[5]

The renal abdomen examination is a single supine abdominal radiograph that must cover from the superior pole of the uppermost (left) kidney to the margin inferior to the symphysis pubis (KUB). On larger patients separate renal and bladder area images may be required. Arrested respiration is vital, as very slight movement unsharpness will obscure small calculi, and larger calculi of lower radio-opacity. The area where calculi are most often overlooked is in the true pelvis overlying the sacrum and sacro-iliac joints, where the background makes it difficult to isolate the radiological appearance of stones.

Computed tomography urography (CTU) (where available) is the most frequent examination to investigate whether an opacity is actually within the urinary tract, or to detect lucent calculi. Otherwise IVU is the examination of choice. The role of ultrasound is very limited as it cannot visualise the ureters. Nuclear medicine can demonstrate the presence and level of ureteric obstruction, but not the cause.

Intestinal obstruction (Fig. 10.4)

Intestinal obstruction may have many causes, but the most common is adhesions due to previous disease or surgery. Tumours (especially in the colon), hernias, and Crohn's disease (especially in the small bowel) are other common causes. The patient may have a previous history, and typically presents with colicky abdominal pain and distension. The bowel sounds on auscultation are said to be high pitched and 'tinkling'.

The supine plain radiograph typically shows abnormally distended bowel loops containing excessive gas. Not infrequently the typical signs are absent, especially if the bowel contains predominantly fluid, and an erect image may then show fluid levels that confirm the diagnosis (in the appropriate clinical setting). Air–fluid levels also occur in a range of conditions, including those not requiring surgery, such as gastroenteritis or jejunal diverticulosis.

Obstruction of the large bowel is differentiated from that of the small bowel mainly by the mucosal patterning of the affected region (houstral folds in the large bowel), physical dimensions and its distribution within the abdomen, thus requiring complete high-detail radiographic coverage of the abdomen.

Gastric outlet obstruction may be seen on supine images (if gas filled) or erect chest or abdomen images if there is more fluid.

CT can demonstrate intestinal obstruction and will often show the cause. Ultrasound can also detect obstruction but less often the cause. Neither is the primary imaging modality.

Fluid collections

Extensive ascites may be seen as a medium opacity band in the paracolic gutters, loss of clarity of the liver edge and medial displacement of the ascending and descending colon or small bowel loops. Ultrasound is far more sensitive and specific and will always be used for diagnosis of this pathology. Loculated fluid collections such as abscess or cyst will have the appearance of a soft-tissue mass, displacing bowel loops. If an abscess contains gas, an air–fluid level may be seen on the erect image. The exact appearance will depend on the location and underlying cause.

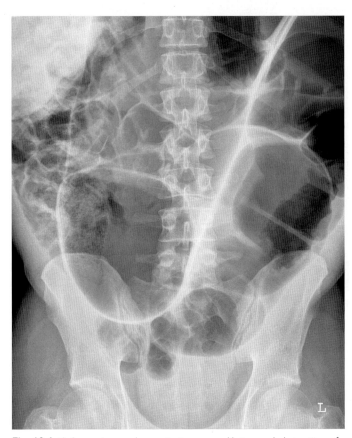

Fig. 10.4 Abdomen image demonstrating gross dilation and obstruction of the large bowel.

Perforation (Fig. 10.5)

Perforation of a hollow abdominal viscus releases free gas into the peritoneal cavity, and this can be sensitively detected by horizontal beam decubitus radiography. As little as 2 ml can be detected.[6]

Common causes are perforated diverticular disease in the large intestine and perforated peptic ulcer. The best investigation is an erect chest radiograph, which will show free gas under one hemi-diaphragm, usually above the liver on the right. If this is not possible, an AP left lateral decubitus projection (right side raised) is a suitable alternative, or a lateral dorsal decubitus (supine) can be obtained. Whichever projection is used, the patient should be left 10 minutes in the intended position to allow the air to rise ensuring no missed diagnosis. The outcome is an image showing a crescent or bubble of gas in the most non-dependent part of the peritoneal cavity.

On supine images free gas may be seen in about 50% of patients by the presence of a double wall sign (coffee bean sign) due to visualisation of the outside of the bowel wall that is not normally seen.

Intraperitoneal air may be demonstrable in over 60% of cases for over 3 weeks after abdominal surgery.

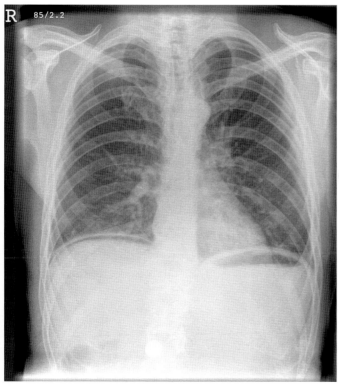

Fig. 10.5 PA chest with air under the right diaphragm, indication of a perforation.

Introduction 10

Radiological considerations (cont.)

Aortic aneurysm

Abdominal aortic aneurysm may be detected by plain radiography, only if there is significant calcification in the wall of the aneurysm. A non-calcified aneurysm may appear as a posterior central soft tissue mass on a lateral projection but is not normally demonstrated on a routine supine abdomen image. A lateral abdominal projection can used to confirm the calcification and the prevertebral location of a mass, but ultrasound will be more useful and diagnostic.

Non-acute aortic aneurysms are normally diagnosed and followed up by ultrasound examinations. In the event of a person presenting with suspected rupture of a previously unknown aneurysm, then urgent surgical treatment is required. The usual procedure would be CT examination en route to theatre. CT is used to determine the extent of the aneurysm and its relationship to the renal arteries, and in some circumstances for assessment of possible rupture.[7]

Retroperitoneal disease

Masses may be seen incidentally on plain images displacing other structures (especially stomach and bowel) or as lack of definition of the psoas muscle outline. Loss of the psoas outline may also occur due to a psoas abscess or haematoma and may also be poorly demonstrated due to spasm caused by renal colic; therefore, this is a suboptimal test for any of these conditions. CT or magnetic resonance imaging (MRI) are the preferred techniques, as ultrasound imaging is too often obscured by bowel gas.

Constipation

This is normally a clinical diagnosis based on frequency and consistency of the stool, change in bowel habit and clinical examination. Radiography should not be requested except to assess secondary obstruction or to determine the residual faecal load (usually in chronic constipation only).[2]

Use in children

As this is a high-dose examination, its use in children should be avoided if possible and an alternative modality, such as ultrasound, used where possible. Radiological indications are discussed in Section 13.

10 Abdomen and pelvic cavity

Antero-posterior – supine (Figs 10.6a, 10.6b)

A table Bucky DDR system is employed or alternatively a 35 × 43 cm CR cassette is selected. In the case of a bariatric patient two exposures in different positions may be necessary to complete the examination.

Position of patient and image receptor

- The patient lies supine on the imaging table with the median sagittal plane at right-angles and coincident with the mid-line of the table.
- The pelvis is adjusted so that the anterior superior iliac spines are equidistant from the tabletop.
- If a CR cassette is selected it is placed longitudinally in the cassette tray (if patient habitus allows) and positioned so that the region below the symphysis pubis is included on the lower margin of the image.
- The centre of the image receptor will be approximately at the level of a point located 1 cm below the line joining the iliac crests. This will ensure that the region inferior to the symphysis pubis is included on the image.

Direction and location of the X-ray beam

- The collimated vertical beam is directed to the centre of the image receptor to include the lateral margins of the abdomen.
- Using a short exposure time, the exposure is made on arrested respiration. Ideally respiration should be arrested on full expiration to allow the abdominal contents to lie in their natural position; however, dependent on the patient's height, respiration may need to be arrested on full inspiration to include the whole abdomen.

Notes

- In the case of a large abdomen/apron an immobilisation/compression band may be applied to reduce patient dose plus the negative effects of scatter upon image quality.
- When using an AEC device, the central and right chambers may be selected simultaneously to avoid the risk of underexposure due to the beam passing through regions containing mainly bowel gas.

Essential image characteristics

- The bowel pattern should be demonstrated with minimal unsharpness.

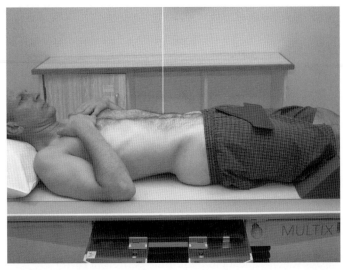

Fig. 10.6a Patient positioning.

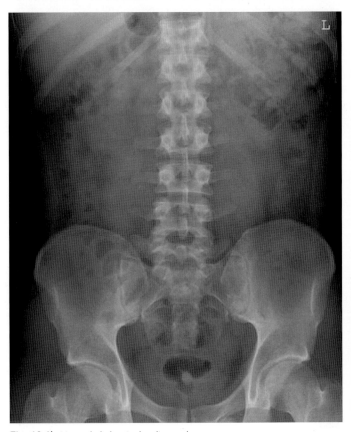

Fig. 10.6b Normal abdominal radiograph.

Abdomen and pelvic cavity 10

Antero-posterior – supine (*cont.*) (Figs 10.7a, 10.7b)

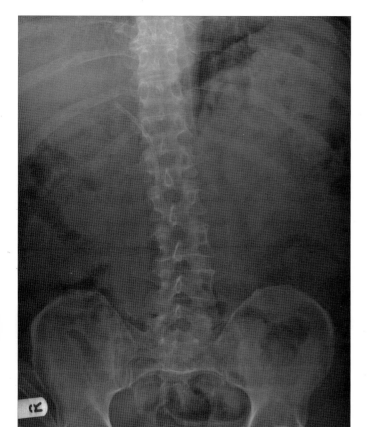

Fig. 10.7a Inadequate/incomplete abdomen radiograph with right ureteric stent lower abdominal margin not visualised.

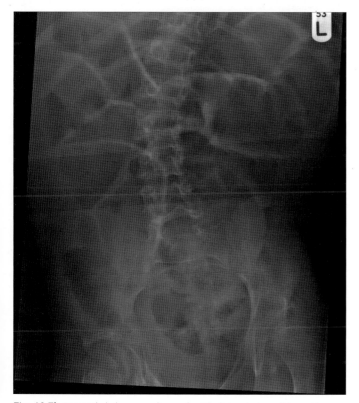

Fig. 10.7b Rotated abdomen radiograph with distended small bowel loops with faecal loading and gas in rectum indicative of small bowel obstruction.

Common faults and solutions

- Failure to include the region inferior to the symphysis pubis and the diaphragm on the same image. This may be due to patient size, in which case two images are acquired, i.e. if using CR the cassettes are placed transversely (landscape) across the abdomen to include upper and lower abdominal regions.
- Failure to visualise the lateral extent of the abdominal cavity including the lateral peritoneal fat stripe may be due to patient size or poor positioning.
- Respiratory movement unsharpness may be reduced by rehearsal of the arrested breathing technique prior to exposure.
- Rotation may be evident when the patient is in pain.
- Underexposure may be caused by patient size or incorrect selection of AECs.
- Presence of artefacts such as buttons or contents of pockets if the patient remains clothed for the examination.

Radiological considerations

- Any cause of movement unsharpness may render small or even medium-sized renal and ureteric calculi invisible.
- Some radiologists state that the erect abdomen is rarely if ever needed to diagnose intestinal obstruction, as subtle signs will nearly always be present on a supine image. In the acute setting however, the erect image can be very valuable to surgical staff who do not have immediate access to an experienced radiologist. In modern practice CT will often be used if obstruction is suspected, and this would render the erect image superfluous.
- Repeated plain abdominal images may be needed to monitor caecal distension in cases of toxic dilatation of the colon. This should be done in close collaboration with the surgical team to ensure adequate patient monitoring while minimising patient radiation dose.
- Perforation of a hollow abdominal viscus requires an erect chest image, or failing that an AP left lateral decubitus image. A supine abdomen image will not usually demonstrate free intraperitoneal air.

Radiation protection/dose

- Strict application of appropriate protocol to determine pregnancy status is imperative in females of child-bearing age.
- For males the correct size of gonad protection should be selected and carefully applied so gonads are shielded and the pelvic region not obscured with lead.

Expected DRL: DAP 2.5 Gy cm^2, ESD 4 mGy.

10 Abdomen and pelvic cavity

Antero-posterior – erect (standing or sitting) (Figs 10.8a–10.8c)

If possible the patient is examined standing or seated against a vertical Bucky, or alternatively may be examined on a tilting table with a C-arm using a large image DDR detector/X-ray tube assembly. If necessary the patient may be examined sitting on a trolley or on a chair using a stationary grid with a 35 × 43 cm CR cassette; however, the resulting image resolution may be compromised.

Position of patient and image receptor

- The patient stands/sits with their back against the receptor/vertical Bucky.
- If standing the patient's legs are placed well apart so that a comfortable and steady position is adopted.
- If seated care must be taken to ensure the flexed knees are not obscuring the lower abdomen.
- The median sagittal plane is adjusted at right-angles and coincident with the midline of the vertical Bucky.
- The pelvis is adjusted so that the anterior superior iliac spines are equidistant from the image receptor.
- The upper edge of the image receptor (DDR detector or 35 × 43 cm CR cassette) is positioned at the level of the middle of the body of the sternum so that the diaphragms are included.
- NB: diverging rays will displace the diaphragms superiorly.

Direction and location of the X-ray beam

- The collimated horizontal beam is directed so that it is coincident with the centre of the receptor in the midline.
- An exposure is taken on normal full expiration.

Position of patient and image receptor (tilting table – postero-anterior)

- This may be undertaken using a tilting table with a C-arm assembly with a large image DDR detector. It is used when undertaking barium examinations of the alimentary tract and other studies requiring an erect image, e.g. IVU to show site of obstruction.
- The patient lies supine on the tilting table with the feet firmly against the step and the detector positioned over the abdomen. The table is slowly moved towards the vertical position until the patient is erect.
- It is not recommended that this procedure should be undertaken if the patient is unwell and unable to stand unaided.
- The upper edge of the image detector is adjusted so that it is at the level of the middle of the body of the sternum in order to include the diaphragms.
- The X-ray tube/C-arm assembly is positioned so that the central ray is horizontal.

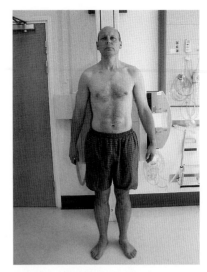

Fig. 10.8a Patient positioning for the vertical Bucky.

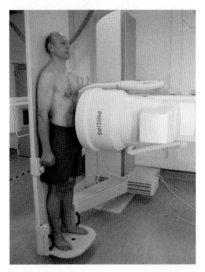

Fig. 10.8b Patient positioning for the C arm system.

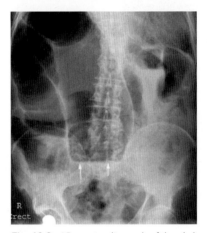

Fig. 10.8c AP erect radiograph of the abdomen showing obstruction and fluid levels (arrows).

- The exposure is made as soon as table movement is stopped. This is preferably when the table is vertical but how near the vertical will depend on the condition of the patient.
- As soon as the exposure has been made, the X-ray tube is moved away and the table moved back into the horizontal position.

Antero-posterior – left lateral decubitus (Figs 10.9a, 10.9b)

This projection is used if the patient cannot be positioned erect to confirm the presence of subdiaphragmatic gas. It should only be undertaken as a specific request when other modalities such as ultrasound/CT cannot be used. It may also be used for confirming a bowel obstruction.

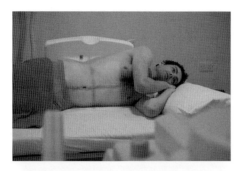

Fig. 10.9a Patient positioning for antero-posterior left lateral decubitus.

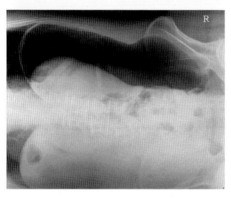

Fig. 10.9b Antero-posterior left lateral decubitus image of the abdomen showing free air in the abdominal cavity.

Abdomen and pelvic cavity 10

With the patient lying on the left side, free gas will rise to be located between the lateral margin of the liver and the right lateral abdominal wall. To allow time for the gas to collect the patient should remain lying on the left side for a short while (e.g. 10 minutes) before the exposure is made.

Position of patient and image receptor

- The patient lies on their left side, on a trolley, with the elbows and arms flexed so that the hands can rest near the patient's head.
- The patient is positioned with the posterior aspect of the trunk against a vertical Bucky DDR system with the upper border of the image receptor high enough to project above the right lateral abdominal and thoracic walls. Alternatively a 35 × 43 cm CR grid cassette is supported vertically against the patients back.
- The patient's position is adjusted to bring the median sagittal plane at right-angles to the image receptor.

Direction and location of X-ray beam

- The collimated horizontal central beam is directed to the anterior aspect of the patient and centred to the centre of the image receptor.

Lateral – dorsal decubitus (supine) (Figs 10.9c, 10.9d)

Occasionally the patient is unable to sit or even be rolled on to their side, thus the patient remains supine and a lateral projection is taken using a horizontal central ray.

Position of patient and image receptor

- The patient lies supine with the arms raised away from the abdomen and thorax.
- A 35 × 43 cm CR grid cassette is supported vertically against the patient's side to include the thorax to the level of mid-sternum and as much of the abdomen as possible. Care should be taken that the anterior wall of the trunk is not projected off the resultant image.
- Alternatively, when using a trolley the patient may be positioned against a vertical Bucky/DDR system utilising the AEC.

Direction and location of the X-ray beam

- The collimated horizontal central beam is directed to the lateral aspect of the trunk at right-angles to the receptor.

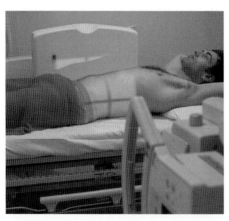

Fig. 10.9c Patient positioning for lateral dorsal decubitus.

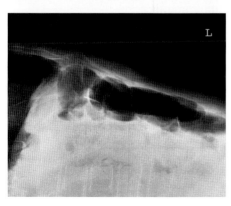

Fig. 10.9d Lateral dorsal decubitus image of the abdomen used to demonstrate free air in a patient who cannot move from supine position.

10 Urinary tract – kidneys–ureters–bladder

Plain radiography of the abdominal and pelvic cavity is undertaken to visualise:

- The outline of the kidneys surrounded by their perirenal fat.
- The lateral border of the psoas muscles.
- Opaque stones in the kidney area, in the line of the ureters and in the region of the bladder.
- Calcifications within the kidney or within the bladder.
- The presence of gas within the urinary tract.
- Any other acute abdominal pathology.

Radiation protection

The 'Pregnancy Rule' should be observed unless permission from the referrer has been given to overrule it in case of emergency. If the whole of the renal tract including bladder is to be visualised then no gonad shielding is applied for females, but for males lead protection can be placed to protect the testes. Other methods previously discussed that reduce radiation dose to the patient should be followed.

Preparation of the patient

The patient should micturate to empty the bladder prior to the examination. If possible, the patient should have a low residue diet during the 48 hours prior to the examination to clear the bowel of gas and faecal matter that might overlie the renal tract. In the case of emergency radiography no bowel preparation is possible. The patient is undressed and wears a gown.

Antero-posterior (Figs 10.10a, 10.10b)

Position of patient and image receptor

- The patient lies supine on the X-ray table with the median sagittal plane of the body at right-angles to and in the midline of the table.
- The patient's hands may be placed high on the chest or the arms may rest by the patient's side slightly away from the trunk.
- The DDR/Bucky detector used should be large enough to cover the region from above the upper poles of the kidneys to the symphysis pubis (or a 35 × 43 cm CR cassette is used).
- The image receptor is positioned so that the symphysis pubis is included on the lower part of the image, bearing in mind the fact that the oblique rays will project the symphysis inferiorly.
- The centre of the image receptor will be approximately at the level of a point located 1 cm below the line joining the iliac crests. This will ensure that the symphysis pubis is included on the image.

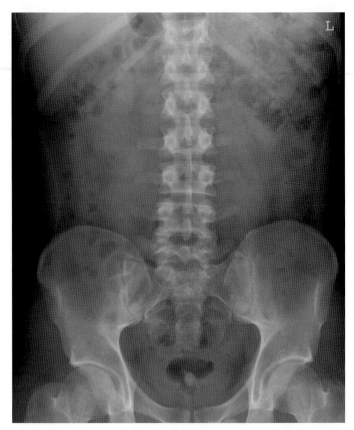

Fig. 10.10a Anterior-posterior KUB abdominal image with adequate demonstration of kidney outline.

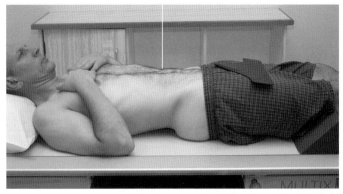

Fig. 10.10b Patient positioning.

Direction and location of the X-ray beam

- The vertical collimated beam is directed to the centre of the image receptor with the lateral margins collimated within the margins of the image receptor.
- The exposure is made on arrested expiration.

Notes

- In some cases it may be necessary to include a collimated kidney area if the superior renal borders are excluded from the full length image.
- For small opacities overlying the kidney, a further image taken on arrested full inspiration will allow differentiation of movement between the opacity and kidney tissue to determine whether it is contained within the kidney.

Urinary tract – kidneys–ureters–bladder 10

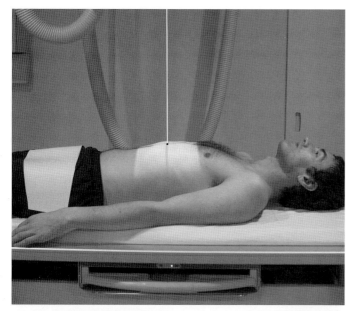

Fig. 10.11a Patient positioning.

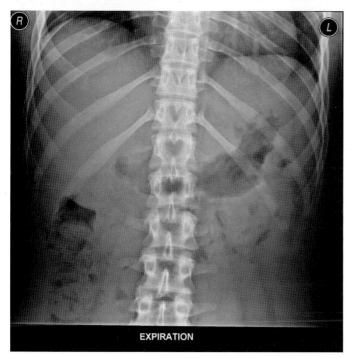

Fig. 10.11b Cross-kidney abdomen taken on expiration.

Urinary tract

Dependent upon the body habitus of an individual patient, the standard CR cassette/receptor size for a KUB radiograph may not be adequate to include the urinary anatomy from superior pole of the left kidney to the anatomical region inferior to the urinary bladder. Thus additional projections may need to be taken to complete the examination.

The KUB should be taken initially and positioned to ensure that the region inferior to the urinary bladder is included. The resultant image is reviewed and the decision for the need to take a cross-kidney AP image is made.

AP cross-kidney (upper abdomen) (Figs 10.11a, 10.11b)

Position of patient and image receptor

- The patient lies supine on the X-ray table with the median sagittal plane of the body at right-angles to and in the midline of the table.
- The patient's hands may be placed high on the chest or the arms may rest by the patient's side slightly away from the trunk.
- The DDR/Bucky detector used should be large enough to cover the region from above the upper poles of the kidneys to the region included superiorly on the incomplete KUB image (or a 35 × 43 cm CR cassette in landscape format is used).
- The appropriate sized cassette/receptor is placed transversely in the Bucky tray and centred in the midline to a level midway between the xiphoid–sternum and iliac crests. If using DDR then adequate collimation to demonstrate this area is required.

Direction and location of the X-ray beam

- The collimated vertical central ray is directed to the centre of the image receptor.

Notes

- The exposure may be taken on expiration to allow for natural positioning of the kidneys.

Expected DRL: DAP 2.5 Gy cm², ESD 4 mGy.

10 Urinary tract – kidneys–ureters–bladder

Additional information about the relationship of opacities to the renal tract may be obtained with further imaging and additional projections. The imaging of choice if an abnormality is demonstrated and the clinical presentation is indicative of renal colic, in some centres, may be a CTU, i.e a CT examination, using IV contrast to demonstrate the function and detailed anatomy of the urinary system. This examination replaces the IVU but is dependent upon CT availability and patient compliance.

The most common supplementary projection to demonstrate an opacity that appears to be in the renal tract or the KUB image is a posterior oblique projection. The right posterior oblique projection shows the right kidney and collecting system in profile and the left kidney en face. Similarly the left posterior oblique projection shows the left kidney in profile and the right kidney enface.

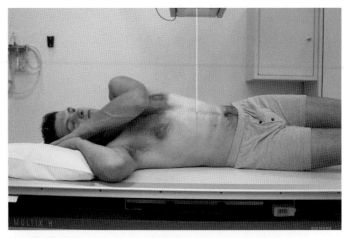

Fig. 10.12a Patient positioning for RPO.

Right posterior oblique (Figs 10.12a, 10.12b)

Position of patient and image receptor

- The patient lies supine on the X-ray Bucky table and then the left side of the trunk and thorax is raised until the coronal plane is at an angle of 15–20° to the table.
- The patient is moved across the X-ray table until the vertebral column is slightly to the left side of the midline and then the patient is immobilised in this position, possibly using radio-opaque pads.
- For the kidney area alone a 24 × 30 cm cassette is placed transversely in the Bucky tray and centred to a level midway between the sterno-xiphisternal joint and umbilicus. If using DDR then adequate collimation to demonstrate this area is required.
- To demonstrate the length of the ureter a 35 × 43 cm cassette might be required and this is centred at the level of the lower costal margin or appropriate collimation if using DDR.

Direction and location of the X-ray beam

- The collimated vertical central ray is directed to the centre of the image receptor/cassette.

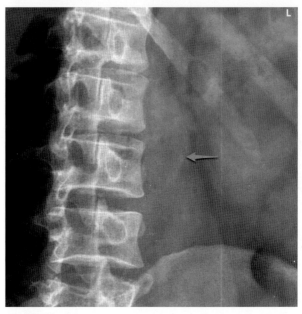

Fig. 10.12b LPO image of the renal area confirming the presence of a small left ureteric calculus at the level of L3. (Copyright [2015] Dr Frank Gaillard; image courtesy of Dr Frank Gaillard and Radiopaedia.org, used under licence.)[8]

Notes

- Over-rotation of the patient will show the right kidney projected overlying the spine.

Left posterior oblique

The positioning is the same as for the right posterior oblique but with the right side elevated.

Calculi within the urinary bladder can move freely particularly if the bladder is full whereas calcification and calculi outside the bladder, e.g. prostatic calculi, are immobile. AP and oblique projections can be taken to show change in relative position of calculi and bladder. To examine the bladder region, caudal angulation is required to allow for the shape of the bony pelvis and to project the symphysis below the apex of the bladder.

Urinary bladder 10

Antero-posterior 15° caudal (Figs 10.13a, 10.13b)

Position of patient and image receptor

- The patient lies supine on the Bucky table with the median sagittal plane at right-angles to, and in the midline of the table.
- A 24 × 30 cm CR cassette is commonly used; this is placed transversely in the tray with its lower border 5 cm below the symphysis pubis. If using DDR then adequate collimation to demonstrate this area is required.

Direction and location of the X-ray beam

- The collimated central ray is directed 15° caudally and centred in the midline 5 cm above the upper border of the symphysis pubis. (e.g. midway between the anterior superior iliac spines and upper border of the symphysis pubis).

Right or left posterior oblique (Figs 10.13c, 10.13d)

Position of patient and image receptor

- From the supine position one side is raised so that the median sagittal plane is rotated through 35°.
- To help stability, the knee in contact with the table is flexed and the raised side supported using a non-opaque pad.
- The patient's position is adjusted so that the midpoint between the symphysis pubis and the anterior superior iliac spine on the raised side is over the midline of the table/receptor.
- A 24 × 30 cm CR cassette is placed longitudinally in the tray with its upper border at the level of the anterior superior iliac spines. If using DDR then adequate collimation to demonstrate this area is required.

Direction and location of the X-ray beam

- The collimated vertical central beam is directed to a point in the midline 2.5 cm above the symphysis pubis.
- Alternatively a caudal angulation of 15° can be used with a higher centring point and the receptor displaced downwards to accommodate the angulation and allow for better demonstration of the apex of the bladder.

Note

The right posterior oblique, i.e. left side raised, will show the right vesico-ureteric junction – a common place for small ureteric calculi to lodge.

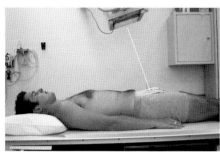

Fig. 10.13a Patient positioning for AP 15° caudal.

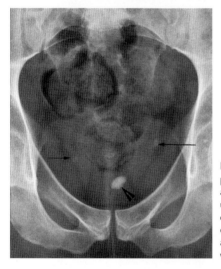

Fig. 10.13b Antero-posterior 15° caudal angulated image of the urinary bladder region demonstrating a bladder calculus (large arrowhead) and small pelvic phleboliths, with lucent centres (arrows).

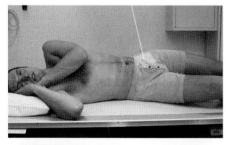

Fig. 10.13c Patient positioning for posterior oblique.

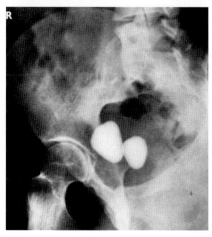

Fig. 10.13d Right posterior oblique image of the bladder area showing large urinary calculi.

10 Biliary system

Ultrasound imaging is the preferred modality to demonstrate the biliary system and further detailed imaging to demonstrate biliary pathologies can be taken using MRI (magnetic resonance cholangiopancreatography [MRCP]). However, plain radiographs of the biliary system may demonstrate opacities including calcifications in the region of the gall bladder and biliary tree.[9]

A low residue diet may be taken during the 2 days prior to the examination to clear overlying faeces and bowel gas. In order to be able to differentiate soft tissues in the region, the radiographic image must have high resolution and have optimal image contrast.

Immobilisation, compression, collimation, short exposure time with high mA are all used to give maximum image quality.

The position of the gall bladder, normally in the middle of the inferior liver margin is variable and it may be more inferior and medial in a thin patient and more superior and lateral in bariatric patients.

For a general survey of the region a left anterior oblique projection is taken. Alternatively a right posterior oblique projection may also be taken.

Left anterior oblique (Figs 10.14a, 10.14b)

The size of the CR cassette, if chosen, is such that a large region of the right side of the abdomen is included.

Position of patient and image receptor

- The patient lies prone on the X-ray table and then the right side is raised rotating the median sagittal plane through an angle of 20°; the coronal plane is now at an angle of 20° to the table.
- The arm on the raised side is flexed so that the right hand rests near the patient's head, while the left arm lies alongside and behind the trunk.
- The patient is moved across the table until the raised right side is over the centre of the table.
- A 24 × 30 cm CR cassette is placed longitudinally in the Bucky tray with its centre 2.5 cm above the lower costal margin to include the top of the iliac crest. If using DDR then adequate collimation to demonstrate this area is required.

Direction and location of the X-ray beam

- The collimated vertical central ray is directed to a point 7.5 cm to the right of the spinous processes and 2.5 cm above the lower costal margin and to the centre of the image receptor.
- The exposure is made on arrested respiration after full expiration.

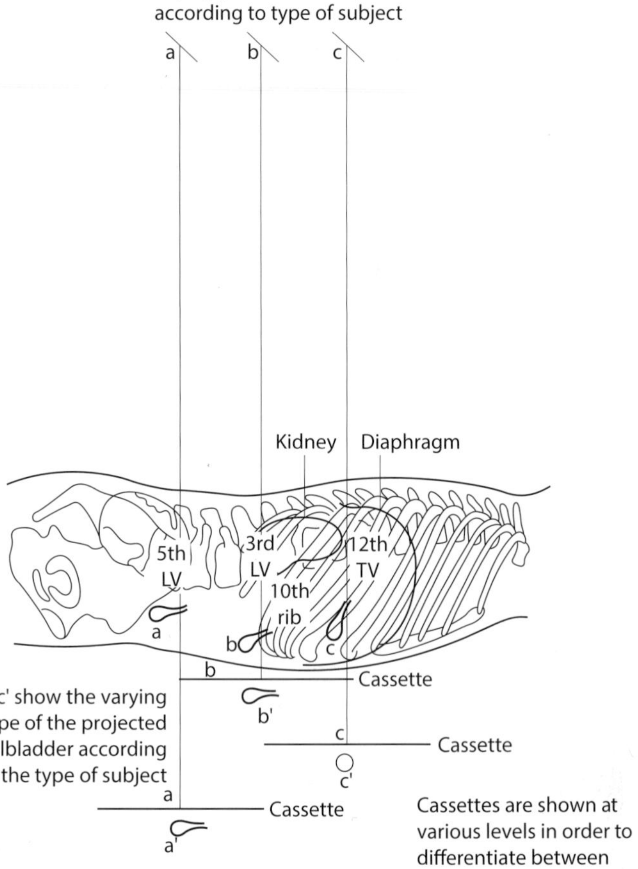

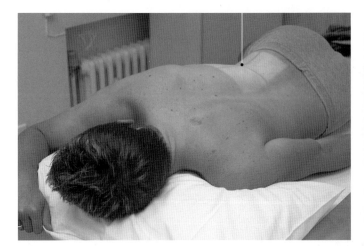

Fig. 10.14a Diagram showing varying shape of the projected gallbladder according to body type of subject.

Fig. 10.14b Patient positioning.

Notes

- An additional image can be taken on arrested respiration after full inspiration to show the relative movement of the gall bladder and overlying calcifications that are suspected to be outside the gall bladder, e.g. within costal cartilages.

Biliary system 10

Right posterior oblique (Fig. 10.15a)

Position of patient and image receptor

- The patient lies supine on the X-ray table and the left side is raised rotating the median sagittal plane through 20°; the coronal plane is now at an angle of 20° to the table and the trunk supported in this position using a non-opaque pad.
- The patient is moved across the table so that the right side of the abdomen is over the centre of the table, and the elbows and shoulders flexed so that the patient can rest their hands under their head.
- A 24 × 30 cm CR cassette is placed longitudinally in the Bucky tray with its centre 2.5 cm above the lower costal margin. If using DDR then adequate collimation to demonstrate this area is required.

Direction and location of the X-ray beam

- The collimated vertical beam is directed to a point midway between the midline and the right abdominal wall 2.5 cm above the lower costal margin, and to the centre of the image receptor.
- Exposure is made on arrested respiration after full expiration.

Radiological considerations (Figs 10.15b–10.15d)

- Many gallstones are not radio-opaque. The pattern of calcification is variable, from an amorphous solid appearance to a concentric laminar structure. Ultrasound is the primary imaging modality for detection and assessment of suspected gallstone disease.
- Calcified stones tend to gather in the fundus of the gallbladder in the prone position. Cholesterol stones in particular are lighter than bile and tend to float, but are not usually radio-opaque.
- Air in the biliary tree may be seen after instrumentation (e.g. sphincterotomy), after passage of calculi or in the normal elderly person with a patulous sphincter of Oddi.[8]

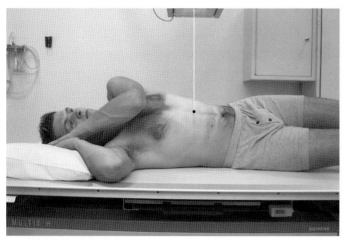

Fig. 10.15a Patient positioning.

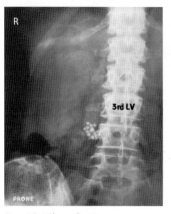
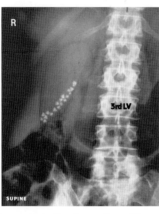

Figs 10.15b and c The images above demonstrate the change in position of the stone-filled gall bladder when the patient is moved from the prone (b) to the supine position (c).

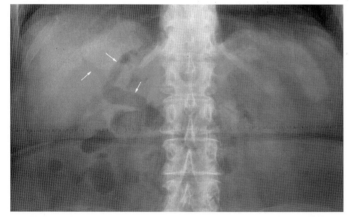

Fig. 10.15d Antero-posterior supine abdomen image of air in the biliary tree.

10 Abdomen and pelvic cavity

Image evaluation – 10-point plan

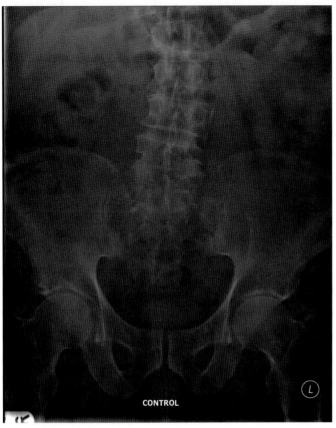

Fig. 10.16a AP abdomen.

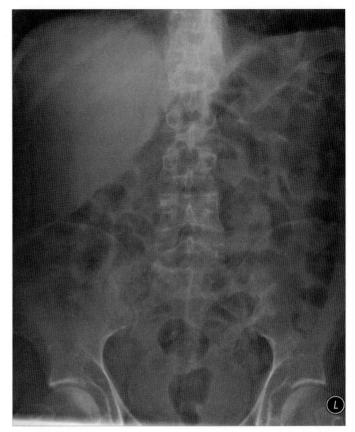

Fig. 10.16b AP abdomen.

IMAGE EVALUATION

AP abdomen (Fig. 10.16a)

The main points to consider are:
- Markers applied pre- and post processing.
- Scoliotic patient but no obvious rotation.
- Too much infrapubic space demonstrated.
- Sub-diaphragmatic region not demonstrated.

Radiographer Comments/Initial report

Additional upper abdomen (cross-kidney) projection required.
No obvious pathology seen.

IMAGE EVALUATION

AP abdomen (Fig. 10.16b)

The main points to consider are:
- Marker applied post processing.
- Symphysis pubis and sub-pubic region not demonstrated.
- Slight rotation demonstrated by vertebral spinous processes.

Radiographer Comments/Initial report

Additional lower abdo projection required.
Note hepatomegaly extending from right hypochondrium into right lumbar region.

Abdomen and pelvic cavity 10

Image evaluation – 10-point plan (cont.)

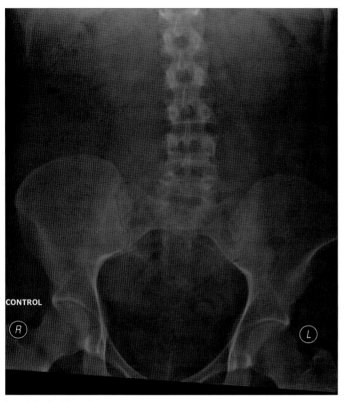

Fig. 10.17a AP abdomen.

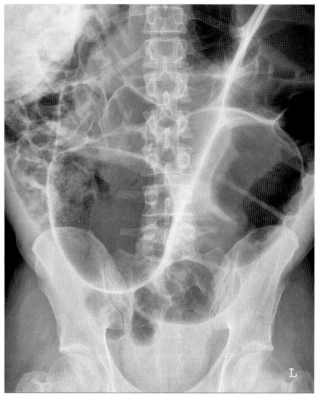

Fig. 10.17b AP abdomen.

IMAGE EVALUATION

AP abdomen (Fig. 10.17a)

The main points to consider are:
- Markers applied post processing.
- Sub-pubic region not demonstrated.
- Slight rotation and scoliosis concave to the patient's right.
- Left kidney outline identified.

Note absence of right kidney outline and psoas muscle indicating muscular spasm, i.e. renal colic on the right side.

Radiographer Comments/Initial report

Image diagnostic with further imaging/examination required to exclude/confirm right renal pathology.

IMAGE EVALUATION

AP abdomen (Fig. 10.17b)

The main points to consider are:
- Sub-pubic region not demonstrated.
- Full abdominal contents not imaged.
- Obvious grossly distended large bowel.

Radiographer Comments/Initial report

Further imaging required to include the whole of the abdomen, incomplete examination but obvious pathology demonstrated.

Section 11
Ward Radiography

CONTENTS

INTRODUCTION	386
Equipment and accessories	388
HEART AND LUNGS	389
Postero-anterior – erect	389
Antero-posterior – erect	390
Postero-anterior or antero-posterior (lateral decubitus)	391
Lateral dorsal decubitus	391
Temporary pacemaker	392
Post-operative radiography	393
CHEST/UPPER ABDOMEN	394
Naso-gastric tube positioning	394
Abdomen	396
Recommended projections	396
Antero-posterior – supine	396
Antero-posterior – erect	397
Antero-posterior supine (left lateral decubitus)	397
Lateral dorsal decubitus – supine	398
CERVICAL SPINE	399
Lateral supine	399
FRACTURED LOWER LIMBS AND PELVIS	400
Antero-posterior	400
FRACTURED FEMUR	401
Lateral	401
Arthroplasty postoperative radiography	401
PAEDIATRIC (GALLOWS TRACTION)	402
Antero-posterior	402
Lateral	402
HEART AND LUNGS – SPECIAL CARE BABY UNIT	403
Antero-posterior	403

11 Introduction

Radiography using mobile X-ray equipment should be restricted to the patient whose medical condition is such that it is impossible for them to be moved to the X-ray department without seriously affecting their medical treatment and nursing care. Such patients may be found in surgical and medical ward environments and in the following areas:

- Intensive care unit (ICU, also known as intensive therapy or treatment units).
- Coronary care unit/Cardiac surgery unit (CCU/CSU).
- High-dependency unit (HDU).
- Special care baby unit (SCBU).
- Resuscitation/major trauma.
- Patients being isolation/barrier or reverse barrier nursed.

Key skills for mobile/ward radiography

- How to use the equipment correctly.
- Effective communication.
- Radiation protection of the staff and patients.
- Infection control.
- Personal preparation.
- Safe practice.
- Production of diagnostic images.
- Team working.

General comments

Examinations are normally complicated by a variety of situations:

- The need to communicate effectively to complete the examination without harming the patients progress/recovery and with minimum disruption to the ward.
- The patient's medical condition, the degree of consciousness and co-operation.
- The patient's treatment and restrictions due to life-support system, drips, and chest or abdominal drains.
- Traction apparatus.
- Physical restrictions due to room size and ability to move mobile or portable X-ray equipment in confined spaces.
- Need to monitor the patient and life-support equipment.

Correct use of the equipment (Figs 11.1a, 11.1b)

- A mobile X-ray unit is selected depending upon the requirement of the radiographic procedure. For example, a mobile X-ray unit may be situated in an area which undertakes mobiles on a routine basis or needs to be taken to the ward.
- For the prevention of infection, the unit selected and image detectors should be cleaned and dried before and after each patient.
- Patient demographics may be entered on the Radiology information system/picture archiving and communication system (RIS/PACS) and exposure parameters adjusted to those required for the examination. The radiographer must be able to assume total control of the situation, and should enlist the help, co-operation and advice of nursing and medical staff before embarking on an examination. A thorough knowledge of the ward is necessary in order that any problems or difficulties can be resolved with the minimum of fuss.
- Any X-ray requests should be checked first to ensure that the examination on the ward is necessary, and that the correct equipment and detectors are obtained for transfer to the wards.
- Patient identification protocols should be correctly applied.
- Detectors used must be clearly marked to avoid double exposure if more than one patient needs examining on the ward.

Advice regarding the patient's medical condition should be sought first, before moving or disturbing the patient. Any disturbance of traction, electrocardiogram (ECG) leads or drains should be undertaken only with the permission of the medical staff. Positioning of the image receptor and movement or lifting of seriously ill patients should be undertaken with the co-operation/supervision of nursing staff.

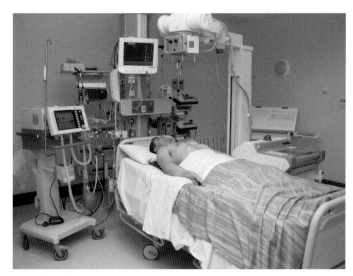

Fig. 11.1a Ward radiography and equipment.

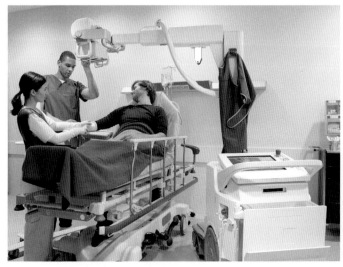

Fig. 11.1b A mobile DDR X-ray machine.

Effective communication

The radiographer must communicate effectively with the ward staff before, during and after the mobile X-ray. The key to a stress-free experience is preparation. It is essential that there is a mechanism for ward staff to communicate effectively and give the radiographer as much notice of all mobile requests. This enables the radiographer to use their time effectively and not be kept waiting due to the patient's or ward management.

The radiographer needs to be informed of the:

- Justification for the examination to be a mobile.
- Urgency of the request.
- Patient's condition and life support.
- Infection status (see opposite).

Following the procedure the radiographer must ensure the ward staff and referrer know when the image will be available on the PACS and when a report is available. All exposure require an evaluation under the IR(ME)R 2000 regulations.

Red flag

If the X-ray examination of the patient demonstrates a 'life threatening' or unexpected appearance the radiographer has a duty of care to the patient and the referrer and ward/clinician should be informed immediately, e.g. a nasogastric tube in the lung rather than the stomach (see page 395).

Radiation protection

This is of paramount importance in the situation where mobile radiography is undertaken. The radiographer:

- Is responsible for ensuring that there is a controlled area of 2 metres during exposure of the patient and that the local rules are adhered to during the examination.
- Must liaise clearly with the ward staff on their arrival on the ward and issue verbal instructions in a clear and distinct manner to staff and patients to avoid accidental exposure to radiation.
- Must be protected adequately from scattered radiation, including those assisting, by the use of personal protective equipment. The use of the inverse square law, with staff standing as far away as possible from the unit and outside the controlled area, should be made when making an exposure.

The patient should also receive appropriate radiation protection. Lead protective shields may be used as backstops when using a horizontal beam to limit the radiation field, e.g. when the absorption nature of room-dividing walls is unknown. Exposure factors used for the examination should be recorded, enabling optimum results to be repeated.

Control of infection

The control of infection plays an important role in the management of all patients, especially following surgery and in the nursing of premature babies.

To prevent the spread of infection, local established protocols should be adhered to by staff coming into contact with patients, e.g. hand-washing before and after every patient and cleaning of detectors and X-ray equipment used for radiographic examination before, between and after each examination. Patients with a known highly contagious infection, and those with a compromised immune system and at high risk of infection, will be isolation-nursed (barrier nursed). In such circumstances, it is important that local protocols associated with the prevention of spread of infection are followed.[1]

The X-ray equipment used in ICU, CSU and SCBU should, ideally, be dedicated units and kept on site. If shared with other areas in the hospital they should be cleaned with disinfectant solution before being moved into infection-controlled units. Equipment is wheeled over dust-absorbent mats at the entrance of such units.

Radiographers should wear gowns or disposable plastic aprons, facemasks and over-shoes before entering these areas.

Image receptors should be cleaned and covered with plastic sheets or clean pillowcases/towels before use. After use, image receptors and all equipment should be cleaned with antiseptic solution. Disposable gloves are worn when touching the patient.

Methicillin-resistant *Staphylococcus aureus* (MRSA) and *Clostridium difficile* (C. difficile) are hospital-acquired bacterial infections that need to be controlled and not spread to other patients. MRSA is resistant to methicillin and many other antibiotics and is a particular threat to vulnerable patients; it can cause many symptoms, including fever, wound and skin infections, inflammation and pneumonia. Both these organisms can be spread readily from an infected patient to others. They are spread mainly from person to person by hand.[2]

When healthcare workers deal with any potentially infected patients, the bacteria may transfer to their hands and can then be passed on to a vulnerable patient. Controls such as effective hand-washing, wearing of gloves and aprons, and the cleaning of the environment and equipment are necessary to prevent spread of the bacteria.

When undertaking radiography on more than one barrier-nursed patient on a ward or ICU, it is important that disposable aprons are changed between patients as well as ensuring that the hands of the operators are washed between patients to prevent the spread of infection. A number of speciality wards use differently coloured aprons per patient bay as a prompt to confine the use of aprons to a specific patient.

Isolation/barrier nursing

Isolation nursing is required to reduce the risk of spreading certain infections or antibiotic resistant germs to other patients and staff. It is also applied to protect patients from infection if they have a weak immune system due to disease, transplant surgery or taking certain drugs.

- Isolation nursing is carried out by placing the patient in a single room or side room.
- Barrier nursing occurs when a patient(s) is kept in a bay and extra precautions are implemented to prevent spread of infection.

NB: there are specific protocols using two members of staff to undertake the X-ray to prevent the spread of infection for patients being isolation/barrier nursed.

11 Introduction

Equipment and accessories

X-ray equipment (Figs 11.2b, 11.2c)

Units fall broadly into two groups – portable and mobile, the broad distinction between the two being the difference in power output and the ability to transfer equipment.

- Portable sets have relatively low mA settings and normally can be dismantled for transfer. Mobile sets have higher power output, are much heavier, and need to be motorised or pushed between locations.
- Mobile X-ray units can be either mains-independent or mains-dependent. Mobile machines are heavy and may be battery-driven to aid transportation around the hospital.
- Older mobile sets, with conventionally powered X-ray generators, require the need of a separate 30 A supply and are connected to socket outlets marked 'X-ray only'. Patients requiring radiography with such machines should be nursed in beds that are within reach of these sockets.
- Modern mains-independent machines can be operated from a standard 13 A supply. These are designed with high-powered battery packs to generate the electrical power for X-ray exposure. Therefore, these units can be moved to areas without electrical mains power or in wards where there is a restriction of mains sockets. They require only access to a 13 A power supply for battery recharging during storage.
- DR mobile X-ray machines have wireless detectors that facilitate image review within seconds of undertaking the examination. Anatomically programmed generators enable optimum exposure setting for any variation in technique. Storage to PACS and availability to the requesting clinician is also almost immediately after the radiographer has checked and accepted image as being diagnostic and meeting with the referrer's request.

In radiography of the chest and abdomen, the use of short exposure times is essential to reduce the risk of movement unsharpness.

Accessory equipment (Fig. 11.2a)

Various aids are available that can assist in positioning both the patient and image receptor. These include foam pads of different sizes and shapes, such as large triangular pads that support the patient and allow the image detector to be inserted in a groove in the pad and magnetic cassette holders.[3] The correct accessories should be selected as part of the equipment needed for the radiographic procedure. A selection of a low ratio 6:1 30 lines per cm parallel stationary grid will reduce the risk of grid cut-off when undertaking conventional radiography.

Heart and lungs

Patients suffering from dyspnoea and severe chest pain are often assessed on the ward. Radiographs are requested to aid

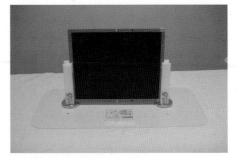

Fig. 11.2a A magnetic lateral cassette holder.

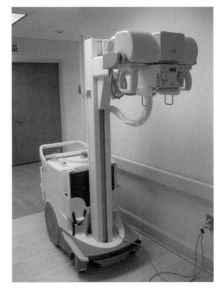

Fig. 11.2b A conventional mobile.

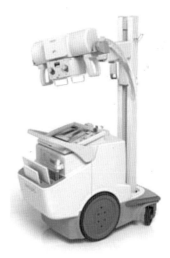

Fig. 11.2c A DR mobile.

in the diagnosis and management of patients. Common conditions include congestive heart failure, coronary heart disease, left ventricular failure, pulmonary oedema, pulmonary embolus, pneumothorax, pleural effusion and pneumonia. Post-operative chest radiography is also often required.

As a general rule, ward radiography should be performed only when it is not possible to move the patient to the X-ray department and when medical intervention is dependent on the diagnosis confirmed on the radiograph. This section should be read in conjunction with Section 7 Thorax and Upper Airway.

Technique and patient position

The choice of erect or decubitus technique is governed primarily by the condition of the patient, with the majority of patients positioned erect. Very ill patients and patients who are immobile are X-rayed in the supine or semi-erect position. With the patient erect, positioning is simplified, control of respiration is more effective as gravitational effect on the abdominal organs allows for the disclosure of the maximum area of lung tissue, and fluid levels are defined more easily with the use of a horizontal central beam.

The postero-anterior (PA) projection is generally adopted in preference to the antero-posterior (AP) when this can be achieved. Erect PA images enable the arms to be arranged more easily to ensure the scapulae are projected clear of the lung fields. Heart magnification is also reduced significantly compared with the AP projection. The radiation dose to the breasts and thyroid is also significantly reduced.

Note

- Patients who are able to undertake a PA chest should of course be evaluated to see if they can go down to the imaging department; however, if being isolation- or barrier-nursed this is not possible.

Images are normally acquired on arrested deep inspiration, which ensures maximum visualisation of the air-filled lungs. The adequacy of inspiration of an exposed radiograph can be assessed by the position of the ribs above the diaphragm. In the correctly exposed image, it should be possible to visualise either six ribs anteriorly or ten ribs posteriorly.

The radiographer must communicate effectively with the patient before, during and after the mobile X-ray. A comprehensive explanation to the patient, along with a rehearsal of the procedure, should ensure a satisfactory result. Respiratory movements should be repeated several times before the performance is considered to be satisfactory. With the patient having taken a deep breath, a few moments should be allowed to elapse to ensure stability before the exposure is made. On inspiration, there is a tendency to raise the shoulders, which should be avoided, as the shadows of the clavicles then obscure the lung apices.

Unconscious patients should be treated in the same way as a conscious patient and the radiographer should explain what they are doing and why they are doing it. If the patient is on a ventilator the radiographer should practice breathing along with the ventilator and ensure they expose the image at full inspiration.

Guide wires, oxygen masks, drains, ECG leads and other life support/monitoring equipment should be arranged so as not to obscure the relevant image. Correct exposures must be recorded to enable comparative images to be taken on subsequent examinations.

It is essential that the correct anatomical and positional markers are included on the image. Any modifications from the standard projection should be noted on the image.

Heart and lungs 11

Postero-anterior – erect (Fig. 11.3)

For cardiac conditions where heart size is a relevant factor and if the patient's condition allows, a PA erect chest should be performed in preference to an AP erect chest.

Position of patient and image receptor

- The patient is positioned with their legs over the side of the trolley/bed facing the image receptor. The image receptor is supported by the patient's arms and pads/pillows. The chin needs to be extended and centred to the middle of the top of the image receptor.
- The median sagittal plane is adjusted at right-angles to the middle of the image receptor. The shoulders are rotated forward and pressed downward in contact with the image receptor. This is achieved by placing the dorsal aspect of the hands behind the image receptor, with the elbows brought cranially allowing the arms to encircle the image receptor.

Direction and location of X-ray beam

- The collimated horizontal central beam is directed at right-angles to the image receptor at the level of the spinous process of T7.
- The surface marking of T7 spinous process can be assessed by using the inferior angle of the scapula before the shoulders are pushed forward.
- Exposure is made in full normal arrested inspiration.

Essential image characteristics

The ideal PA chest radiograph should demonstrate the following:

- Full lung fields with the scapulae projected laterally away from the lung fields.
- The clavicles symmetrical and equidistant from the spinous processes and not obscuring the lung apices.
- The lungs well inflated, i.e. it should be possible to visualise either six ribs anteriorly or ten ribs posteriorly.
- The costo-phrenic angles and diaphragm outlined clearly.
- The mediastinum and heart central and defined sharply.

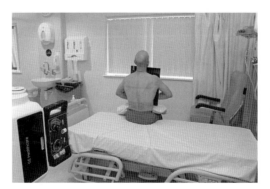

Fig. 11.3 The technique for a postero-anterior mobile chest X-ray.

11 Heart and lungs

Antero-posterior – erect (Figs 11.4a–11.4c)

Where an erect PA image is not possible, the patient should be X-rayed sitting erect and facing the X-ray tube. If an AP erect is not possible, the patient should be positioned supine as the semi-recumbent position is not favoured as the degree of recumbence is not reproducible across a series of images.

A 35 × 43 cm computed radiography (CR) cassette or portable direct digital radiography (DDR) detector is selected for all the projections described.

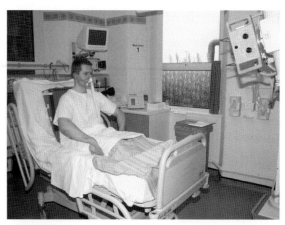

Fig. 11.4a Patient positioning – AP erect.

Position of patient and image receptor

- The patient should be sitting erect and facing the X-ray tube with the image receptor supported against the back of the patient, using pillows or a large wedge-shaped foam pad, with its upper edge above the lung fields.
- If an AP erect is not possible, the patient may be positioned supine.
- The median sagittal plane is adjusted at right-angles to, and in the midline of, the 35 × 43 cm image receptor.
- Rotation of the patient is prevented by the use of foam pads. Rotation produces a range of artefacts and must be avoided or minimised. If possible, the arms are rotated medially, with the shoulders brought forward to bring the scapulae clear of the lung fields.

Direction and location of the X-ray beam

- Assuming the patient can sit fully erect, the collimated X-ray beam is directed first at right-angles to the image receptor and towards the sternal angle.
- The collimated X-ray beam is then angled until it is coincident with the middle of the image receptor, thus avoiding unnecessary exposure to the eyes.
- The use of a horizontal central ray, however, is essential to demonstrate fluid, e.g. pleural effusion or any air under the diaphragm. If the patient is able to sit erect, direct the collimated X-ray beam at right-angles to the middle of the image receptor. The clavicles in the resultant radiograph, however, will be projected above the apices.
- If the patient is unable to sit erect, fluid levels are demonstrated using a horizontal ray with the patient lying down in the positions (described on page 391).

Notes

- Where possible, a high-powered mobile is used to enable a 180 cm focus-to-receptor distance (FRD) for erect positioning of the patient.
- For supine images, the FRD may be restricted due to the height of the bed and the height limitations of the X-ray tube column. The FRD should be higher than 120 cm, otherwise image magnification and unsharpness will increase.

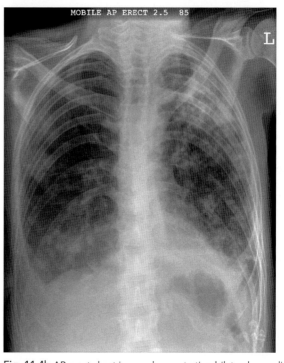

Fig. 11.4b AP erect chest image demonstrating bilateral consolidation with a right pleural effusion (in this case due to tuberculosis).

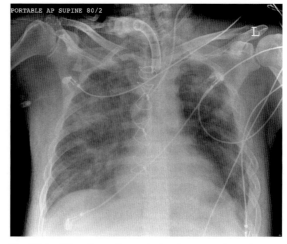

Fig. 11.4c AP supine radiograph showing extensive pulmonary oedema and haemorrhage after trauma, with multiple left-sided rib fractures. Sternal wires indicate previous cardiac surgery. Note left jugular central line and tracheostomy. It is not possible to exclude pleural effusion or pneumothorax on an AP supine image.

Patients who are too ill to sit erect may be examined whilst lying down. The use of a horizontal central ray is essential to demonstrate fluid levels, e.g. hydropneumothorax.

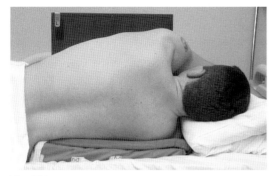

Fig. 11.5a Patient positioned for a PA chest (lateral decubitus) projection.

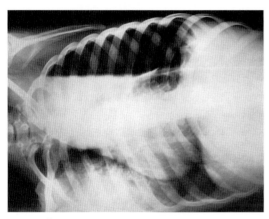

Fig. 11.5b PA radiograph in a lateral decubitus position demonstrating a plural effusion with a pneumothorax.

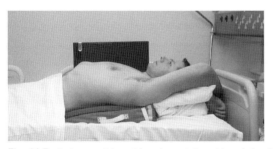

Fig. 11.5c Patient positioned for a lateral chest (dorsal decubitus) projection.

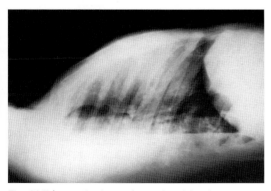

Fig. 11.5d Lateral radiograph in a dorsal decubitus position demonstrating a plural effusion with a pneumothorax.

Heart and lungs 11

Postero-anterior or antero-posterior (lateral decubitus) (Figs 11.5a, 11.5b)

This projection is used to confirm the presence of fluid. Moving the patient into a different position causes movement of free fluid, so that location is also detected. It may also be used to demonstrate the lateral chest wall of the affected side clear of fluid, and to unmask any underlying lung pathology.

Position of patient and image receptor

- The patient is turned on to the unaffected side and, if possible, raised on to a supporting foam pad.
- A 35 × 43 cm CR cassette or DDR detector is supported vertically against the anterior chest wall, and the median sagittal plane is adjusted at right-angles to the detector.
- The patient's arms are raised and folded over the head to clear the chest wall.

Direction and location of the X-ray beam

- The collimated horizontal X-ray beam is directed at right-angles to the image receptor and centred at the level of the 8th thoracic vertebra.
- Alternatively, an AP projection may be taken, with the detector supported against the posterior aspect of the patient.

Lateral dorsal decubitus (Figs 11.5c, 11.5d)

This projection will show as much as possible of the lung fields, clear of a fluid level, when the patient is unable to turn on their side.

Position of patient and image receptor

- The patient lies supine and, if possible, is raised off the bed on a supporting foam pad.
- The arms are extended and supported above the head.
- A 35 × 43 cm CR cassette or DDR detector is supported vertically against the lateral aspect of the chest of the affected side and adjusted parallel to the median sagittal plane.

Direction and location of the X-ray beam

- A horizontal collimated X-ray beam is directed at right-angles to the image receptor and centred to the axilla.

Notes

- Further projections may be taken with the patient lying on the affected side or in the prone position to disclose further aspects of the lung fields not obscured by fluid.
- A stationary grid may have to be used if the depth of the thorax is likely to produce an unacceptable amount of secondary radiation.

11 Heart and lungs

Temporary pacemaker

Patients suffering from heart block are often treated with an electrical pacemaker, which regulates the heart rate. A temporary cardiac electrode is used consisting of a bipolar wire 100 cm long, covered in Teflon, and terminating in a platinum tip electrode separated from a second electrode, which encircles the wire. At the other end, two wires are connected to a battery pacemaker.

The electrode is usually passed into the right subclavian vein and directed into the right ventricle, where the tip is lodged against the endocardial surface near the lower part of the interventricular septum. An electrical impulse is generated across the endocardial surface and adjusted to the required heart rate.

This procedure may be performed in a cardiac catheter laboratory, if available, or in a side ward or dedicated pacing room adjacent to a coronary care facility. Whist screening takes place the area becomes a 'controlled area' and local radiation rules must be applied, i.e.:

- Restricted access to only staff involved in the procedure.
- Staff wear personal protective equipment during the procedure.
- A mobile lead screen may be advisable if this procedure is undertaken on a frequent basis.
- The door to the room is closed and a sign displayed to prevent access during screening.

The procedure described below, using a mobile C-arm fluoroscopy unit (Image intensifier/solid state detector), is typical of an insertion of a temporary pacemaker in a side ward dedicated for this procedure.

Mobile C-arm fluoroscopy (Figs 11.6a, 11.6b)

- A mobile C-arm (23 or 31 cm field of view ideally) is selected. As insertion of the electrodes may be prolonged, it is important that the set is equipped with 'last image hold' and pulsed fluoroscopy in order to reduce patient and staff dose.
- The patient lies on a trolley or bed with a radiolucent top, which can accommodate the C-arm of the intensifier.
- The intensifier is positioned on the opposite side of the operating position, with the long axis of the machine at right-angles to the bed or trolley and with the intensifier face above and parallel to the patient's upper thorax.
- The wheels of the image intensifier are rotated in order to allow free longitudinal movement of the device, with the cross-arm brakes released to facilitate movement across the patient.

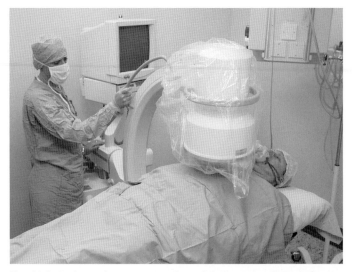

Fig. 11.6a Radiographer positioning the mobile C-arm image intensifier prior to the pacemaker wire insertion via the left subclavian approach.

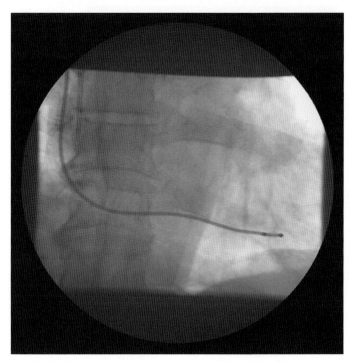

Fig. 11.6b Fluoroscopic image demonstrating the location of the pacemaker wire.

- During the procedure, the C-arm is 'panned' so that the advancement and direction of the tip are observed until the tip of the electrode is located correctly within the right ventricle.
- Control of the screening factors, screening time and radiation protection is the responsibility of the radiographer.
- As the procedure is performed under aseptic conditions, a sterile protective cover is normally secured to the image intensifier housing.

Heart and lungs 11

Post-operative radiography (Figs 11.7a–11.7c)

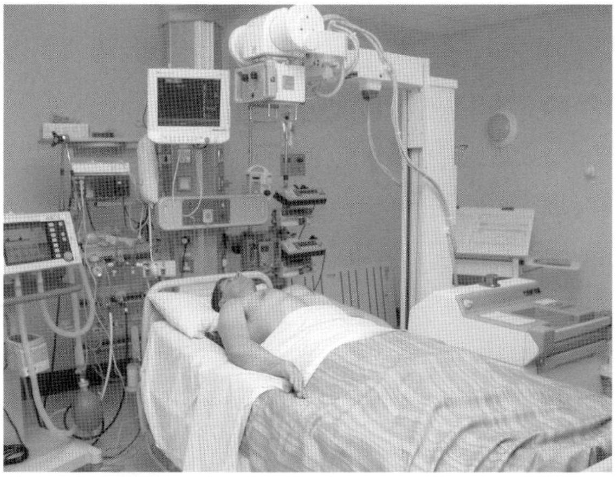

Patients who have undergone major cardiac or thoracic surgery are invariably nursed intensively in either a CSU or ITU, depending on the type of surgery performed. Such patients can be connected to an assortment of catheters and tubes for monitoring purposes and chest drainage, e.g. following cardiac or thoracic surgery for drainage of the thoracic cavity of fluid and connections to underwater seals may be necessary to keep the lungs inflated. Strict control of infection procedures must be followed to ensure that the patient is not exposed to infection. A series of radiographs may be required during postoperative care, the first shortly after surgery. The first radiograph, and for a few days until the patient is fit to sit erect, is usually taken with the patient supine. The same principles of consistent radiographic positioning and exposure are applied to enable accurate comparisons of radiographs over a period of time. The positioning of the patient should be carried out using a rehearsed procedure to reduce patient movement and undue back strain for everyone involved in handling the patient. Care should also be taken to expose on full inspiration when the patient is connected to a ventilator.

Endotracheal tube

The position of an endotracheal tube can be assessed from an AP projection of the chest, which must be exposed with enough penetration to show the trachea and carina. The position of the tube is checked to ensure that its distal end is not lying in the right bronchus.

Central venous pressure line

A fine catheter is positioned in the superior vena cava in seriously ill patients as a means of measuring central venous pressure and injecting drugs. The catheter may be introduced via one of the jugular or subclavian veins, or a peripheral vein. The position of a catheter or line can be assessed from the AP projection of the chest exposed with enough kilovoltage to penetrate the mediastinum. The position of the catheter is checked to ensure that its distal end has not been directed into the right internal jugular vein or the right atrium of the heart. The root of the neck should be included on the radiograph. There is a risk of inducing a pneumothorax with this procedure and therefore it is important that the chest image includes the apex of the lung.

Chest drain insertions

Chest drains are used for drainage of a pneumothorax or pleural effusion, whether spontaneous or following cardiac or thoracic surgery. If the drain is connected to an underwater seal chamber, care must be taken not to elevate the chamber above the level of the drain, or water may siphon back into the thorax. An AP erect image is required to show the position of the tube and to show any residual air within the thorax.

Fig. 11.7a The technique for a supine chest.

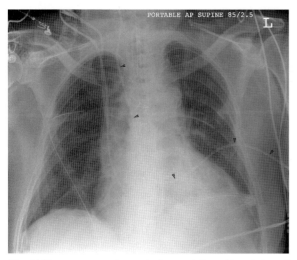

Fig. 11.7b AP supine radiograph showing bilateral basal chest drains, endotracheal tube, right jugular central venous catheter and a pulmonary artery catheter (in this case unusually passing to the left pulmonary artery rather than the right). NB: to avoid confusion the extracorporeal part of the pulmonary artery catheter (arrowheads) should have been positioned out of the field of view.

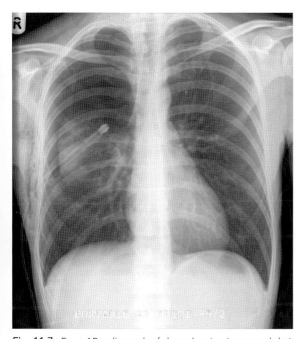

Fig. 11.7c Erect AP radiograph of chest showing intercostal drain in situ for pneumothorax.

11 Chest/upper abdomen

Naso-gastric tube positioning (Figs 11.8a, 11.8b)

A now common examination, which is becoming routinely requested for in-patients, is a chest/upper abdomen X-ray specifically for naso-gastric tube (NGT) positioning post insertion. This follows national guidelines in the UK following a number of incidents that resulted in serious harm or death.[4]

The NGT is a long polyurethane or silicone tube passed via the nostril with the tip located in the lower stomach. It has three specific uses:

- Allow drainage of stomach contents.
- Allow removal of air.
- Provide a safe access route to the gastrointestinal tract (GIT) for the administration of fluids, medicines and/or nutrients.

Radiographic check images of tube placement continues to be the gold standard, although inexperience in image interpretation can lead to misreading of the tube position. Therefore, standardised training and specific guidelines for insertion of the NGT must be undertaken by the doctor or other health professionals caring for that patient. The patient must be assessed prior to administration using national guidelines and local protocols. Only when these protocols have been followed and the correct positioning of the tube has been verified can any feeding/drainage begin.

The vast majority of naso-gastric intubations are uncomplicated and dealt with by suitably trained practitioners within the ward environment measuring the pH of gastric aspirate. Only if the first-line ward tests fail should check X-rays be undertaken. The tube position assessment in therefore the second-line test method (i.e. when pH test is not conclusive). The exposure and image receptor positioning must be optimised to demonstrate the NGT. Interpretation of the image prior to feeding the patient through the NGT must be by specific medical personnel only, trained to the level required by national guidelines.

Radiographers have been shown to be able to provide a sustainable check image interpretation service including removing and resisting tubes as required.[5] With this service suitably trained and competent radiographers have the chance to play a major role in improving patient safety.[6]

Imaging procedure

The same procedure is carried out as for an AP CXR either in the erect position or supine as on pages 242, 243 should be followed with the following specific modifications:

The exposure must be adjusted to ensure that the contrast and density are adequate to identify the tip of the NGT in the stomach

- The location of the collimated X-ray beam is adjusted more inferior to normal chest X-ray positioning to demonstrate the upper abdomen below the diaphragm.
- As a guide, the cardio-phrenic angles should be approximately half way down the image receptor.

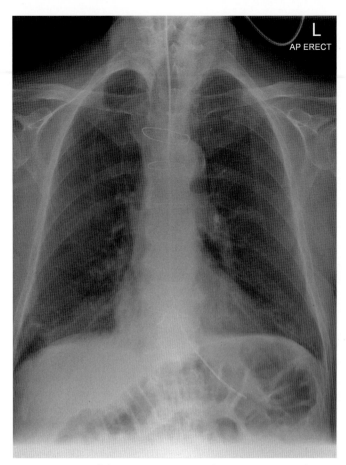

Fig. 11.8a Image of chest x-ray examination demonstrating correctly positioned NGT.

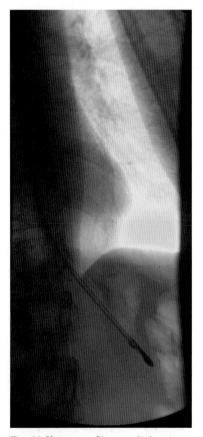

Fig. 11.8b Image of 'inverted' chest/upper abdomen demonstrating correctly positioned NGT.

Notes

- Of particular importance is the tube appearance at the level of the carina and whether the tube has passed to the left or right suggesting it has passed into the lung. See Fig. 11.9a, which demonstrated a NGT in the right lung.
- The resultant image may be post processed to optimise visualisation of the NGT.
- The NGT may be more readily identified radiologically by inverting the image (see Fig. 11.8b).
- All post processed images should be saved as additional images and annotated as such with the original identified in the patient's folder.

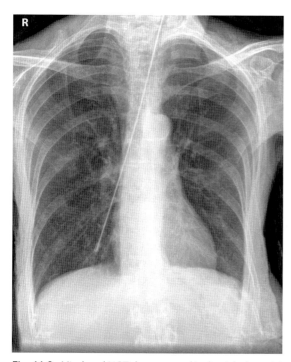

Fig. 11.9a Misplaced NGT demonstrated in the right lower lobe.

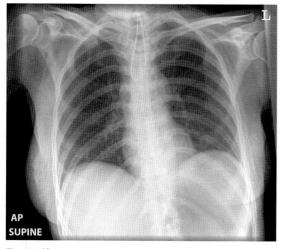

Fig. 11.9b Misplaced NGT demonstrated – note the tube curls backwards in the opposite direction.

Chest/upper abdomen 11

Naso-gastric tube positioning (cont.) (Figs 11.9a–11.9c)

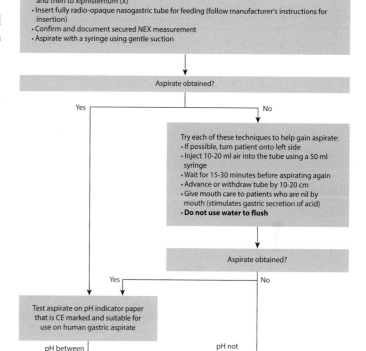

A pH of between 1 and 5.5 is reliable confirmation that the tube is not in the lung. However, it does not confirm placement in the stomach as there is a small chance the tip of the tube may sit in the oesophagus, where it carries a higher risk of aspiration. If this is any concern, arrange radiography to confirm tube position.

If pH readings are between 5 and 6 it is recommended that a second, competent person checks the reading or retests.

Fig. 11.9c Algorithm for checking placement of nasogastric tubes in adults. Adapted from National Patient Safety Agency.[6]

11 Chest/upper abdomen

Abdomen

Mobile radiography of the abdomen may be required in cases of acute abdominal pain or following surgery, when the patient is unstable, to determine whether any of the following are present:

- Gaseous distension of any part of the GIT.
- Free gas or fluid in the peritoneal cavity.
- Fluid levels in the intestines.
- Localisation of radio-opaque foreign bodies.

Recommended projections

Typical imaging protocols are described in Section 10. Below is a summary of some of projections used for the conditions listed.

Gaseous distension	AP abdomen, patient supine
Free gas in the peritoneal cavity	AP chest, patient erect AP abdomen, patient supine AP/PA left lateral decubitus
Fluid levels	AP abdomen, patient erect
Radio-opaque foreign bodies	AP abdomen, patient supine

AP, antero-posterior; PA, postero-anterior.

Antero-posterior – supine (Figs 11.10a–11.10c)

Position of patient and image receptor

With the patient supine, a stationary grid is used in conjunction with a 35 × 43 cm CR cassette or a portable DDR detector and is carefully positioned under the abdomen. The patient may be lifted by using a well-rehearsed and safe lifting technique whilst the image receptor is slipped beneath them. Care should be exercised to avoid hurting the patient by forcing the image receptor into position, or using a cold cassette, which might shock the patient.

The grid and image receptor should be positioned to include the symphysis pubis on the lower edge of the image. The image receptor should also be in a horizontal position on the bed and not lying at an angle. If the stationary grid is not flat, there may be grid cut-off of the radiation beam, which may give the appearance of a lesion of increased radio-opacity, such as an intra-abdominal mass due to loss of image density.

Direction and location of the X-ray beam

- A collimated vertical X-ray beam is directed at right-angles to the image receptor and centred in the midline at the level of the iliac crests.
- Exposure is made on arrested expiration.

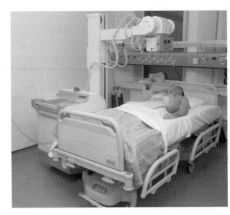

Fig. 11.10a Photograph of technique for a supine abdomen.

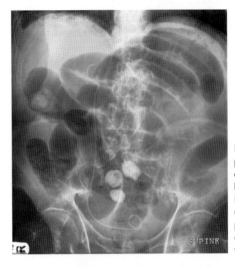

Fig. 11.10b Supine portable abdomen that demonstrates a small bowel obstruction. NB: patient has a right ureteric pigtail stent as patient had transitional cell carcinoma of the bladder.

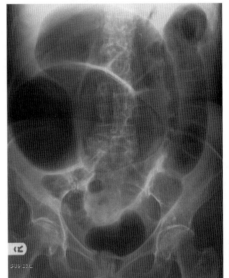

Fig. 11.10c Supine portable radiograph of abdomen showing distal colonic obstruction.

Notes

- Radiographs may be taken using a high kV technique to shorten the exposure time and reduce movement blur.
- Foam pads may be used to prevent rotation of the patient.
- Correct anatomical side and positional markers must be included on the image.

Chest/upper abdomen 11

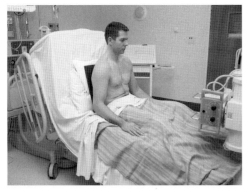

Fig. 11.11a The technique for an erect abdomen.

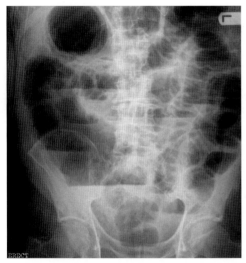

Fig. 11.11b AP erect radiograph of abdomen showing small bowel obstruction, with gas in the bowel wall (right upper quadrant) indicating impending perforation.

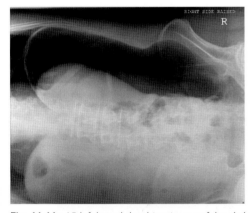

Fig. 11.11c AP left lateral decubitus image of the abdomen showing free air in the abdominal cavity (above) and technique opposite.

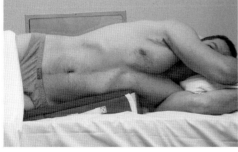

Fig. 11.11d The technique for AP left lateral decubitus of the abdomen.

Antero-posterior – erect (Figs 11.11a, 11.11b)

The mobile unit is positioned to enable horizontal beam radiography necessary for the demonstration of fluid levels.

Position of patient and image receptor

- Depending on the patient's medical condition, the patient's bed is adjusted to enable the patient to adopt an erect or semi-erect position. If necessary, a number of pillows or an alternative supporting device is positioned behind the patient to aid stability.
- The patient's thighs are moved out of the beam to ensure that they are not superimposed on the image.
- A 35 × 43 cm CR cassette or a portable DDR detector with a stationary grid attached is placed against the posterior aspect of the patient, with the upper border of the image receptor positioned 2–3 cm above the xiphisternal joint to ensure that the diaphragm is included on the image to enable demonstration of free air in the peritoneal cavity.

Direction and location of the X-ray beam

- A collimated horizontal X-ray beam is directed to the centre of the image receptor using a 110 cm FRD that will avoid grid cut-off.

Antero-posterior supine (left lateral decubitus) (Figs 11.11c, 11.11d)

This projection, which uses a horizontal central ray, is selected as an alternative to the AP erect projection when the patient is unable to sit. It is also useful in demonstrating free air in the peritoneal cavity.

Position of patient and image receptor

- The patient is turned on to the left side, ideally for 20 minutes prior to the exposure, allowing any free air in the abdominal cavity to rise toward the right flank to avoid the problem of differential diagnosis when air is present on the left side of the abdomen within the region of the stomach.
- The grid and image receptor are supported vertically at right-angles to the horizontal central ray, and is positioned against the posterior aspect of the patient to include the right side of the diaphragm.

Direction and location of the X-ray beam

- A collimated horizontal X-ray beam is directed to the centre of a 35 × 43 cm CR cassette or portable DDR detector with a stationary grid attached.

11 Chest/upper abdomen

Lateral dorsal decubitus – supine (Figs 11.12a–11.12c)

This projection is selected as an alternative to the AP (left lateral decubitus) projection when the patient is too ill to move. It is also used to demonstrate calcification of the abdominal aorta. Abdominal aortic calcification is variable, even in the presence of an aneurysm, and in modern practice it would be more usual to perform ultrasound to assess the size of the aorta and the possibility of abdominal aneurysm. Ultrasound can be done in the emergency room. Computed tomography (CT) scanning offers a greater possibility of demonstrating leak from an aneurysm if the patient is sufficiently stable.

Position of patient and image receptor

- The mobile set is positioned so as to enable horizontal beam radiography.
- The patient lies supine and, if possible, is raised off the bed on to a supporting foam pad.
- The arms are extended and supported above the head.
- A stationary grid and image receptor are supported vertically against the lateral aspect of the abdomen and adjusted parallel to the median sagittal plane.
- The image should include the dome of the diaphragm, the anterior abdominal wall and the vertebral bodies.

Direction and location of the X-ray beam

- A collimated horizontal X-ray beam is directed to the centre of a 35 × 43 cm CR cassette or portable DDR detector.

Radiation protection

- The radiographer should stand at least 2 metres behind the X-ray tube.
- A mobile radiation protection barrier should be positioned behind the patient to confine the primary radiation field.

Notes

- Free air in the peritoneal cavity can sometimes be demonstrated on a conventional AP radiograph.
- In the example opposite, free gas is demonstrated by the presence of a double wall sign. In this image both the inside and outside of the bowel wall are seen, as compared with just the lumen side normally, as the result of air both within the lumen of bowel and free in the peritoneal cavity surrounding the section of bowel.
- Correct anatomical side and positional markers must be included on the image.

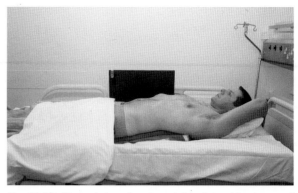

Fig. 11.12a The technique for a lateral dorsal decubitus image of the abdomen.

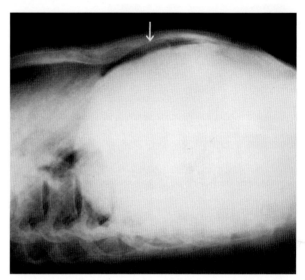

Fig. 11.12b Lateral dorsal decubitus image of the abdomen showing free air in the peritoneal cavity lying adjacent to the anterior abdominal wall.

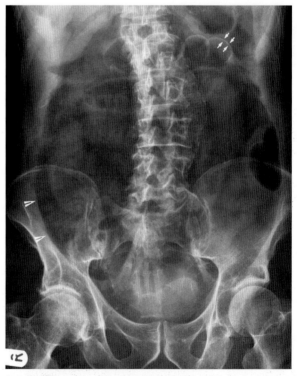

Fig. 11.12c AP radiograph of abdomen showing extensive free air in the peritoneal cavity (arrowheads) and double lumen effect demonstrated in left upper abdomen (arrows).

Cervical spine 11

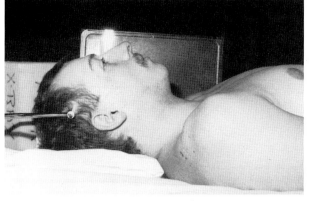

Fig. 11.13a Patient positioned for a lateral cervical spine projection.

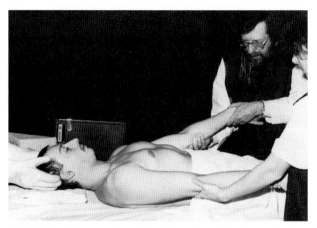

Fig. 11.13b Patient positioned for a lateral cervical spine projection with traction applied.

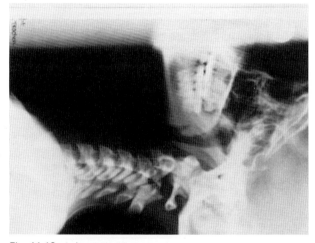

Fig. 11.13c 1 day on traction.

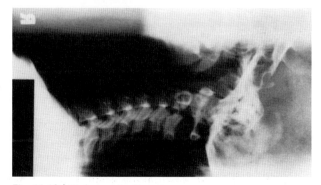

Fig. 11.13d 30 days on traction.

A patient with a spinal fracture dislocation is commonly nursed with skull traction and weights. This is applied by means of a skull calliper secured to the outer table of the parietal regions of the skull. Necessary weights in the early stages of traction may be more than those that are required to maintain realignment of the vertebrae. Traction is continued until there is consolidation.

Lateral projections of the cervical vertebrae, over several weeks, are necessary to assess the effectiveness of the traction and demonstrate the alignment of the vertebrae in relation to the spinal cord. Each radiograph is marked with the weight of the applied traction.

Lateral supine (Figs 11.13a–11.13d)

Position of patient and image receptor

- The mobile set is positioned so as to enable horizontal beam radiography.
- With the patient in the supine position, a 24 × 30 cm CR cassette or suitably sized portable DDR detector is supported vertically against the shoulder, parallel to the cervical vertebrae and centred at the level of the prominence of the thyroid cartilage.
- The image receptor is secured in position using a cassette holder or sandbags.
- The patient's shoulders must be depressed by the supervising clinician gripping the patient's wrists and pulling the arms caudally.

Direction and location of the X-ray beam

- A collimated horizontal X-ray beam is directed to a point vertically below the prominence of the thyroid cartilage at the level of the mastoid process through the 4th cervical vertebra.

Note

- In the radiographs opposite, part of the skull has been included on the image to show where the skull calliper is secured to the parietal regions.

Radiation protection

- A mobile radiation protection barrier should be positioned behind the patient to confine the primary radiation field.
- The person applying the traction must be medically supervised and wear a radiation protection lead-rubber apron and ensure that the X-ray beam is collimated to the area of interest.

11 Fractured lower limbs and pelvis

Orthopaedic radiography may be required to be undertaken on the ward immediately following surgery or following the application of traction. For the limbs, two radiographs are taken at right-angles to each other to check on the position and alignment of fractured bones. Examination of the patient will be made difficult if a suspension system is used, which will include weights and a metal pulley rope structure that is connected to the patient's bed. Great care should be exercised not to disturb these appliances, as they may disturb the position of the fractured bones and add to the patient's pain. A heavy patient may tend to sag into the mattress of the bed, which complicates matters when positioning for projections of the upper femur. The patient may be able to lift their bottom off the bed using the overhead hand grip so that a support pad or cassette tunnel device can be introduced under the buttocks.

Antero-posterior (Figs 11.14a–11.14d)

Position of patient and image receptor

- The mobile set is positioned carefully relative to any overhead bed supports, with adjustment being made with help of the nursing staff.
- A suitably sized image receptor is selected and carefully positioned under the femur or lower leg to include the joint nearest the fracture and as much of the upper or lower limb as possible to enable bone alignment to be assessed.
- The image receptor is supported parallel to the femur or lower limb by the use of non-opaque pads.
- For fractures of the neck of femur or pelvis, a careful process using slide sheets should be used to minimise disturbance to the patient. There are 'cassette tunnel devices' which may be used and only need one major disturbance to the patient. Once in position, an image receptor may be positioned without any further disruption to the patient. This also serves in aiding the positioning for the lateral projection when the patient is raised, allowing adequate demonstration of the femur.

Direction and location of the X-ray beam

- A collimated vertical X-ray beam is directed at right-angles to the middle of the image receptor with the central ray at right-angles to the long axis of the bones in question, in accordance with the techniques previously described in Section 4 Lower limb.

Note

Repeat examinations will be required over a period of time to assess the effectiveness of treatment; therefore, careful positioning and exposure selection are required to ensure that images are comparable. Exposures and adapted technique should be written down for future examinations.

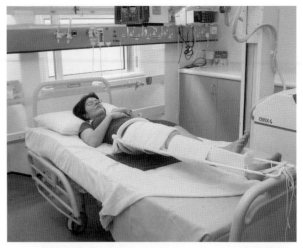

Fig. 11.14a Patient positioned for AP femur (hip down) following the application of a Thomas's splint.

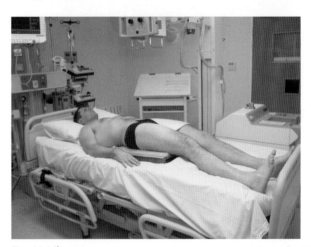

Fig. 11.14b Patient resting on a wooden cassette tunnel device for AP pelvis.

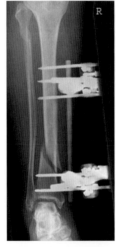

Fig. 11.14c AP image of tibia and fibula showing external fixation device.

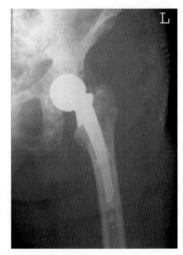

Fig. 11.14d AP post-operative image of hip joint following arthroplasty.

Radiation protection

- Radiation protection is particularly important and gonad shields should be used.
- A mobile radiation protection barrier should be positioned behind the patient when undertaking lateral projections.

Position of patient and image receptor

- The mobile X-ray equipment is carefully repositioned to enable horizontal beam radiography.
- When the examination is for the distal 2/3 of the femur, the image receptor may be positioned vertically against

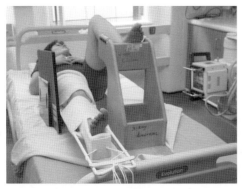

Fig. 11.15a Patient positioned for lateral femur (knee up) following the application of a Thomas's splint.

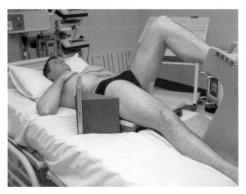

Fig. 11.15b Patient positioned for lateral hip with pelvis raised resting on a cassette tunnel device.

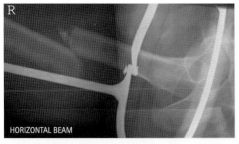

Fig. 11.15c Lateral image of a right fractured femur in a Thomas's splint.

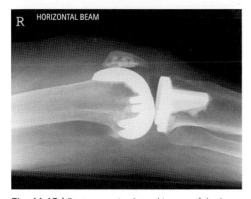

Fig. 11.15d Post-operative lateral image of the knee using a horizontal beam following joint replacement.

Fractured femur 11

Lateral (Figs 11.15a–11.15c)

the medial side of the thigh and the horizontal beam directed latero-medially.

- When the proximal part of the shaft or the neck of the femur is being examined, the image receptor is positioned vertically against the lateral side of the thigh and the beam is directed medio-laterally, with the opposite leg raised on a suitable support so that the unaffected thigh is in a near-vertical position.
- For the neck of femur, a stationary grid and image receptor are positioned vertically, with one edge against the waist above the iliac crest on the side being examined and adjusted with its long axis parallel to the neck of femur.
- To demonstrate fractures of the upper femur, it is essential that the patient is raised off the bed on a suitable rigid structure, such as a firm foam pad or a cassette tunnel device.

Direction and location of the X-ray beam

- For the neck of femur a collimated X-ray beam is directed to the distal 2/3 of the femur, the horizontal central ray is centred to the middle of the stationary grid and image receptor and parallel to a line joining the anterior borders of the femoral condyles.
- To demonstrate the neck of femur, which will include the hip joint, a collimated X-ray beam is directed midway between the femoral pulse and the palpable prominence of the greater trochanter, with the central ray directed horizontally and at right-angles to the detector.

Note

When using a stationary grid, it is essential that the image receptor remains vertical to avoid grid cut-off.

Arthroplasty postoperative radiography (Fig. 11.15d)

An AP projection of the hip is taken within 24 hours of surgery to include the upper 1/3 of the femur to demonstrate the prosthesis and the cement restrictor, which is distal to the prosthesis. This may be highlighted by a radio-opaque marker in the form of a ball-bearing, which should appear in all subsequent follow-up images of the hip joint if it has been used.

Loosening of the prosthesis can occur by impaction of the femoral shaft of the prosthesis into the native femur. This is detected most easily by observing a reduction in the distance between the cement restrictor and the tip of the prosthesis. It is therefore most important that the first image includes the cement restrictor. The patient management is also determined on confirmation that the hip joint has not dislocated.

AP and lateral projections are again often acquired of the knee joint the day following knee joint replacement.

11 Paediatric (gallows traction)

This type of traction is used on children from birth to 12 months. Two projections, AP and lateral, are taken to assess bone alignment and new bone formation. The application of gonad protection and careful collimation of the X-ray beam are essential. Great care should be exercised to avoid disturbing the traction; however, it is still usually possible to maintain traction and rotate the child so that the front of the suspended legs are facing the side of the cot, which can be lowered during exposure to avoid superimposition of the cot's vertical bars.

Antero-posterior (Figs 11.16a, 11.16c)

Position of patient and image receptor

- The child lies supine, with both legs suspended vertically, an image receptor is supported against the posterior aspect of the affected leg using foam pads or an L-shaped plastic image receptor support device.
- The image receptor is positioned to enable full coverage of the femur, including the knee and hip joints.

Direction and location of the X-ray beam

- A collimated horizontal X-ray beam is directed to the middle of the anterior aspect of the femur and at right-angles to the image receptor.

Lateral (Figs 11.16b, 11.16d)

Position of patient and image receptor

- To avoid superimposition of the unaffected femur, the sound limb is carefully removed from the traction by the medical officer and held in a position outside the radiation beam.
- Alternatively, the traction may be adjusted and the sound limb supported temporarily in a different position.
- The medical officer or health professional must wear a lead-rubber apron and lead-rubber gloves.
- An image receptor is supported vertically against the lateral aspect of the affected leg and adjusted parallel to the femur.

Direction and location of the X-ray beam

A collimated horizontal X-ray beam is directed to the middle of the medial aspect of the femur and at right-angles to the image receptor.

Note

- Correct anatomical side marker must be included on the image.

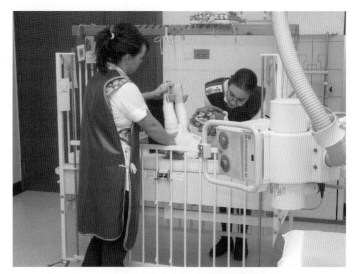

Fig. 11.16a Child in the process of being positioned for AP femur.

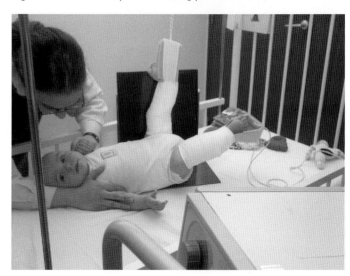

Fig. 11.16b Child in the process of being positioned for lateral femur.

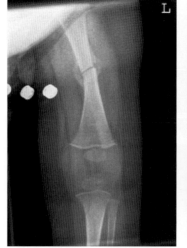
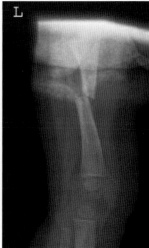

Fig. 11.16c and d AP (left) and lateral (right) images of left femur 2 weeks post trauma.

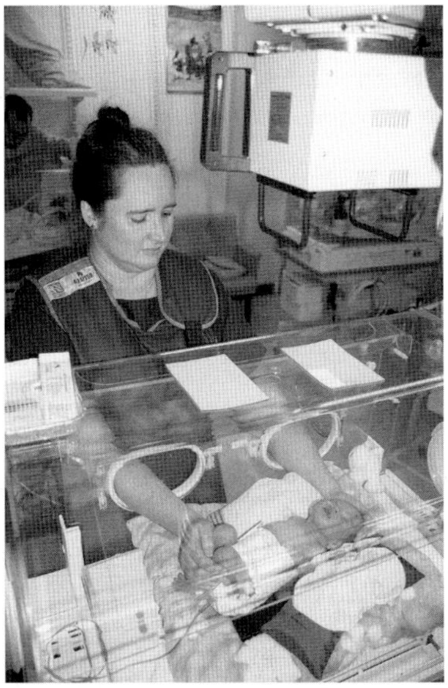

Heart and lungs – special care baby unit 11

The baby will be nursed in an incubator and may be attached to a ventilator. The primary beam is directed through the incubator top, with care being taken to avoid any opacity or cutouts in the incubator top falling within the radiation beam.

Different designs of incubators are available, with many requiring the image receptor to be placed within the incubator. However, a number are designed to facilitate positioning of the image receptor on a special tray immediately below and outside the incubator housing.

Antero-posterior (Figs 11.17a–11.17d)

When placing the image receptor inside the incubator an 18 × 24 cm CR cassette or suitably sized DDR receptor that has just been cleaned and is at room temperature is used. Disposable sheets should also be placed between the baby and the receptor.

Position of patient and image receptor

- The baby is positioned supine on the receptor with the median sagittal plane adjusted perpendicular to the middle of the receptor ensuring that the head and chest are straight with shoulders and hips being level.
- The head may need a sandbag for support on either side.
- A 10° covered foam pad should be placed under the shoulders to lift the chin and to avoid it obscuring the lung apices.
- Arms should be on either side, slightly abducted from the trunk to avoid being included in the radiation field.
- Arms can be immobilised with Velcro bands and/or small sandbags.
- Baby requiring holding- see page 435.

Direction and location of the X-ray beam

- The vertical collimated beam is centred in the midline just below the level of the axillary folds (intermammillary line).
- Consistent maximum FRD should be used.
- Although some incubators have cassette trays placing the cassette under the baby is recommended as routine, to avoid magnification and change of exposure factors.

Notes

- Very short exposure times are required for these procedures and modern equipment can deliver an exposure time as low as 0.003 seconds.
- Lead-rubber can be applied on the top of the incubator to the edges of the X-ray beam to enhance collimation.
- Optimised exposure factor details should be recorded for subsequent imaging, with positioning legends recorded on the image to allow comparisons with future images.

Fig. 11.17a Baby positioned for AP chest and abdomen.

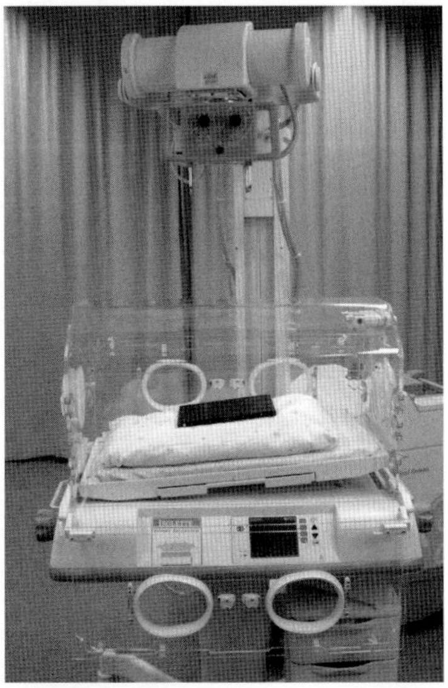

Fig. 11.17b Equipment positioned for an AP chest demonstrating angulation of the incubator tray.

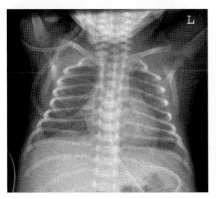

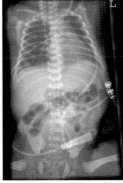

Fig. 11.17c AP supine image of the chest in a neonate of 28 weeks gestation.

Fig. 11.17d AP supine image of the chest and abdomen showing position of an arterial line, which has been enhanced using contrast media.

A full account of neonatal radiography is given in Section 13.

Neonates suffering from respiratory distress syndrome are examined soon after birth to demonstrate the lungs, which are immature and unable to perform normal respiration.

Section 12
Theatre Radiography

CONTENTS

INTRODUCTION	406
Key skills	406
Radiation protection	407
Sterile areas/infection control	408
Equipment	408
NON-TRAUMA ORTHOPAEDIC SURGERY	409
TRAUMA ORTHOPAEDIC SURGERY	410
DYNAMIC HIP SCREW INSERTION	413
Imaging procedure	413
Surgical procedure	414
INTERVENTIONAL PROCEDURES	415
Retrograde pyelography	415
Percutaneous nephrolithotomy	416
OPERATIVE CHOLANGIOGRAPHY	417
Imaging procedure	417
PAIN MANAGEMENT	418
Introduction	418
Imaging procedure	418
EMERGENCY PERIPHERAL VASCULAR PROCEDURES	419
Introduction	419
Imaging procedure	419

12 Introduction

Theatre radiography plays a significant role in the delivery of surgical services. The following settings are typical examples where the radiographer is required:

- Aid in the diagnostic or therapeutic pathway of the patient.
- Demonstrate the location/position of anatomy/surgical equipment.
- Pins and plates.
- Interventional catheters.
- Guide the positioning of equipment.
- Dynamic screwing.
- Kyphoplasty.
- Demonstrate function.
- Arthrogram.
- Dynamic movement.
- Trauma surgery.
- Interventional procedures.
- Emergency peripheral vascular procedures, e.g. stent insertion; however, this may be performed in dedication X-ray suites.

Key skills

Radiographers should consider themselves part of the inter-professional team in theatre and communicate effectively with other healthcare professionals and the nursing staff. The radiographer must be familiar with the layout and protocols associated with the theatre to which they are assigned. They should demonstrate a working knowledge of the duties of each person in the operating theatre, and ascertain the specific requirements of the surgeon who is operating.

They should be comfortable discussing the procedure and image appearance with the surgeon to be able to locate anatomical landmarks or the position of guide wires and surgical instruments.

Key skills for theatre include:[1]

- How to use the equipment correctly.
- Effective communication.
- Personal preparation.
- Safe practice.
- Production of diagnostic images.
- Radiation protection of the staff and patients.
- Infection control.
- Team working.

Effective use of equipment

- A mobile X-ray unit or mobile image intensifier (II) is selected depending upon the requirement of the radiographic procedure. For example, a mobile X-ray unit may be used for plain chest radiography or a mobile image fluoroscopy unit for the screening of orthopaedic procedures, such as hip pinning.
- For the prevention of infection, the unit selected should be cleaned and dried after each patient. Where appropriate protective plastic coverings can be used to reduce blood contamination during surgical procedures. When blood or other bodily fluids do come into contact with the imaging equipment, an appropriate cleaning solution e.g. Haztab should be used.
- Before the procedure an image intensifier should be connected to picture archiving and communication system (PACS) if available, assembled and tested ahead of the procedure to ensure that it is functioning effectively prior to patient positioning. The field of irradiation should be collimated to the predicted area of interest.
- Patient demographics entered on the PACS system and exposure parameters are adjusted to those required for screening or image recording. Ideally half-dose or pulsed settings should be used to minimise the radiation dose.
- Equipment is covered in sterile covers if required (Fig. 12.1).

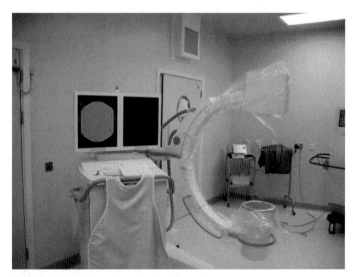

Fig. 12.1 Image intensifier prepared ready for the procedure.

Effective communication

The radiographer must communicate effectively with the theatre staff before, during and after the theatre procedure. The key to a stress-free experience is preparation. It is essential that there is a mechanism for theatre staff to communicate effectively and give the radiographer prior notice of all cases requiring their attendance. This enables the radiographer to arrive early, change into their theatre clothes and justify the request card prior to the start of the procedure.

Important checklist

Personal preparation is the first concern of the radiographer prior to entering an aseptic controlled area.

The uniform and any jewellery is removed and replaced by theatre wear. The hair is completely covered with a disposable hat. Theatre shoes or boots are worn and a facemask is put on (when required). In addition, a dose-monitoring badge is pinned to theatre garments.

Special attention is made to washing the hands using soap, ensuring that the hands are washed prior to and after each patient. If the skin has an abrasion this should be covered with a waterproof dressing.

Before the procedure the radiographer should determine:

- The procedure(s) being undertaken and the surgeon operating, as surgeons may have variable requirements.
- The equipment required and the preparation necessary for the procedure.
- The patient demographics so they can be entered on the Radiology information system (RIS)/PACS and imaging equipment.
- Open the patient's folder with the patient's previous images/reports for the surgeon to view.

Time out

It is now common practice in operating theatres to call a 'time out'[2] with the operating team before the operation starts. The procedure is used to stop any errors being made in the procedure and discuss any issues or anticipated safety concerns, e.g. patient allergies or anticipated complications. The following areas are checked in the presence of the surgeon, operating nurse, anaesthetist and radiographer. It is usual to have the signed consent form from the patient and a wristband on the patient as a reference point. Pre-operative checks include:

- Patient identification.
- Signed consent for the procedure.
- The operation being undertaken and the relevant anatomical side.
- Methicillin resistant *Staphylococcus aureus* MRSA check.
- Pregnancy check if appropriate.
- Previous radiographic images on PACS.

The radiographer has a duty:

- To ensure the image required is displayed appropriately on the monitor, the surgeon can see the monitor clearly and the image quality is maintained.

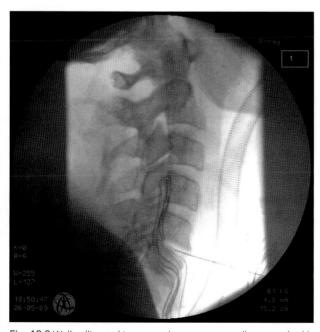

Fig. 12.2 Well collimated image to demonstrate needle at vertebral level C5/C6.

Introduction 12

Key skills (*cont.*)

- To provide effective radiation protection of all staff (only necessary staff should be present when screening).
- To know when the examination is concluded so they can leave the theatre and what follow up is required for the patient.

After the procedure the radiographer will take steps to:

- Record radiation dose information.
- Ensure images are recorded on PACS.
- Ensure the imaging equipment and protective clothing is cleaned and stored away effectively.

Radiation protection

Radiation protection is the responsibility of the radiographer operating the X-ray equipment. Therefore, the radiographer should ensure that radiation monitoring badges, lead protective aprons and thyroid shields are worn by all staff when in the controlled area (2 metres from the X-ray tube). Furthermore, as soon as the imaging equipment is switched on, a controlled area exists.[3] Therefore, all doors, which have access to the controlled area, must display radiation warning signs and personnel not required must leave the theatre (see Fig. 12.3c).

- Patient identification must be confirmed with either the Anaesthetist or an appropriate member of the theatre team, prior to commencement of image acquisition or the patient if they are awake.
- The radiographer should not be surprised if the surgeon wants to screen whilst rotating the limb or during a dynamic screwing. Fluoroscopy is a dynamic process and if plain images are adequate it would be better to use a digital mobile X-ray unit as the image quality is better.
- Intelligent collimation to the area of interest when using fluoroscopy will reduce radiation dose and scatter to improve image quality (Fig. 12.2).
- The inverse square law principle must be applied in the theatre environment. Therefore, staff must be standing at the maximum distance from the source of radiation, and outside the path of the radiation field during exposure.
- The radiographer must minimise the dose to the patient and staff by use of dose-saving facilities (half-dose/pulsed beam) and minimise fluoroscopy times. Fluoroscopy should only be undertaken when the surgeon indicates that it is required and following further surgical intervention, i.e. to check the position of a needle inserted into a joint space.
- The radiographer must give clear instructions to staff before any exposures are made regarding their role to reduce the risk of accidental exposure.
- It is a legal requirement to record the screening time and radiation dose for each patient examination. This should be regularly monitored to ensure the doses are as low as reasonably practicable.

12 Introduction

Sterile areas/infection control

Equipment used in operating theatres must be kept clean and stored in the theatre environment. It must be cleaned regularly and prior to and after every case. The radiographer should dress in scrubs, wear approved footwear, theatre hats and masks if required. Not all theatre cases require full sterile protection so the equipment should be protected appropriately and covered to protect the patient from infection and the equipment from damage.

Where a sterile procedure is required and in all invasive procedures where the skin is pierced, the mobile fluoroscopy unit must be covered appropriately by sterile plastic coverings or drapes. Sterile procedures are an everyday occurrence for the theatre staff so their help and guidance can easily be sought.

The radiographer should avoid the contamination of sterile areas. Ideally, equipment should be positioned before any sterile towels are placed in position, and care should be exercised not to touch sterile areas when positioning the C-arm or moving equipment during the operation unless it is draped (Figs 12.3a, 12.3b).

Darkroom facilities/PACS connectivity

If using screen/film systems to record a permanent image the film will need to be processed using chemical processing. Unless there is a substantial workload the film should be processed in the main department as developing film occasionally will lead to poor processing of the image or a need to change the chemistry too frequently to make the process economical.

Modern hospitals do not use screen/film for theatre but have direct connectivity to the RIS and PACS in the radiology department. The patient is imaged digitally and sent to the appropriate patient folder. There may be the facility to record images from the monitor using thermal transparency film. Thermal film is not light sensitive so may be loaded in daylight and records directly from the primary monitor via a screen 'grab' process. Images on the secondary monitor need to be transferred to the primary one before recording can take place.

Accessory equipment

All accessory equipment should ideally be stored and used only in the theatre environment. The radiographer must be familiar with the accessory equipment and its function.

Equipment

A mobile X-ray unit or mobile II/solid state detector is selected depending upon the requirement of the radiographic procedure. For example:

- A mobile X-ray unit may be used for plain image chest radiography postoperatively.
- A mobile image intensifier for the screening of orthopaedic procedures, e.g.:
  - Open reduction and internal fixation (ORIF).
  - Dynamic hip pinning.

- For the prevention of infection, the unit selected should be cleaned and dried after each patient. Where appropriate protective plastic coverings can be used to reduce blood contamination during surgical procedures. When blood or other bodily fluids do come into contact with the imaging equipment, an appropriate cleaning solution, e.g. Haztab should be used.
- Before use, an image intensifier should be assembled and tested ahead of the procedure to ensure that it is functioning effectively prior to patient positioning.
- Exposure parameters are then adjusted to those required for screening or image recording on image receptor.

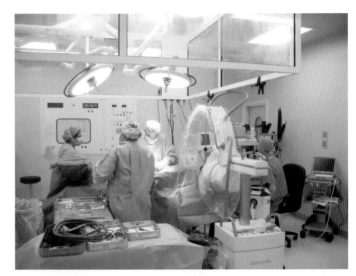

Fig. 12.3a Image intensifier draped for surgery.

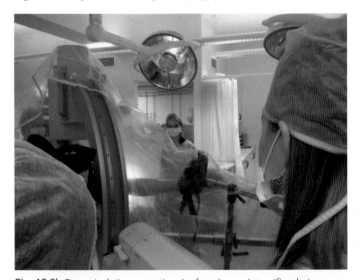

Fig. 12.3b Drape isolating operative site from image intensifier during orthopaedic hip surgery.

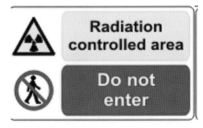

Fig. 12.3c Radiation protection sign.

Non-trauma orthopaedic surgery 12

The radiographer plays a significant role as part of the orthopaedic theatre team, where imaging control is required for an operative procedure.

Fluoroscopic imaging during the procedure is most frequently required to aid in trauma orthopaedic surgery. However, in a small number of cases it is also required for non-trauma corrective orthopaedic surgery. In both instances however, the radiographer will be required to work in a theatre environment primarily using a mobile C-arm image intensifier/solid state detector, equipped with an image memory device (Fig. 12.4a).

There is currently an endless list of non-trauma corrective orthopaedic procedures being performed throughout the world. The majority of these involve the replacement of joints as a result of chronic bone or joint disease.

For example severe osteoarthritis (OA) of the hip can be corrected using the implantation of a prosthetic total hip joint replacement. These procedures however no longer require the aid of imaging control due to the advancements of surgical techniques. Nevertheless, more complex paediatric operative procedures do require imaging control, namely osteotomies, which are carried out in order to correct defects in bone and joint alignment. Such procedures vary in complexity in terms of corrective surgery and will involve the use of fixation plates (Fig. 12.4b).

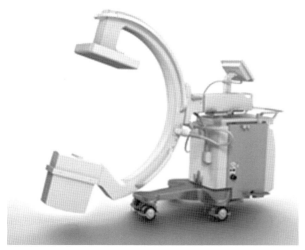

Fig. 12.4a Example of a mobile fluoroscopy unit – solid state detector.

Common corrective orthopaedic operative procedures include:

Pathology	Operative procedure
• Congenital dislocation of the hip (CDH) • Perthes disease • Hip dysphasia	• Salter pelvic osteotomy
• Persistent femoral antiversion	• Deviation femoral osteotomy
• Vargus deformity of the knee	• Proximal tibial osteotomy

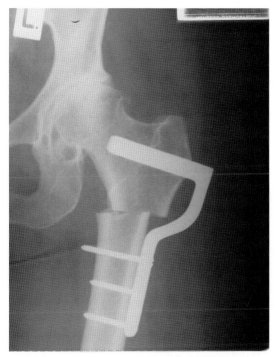

Fig. 12.4b Example of hip osteotomy.

12 Trauma orthopaedic surgery

As described, some orthopaedic surgical procedures are necessary to correct growth defects in bone and joint alignment. However, the majority of the radiographer's workload in the theatre environment will focus on trauma orthopaedic surgery, assisting in the:

- Successful reduction of fractures (Figs 12.5a–12.5c).
- Implantation and removal of internal or external fixing devices.

There are various trauma orthopaedic procedures where radiographic imaging is required. The adjacent table provides examples of familiar trauma operative procedures in relation to fracture types. Image examples and important factors to note during the imaging procedure are provided on this and subsequent pages.

In addition, a more extensive explanation of the typical dynamic hip screw (DHS) surgical and imaging procedure can be found on page 413.

Common trauma orthopaedic operative procedures

Fracture type	Operative procedure
Hip fractures	
INTRACAPSULAR	
• Sub-capital or transcervical – displaced.	• Reduction and internal fixation
• Sub-capital or transcervical – undisplaced	• Femoral head replacement
	• Cancellous hip screws
EXTRACAPSULAR	
• Intertrochanteric or basal fractures	• DHS or gamma nail
• Sub-trochanteric fractures	• DCS or gamma nail
Fractures of the upper & lower extremities	
• Simple fractures of the fingers, hands, wrists, elbow and feet	• MUA
	• Kirschner ('K') wire insertion
• Complicated fractures of the ankle, elbow, wrist and forearm	• ORIF with compression plates & screws
• Comminuted fracture	
	• External fixation
• Open fractures of the tibia or femur with significant soft tissue involvement	• External fixation
	• Unreamed intramedullary nail insertion with proximal and/or distal locking
• Closed fractures of the tibia or femur	• Reamed intramedullary nail insertion with proximal and/or distal locking
• Fractures of the humerus	• Intramedullary rod
• Olecranon & patella fracture/displacement following trauma	• Tension band wiring

DCS, dynamic condylar screw; DHS, dynamic hip screw; MUA, manipulation under anaesthetic, ORIF, open reduction and internal fixation.

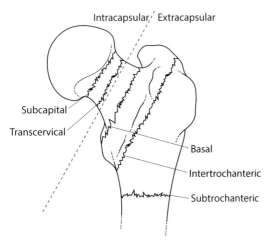

Fig. 12.5a Diagram illustrating types of intracapsular and extracapsular hip fractures.

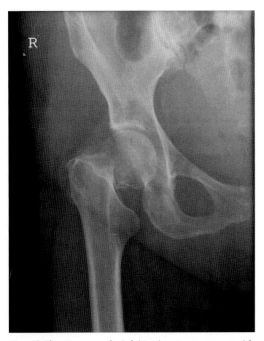

Fig. 12.5b AP image of a left hip showing transcervical fracture.

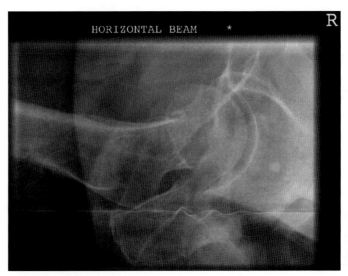

Fig. 12.5c Lateral image of a left hip showing impacted subcapital fracture.

Trauma orthopaedic surgery 12

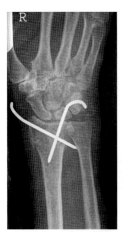 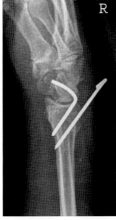

Figs 12.6a and b Examples of Kirschner wire insertion.

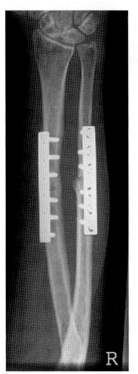 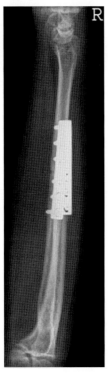

Figs 12.6c and d Examples of internal plates and screws following an open reduction and internal fixation (ORIF).

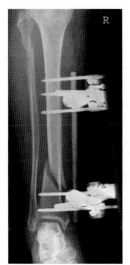 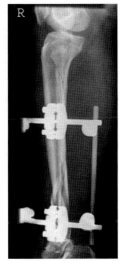

Figs 12.6e and f Examples of external fixation of the tibia and fibula.

The Kirschner wire insertion is performed mostly in corrective simple fracture extremity surgery. It is important to ensure when positioning the image intensifier for this surgical procedure, that the C-arm is rotated through 180°, therefore, placing the affected limb closest to the detector as this reduces magnification and improving image quality.

Open reduction and internal fixations (ORIFs) are performed mostly in complicated fractures where the fracture cannot be satisfactorily held by any other means, i.e. mid-shaft forearm fractures can be stabilised using compression plates and screws. Again the image intensifier must be positioned with the affected limb closest to the detector allowing minimum magnification and distortion of the image. This also facilitates the surgeon ease of movement when positioning for both the AP and lateral images.

Imaging control is often required at the beginning of the operation and at the end of this procedure as the surgeon can often visualise the fracture site during the operation and can directly visualise the fracture and fixation devices (Figs 12.6a–12.6d).

Hints and tips

- Intelligent collimation to the area of interest with reduce scatter and improve image quality.
- If repeated images are being taken with movement of the limb between the AP and lateral it may be a good idea to draw a big X on the drapes at the centre of the 'field of view'. This helps repositioning and avoids missing the area of interest.
- External fixation and Steinmann pin insertions for traction, often require imaging control to visualise the progress of the surgical procedure. Various external fixators are in use from the Ilizarov (ring fixator) to the AO (Arbeitsgemeinschaft für Osteosynthesefragen) tubular system. In either instance, image guidance is often required to demonstrate the true position of the screw or pin during surgical positioning and to aid in the reduction/manipulation of the fracture site when the fixator is in place (Figs 12.6e, 12.6f).
- Tension band wirings like ORIFs, are essentially an open surgical procedure. In these instances imaging control to assist the surgeon is often kept to a minimum and is upon his/her request (Figs 12.6g, 12.6h).

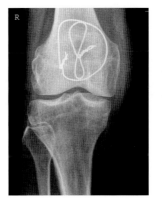 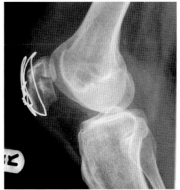

Figs 12.6g and h Example of tension band wiring.

12 Trauma orthopaedic surgery

Intramedullary nailing requires intermittent imaging control throughout the majority of the surgical procedure, not only to assist the surgeon in visualising the nail as it passes through the medulla of the long bone but more importantly to assist in the proximal and distal locking of the nail with cortex screws.

During the proximal and/or distal locking of the surgical procedure, the radiographer must aim to image the nail within the medulla of the long bone demonstrating the circular holes within the nail en.face, thus allowing the surgeon to insert the cortex screws with ease (Figs 12.7a–12.7d).

Hints and tips

To minimise magnification:

- Keep the X-ray tube as far away from the patient as possible to minimise magnification.
- Keep the image detector (II or solid state detector) as close to the patient as possible.
- Ensure you can image the patient in both the AP and lateral projection with minimal changes to the C-arm, e.g. without altering the height.
- Keep screening doses to a minimum and only image the patient if the surgeon has made a significant change to the procedure, e.g. inserted the nail further into the limb.
- Remember to save the previous image and transfer to the secondary screen when changing from an AP to lateral projection.
- Laser guidance facilities are available on some image intensifiers to assist in this procedure; unfortunately the theatre light need to be extinguished to see the laser lights.

Mean effective doses from orthopaedic procedures

Procedure	Mean effective dose (mSv)	Equivalent number of PA chest radiographs (each 0.02 mSv)
Knee[4]	0.005	0.25
Shoulder[4]	0.01	0.5
Arthrograph[5]	0.17	8.5
Cervical Spine[4]	0.2	10
Lumbosacral joint[5]	0.34	17
Pelvis[4]	0.6	30
Hip[4]	0.7	35
Thoracic aortography[5]	4.1	205

Cancellous hip screws are used mostly for undisplaced subcapital or transcervical fractures. The imaging procedure for this technique is similar to the DHS procedure, which will be discussed in more detail in the following section (Figs 12.7e, 12.7f).

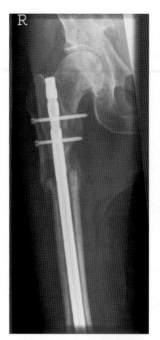
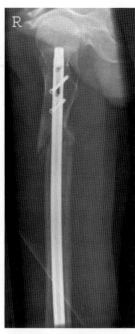

Figs 12.7a and b Examples of an intramedullary nail insertion of the femur (hip down).

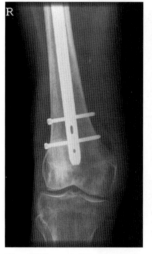
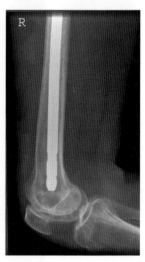

Figs 12.7c and d Examples of an intramedullary nail insertion of the femur (knee up) showing distal locking.

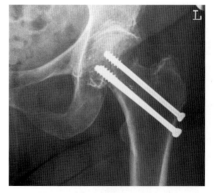
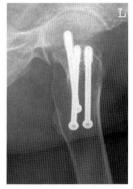

Figs 12.7e and f Example of cancellous screws in different patients.

Dynamic hip screw insertion 12

The procedure described for a dynamic hip screw (DHS) insertion is typical of that employed in an orthopaedic theatre. Surgeons, however, use a variety of approaches, and the radiographer should be aware of the technique employed in their own hospital.

The technique described employs the use of a sterile protective barrier, which separates the image intensifier from the surgeon and the operative field.

During the operative procedure images of the hip and neck of femur are taken at right-angles at various stages. Care should be taken therefore when moving the imaging intensifier into these required imaging positions to ensure that the sterile field is not comprised.

Imaging procedure

A mobile C-arm image intensifier/digital detector is preferred for this procedure as it provides a real-time image to assist the surgeon in positioning the guide wire and subsequent DHS internal fixator. Ideally, all equipment in use should be equipped with a memory device that gives an immediate play-back of the image last seen on the screen.

Using a system equipped with a memory device helps reduce the radiation dose to the patient, as the surgeon is able to study an image without further irradiating the patient. Furthermore, it also allows storage of the last image so that comparisons can be made of any alterations to the position and direction of the guide wire or DHS. In addition, hard copy images can be taken at the end of the operation to help demonstrate the completed procedure and act as a permanent record of the procedure.

Before the operation commences, the patient, whilst anaesthetised is transferred to a special orthopaedic operating table with leg supports. The patient is positioned with the unaffected leg raised, flexed and in abduction, and the affected leg extended and in medial rotation. Traction is applied to the affected limb enabling manipulation and alignment of the fracture site.

At this stage the mobile image intensifier/digital detector is positioned to enable screening of the hip in both the PA and lateral directions. The long axis of the C-arm is positioned between the patient's legs and adjacent to the unaffected limb, enabling the C-arm to be rotated through 90°, parallel to the neck of the femur. Once positioned correctly the image intensifier is locked into position and checked to ensure that the C-arm rotates freely from the PA to lateral screening positions and that the femoral neck is imaged in the middle of the image intensifier face (Figs 12.8a, 12.8b).

As the C-arm is positioned on the opposite side of the sterile protective barrier a sterile cover over is not required. However, a plastic protective cover is placed over the X-ray tube housing to protect the tube covering in the event of blood spillage from the operative site.

During the surgical/imaging procedure the radiographer makes appropriate alterations to exposure factors and orientation controls. A record is made of the total screening time and radiation dose employed during the operation.

It is important to note at this stage, that a device similar to 'Sampath's clock face' can prove to be an invaluable tool to assist the radiographer in the orientation process (Figs 12.8c, 12.8d).

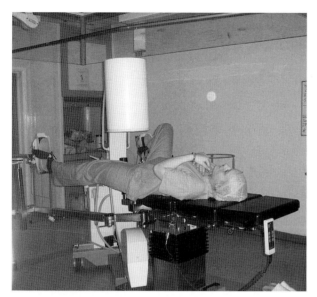

Fig. 12.8a Image intensifier and theatre table with II in PA position.

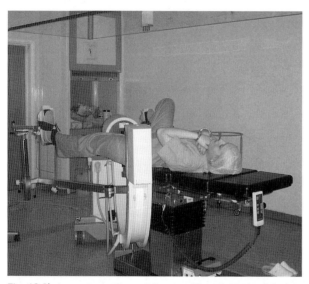

Fig. 12.8b Image intensifier and theatre table with II in lateral position.

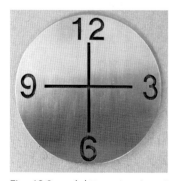
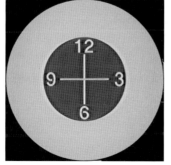

Figs 12.8c and d Examples of a radio-opaque clock device used for orientation of an image intensifier and an X-ray image of the device.

12 Dynamic hip screw insertion

Surgical procedure

The diagrams opposite illustrate the typical images that are acquired during an operative procedure using the DHS.

For this procedure a DHS guide wire and angle guide are first required. The guide wire is positioned through the centre of the neck of femur and an appropriate triple reamer is placed over the guide wire to allow a channel to be reamed for the insertion of a lag screw. When the channel is completed, the lag screw is inserted with the threaded tip lying approximately 10 mm from the joint surface. A DHS plate is then placed over the distal end of the lag screw assembly and positioned until it is in contact with the lateral cortex of the proximal femur. Cortex screws are then used to secure the DHS plate in position.

The diagrams (Figs 12.9a–12.9d) demonstrate:

- The reduced fracture.
- The fracture reduced with the angle guide and guide wire during positioning.
- The reaming of a channel prior to the insertion of the lag screw.
- Insertion of the lag screw and DHS plate.
- Completed operation with a DHS inserted to stabilise the fracture site.

As outlined earlier, there are a variety of other operative procedures for the treatment of intertrochanteric and femoral neck fractures. Common to each technique adopted, is the placing of guide wires along the femoral neck and into the head of the femur, prior to the insertion of screws or securing plates.

Whist acquisition of images during these operative procedures is a dynamic process, with images acquired at each stage in the PA and lateral planes, permanent images are recorded at the end of the procedure and transferred onto PACS (Figs 12.9e, 12.9f).

These images are best acquired using the image intensifier/solid state memory device as this reduces radiation dose to the patient and staff. It is important however, that the hip joint and proximal end of the femur are demonstrated to ensure that the full extent of fixation plates, wires or screws can be seen on these images.

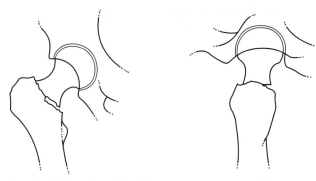

Fig. 12.9a PA and lateral hip diagram showing a reduced fracture.

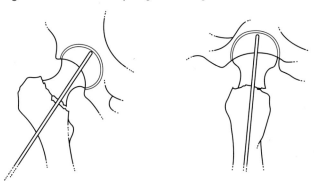

Fig. 12.9b PA and lateral hip diagram showing a guide wire positioned through the centre of the neck of the femur.

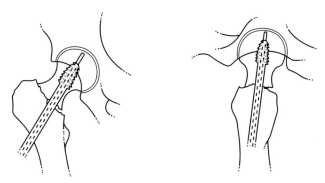

Fig. 12.9c PA and lateral hip diagram showing insertion of the lag screw.

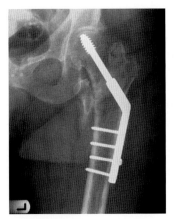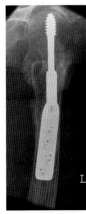

Figs 12.9e and f AP and lateral images of the hip demonstrating a DHS implant.

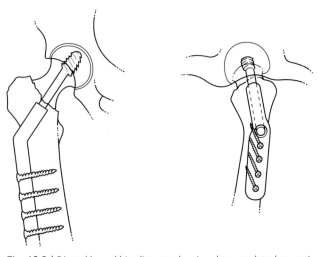

Fig. 12.9d PA and lateral hip diagram showing the completed operation with lag screw and DHS plate secured in position.

Interventional procedures 12

Interventional urology plays an important role in the theatre setting, particularly for those patients who require general anaesthesia. Patients who undergo the following procedures are typical examples:

- Retrograde pyelography.
- Percutaneous nephrolithotomy.

Retrograde pyelography (Figs 12.10a–12.10d)

Retrograde pyelography, also known as ascending pyelography, involves a mechanical filling procedure to demonstrate the renal calyces and pelvis with a suitable organic iodine contrast agent.

Cystoscopy is first performed to locate a catheter in the affected kidney. A mobile C-arm image intensifier/solid state detector and a radiolucent theatre table suitable for cystoscopy are usually selected for this procedure. Combined, this selection provides a real-time image to the surgeon of the flow of contrast media through the ureter and pelvi–calyceal system whilst simultaneously allowing cystoscopy to be performed.

Imaging procedure

- The patient is positioned supine. The mobile C-arm is positioned at 90° to the patient to provide a PA projection of the abdomen. The patient is positioned on the table and the manoeuvrability of the C-arm is assessed prior to commencement of surgery, ensuring full visualisation of the urinary tract is feasible without collision with the table's main support pillar.
- During fluoroscopy, 5–20 ml of 150 mg I/ml strength contrast agent is introduced via the ureteric catheter into the affected renal pelvis.
- Permanent images are acquired of the contrast filled calyces and ureters, using the last image hold facility or using a single exposure technique.
- The catheter is withdrawn using fluoroscopy to observe the emptying of the contrast into the bladder.
- Images are acquired as and when required by the surgeon to record any abnormalities.

Notes

This procedure may be undertaken in the imaging department as part of a two staged procedure with the patient having had the cystoscopy in theatre under anaesthetic first.

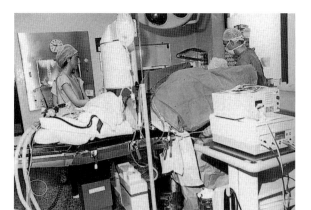

Fig. 12.10a The procedure in theatre.

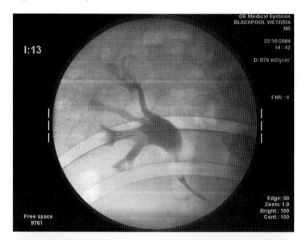

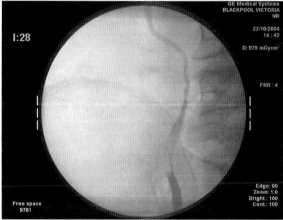

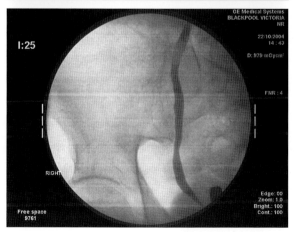

Figs 12.10b–d A contrast filled collecting system and ureter acquired using a mobile C-arm intensifier and digital image capture device.

12 Interventional procedures

Percutaneous nephrolithotomy

Percutaneous nephrolithotomy (PCNL) is an interventional procedure used to remove renal stones directly via a nephrostomy tract.

A mobile C-arm and a radiolucent theatre table suitable for cystoscopy are usually selected for this procedure. Combined, this selection provides a real-time image to the surgeon of the flow of contrast media through the urinary system whilst simultaneously allowing cystoscopy to be performed. Small stones less than 1 cm that have proved unsuitable for treatment by lithotripsy are removed by special instruments in conjunction with cystoscopy. Larger stones, e.g. staghorn calculus, require first to be disintegrated by electrohydraulic lithotripsy or ultrasound shock waves (Fig. 12.11a).

Imaging procedure (Figs 12.11b–12.11d)

With the patient supine on the operating table for cystoscopy, a retrograde catheter is placed in the renal pelvis or upper ureter on the affected side. This facilitates contrast medium (150 mg I/ml) or methylene blue solution to be injected into the renal pelvis throughout the procedure. The patient is then carefully turned into the prone oblique position, with the affected side uppermost.

After opacification of the collecting system with contrast and methylene blue solution, the posterior calyx of the lower calyceal group is punctured with an 18-gauge needle cannula. Imaging is frequently performed during this procedure with the C-arm vertical and angled obliquely across the long axis of the body to aid localisation of the kidney.

Following removal of the central needle and aspiration of the mixture of urine, contrast and methylene blue to ensure accurate position within the collection system, a soft J-wire and then a stiff wire are passed in an antegrade manner into the kidney. The tract is then dilated up to a 30F size (1 cm) using either a series of plastic dilators or alternatively a combination of dilators and a dilation balloon. A 1 cm sheath is then placed over the largest dilator or dilated balloon directly into the renal pelvis.

A nephroscope, with its light source, is passed through the sheath to visualise the collecting system and facilitate the passing of instruments required to disintegrate and remove the calculus. During the procedure an irrigation system, incorporated into the nephroscope, will wash clear any calculus fragments from the renal pelvis. Attention should be paid that any access water from this process does not come in contact with the image intensifier.

At the end of the procedure a 6F pigtail catheter is left in the renal pelvis to allow antegrade drainage of the kidney and to perform antegrade contrast studies if required to check for residual stone fragments.

Careful collimation of the X-ray beam should be employed during this long imaging procedure. Permanent images are acquired of the contrast filled calyces using the machines last image hold facility or using an exposure technique.

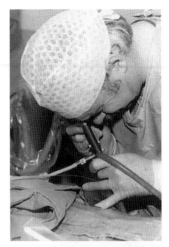

Fig. 12.11a Surgeon with nephroscope and irrigation tube.

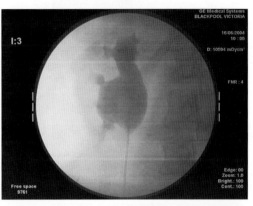

Fig. 12.11b Image showing retrograde filling of kidney.

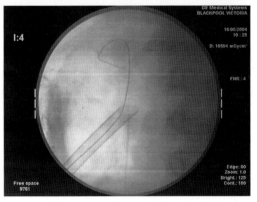

Fig. 12.11c Image showing sheath situated in the renal pelvis.

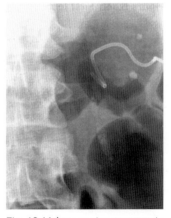

Fig. 12.11d Image showing pigtail catheter left in situ.

Cholangiography refers to the demonstration of the hepatic, cystic and bile ducts by direct injection into the biliary tree. The examination may be requested during cholecystectomy to demonstrate the presence of any gallstones within the biliary ducts. The patient is positioned supine during the operation.

Operative cholangiography 12

A mobile C-arm image intensifier/solid state detector and a theatre table with a radiolucent table top are often selected for this procedure as combined this provides a real-time image for the surgeon to assess the flow of contrast media through the biliary tree.

Alternatively, the examination is performed using a specially adapted theatre table with a radiolucent tabletop, a device commonly known as a 'Baker's tray' and a mobile X-ray machine. A 24 × 30 cm grid computed radiography (CR) image receptor is usually selected (Fig. 12.12a).

This method does have disadvantages unless a direct digital radiography (DDR) wireless detector is used, as the CR receptor has to be processed thereby adding a delay in the operation.

Imaging procedure

Mobile C-arm

When a mobile C-arm is employed the base is positioned on the opposite side of the table to which the surgeon is operating and moved into position over the operation site to adopt a PA projection of the abdomen. It is preferred that the equipment and patient are positioned on the table before the operation commences to ensure that the C-arm will move into position without being obstructed by the table's main support pillar.

Under carefully controlled conditions, 20–30 ml of a water-soluble organic iodine compound (150 mg I/ml) is injected, without bubbles, by the surgeon into the biliary tract. The contrast is observed as it flows through the biliary tree into the duodenum.

Images of the contrast filled biliary tree are acquired using the machines last image hold facility or using a single exposure technique (Fig. 12.12c).

Mobile X-ray machine

When an image detector tray (Baker's tray) mechanism is employed, an initial antero-posterior (AP) projection of the right upper abdomen may be taken prior to the operation. The image receptor is positioned on the tray mechanism, off-set relative to the centre to coincide with the right side of the abdomen. It is then moved using a long handle to a position along the table to coincide with the operation field, which should include the biliary tree and the duodenum. A note is made of the correct detector position.

When required AP projections of the abdomen are taken during and at the termination of the injection of contrast to ensure that any filling defect is constant, and that contrast medium is seen flowing freely into the duodenum. A 24 × 30 cm grid (6:1 or 8:1 grid ratio) is used with an image receptor combination. Exposure is made using a high kilovoltage technique of approximately 85–90 kV in order to minimise surface entry dose and movement unsharpness. Movement blur may also be eliminated by the anaesthetist arresting the patient's respiration during the exposure (Fig. 12.12b).

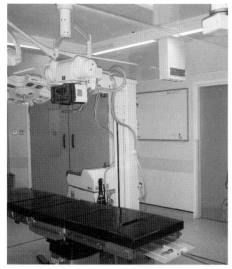

Fig. 12.12a Mobile and theatre table with Baker's tray.

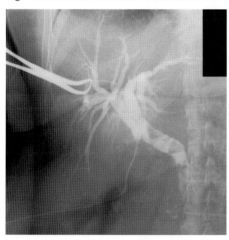

Fig. 12.12b Image of operative cholangiogram using a conventional mobile X-ray unit and 'Baker tray'.

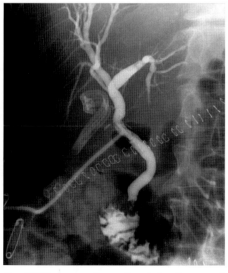

Fig. 12.12c Image of operative cholangiogram using a mobile C-arm intensifier and digital image capture device.

12 Pain management

Introduction

Interventional procedures for the management of pain have evolved with advancements in the widespread use of image-guided techniques utilising C-arm fluoroscopy and contrast medium. This change has improved the delivery of medications to the area of pathology. The key skills of the radiographer remain the same as for other fluoroscopic examinations.

The objective of the examination is to establish accurately and monitor the site of injection, with the minimum radiation dose to the patient and staff. This is whilst maintaining a sterile environment and preventing any cross infection.

Common procedures include:

- Injections of steroid or local anaesthetic into:
  - Joint spaces.
  - Epidural.
  - Facet joints.
  - Sacro-iliac joints
- Spinal surgery:
  - Lumbar decompression.
  - Discectomy.
  - Laminectomy.
  - Balloon kyphoplasty.
  - Anterior cervical disc fixation.
- Transforaminal epidural steroid injection.
- Coeliac plexus nerve blocks.
- Selective nerve root block.
- Lumbar sympathetic block.
- Cervical epidural.

Imaging procedure

Mobile C-arm

When a mobile C-arm is employed the base is positioned on the opposite side of the table to which the surgeon is operating and moved into position over the operation site. The image intensifier needs to be protected from spills of blood from the injection site.

Hints and tips

Always make sure you are present in the theatre when the patient is being transferred onto the operating theatre. This will enable you to make sure the patient is positioned to facilitate screening without artefacts from the operating table. It also helps to position the imaging monitors in the best position for the surgeon to see the images without moving from their operating position. It is also possible to make sure the shoulders are 'pulled down' demonstrate the lower cervical vertebrae to adequately.

Intelligent collimation to the area of interest will reduce scatter and improve image quality (Figs 12.13a–12.13c). Whilst both

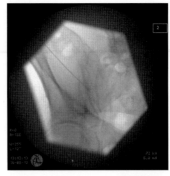

Fig. 12.13a Well-collimated image demonstrating an injection into left sacro-iliac joint.

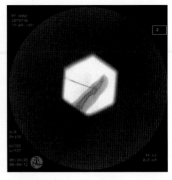

Fig. 12.13b Well-collimated image demonstrating an injection into distal interphalangeal joint.

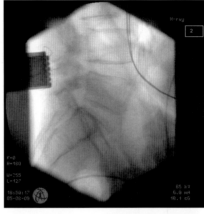

Fig. 12.13c Image 1: well-collimated image – L4–L5 disc space.

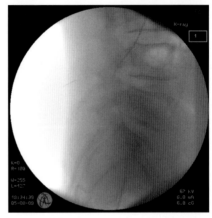

Fig. 12.13d Image 2: poor/no collimation – L4–L5 disc space.

images 12.13c, 12.13d answer the diagnostic question, i.e. what vertebral level is being imaged (L4–L5 disc space), the well collimated image also has a much lower radiation dose.

Keep screening doses to a minimum using pulse mode and only image the patient if the surgeon has made a significant change to the procedure, e.g. inserted the needle further into the joint.

Remember to save the previous image and transfer to the secondary screen when changing from an AP to lateral projection or injecting contrast agent to show filling within the joint.

The lateral vertebral images of L4–L5 disc space demonstrate the differences in quality of theatre images. Figure 12.13c is done with intelligent collimation to the area of interest, whilst Figure 12.13d is acquired with no collimation prior to exposure and is centred posteriorly to the vertebral bodies, which could lead to errors due to the poor quality of the image.

Emergency peripheral vascular procedures 12

Introduction

Emergency angiography is sometimes performed in the theatre environment as part of corrective surgery to vessels following major trauma or bypass grafting to assess the patency of vessels.

A mobile C-arm image intensifier/solid state detector and a theatre table with a radiolucent tabletop are usually selected for this procedure. The C-arm will provide the surgeon with a real-time image of the flow of contrast media through the vessels. The procedure is best undertaken with a relatively large image intensifier with a generator capable of rapid image acquisition, subtraction, road-mapping and last image hold facilities and with two television monitors, one giving real-time display of imaging and the other showing post-processed images of the vessels in normal or subtracted modes.

The patient is positioned supine during the operation. An arterial catheter is inserted, usually by Seldinger technique as described in *Clark's Special Procedures in Diagnostic Imaging*.[6]

Imaging procedure

When a mobile C-arm is employed, the intensifier is positioned to adopt a PA projection of the affected area. The image intensifier/solid state detector face is positioned as close as possible to the skin surface to reduce magnification. For the lower limb, for instance, the patient is positioned on the table before the operation to ensure that the intensifier will move into position without being obstructed by the table's main support pillar. The intensifier should be positioned with its wheels adjusted such that the intensifier can be moved, if necessary, along the length of the limb to follow the flow of contrast.

For subtraction angiography, the image intensifier is positioned over the region of interest, with the region screened to check for collimation of the X-ray beam. With the subtraction technique, selected fluorography is activated, following which up to 20 ml of a contrast agent (300 mg I/ml) is injected into the blood vessel (proximal to the affected site) and images are acquired as directed by the intensifier image acquisition software.

Continuous filling of the blood vessels with contrast agent is observed in the subtracted mode, showing the patency and any pathology of the affected vessel. An image acquisition rate of 1–2 frames/s (fps) is selected and run time is determined visually.

If necessary, a road-map technique may be performed, which facilities the accurate positioning of a catheter/guide wire under fluoroscopic control after first acquiring an image of the area of interest and then superimposing this image on the real-time fluoroscopic image (Figs 12.14a–12.14d).

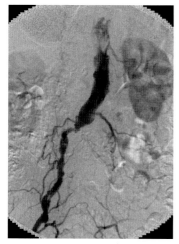

Fig. 12.14a Angiogram of aorta showing complete occlusion of the left common iliac artery.

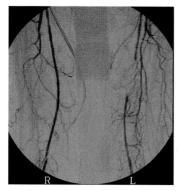

Fig. 12.14b Angiogram of femoral arteries on 12 inch image intensifier, showing short segment occlusion of the left superficial femoral artery.

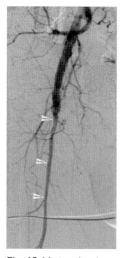

Fig. 12.14c Localised angiogram of right common femoral artery showing flow into the profunda (deep) branch (arrowheads), and occlusion of the superficial femoral artery.

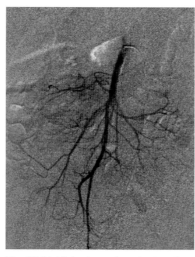

Fig. 12.14d Selective catheterisation of the mesenteric circulation looking for a source of intestinal haemorrhage. This examination is normal.

Section 13
Paediatric Radiography

CONTENTS

INTRODUCTION	423	ABDOMEN	444
General comments	423	Referral criteria	444
Legislation	423	Recommended projections	444
Justification	423	Antero-posterior	445
		Modifications in technique	447
THE PATIENT	425		
Psychological considerations	425	SKULL	449
Child development	425	Referral criteria	449
Anatomical differences between		Recommended projections	450
children and adults	426	Fronto-occipital	451
Approach to a paediatric patient,		Fronto-occipital 30° caudal	452
preparation and sedation	426	Lateral – supine	453
Non-accidental injury	427		
Pregnancy	428	SINUSES	454
Children with special needs	428	Occipito-mental – erect	454
Environment – dedicated paediatric areas	428	Referral criteria	454
IMAGING EQUIPMENT	429	POST-NASAL SPACE	455
		Lateral supine	455
IMAGE QUALITY, RADIATION		Referral criteria	455
PROTECTION MEASURES AND			
DOSIMETRY	431	DENTAL RADIOGRAPHY	456
		PELVIS/HIPS	457
COMMON PAEDIATRIC EXAMINATIONS		Referral criteria	457
AND CHEST – NEONATAL	434	Recommended projections	457
Common paediatric examinations	434	Antero-posterior	458
Chest – neonatal	434	Antero-posterior – erect (weight-bearing)	459
Referral criteria	434	Hips – lateral both hips (frog projection)	460
Recommended projections	434		
Antero-posterior – supine	435	SPINE – SCOLIOSIS	461
		Referral criteria	461
CHEST – POST-NEONATAL	438	Recommended projections	462
Referral criteria	438	Postero-anterior – erect	462
Recommended projections	439	Lateral	464
Postero-anterior – erect	440		
Antero-posterior – erect	440	SPINE – CERVICAL, THORACIC	
Antero-posterior – supine	442	AND LUMBAR	466
Lateral	443	Referral criteria	466
Cincinnati filter device	443	Cervical spine	466

LEG LENGTH ASSESSMENT	468
Single exposure CR method	470
DDR method	471
Localised exposure method	471
ELBOW	472
Lateral (alternative positioning)	472
Antero-posterior (alternative positioning)	473
BONE AGE	475
Referral criteria	475
Recommended projections	475
FEET – SUPPORTED/WEIGHT-BEARING	476
Referral criteria	476
Recommended projections	476
Dorsi-plantar – weight-bearing	476
Lateral – weight bearing	477
SKELETAL SURVEY FOR NON-ACCIDENTAL INJURY	480
Rationale for projections	480
Referral criteria	480
Recommended projections	480
Consent	480
SKELETAL SURVEY FOR SYNDROME ASSESSMENT	484
IMAGE EVALUATION	486
APPENDIX	492
NAI consent form	492
ACKNOWLEDGEMENTS	494

General comments

A range of common paediatric X-ray examinations are described that differ in approach and technique to those performed on adults. Achieving diagnostic quality radiographs whilst minimising patient dose is the goal of any imaging department, and this is no more important than in paediatrics. Children are special cases, since they have a two to four times higher risk of late manifestations of the detrimental effects of radiation. The use of radiological and radiographic imaging techniques is increasing. UNSCEAR compared dose surveys undertaken in 1991–1996 and 1997–2007 and found a 70% increase in the worldwide collective effective dose for medical diagnostic procedures. For the first time this has resulted in a situation where the annual collective dose per capita is higher than the background dose in several developed countries.[1] More frequent radiological examinations are being undertaken, which contributes to an accumulative lifetime risk and which makes the adverse effects of radiation exposure more likely to manifest in children.

Therefore, it is vitally important that careful attention to every aspect of the imaging chain be scrutinised and dose reduction measures used wherever reasonably practicable, complying with the principle of 'as low as reasonably possible' (ALARP) and the philosophy of radiation protection. Any residual risk as a result of a procedure should be 'as low as reasonably practical'.[2]

Staff working with children need skill and experience in order to gain their patients' confidence and co-operation. A clear commitment to paediatrics is essential and a dedicated core group of staff responsible for children and for advising others is vital. In this way there can be an understanding of a child's needs, development, psychology and range of pathology.

Dedicated paediatric areas, rooms, equipment and staff all lead to a far higher likelihood of a high-quality examination, at an achievable low dose, without protracted investigation times and without causing undue stress to the child, parent or staff.

Legislation

An environment of quality and safety within diagnostic imaging departments has been progressively promoted and encouraged throughout the European Community for many years. The Commission of European Communities has provided support by establishing legal requirements for the radiation protection of the patient and it has been recognised clearly that particular emphasis must be placed on paediatrics.[3] The key to the optimisation of paediatric imaging is to produce a radiograph that is of sufficient quality for a radiological diagnosis, at the lowest achievable dose. The need for specific recommendations with regard to defining quality objectively led to the publication of *European Guidelines on Quality Criteria for Diagnostic Radiographic Images in Paediatrics* in 1996.[4] The guidelines contain image quality criteria and entrance surface doses for a standard 5-year-old child, with examples of good technique that would allow these criteria to be met. The criteria given in this chapter are based on the recommendations of the European text but are separated into two categories so that

Introduction 13

problems due to technique can be differentiated from those arising from varying physical parameters (e.g. kV, grid).

National diagnostic reference levels (DRLs) are produced and published by the National Radiological Protection Board (NRPB) now the Health Protection Agency (HPA) of the UK.[5] These are based on rounded 3rd quartile values of a national survey and are reviewed every 5 years.[6] Local current diagnostic reference levels are included for the trunk examinations. These can be used to establish other local DRLs in combination with the UK National diagnostic reference levels for plain radiographs, and as recommended by the Ionising Radiation Medical Exposure Regulations (IRMER) 2000.[7]

In children, meaningful reference doses require consideration of size. This can be addressed by use of NRPB normalisation factors, which can be applied to reference doses for five standard sizes (0, 2, 5, 10 and 15 years),[8] or by the use of callipers to measure patient body thickness.[9]

Justification

The dose reduction measures achieved by improving radiographic practice are insignificant compared with the doses saved from not performing the examination at all. Justification is the essential first step in radiation protection, and it is the duty of all radiographers, radiologists and referrers to ensure that every investigation performed is the correct examination and is essential in the management of the patient.

As recommended by the International Commission on Radiological Protection (ICRP),[10] radiographic and radiological procedures must be justified.

- The use of a radiological examination must do more good than harm.
- The specific radiological examination when required for a specific disease and age group must have a specified objective that should improve the diagnosis and treatment or will provide necessary information about the exposed individual.
- The examination must be required for that individual.

It should also be clear that the necessary result could not be achieved with other methods, which would be associated with a lower risk to the patient. The use of alternative modalities such as ultrasound and magnetic resonance imaging (MRI), which do not use ionising radiation, should be considered. This is particularly in children where repeated studies are required. Advances in these two imaging areas have resulted in a wider range of imaging possibilities, for example the use of ultrasound in anal atresia and the use of MRI urography in the demonstration of an ectopic ureter.

The Royal College of Radiologists' evidence-based referral guidance iRefer[11] addresses the need for advice on justification and also give recommendations regarding appropriate imaging pathways in paediatrics. The most appropriate diagnostic imaging is suggested to answer a variety of frequent clinical questions.

13 Introduction

Justification (cont.)

Referral criteria should include not only when investigations are justified but importantly, when investigations should not be performed and when a more senior clinical referral is required. For example, an abdominal radiograph in non-specific abdominal pain is unlikely to demonstrate pathology in the absence of loin pain, haematuria, diarrhoea, a palpable mass, abdominal distension or suspected inflammatory bowel disease; a follow-up chest X-ray (CXR) is not required routinely for follow up of simple pneumonia in a clinically well child; and some radiographs should not be performed routinely before there has been development of certain normal structures, e.g. sinuses (6 years), nasal bones (3 years), scaphoids (6 years). Careful justification has been shown to reduce significantly the number of radiological and radiographic procedures undertaken. Referral criteria are provided for each of the selected imaging areas below.

Optimisation

Once it has been decided that an investigation needs performing, choice of the most appropriate technique is essential (Figs 13.1a–13.1c). In view of the plethora of imaging techniques now available, radiologists and radiographers are best placed to give clinicians advice.

However, due to the pressures on most departments, individual advice is not possible for every case, and agreed written guidelines between clinicians and X-ray staff should be compiled. Justification and optimisation need good clinico-radiological co-operation.

Examples of optimisation include the use of faster image acquisition systems for follow-up studies, using a lower kV/ higher mAs to optimise bony definition in non-accidental injury (NAI) CXR examination, and the use of additional lateral coning devices to protect the developing breast in follow-up studies of scoliosis in the adolescent female (Fig. 13.1d).

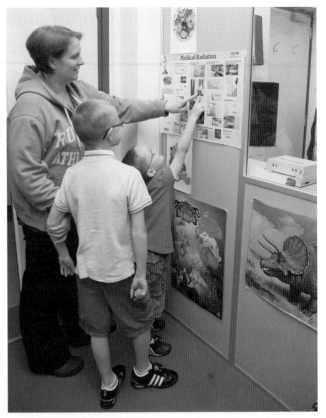

Fig. 13.1b Information notices in an X-ray room.

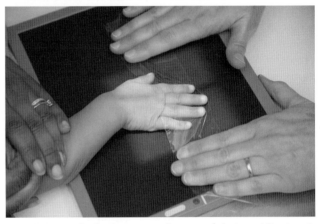

Fig. 13.1c Use of cellophane, non adhesive tape for immobilisation of the hand. Skin wrinkling should be avoided.

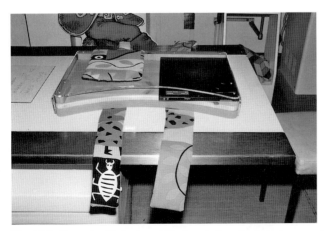

Fig. 13.1a Example of baby immobilisation device – the baby is secured by Velcro strapping with the cassette inserted under a Perspex sheet.

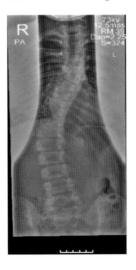

Fig. 13.1d Image of the whole spine in an 11-year-old girl with a scoliosis due to congenital fusion of the 5th and 6th thoracic vertebrae. Iliac crest apophyses not yet present. Lateral breast cones used.

Psychological considerations

Children are not 'mini adults'. There are significant differences in the way children of various ages and ability will react in X-ray departments. Young children are sometimes unable to comprehend fully explanations given and can misinterpret well-meaning intentions of staff. Children also do not have a clear perception of time, staying still for a few minutes to them, can seem like hours. Ill children in particular can become disorientated and have even greater difficulty in co-operating; pain, fear and anxiety can all be exaggerated. Illness can also cause emotional withdrawal, leading to lack of interest and loss of confidence. A sympathetic, kind but firm approach here is essential.

Parents usually bring their children for investigations but, sometimes, another member of the family or a care worker is in attendance and it is important to understand the relationship of the accompanying persons from the beginning.

Parental/carer participation is vital. It does not matter how empathic the staff are, children feel at their most comfortable with their parents and in surroundings they might consider familiar. Parents can be encouraged to be as supportive as possible and to bring the child's favourite toy or special blanket or books. It is preferable for staff initially to direct all their explanations to the child and the parents can listen in. Great care must be taken to talk slowly, clearly and in short succinct sentences. Children and parents can misunderstand and, for complex procedures, they are advised to visit the department beforehand. Written handouts are very helpful so that both parent and child can be as aware as possible of the nature of various procedures (Fig. 13.2).

Sometimes parents are extremely distressed. It is essential to be calm and behave in a completely professional manner at all times. Escorting the parents and any disconcerted child to a private area is advisable so that other children and parents do not become upset. Sometimes a more senior member of the department or radiologist may be needed to discuss any significant problems.

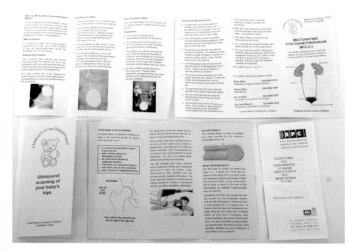

Fig. 13.2 Examples of patient information leaflets.

The Patient 13

Child development

In the context of diagnostic imaging, childhood can be divided into six main age groups, each of which has different needs and capabilities:

- Birth to 6 months.
- Infancy (6 months to 3 years).
- Early childhood (3–6 years).
- Middle childhood (6–12 years).
- Early adolescence (12–15 years).
- Late adolescence (15–19 years).

A different level of understanding and communication is required for each age group.

In the age group birth to 6 months, it is relatively easy to examine a child, as such children are not yet fearful of strangers. They sleep easily and can usually be quietened by a simple bottle-feed.

At 6 months to 3 years, children become increasingly fearful of strangers and cling to their parents. Communication with children of this age may be particularly difficult. Parents will usually have to maintain very close body contact with their child. The use of flashing or musical toys, blowing bubbles, simple rattles or bells may be useful in distracting children of this age. It may also be useful to allow some time for the child and their parents to become familiar with new surroundings before a procedure is undertaken (Fig. 13.4c).

At 3–6 years, communicating is easier but should be limited to simple, child-friendly terminology. Children of this age will often be more co-operative if there is an element of play involved, e.g. describing various pieces of equipment as space ships, seesaw rides, etc. They also have an awareness of modesty, and allowing them to leave on some of their normal clothes can be helpful. Children of this age are often extremely physically active and often do not respond well to attempts at physical restraint. If close parental involvement is not helpful, then swaddling young children in cotton blankets or towels can be useful for some examinations. Televisions, DVD players or computer tablets can be very useful distractors.

Children aged 6–12 years are of school age and have a growing capacity to understand what degree of co-operation is required of them and how the results of any tests will be helpful in treating their problems. An awareness of the most fashionable popular toys is very useful. It is also essential that any posters, books, games, etc. in the department are as up-to-date as possible to maintain credibility.

At 12–19 years, children become increasingly embarrassed and aware of their bodies and their development. It is essential at this age that communication and explanation should match their level of maturity. Their right to privacy must be respected at all times. This may include ensuring that there are assigned areas of the department where confidentiality can be maintained, which may involve discussions without the parents being present if the adolescent so desires. If there is a male radiographer, it is advisable that a parent or carer accompanies a female child.

13 The Patient

Anatomical differences between children and adults

Not only are children smaller, their bodies are different, e.g.:

- Young babies have thin skull vaults and vascular markings are not present before 1 year.
- The nasal bones are not ossified before 3 years of age.
- Paranasal sinuses are not normally pneumatised until 6 years of age.
- Scaphoid bone is not ossified before 6 years of age.
- The smaller depth of the thorax (antero-posterior [AP] diameter) results in less enlargement of the heart, due to magnification, on AP projections of the chest compared to adults.
- The thymus contributes to the cardiomediastinal shadow in young children and its variable presentations can mimic pathology.
- Multiple ossification centres at various sites can cause confusion and reference texts should always be available, which in combination with high quality images will aid interpretation.
- Faster heart and respiratory rates.
- More radiosensitive red bone marrow is more widespread in children and is present in almost all bones of a neonate.

These anatomical differences should be taken into account when optimising techniques in paediatric radiography.

Approach to a paediatric patient, preparation and sedation (Figs 13.3, 13.4a–13.4e)

Staff should always introduce themself to a child and parent in a friendly and capable manner. The child's name, age and address should be verified and it is important to bend down to speak to the child at their level. A firm but kindly approach is required and the child should be escorted into the already prepared imaging room. It is preferable for the X ray tube to be in the correct position. Adjusting its height over the child can be disconcerting. Usually only one parent is asked to accompany the child into the room. This complies with radiation protection guidelines. Both parents are sometimes required for assisting with immobilisation of the child.

A very encouraging reassuring attitude has to be adopted and an enormous amount of praise should be given for every single act of co-operation e.g., "You are the best child at keeping still we have had all day!" or "you are so clever!"

Always be honest in answering any questions; keeping one's credibility is essential in maintaining rapport with children. Allow the child to see the effect of switching on the light beam diaphragm or riding on a chair or table beforehand if necessary.

Rewards of stickers, balloons and bravery certificates are a must (Fig. 13.4d). If a child's first experience of an X-ray department is a pleasant one, any future attendances will be far easier.

Given the right approach and surroundings most children are co-operative. However, there are some who become physically aggressive and abusive, throwing temper tantrums at every suggestion. In these situations, it is better to get on with the procedure as quickly as possible, a firm approach and a range of simple, well tried immobilisation devices are recommended. Lots of cuddles with the parents/carer afterwards will soon calm the child.

Children admitted as inpatients need more specific preparation, including liaising with the ward nursing staff and arranging a nurse escort where necessary. Planning of any radiograph should allow for the presence of any intravenous (IV) lines, drainage tubes, stomas etc. It should be ascertained whether the patient would have adequate oxygen supply or IV fluid before arranging the examination.

If any patient has a contagious disease, barrier methods of handling must be instituted. A decision should be made as to whether the patient should be brought to the department or whether the examination should be performed with bed/cot side mobile equipment. In addition, careful timing of the examination in order to avoid close proximity with other vulnerable patients is recommended (e.g. those who are immunocompromised or neonates). Plastic aprons, gloves and careful handwashing are required of all attendants. Masks or eyewear are only necessary if spraying of any body fluids is likely. All items contaminated by body fluids should be disposed of carefully according to local Health and Safety Rules. All equipment that comes into contact with the child should be disinfected with the recommended cleaning agent for that equipment.

As in Outpatients, other specific preparation for simple radiographs is rarely required. However, a prone invertogram for assessment of imperforate anus should not be performed in less than 24 hours after birth to allow more distal bowel to be delineated and should be taken after the patient has been kept in the prone position for 15 minutes.

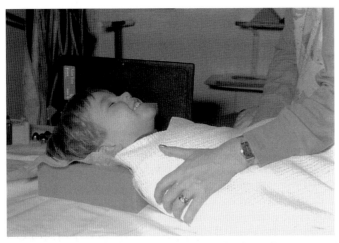

Fig. 13.3 Child swaddled in cotton blanket for skull radiography.

The Patient 13

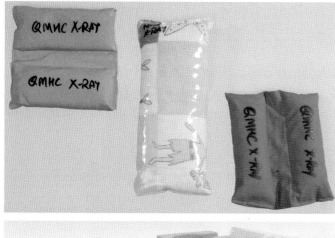

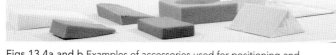

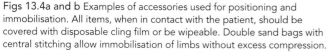

Figs 13.4a and b Examples of accessories used for positioning and immobilisation. All items, when in contact with the patient, should be covered with disposable cling film or be wipeable. Double sand bags with central stitching allow immobilisation of limbs without excess compression.

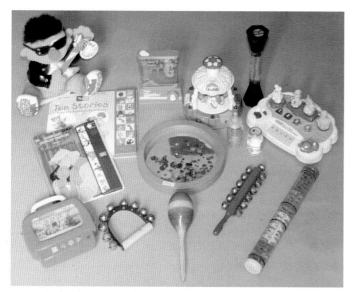

Fig. 13.4c Examples of toys useful to distract the child.

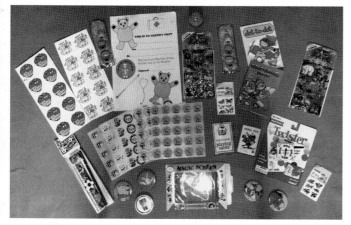

Fig. 13.4d Examples of certificates and rewards.

Non-accidental injury

The imaging of children for suspected NAI could be stressful for all concerned because of the implications. Anyone working with children has a professional duty to safeguard and promote the welfare of children when doing their jobs.[12] These children are some of the most vulnerable attending imaging departments. They may already have multiple injuries, be in pain, be wary of adults and it may be difficult to obtain their co-operation. A skeletal survey should be performed with great patience, understanding and skill. Radiographs of the highest diagnostic quality are required. The process can be daunting for any child's parent or carer to observe and there have been cases where a carer has raised concern that fractures could have been caused during the examination or positioning of their child by hospital staff.

The joint RCR and RCPCh Standards for Radiological Investigation of Suspected Non-Accidental Injury (2008)[13] are comprehensive; there is also a joint addendum to the guidance issued by the RCR and SCoR (2012)[14] emphasising that positioning for NAI skeletal surveys should be by simple extension, flexion or rotation of limbs and holding. No twisting movement should be necessary.

It is important to assess the degree of gentle immobilisation that will be required and to ensure that the parent or carer fully understands and gives consent for the degree of immobilisation and use of any accessories that will be required. It is extremely important for at least three hospital staff to be present during the examination and their presence recorded. (two radiographers and one trained paediatric care worker with experience in immobilisation techniques). If at any time a carer becomes concerned that their child is overly distressed, then further explanations or review of alternative measures should be undertaken before proceeding.

In cases where sedation is being given for computed tomography (CT) of the brain, then the NAI skeletal survey could be co-ordinated to make best use of the sedation given. Chloral hydrate and midazolam are suitable alternatives.

It is essential that all those involved in the sedation of children are well trained and updated in resuscitative techniques.

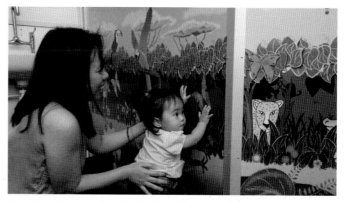

Fig. 13.4e Example of child friendly lead screen with animal mural.

13 The Patient

Pregnancy

This can be a difficult issue but the guidelines of the Royal College of Radiologists state that the possibility of pregnancy should be broached in all female patients who have started menstruating (approximately over the age of 12 years).[11] Discretion is essential, honest answers are more likely if the child is not with her parents. It is preferable for the child to be taken into the imaging room on her own and then tactfully asked if she is menstruating and whether she might be pregnant. The choice of a female radiographer or radiologist may be more acceptable. As in adults, the 28 day rule applies for examinations that directly include the abdomen or pelvis. The 10 day rule applies for fluoroscopic examinations of the abdomen, abdominal CT and intravenous urograms (IVUs). A clear explanation of the risk of radiation to any unborn baby is necessary.

It is also important to ensure that all those providing restraint are not pregnant.

Children with special needs

It is important to ascertain or make an assessment as to whether children have one or both handicaps. It is so easy to assume that a physically disabled child also has a learning disability. Whatever the degree of disability, all children should be given the opportunity to be spoken to directly and to listen to explanations. The parents and carers are very dedicated to their children and their presence is usually invaluable. They are usually the best in describing which is the best way to approach physical needs such as lifting or transferring onto the X-ray table or introducing oral contrast. In some cases, it may be preferable to examine the child in their normal position, e.g. still in the wheelchair.

Environment – dedicated paediatric areas

Waiting area (Fig. 13.5a)

The reception area is the child's and the parent's first contact with the X-ray department. It is essential that the staff and the environment put the child and parents at their ease as quickly as possible. Working with children requires a child-friendly approach from all individuals involved.

The waiting area should be as well equipped as possible. It does not have to involve much expense, but toys and games aimed at all age groups should be available. More general departments could consider having video/computer games available in the paediatric area, even if this is shared with other paediatric departments.

More specialised departments may be able to employ a play therapist. This is particularly useful in gaining children's confidence for more complex procedures. Drawing and colouring activities are often appreciated, and children love donating their own compositions to the department's decor.

Imaging room (Fig. 13.5b)

The room should already be prepared before the child enters. It is preferable to keep waiting times for examinations to a minimum, as this will significantly reduce anxiety. The room must be immediately appealing, with colourful decor, attractive posters and stickers applied to any equipment that may be disconcerting. Soft toys undergoing mock examinations are also helpful.

A fairly low ambient lighting is preferred, unless fluoroscopy equipment, for example, can be operated in normal daytime lighting. This avoids darkening the room later, which may frighten a child.

As mentioned already, time can appear to pass very slowly for some children. If they can be distracted with music (CD/tape) or moving images (projectors/DVD players), they are far less likely to need physical restraint. Any devices, e.g. syringes, which may upset the child, should be kept out of view until they are needed.

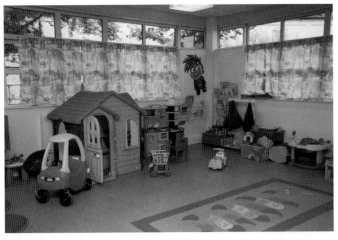

Fig. 13.5a A child friendly waiting area, appropriately decorated and suitable for a paediatric service.

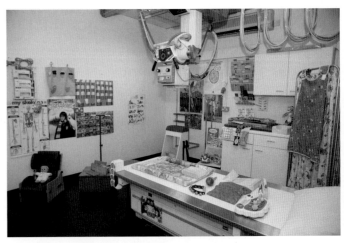

Fig. 13.5b A child-friendly imaging room.

Imaging equipment 13

X-ray generators

As has already been described above, children have faster heart/respiratory rates and they generally have difficulty in staying still. Very short exposure times are required and a nearly rectangular voltage waveform and a minimal amount of ripple are desirable. Only high-frequency generators can provide this. Similarly mobile equipment should have converter generators.[4]

The timers should also be very accurate. Meticulous quality control programmes should be in place to ensure that the chosen radiographic voltage matches the effective voltage. Inconsistencies can arise at short exposure settings.[4] In order to keep exposure times to a minimum, the cable length between the transformer and the tube should be as short as possible and all equipment being used for paediatrics should be able to accurately reproduce exposure times of <1 ms.

The radiation emitted takes some time to reach its peak voltage. This is not significant in the longer exposure of adults but in children long pre-peak times may result in a lower effective voltage. Equipment should be used which has short pre-peak times or the addition of added filtration should be considered to eliminate any unnecessary low kV radiation.

Selection of tube potential

Several publications have recommended selection of a high kV technique as a dose saving measure.[4,15] The Commission of European Communities (CEC) Guidelines[4] for example, recommend a minimum kV of 60 for neonatal radiographs. Selection of kV should be as high as possible consistent with desired image quality. This does result in less contrasted radiographs and a radiological preference for these types of images should be developed.

Focal spot

A focal spot size of 0.6–1.3 mm is acceptable for paediatrics. A change in focal spot size does not affect the dose but a smaller size improves the image quality at a cost of increased tube loading and possibly longer exposure times.

Additional filtration

Most X-ray tubes have an inherent filtration of 2.5 mm of aluminium. The CEC Guidelines[4] recommend the additional use of 0.1 mm of copper or up to 3 mm of additional aluminium and several authors have demonstrated the dose saving advantage of additional copper filtration whilst maintaining diagnostic quality.[16] Additional filtration further removes the soft part of the radiation spectrum, which is completely absorbed by the patient, uselessly increasing the dose, but not contributing to the production of the radiographic image. In our experience, 0.1 mm of additional copper with an initial inherent filtration of 2.5 mm. Aluminium leads to an entrance dose reduction of 20% with no significant loss of quality in the majority of examinations.

A reduction in image quality has only been noticed in low kV techniques of small children's peripheries (e.g. for NAI and on Special care baby unit [SCBU]) and in order to take this into account easily removable added filtration may be advisable so that it can be removed when appropriate. In order to avoid confusion of exposure factors some equipment may be left without added filtration should more than one piece of equipment be available.

It is generally not recommended to have additional filtration on mobile equipment for SCBU if avoidable, due to the noticeable reduction in quality.

Antiscatter grid

An antiscatter grid is not always required in children. An antiscatter grid results in an increase in dose of approximately 100%, and its use should always be justified by the need for an increase in image quality. Antiscatter grids are not used for examination of the chest. Skull radiographs less than 1 year of age, and pelvis, abdominal and spine radiographs under the age of 3 years, do not routinely require the use of an antiscatter grid and can also be avoided in older children of small size. The experience of the radiographer is essential here. If a grid is to be used, then a grid ratio of 8:1 and a line number of 40/cm are recommended. The grid should contain low-attenuation materials such as carbon fibre, and the correct focus-to-receptor distance (FRD) for a focused grid should be used.

Focus-to-receptor distance

Increasing the FRD necessitates an increase in exposure factors but the overall effective dose to the patient is reduced and the blurring due to magnification effect is also reduced. A maximum FRD should be used, a minimum of 100 cm for over couch tubes and a minimum of 150 cm for vertical stands in chest and spinal radiography. If designing new departments, consideration should be given to allow for long FRDs (e.g. over 200 cm), which can be useful for reducing magnification and for using an air-gap technique.[17–19]

Automatic exposure control

Very few automatic exposure chambers have been made specifically for children, and therefore they are not always able to compensate fully for the wide range of body sizes in children. Usually, use of automatic exposure control (AEC) devices lengthens the minimal exposure time and can result in higher doses in paediatric practice. Well-tried and structured exposure charts are more likely to produce higher-quality images at lower doses.

Exposure charts are normally based on children's ages, although size is more accurate, and this means that radiographic experience and training is vital in selecting appropriate exposure factors.

AEC chambers are also usually built behind the grid. Therefore, an examination using an AEC in these conditions also necessitates using the grid if they can't be removed.

13 Imaging equipment

Film/intensifying screen combinations

Whilst digital imaging systems are now commonplace, film and film processing continue to be used in some situations. High-speed screen/film systems, high kV techniques and the deselection of a grid have been found to be the most important methods of reducing dose in radiographic practice.

In our experience, high resolution, 200 speed screen/film systems should be limited to peripheries. Most examinations can be performed with rare earth or equivalent screens, i.e. speed classes of 400–600. Many follow-up examinations and radiographs for swallowed foreign bodies can be performed with very fast screen/film systems (700–800).

It should be recognised that various manufacturers do not have the same effective speed of screen/film system for the same numerical description and the speed of the system can also vary with the kV. Thus optimum kV for the system chosen should be used.

Film processing and viewing conditions

As in adults, the gains obtained in perfecting radiographic practice are lost if simple measures are not taken to ensure that both film processing and lighting conditions for viewing radiographs are not fully optimised.

Film processing should be the subject of daily quality assurance assessment and the brightness of a film viewing box should be 2000–4000 cd/m for films in the density range of 0.5–2.2 and a low level of ambient light in the viewing room is essential as described in the CEC guidelines.[4]

Digital radiography

Significant advances have been made in digital imaging.[20,21] Computed radiography (CR) and direct digital radiography (DDR) are now far more widely available and, if used appropriately, allow a significant reduction in radiation dose whilst improving image quality. However, maximising the benefits of CR and DDR in children is still a challenge and their use does not automatically result in lower doses. Sanchez Jacob et al. found that there was a considerable range of dose level in CR that still produced a diagnostic image and that there was no significant correlation between dose levels and image quality across a wide range.[22]

The most important advantage of CR/DDR is that it maintains its detective quantum efficiency (DQE) over a much wider range than screen/film. This wider latitude significantly reduces the risk of requiring a repeat image to be taken for an incorrect exposure. However, excessive doses can be delivered without realising that this is the case because the resultant image is not overexposed and post-processing techniques can mask high-dose examinations. Concern has been raised that "If careful attention is not paid to the radiation protection issues of digital radiography, medical exposure of patients will increase significantly and without concurrent benefit".[23]

Underexposed CR/DDR images are noisy and grainier, whilst overexposed images are sharper and appear of higher quality. This can result in the acknowledged effect of 'dose creep', which results in higher doses due to misguided attempts to produce a higher quality image than is necessary or to reduce the possibility that an image could be undiagnostic and may need to be repeated.

If departments are aware of these issues then there are distinct benefits; when used optimally, it has been shown that there can be dose savings of up to 60% when comparing a 1000 speed CR system with the commonly used 400 speed systems used in most departments.[24]

The many advantages of digital imaging were outlined in the second ALARA conference organised by the Society of Paediatric Radiology in Texas 2004[25] and recommendations are also given in publications such as Practical applications of CR in Paediatric Imaging.[26]

Advantages of CR/DDR include contrast being independent of kV through adjustment of window width and brightness being independent of mA by adjustment of window level. There is also a wide range of post-processing possibilities, tubes and lines are more easily demonstrated and there is a wide grey scale of soft tissue and bony structures. Labelling and transmission of data are also easier.

Use of the exposure index of digital systems has not been as well-developed in children as in adults. Their aim is to provide a dose indication. However, there is no standardisation of these dose indicators, they need to be expertly calibrated and they are subject to interference. It is preferable not to rely on this index but to produce specific radiographic exposure charts that take into account patient size. When a new CR/DDR system is installed, well-established exposure charts should first be used to select the optimum exposure factors to produce the best diagnostic image at the lowest practicable dose. However, the dose parameters should still be monitored using the exposure index of the digital system.[27] The exposure factors and dose readings should be either printed on the images or recorded in the radiology information system for every individual patient.

Accessories including immobilisation devices (Figs 13.6, 13.1c, 13.4a, 13.4b)

The hallmark of successful paediatric imaging is by the use of accessories, which, in the main, are simple and inexpensive. Most important is to have an adequate range to comply with the needs of a wide range of body sizes. The various accessories are described in the following text according to the anatomical area and corresponding radiographic technique. Positioning aids can cause more artefacts in CR/DDR imaging and this should be taken into account when planning any immobilisation.

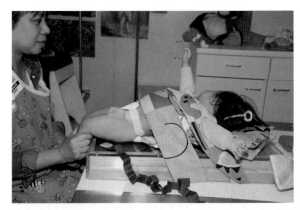

Fig. 13.6 A baby immobilisation device for infant supine antero-posterior pelvis. It enables immobilisation by one holder. Infant is secured with Velcro strapping and cassette is inserted under a Perspex sheet.

Essential image characteristics

The essential image characteristics that should be demonstrated in any of the projections described in this chapter are found by reference to the publication of the Commission of European Communities (CEC) title *European Guidelines on Quality for Diagnostic Images in Paediatrics*. This publication provides guidance on technique, representative exposure factors and corresponding patient doses by age. Visibility of a structure is described in three grades, as follows:

Visualisation	Characteristic features are detectable but only just visible
Reproduction	Anatomical details are visible but not clearly defined
Visually sharp reproduction	Anatomical details are clearly defined

Image quality assessment

Unharmonised, and in many places unoptimised, examination techniques have been shown to produce a great variation in the absorbed dose to children examined,[28] and many dose surveys have demonstrated wide dose ranges.[29,30]

As described above, image quality criteria for paediatrics have been introduced by the CEC to address this situation.[4] These image criteria are an attempt to assess objectively a radiograph and determine diagnostic quality.

However, it is stated clearly in the guidelines that under no circumstances should an image which fulfils all clinical requirements but does not meet all image criteria ever be rejected. This is an important point, as although one should always strive for excellence, the aim is always for a diagnostic image that answers the clinical question. Unnecessarily high quality that results in higher doses should be avoided.

The quality criteria consist of those that depend on correct positioning of the patient and those that depend on the physical parameters that reflect the technical performance of the imaging system.

There is still a subjective element to the criteria. However, several authors have explored the value of the CEC criteria and have found that they allowed a reduction in effective dose by up to 50% without a significant reduction in diagnostic image quality.[31–33]

Dose is influenced most by a choice of physical parameters, such as kV, speed of screen/film system, selection of the sensitivity of a CR system and the use of an antiscatter grid. However, image quality is far more dependent on radiographic technique.

Image quality, radiation protection measures and dosimetry 13

Audit and quality assurance

In an X-ray department this is a complex activity and all staff should be involved. There are strict regulations with regard to health and safety and radiation protection measures and close involvement of medical physicists is advised.

It is recommended that there should be at least one radiographer with additional specialised paediatric training in each general imaging department. Reject analysis should include:

- Anatomical cut off.
- Movement unsharpness.
- Degree of under- or overexposure.
- Use of post processing.
- Number of repeats.
- Artefacts.

Coning devices and gonad protection (Figs 13.7a, 13.7b, 13.8a–13.8c)

Careful collimation is an important tool in dose reduction and also improves image quality; primary and scattered radiation is also reduced. All radiographs should show all four diaphragm edges or circular cones, and the collimation should be limited strictly to the region of interest. The maximum field size at each edge should not exceed 1 cm beyond the region of interest in neonates and 2 cm for older children.[4]

It is important when using additional devices that the light beam diaphragm is coned initially, before inserting the additional device. The latter alone is not sufficient protection if the primary cones are left widely open. Shaped additional coning such as window protection for hips can be used for either male or female patients, being inverted for the latter.

Poor coning technique can be disguised by using post-processing digital cones in CR and DDR systems. Any audit of image quality should include an assessment of native images on the CR/DDR console before they are post processed and sent to a picture archiving and communication system (PACS) system.

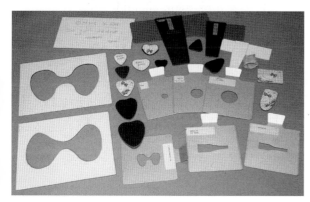

Fig. 13.7a Variety of paediatric gonad shields and coning devices.

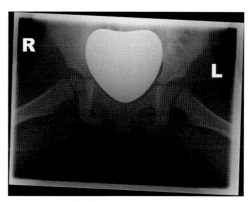

Fig. 13.7b Frog lateral both hips with female gonad protection.

13 Image quality, radiation protection measures and dosimetry

A wide range of gonad protection is required in various sizes and shapes (Figs 13.8a–13.8c). Gonad protection should be applied even in the erect position. It can be secured in position with sticky tape. Lead protection on the patient next to the primary beam, if used correctly, is important in reducing exposure to tube-scattered radiation. However, current X-ray equipment allows very precise collimation of the X-ray beam resulting in very little tube scatter. Therefore, in examinations such as erect CXR, it is considered to be more important to ensure good collimation and to produce a diagnostic quality radiograph at the first attempt. With larger patients the effect of backscatter from the lead protection next to the primary beam reduces its beneficial effect of reducing tube scatter. However, although the dose protection effect is small, if used correctly, it has a reassuring effect on parents.

If lead protection is used to reduce tube scatter to the patient, it should not obscure essential anatomical detail and should not be in the primary beam. It should also be noted that there is more artefact from positioning aids in CR/DDR imaging.

Dose measurement

All radiographic equipment, including mobile and fluoroscopy equipment, should have dose–area product (DAP) meters in place. DAP meters are placed beneath the X ray beam collimators and intercept the whole X-ray beam. The DAP is a multiplication of the dose and the area of the X-ray beam. It is expressed in $cGy\,cm^2$ or $mGy\,cm^2$. DAP meters do not give a precise measurement of dose but have been shown to provide a sensitive, convenient and simple method of monitoring and recording doses in paediatric radiography.[34] They need to be of a high specification for children, otherwise the dose readings will not be accurate, and need to be regularly recalibrated. Careful monitoring and recording of these DAP meter readings is essential in providing feedback to staff. In due course, a record of accumulative dose in children will become a legal requirement.

Balancing dose and image quality

An attempt should always be made to obtain the best-quality radiograph at the first attempt. Careful preparation is the key.[35] Radiographs should be repeated only at a radiologist's request or if they fail to answer the clinical question.

Comparison should be made with available DRLs. However, the National Reference Doses[5] are those above which corrective action should be taken; they are set at the 3rd quartile level and may be considered high. In addition to the National Reference Doses, therefore, local DRLs should be derived from local dose audit.

Note

The measurement of dose should be an integral part of imaging. UK DRLs are based on 3rd quartile values following national surveys, i.e. 25% of hospitals exceeded the reference levels in the surveys. The aim is for local DRLs to be lower than the national DRLs. UK radiographic DRLs for children were last published in 2000. Therefore, local DRLs from our non-specialist department are provided based on age, DAP meter readings and the use of CR. They should be used for reference only as these local DRLs may not be representative of wider general practice. Lower doses may be achieved with different techniques including optimised (avoiding dose creep) DDR, whereas use of screen/film combinations may result in higher doses. Entrance surface dose reference levels from the UK national survey in 2000 are also included and these would have been based on the use of screen/film.

There is known to be a wide variation in size for age and concerns have been expressed that there has been a progressive increase in children's sizes over the past few decades. Therefore, exposures based on patient body thickness are also recommended. The results of a hospital survey of paediatric chest doses in Finland based on patient body thickness has been published[36] and the dose curves are available on the Finland Radiation Safety and Nuclear Authority web site.[9]

The aim is always to obtain a diagnostic image at the lowest dose, compatible with the ALARP principle.[2]

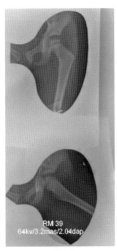

Fig. 13.8a Male window gonad protection used for follow-up radiograph of left hip with Perthes' disease.

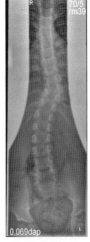

Fig. 13.8b Breast shielding for a postero-anterior erect spine in a patient with a congenital scoliosis. Note butterfly and block vertebrae.

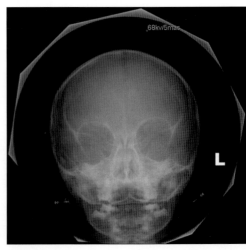

Fig. 13.8c Circular cones for antero-posterior skull radiograph. Earrings should be removed when possible.

Image quality, radiation protection measures and dosimetry 13

The tables demonstrated are of current local DRLs as used at the authors' hospital (a general hospital) and are based on CR imaging with tube filtration of 2.5 mm of inherent aluminium and 0.1 mm of additional copper filtration No additional copper filtration is used for the neonatal images. The local DRLs have been derived by calculating the mean at each specific age (up to 1 year, 1, 5, 10 and 15 years) after excluding significantly undersized and oversized patients. Levels of 20% above have been set as a trigger for investigation and remedial action when these levels are consistently exceeded. When lead gonad protection is placed on the patient, particularly for the AP pelvis or a circular cone is used for skull radiography, the true DAP would be lower than indicated.

Patient body thickness is considered to be a more appropriate method of analysing dose in children and is now being measured at our hospital. Below is the Radiation and Nuclear Safety Authority of Finland (STUK) dose graph for a frontal examination of the chest based on patient body thickness and an example of our calliper used as a measuring device (Figs 13.9a, 13.9b).[9]

Exam	Age y	Local DRL (2014) cGy cm²	Investigation Level (LDRL +20%)	NRPB 2000 data ESD (mGy)
Chest	Neonate (1–3.5 kg)	0.04	0.05	
	0	0.5	0.6	0.05
	1	0.61	0.73	0.05
	5	0.81	0.97	0.07
	10	1.72	2.1	0.12
	15	2.45	2.94	0.12

Exam	Age y	Local DRL (2014) cGy cm²	Investigation Level (LDRL +20%)	NRPB 2000 data ESD (mGy)
Skull AP/PA	0–1 mo	1.1	1.4	0
	1	1.5	1.9	0.8
	5	3.3	3.9	1.1
	10	–	–	1.1
	15	–	–	1.1

Exam	Age y	Local DRL (2014) cGy cm²	Investigation Level (LDRL +20%)	NRPB 2000 data ESD (mGy)
Pelvis AP	0	0.5	0.6	0
	1	0.6	0.7	0.5
	5	1.8	2.2	0.6
	10	8.9	10.6	0.7
	15	19.7	23.7	2

Exam	Age y	Local DRL (2014) cGy cm²	Investigation level (LDRL +20%)	NRPB 2000 data ESD (mGy)
Abdomen	Neonate (1–3.5 kg)	0.04	0.05	
	0	0.8	0.96	0
	1	1.7	2.00	0.4
	5	3.6	4.30	0.5
	10	18.1	21.7	0.8
	15	28.9	34.6	1.2

Exam	Age y	Local DRL (2014) cGy cm²	Investigation Level (LDRL +20%)
Whole PA spine for scoliosis	0	–	–
	1	–	–
	5	–	
	10	3.8	4.6
	15	5.7	6.8

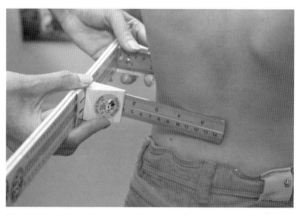

Fig. 13.9a Calliper for measuring body thickness.

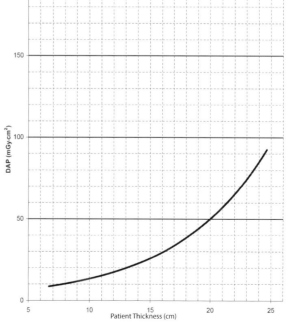

Fig. 13.9b Graph of patient thickness and dose for frontal chest radiograph.

13 Common paediatric examinations and chest – neonatal

Common paediatric examinations

A range of common paediatric X-ray examinations are described that differ in approach and technique to those performed on adults. Those described are:

- Chest – neonatal.
- Chest – post-neonatal.
- Skull.
- Sinuses and post-nasal space (PNS).
- Dental.
- Abdomen.
- Pelvis and hips.
- Spine for scoliosis.
- Spine.
- Leg length assessment.
- Elbow.
- Bone age, hand and knees.
- Feet for talipes assessment.
- Skeletal survey for NAI.
- Skeletal survey for syndrome assessment.

Chest – neonatal

Chest radiographs are the most common requests on the SCBU/Neonatal unit (NNU), with the infant nursed in a special incubator.

All requests should be strictly justified. Image acquisition just before insertion of lines or catheters should be avoided when a post-line insertion image is anticipated. Good-quality technique is essential. The range of diagnoses possible in neonatal chest radiography is fairly limited, and differing pathologies can look similar. Correlation with good clinical information is essential. Study of a sequence of radiographic images over a period may be necessary for correct interpretation, and therefore accurate recording and reproduction of the most appropriate radiographic exposure are essential for comparisons to be made. The shape of the thorax and layout of corresponding cardio-respiratory structures differs from that of the adult and the radiographic technique must be applied to reflect these differences.

Chest radiographs are the most common requests for neonates. Serial radiographs are often undertaken and consistency in technique is required for comparisons to be made.

Referral criteria

These include:

- Respiratory difficulty.
- Infection.
- Meconium aspiration.
- Chronic lung disease.
- Pleural effusion/pneumothorax.
- Position of catheters/tubes.
- Heart murmur/cyanosis.
- Oesophageal atresia.
- Previous antenatal ultrasound abnormality suspected.
- Thoracic cage anomaly.
- As part of a skeletal survey for syndrome/NAI.
- Postoperative.

A request for chest and abdomen on one radiograph, with centring to the chest, is sometimes indicated in the following:

- Localisation of tubes or catheters.
- Suspected diaphragmatic hernia.
- Suspected abdominal pathology causing respiratory difficulty.

Recommended projections

Examination is performed by means of the following projections:

Basic	AP – supine
Alternative	PA – prone
Supplementary	Lateral

AP, antero-posterior; PA, postero-anterior.

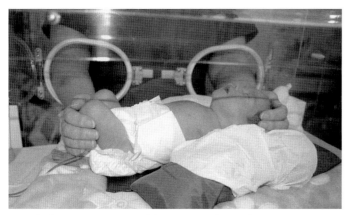

Fig. 13.10a Neonate positioned for AP supine chest radiograph.

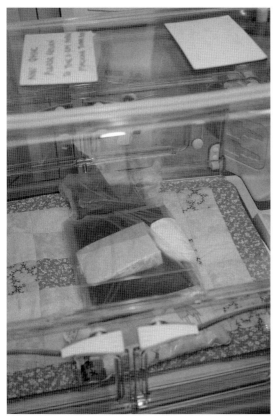

Fig. 13.10b Foam pad used to tilt baby to avoid lordotic projection. Lead pieces on top of incubator to exclude contralateral limb in assessment of vascular lines.

Common paediatric examinations and chest – neonatal   13

Antero-posterior – supine (Figs 13.10a, 13.10b)

An 18 × 24 cm CR cassette that is at body temperature is selected. A single use disposable plastic bag should be used to cover the cleaned image cassette. Modern incubators with cassette trays may be used to avoid disturbance of a very sick baby (see below).

Position of patient and image receptor

Sleeping baby

- The baby is positioned supine on the cassette with the median sagittal plane adjusted perpendicular to the middle of the cassette, ensuring that the head and chest are straight with shoulders and hips being level.
- The head may need a sandbag for support on either side.
- A 10° covered foam pad should be placed under the shoulders to lift the chin and to avoid it obscuring the lung apices.
- Arms should be on either side, slightly abducted from the trunk to avoid being included in the radiation field.
- Arms can be immobilised with Velcro bands and/or small sandbags.

Baby requiring holding

Positioning is the same as that described for the sleeping baby but can be performed by a single assistant with the following adaptations:

- The arms should be held flexed on either side of the head.
- Alternatively, the baby's head can be held from the top with the arms at the sides abducted from the trunk and immobilised by the use of small double sandbags.
- Legs should be held straight above the knees to keep the pelvis straight.

Direction and location of the X-ray beam

- The vertical collimated beam is centred in the midline just below the level of the axillary folds (intermammillary line).
- Consistent maximum FRD should be used.
- Although some incubators have cassette trays placing the cassette under the baby is recommended as routine, to avoid magnification and change of exposure factors.

13 Common paediatric examinations and chest – neonatal

Antero-posterior – supine (cont.)

Essential image characteristics (Figs 13.10c, 13.11a, 13.11b)

- Peak inspiration to include 8–9 posterior ribs (4–5 anterior ribs).
- No rotation, the anterior rib ends should be equidistant from the spine and the medial ends of the clavicles should overlap the transverse processes of the spine.
- No tilting; the medial ends of the clavicles should overlie the lung apices.
- Superior/inferior coning should be from cervical trachea C6/C7 to T12/L1 including the diaphragms.
- Lateral coning should include both shoulders and ribs but not beyond proximal 1/3 of humeri.
- Reproduction of the vascular pattern in the central 2/3 of the lungs.
- Reproduction of the trachea and major bronchi.
- Visually sharp reproduction of the diaphragm and costophrenic angles.
- Reproduction of the spine and paraspinal structures.
- Visualisation of retrocardiac lung and mediastinum.
- Visually sharp reproduction of the skeleton.

Common faults and solutions

- Classically, incubator porthole of must not overlie chest (see Fig. 13.11c).
- All extraneous tubes and wires should be repositioned away from the chest area.
- Exposure should be in inspiration. Watching for full distension of the abdomen rather than the chest best assesses this. Expiratory images mimic parenchymal disease.
- Arms should not be fully extended above the head as this can lead to the upper ribs pointing upwards and the anterior diaphragm obscuring the lung bases.
- Arms, if positioned by the side of the patient, should not be too close to the chest as this can cause vertical skin creases which give a false impression of a pneumothorax.
- Minimal exposures of less than 0.02 seconds should be used to avoid motion artefact.
- Rotated images should be avoided, as this can cause misinterpretation of mediastinal shift and lung translucency. The separate ossification centres of the sternum, projected over the lungs can also cause confusion (Fig. 13.10d).
- In neonatal work, for the departments who still use film/cassette the label should not obscure any of the anatomical detail. (This is not applicable to CR and DDR systems.)

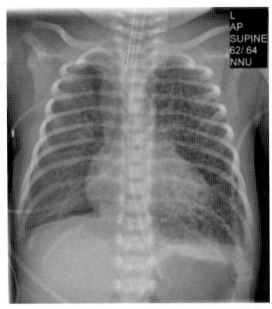

Fig. 13.10c AP supine chest radiograph of a 4-day-old premature neonate demonstrating a right pneumothorax and pulmonary interstitial emphysema in the left lung.

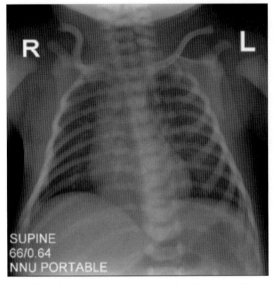

Fig. 13.10d AP supine chest radiograph of a 1-day-old neonate. Patient is rotated to the right and the ossification centres of the manubrium overlie the right hemithorax, which could be misinterpreted as rib fractures.

- Taking a radiograph when a baby is crying should be avoided, as this can cause overexpansion of the lungs, which may mimic pathology.
- Image acquisition just prior to insertion of tubes/lines when a post line insertion image is anticipated.
- The shape of the thorax and layout of corresponding cardio-respiratory structures differs from that of adults; the radiographic technique must be applied to reflect these differences.

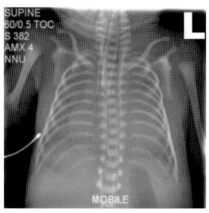

Fig. 13.11a AP supine chest radiograph of a 1-day-old neonate demonstrating severe respiratory distress syndrome with endotracheal tube wrongly positioned down the right main bronchus.

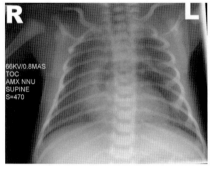

Fig. 13.11b AP supine chest radiograph of a 4-day-old neonate demonstrating a pneumomediastinum.

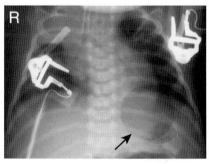

Fig. 13.11c AP supine neonatal chest radiograph with shadow of incubator porthole superimposed on the lungs.

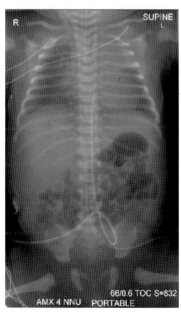

Fig. 13.11d AP supine chest and abdominal radiograph combined of a 1-day-old neonate. Demonstration of UVC and UAC. UVC has entered the right portal vein instead of crossing the ductus venosus into the IVC and should be repositioned or withdrawn. Prominent normal left lobe of thymus obscures the upper lobe of the left lung.

Common paediatric examinations and chest – neonatal

13

Antero-posterior – supine (*cont.*)

Radiological considerations

- If the baby is intubated, great care must be taken not to dislodge the endotracheal tube (ETT). Even small movements of the head can result in significant movement of the tip. In a very premature baby it is best to leave the head in a sideways position to avoid any movement of the ETT. The ETT tip should lie in the lower 1/3 of the trachea, approximately between T1 and the carina (Figs 13.11a, 13.10c).
- An umbilical arterial catheter (UAC) follows the umbilical artery down inferiorly to either internal iliac artery and then via the iliacs to the aorta. This catheter is usually finer and more radio-opaque than an umbilical venous catheter (UVC). The former should ideally be placed with its tip in the mid-thoracic aorta between T4 and T9, which avoids the risk of causing thrombosis if the tip is opposite the origins of any of the abdominal vessels. Some UACs can be left with their tips in the lower abdominal aorta, below the level of L2, if there has been difficulty with advancing them. The UVC passes directly upwards through the ductus venosus in the liver and should lie with its tip in the inferior vena cava or right atrium. If lines are only faintly radio-opaque, then ultrasound can also be used for localisation (Fig. 13.11d).

Notes

- Minimal handling and the avoidance of heat loss from any incubator are essential. Babies are very vulnerable to infection, and therefore strict hygiene rules and hand washing are paramount.
- All the cassettes and foam pads inserted into an incubator should be wipeable.
- All nurses must be trained, experienced and confident in holding babies for immobilisation techniques.
- All preparation of the X-ray equipment should be performed before placing the X-ray cassette under the baby.

Radiation protection

- Accurate collimation of the X-ray beam is vital.
- Holder's hands should not in be the direct beam.
- Additional lead masking can be used to protect contralateral limbs in the assessment of vascular lines.
- The abdomen should be included on a CXR only if assessment of catheters or relevant pathology is present. In this case, male gonads should be protected.
- All mobile equipment on SCBU should have short-exposure capability to allow kV selection of over 60 kV as a dose-reduction measure. If this is not possible, then additional filtration can be considered, but this can affect the quality of the image.
- An accurate exposure chart according to infant weight should be available.
- All mobile equipment should have a DAP meter.[37]

13 Chest – post-neonatal

Referral criteria

Specific technique depends on the clinical referral, as follows:

Congenital heart disease

A CXR is rarely useful in children with an asymptomatic murmur but can distinguish non-cardiac from cardiac disease,[11] and echocardiography is normally recommended. It has been demonstrated that there is only 58% sensitivity, although 92% specificity, of a CXR predicting cardiac enlargement on echo.[38]

However, a CXR can demonstrate, mediastinal configuration and pulmonary vascularity (Fig. 13.12c).

The dimensions of the small paediatric chest are such that the choice of PA/AP projection does not have such an influence on the impression of cardiac size, unlike in adults. However, in some cases of known congenital heart disease, it may be advisable to use the same projection for initial and follow-up studies.[39]

The variations in the appearance of the normal thymus (Fig. 13.12a) often cause confusion.

Wheeze

A CXR will commonly show hyperinflation and bronchial wall thickening due to asthma or a viral infection such as bronchiolitis. A CXR is indicated if there is clinical suspicion of underlying pneumonic infection or secondary pneumothorax. The radiographs of children with hyperinflated lungs often demonstrate a lordotic position and measures should be taken (see pages 440, 442) to avoid this and to avoid the lung bases being obscured.

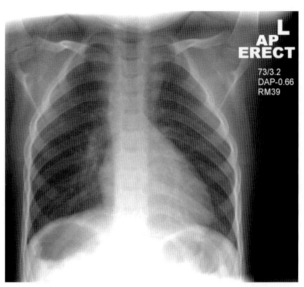

Fig. 13.12c AP erect chest radiograph of a 4-year-old child with double outlet right ventricle shows wide superior mediastinum, laevocardia, horizontal fissure on the right, left azygous fissure and stomach on the right. Being able to identify these features is important in the full evaluation of complex congenital heart disease.

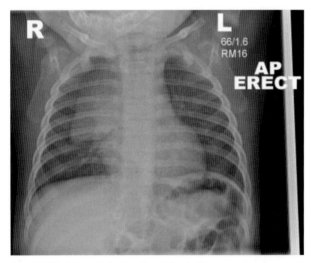

Fig. 13.12a AP erect chest radiograph of a 7-month-old infant demonstrating a normal prominent right lobe of thymus.

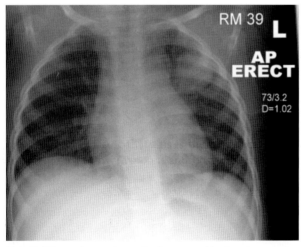

Fig. 13.12b AP chest radiograph of a 1-year-old infant demonstrating a round pneumonia in the upper lobe of the left lung.

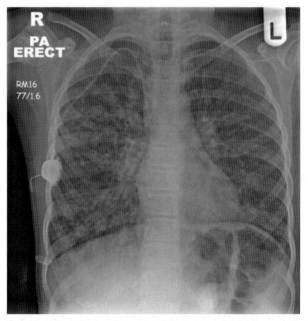

Fig. 13.12d PA chest radiograph of a 9-year-old child with cystic fibrosis and secondary pneumonia in the right middle lobe and lingula. Hickman line in a satisfactory position overlying the superior vena cava. Button artefacts should be avoided where possible.

Inhaled foreign body

A high index of suspicion is required. CXRs are often normal. As air trapping is the most common sign, if not evident on a radiograph, mediastinal shift can be demonstrated on fluoroscopy. An expiratory radiograph can also be considered if the child is able to co-operate. If clinical suspicion remains high, bronchoscopy would still be indicated. In low suspicion cases, a low dose multidetector CT (MDCT) of the bronchial tree could be considered to avoid any unnecessary bronchoscopy.[11]

An AP image of the chest using a Cincinnati filter can also be considered to demonstrate the trachea, main bronchi, mediastinum and any mediastinal shift. All images should include the pharynx, trachea, major bronchi and lungs and should be as straight as possible, to allow assessment of mediastinal shift.

Oesophageal pH probe for reflux study

An AP projection supine rather than a lateral projection is preferred as it gives a lower dose. It should be coned from C7 to T12 and laterally to the mediastinum. The tip of the probe should be at T7/T8.

Acute stridor

Stridor from birth is most commonly due to a 'floppy larynx'. A CXR is not usually indicated. However, if a vascular ring is suspected, a CXR may demonstrate the position of the aortic arch and an oesophagogram would be indicated. A Cincinnati radiograph or low dose MDCT can demonstrate any tracheal narrowing.

New-onset acute stridor is usually due to a viral infection such as croup or a bacterial infection such as epiglottitis. Care must be taken in ensuring that the patient has a stable airway before undertaking any examinations of the latter.

A lateral neck radiograph would be indicated and in some specific circumstances, e.g. a suspected tracheal foreign body (FB), a CXR could be performed. A patient with a tracheal FB should have urgent bronchoscopy and measures taken to ensure that the FB does not get dislodged into a more hazardous position.

Acute chest infection

A CXR is not normally required as most infections only affect the bronchi as bronchitis. A CXR is indicated for a suspected pneumonia.

Unlike adults, when a tumour may underlie a pneumonia, follow-up radiographs are not required if a child makes a clinical recovery. Follow-up radiographs can be considered if there is a round pneumonia (Fig. 13.12b), extensive lobar or sub-lobar pneumonia, adenopathy or pleural effusion present. This should usually not be performed less than 3 weeks after the clinical event as radiological resolution lags behind clinical resolution.

However, any deterioration in a clinical condition should be imaged promptly. A repeat radiograph is also indicated after treatment to ensure that there has been re-expansion of any areas of collapse.

Recurrent cough

Recurrent cough can be due to underlying asthma or a cardiac anomaly. A CXR is only indicated if a child has not responded

Chest – post-neonatal 13

Referral criteria (*cont.*)

to treatment, a child is clearly unwell or has a known underlying condition such as cystic fibrosis (Fig. 13.12d), chronic lung disease, an immune deficiency or congenital heart disease.

Acute chest pain and shortness of breath can also be due to a pneumothorax and a CXR is indicated if this is suspected.

Trauma

Radiographs may need to be taken supine and a horizontal beam may be required to demonstrate a pneumothorax or pleural effusion.

Others

- Suspected malignancy.
- Swallowed foreign body – see abdomen, page 447.
- Tuberculosis (TB) contact, Heaf test >grade 2.
- Acute abdominal pain, lower lobe pneumonia can masquerade as abdominal pain.
- Fever of unknown origin.
- Exacerbation of known chronic lung disease.
- Smoke inhalation.
- Near drowning.
- Haemoptysis. More likely to be due to upper airways infection in children.
- Acute chest pain.

Recommended projections

Examination is performed by means of the following projections:

Basic	PA – erect
Alternative	AP – erect AP – supine
Supplementary	Lateral AP with Cincinnati filter

AP, antero-posterior; PA, postero-anterior.

There is some controversy as to whether CXRs of children beyond the neonatal period should be taken supine or erect and PA or AP.

It is recommended that a PA erect projection should be adopted when a child can stand or when age allows, usually when over the age of 3 years. This results in a lower breast dose. An erect projection also allows better expansion of the lungs and demonstration of pleural effusions and pneumothoraces. However, if this is not possible, then supine projections are taken. For all projections, it is important that the child should be straight, with no rotation and distal 2/3 of humeri excluded.

13 Chest – post-neonatal

Postero-anterior – erect (Fig. 13.13a)

The key to erect chest radiography is to use a specifically designed paediatric seat and an image receptor holder/vertical chest stand, which allow a parent or carer to hold their child easily. A CR cassette or DDR detector is selected relative to the size of the child.

Position of patient and image receptor

- Depending on the child's age, the child is seated or stood facing the cassette, with the chest pressed against it.
- The arms should not be extended fully but should be raised gently, bringing the elbows forward.
- The parent or carer should hold the flexed elbows and head together then pull the arms gently upwards and slightly forward to prevent the child from slumping backwards.

Direction and location of the X-ray beam

- The collimated horizontal beam is directed at right-angles to the receptor and centred at the level of the 8th thoracic vertebra (spinous process of T7).

Antero-posterior – erect (Figs 13.13b, 13.13c)

This is done when the PA projection is not possible.

Position of patient and image receptor

- The child is seated with his or her back against the image receptor, which is supported vertically, with the upper edge of the image receptor above the lung apices.
- Place a 15° foam wedge behind the shoulders to prevent the child from adopting a lordotic position.
- The arms should be raised gently, bringing the elbows forward. The arms should not be extended fully.
- The parent or carer should hold the flexed elbows and head together with their fingers on the forehead, to prevent the child's chin from obscuring the upper chest.
- The holder should pull the forehead gently upwards to prevent the child from slumping forward.

Direction and location of the X-ray beam

- The collimated horizontal central beam is angled 5–10° caudally to the middle of the image receptor at the level of the 8th thoracic vertebra, approximately at the midpoint of the body of the sternum. This is particularly important in children with hyperinflated chests due to diseases such as bronchiolitis, which predisposes to lordotic projections.
- The radiation field is collimated to the ribcage thus avoiding exposure of the eyes, thyroid and upper abdomen.

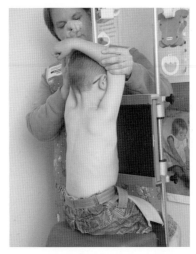

Fig. 13.13a Child positioned for PA erect chest radiograph.

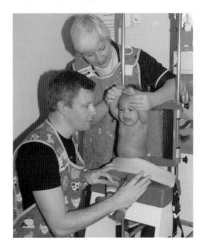

Fig. 13.13b Child positioned for AP erect chest radiograph. Holder's fingers should be placed on the child's forehead to prevent the head rolling forward and the chin obscuring the upper chest.

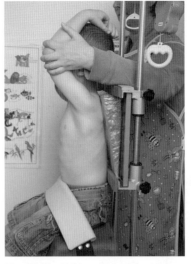

Fig. 13.13c Child positioned for AP erect radiograph with a wedge foam pad used to avoid a lordotic projection.

Notes

- A comfortable seat, with Velcro straps encased in foam that can be applied over the thighs, is extremely useful.
- Mobile lead shielding is optional.

Chest – post-neonatal 13

Antero-posterior – erect (cont.)

Correct interpretation of paediatric chest radiographs requires images taken in maximum inspiration without rotation or tilting. The radiographer should watch the child's chest/abdominal movements to obtain a maximum inspiration.

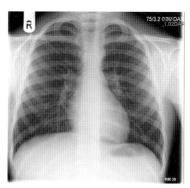

Fig. 13.14a PA erect chest radiograph of a 9-year-old child. Normal appearances, TB contact.

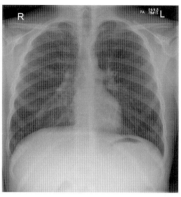

Fig. 13.14b PA erect chest radiograph of a 5-year-old child with cystic fibrosis right middle lobe (RML), pneumonia and tip of right central line overlying the left axillary vein.

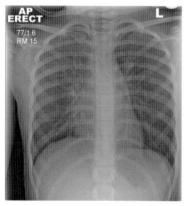

Fig. 13.14c AP erect chest radiograph of a 7-year-old child with acute asthma demonstrates hyperventilation of the lungs, elevation of the horizontal fissure due to volume loss in the right upper lobe and pneumonic consolidation in the right middle lobe.

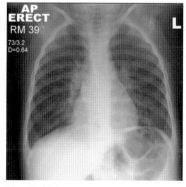

Fig. 13.14d AP erect chest radiograph of a 1-year-old child with right middle lobe pneumonia, widespread peribronchial opacity and small bilateral pleural effusions. Erect chest radiographs are preferred whenever possible, as small effusions or pneumothoraces can be missed on supine radiographs.

Common faults and solutions

- Incorrect density – needs radiographer experience in assessing the size of the child and careful exposure charts. The kV should not be less than 70.
- Thorax tilted backwards (AP projection), with clavicles shown high above the lung apices. This lordotic projection results in the lower lobes of the lungs being obscured by the diaphragms. Pneumonia and other lung pathology can be missed. See 'Position of patient and image receptor' for how to correct this fault.
- Holder's hands on the shoulders on the shoulders should be avoided and a child's arms, skull and abdomen (beyond the diaphragms) should be excluded from the primary beam by tight collimation.

Essential image characteristics

AP/PA projection:

- Peak inspiration (PA, six anterior ribs, 5/6 for AP; nine posterior ribs above the diaphragm).
- Whole chest from just above the lung apices to include the diaphragms and ribs.
- No rotation (medial ends of clavicles or 1st ribs should be equidistant from the spine).
- No tilting (clavicles should overlie lung apices). Anterior ribs should point downwards.
- Reproduction of trachea, proximal bronchi and vascular pattern in central 2/3 of the lungs
- Visually sharp reproduction of the diaphragm and costophrenic angles.
- Reproduction of the spine and paraspinal structures and visualisation of the retrocardiac lung and mediastinum.

Radiological considerations (Figs 13.14a–13.14d)

- CXRs are not routinely required for simple chest infections.
- Follow-up chest images are not routinely required if there has been a good response to treatment unless the initial chest image showed lobar pneumonia, extensive sub-lobar pneumonia involving several segments, pneumatoceles, adenopathy or pleural effusion.
- Prompt follow-up CXR is required following physiotherapy and antibiotics for areas of collapse to confirm re-expansion. Otherwise follow-up radiographs should not be taken for less than 3 weeks as radiological resolution lags behind clinical resolution. Repeat images are required earlier if there is any deterioration.

13 Chest – post-neonatal

Antero-posterior – supine
(Figs 13.15a–13.15d)

The AP (supine) projection is performed as an alternative to the erect position when the latter is not possible.

Special attention is required when imaging a baby's chest. As the chest is conical in shape, positioning a baby supine with the back against a cassette results in a lordotic projection, with the clavicles projected above the apices and a large part of the lower lobes superimposed on the abdomen. The heart also appears foreshortened. In a correct projection, the anterior rib ends will be projected inferiorly to the posterior rib ends, and the clavicles will be seen superimposed on the lung apices. This can be accomplished either by leaning the baby forward or by angling the X-ray tube caudally, or both.

The projection is often performed as part of a mobile X-ray examination on children of all ages.

A cassette size is selected depending on the size of the child.

Position of patient and image receptor

- The child is positioned supine on the image receptor, with the upper edge positioned above the lung apices.
- When examining a baby, a 15° foam pad is positioned between the thorax and the cassette (thick end under the upper thorax) to avoid a lordotic projection. A small foam pad is also placed under the child's head for comfort.
- The median sagittal plane is adjusted at right-angles to the middle of the cassette. To avoid rotation, the head, chest and pelvis are straight.
- The child's arms are held, with the elbows flexed, on each side of the head. Alternatively, the arms are extended and abducted from the trunk, immobilised with sand bags.
- A suitable appliance, e.g. Velcro band, is secured over the baby's abdomen and sandbags are placed next to the thighs to prevent rotation.

Direction and location of the X-ray beam

- The collimated vertical beam is directed at right-angles to the receptor and centred at the level of T8 (mid-sternum).
- For babies with a very hyperinflated barrel chest (due to bronchiolitis or asthma), the tube is also angled 5–10° caudally to avoid a lordotic projection.

Common faults and solutions

- Care should be taken not to have the lung apices obscured by the chin or excluded from the image.
- An excessive lordotic projection results in the lower lobes of the lungs being obscured by the anterior diaphragms. Pneumonia and other lung pathology can thus be missed. This can be avoided by adopting the positioning described above.

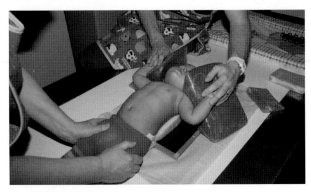

Fig. 13.15a Patient positioned for AP supine chest radiograph.

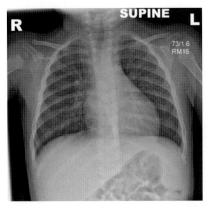

Fig. 13.15b AP supine chest radiograph of a 9-month-old infant with bronchiolitis.

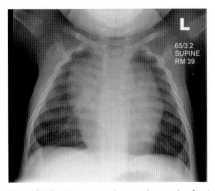

Fig. 13.15c AP supine chest radiograph of a 4-month-old infant with prominent normal thymus. Some thymic glands can be particularly large.

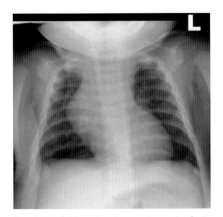

Fig. 13.15d AP supine chest radiograph of a 2-month-old infant demonstrating normal right lobe of thymus and skin creases that could be avoided by moving the right arm laterally. Skin creases can mimic lung margins of a pneumothorax.

Chest – post-neonatal 13

Lateral (Figs 13.16a, 13.16b)

This supplementary projection is undertaken to locate the position of an inhaled or swallowed FB, to evaluate middle lobe pathology or to localise opacities demonstrated on the PA/AP projection. A CR cassette is selected.

Position of patient and image receptor

- The erect patient is turned to bring the side under investigation towards the image receptor. The median sagittal plane is adjusted parallel to the cassette.
- The outstretched arms are raised and held above the head and supported.
- The mid-axillary line is coincident with the middle of the cassette, and the cassette is adjusted to include the apices and the inferior lobes.

Direction and location of the X-ray beam

- The collimated horizontal beam is directed at right-angles to the receptor.
- Exposure is made on peak inspiration.

Essential image characteristics

- Peak inspiration (six anterior ribs above the diaphragm).
- Whole chest from C7 to L1.
- Sternum and spine to be included and to be true lateral.
- Visualisation of whole trachea and major bronchi.
- Visually sharp reproduction of the whole of both domes of the diaphragm.
- Reproduction of the hilar vessels.
- Reproduction of the sternum and the thoracic spine.

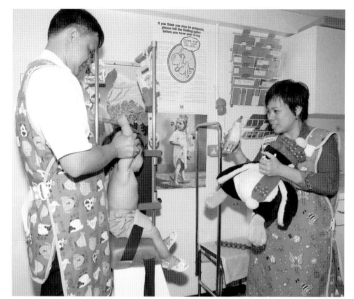

Fig. 13.16a Infant positioned on a special seat against the chest stand for a lateral projection. Distraction aids being employed.

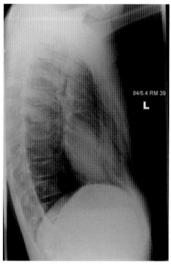

Fig. 13.16b Lateral erect chest radiograph of a 5-year-old child demonstrating a significant pectus deformity.

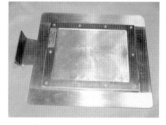

Fig. 13.16c Cincinnati filter device.

Cincinnati filter device (Figs 13.16c, 13.16d)

The use of this filter device is employed in cases of suspected inhaled FB or to demonstrate the trachea and major bronchi. An AP image of the chest is acquired with the child lying supine.

The Cincinnati filter is composed of 2 mm of aluminium, 0.5 mm of copper and 0.4 mm of tin inserted into the collimator box so that the copper layer is towards the X-ray tube. Exposures used are in the range of 125–140 kV and 10–16 mAs, using a CR cassette and grid system.

On the exposed radiograph, bone detail is effaced to a considerable degree, allowing soft tissue and air interfaces in the mediastinum and adjacent lung to be seen. The trachea and proximal bronchial anatomy are demonstrated well.

A low-dose CT can be considered as an alternative and all patients with suspected aspirated FB should be referred for bronchoscopy.

Careful handling is always advisable in children suspected to have an inhaled FB, as dislodgement can result in total airway obstruction.

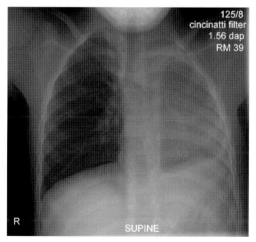

Fig. 13.16d AP supine chest radiograph of a 6-year-old child with Cincinnati filter showing no air in the left upper lobe bronchus or lobe – congenital left upper lobe (LUL) sequestration.

13 Abdomen

Abdominal radiography is not routinely indicated for imaging of the acute abdomen in children and is performed in conjunction with abdominal ultrasound.

Referral criteria

- Non specific abdominal pain
- Ultrasound should be performed first.
- Abdominal radiography may be indicated if following are present:
  - Loin pain.
  - Haematuria.
  - Diarrhoea.
  - Palpable mass.
  - Abdominal distension.
  - Suspected new-onset inflammatory bowel disease. (Patients with known Crohn's disease should have ultrasound to assess any exacerbation but a radiograph would be indicated in those with known ulcerative colitis.)

Acute abdominal pain

- Ultrasound is again the first investigation of choice.
- However, an abdominal radiograph should be performed if malrotation, volvulus or intestinal obstruction is suspected.
- An intussusception or appendix mass is better demonstrated on ultrasound, but an abdominal radiograph can demonstrate any small bowel obstruction, evidence of perforation or an appendicolith.

Constipation

- There is a wide variation in the normal amount of faecal residue seen on an abdominal radiograph.
- Ultrasound should be used to demonstrate the degree of faecal distension in the rectum and its impression on the posterior bladder wall. Radiographs are reserved for those with intractable constipation who have not responded to treatment. (See Radiological considerations page 447.)
- There should be a higher suspicion of Hirschsprung's disease in those under 2 year of age and an abdominal radiograph is indicated if this is the clinical concern.

Suspected swallowed foreign body

(See Radiological considerations, page 447.)

Urinary tract infection

- Ultrasound is the investigation of choice.
- An abdominal radiograph may be indicated if haematuria, severe loin colic or a previous history of calculi is present.
- A radiograph may also be indicated if recurrent urinary tract infections are associated with enuresis that has not responded to treatment. An assessment of faecal loading and the exclusion of a spinal abnormality is required.

Palpable mass

- Ultrasound should be performed first.
- A radiograph may demonstrate additional features such as the confirmation of calcification, secondary bowel obstruction or any spine/bony involvement.

Other

- Trauma: when intestinal perforation is suspected.
- Failure of passage of meconium.
- Imperforate anus: ultrasound of the perineum is now the preferred examination for assessment of anal atresia as it is more likely to identify correctly the level of atresia. However, plain radiographs can still be performed as below.

Recommended projections

Examination is performed by means of the following:

Basic	AP – supine (Fig. 13.17)
Alternative	PA – prone
Supplementary	Lateral PA – left lateral decubitus AP – erect

AP, antero-posterior; PA, postero-anterior.

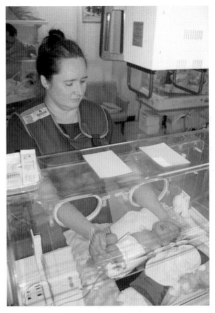

Fig. 13.17 AP supine combined chest and abdomen in a neonate to show position of intravascular lines.

Abdomen 13

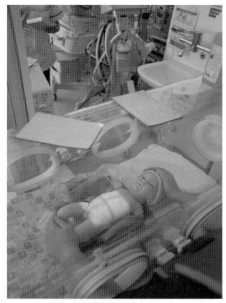

Fig. 13.18a AP supine of baby abdomen with legs straight to ensure no loss of detail in the pelvis. Corner of rubber lead on top of incubator used to protect gonads.

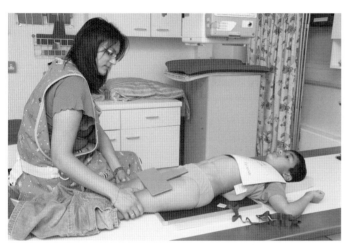

Fig. 13.18b Older child positioned on an imaging table for AP supine abdomen. Lead-rubber on chest can be used to exclude tube scatter but primary collimation is most important.

Antero-posterior (Figs 13.18a–13.18d)

A DDR detector system is employed without the use of a grid or alternatively an appropriately sized CR cassette is selected depending on the size of the patient.

Position of patient and image receptor

- The child lies supine on the X-ray table or in the incubator in the case of a neonate, with the median sagittal plane of the trunk at right-angles to the middle of the image receptor.
- To ensure that the child is not rotated the anterior superior iliac spines should be equidistant from the image receptor.
- The image receptor should be large enough to include the symphysis pubis and the diaphragm.

Direction and location of the X-ray beam

- The collimated vertical beam is centred to the middle of the cassette.

Notes

- All acute abdominal radiographs should include the diaphragms and lung bases. Lower lobe pneumonia can often masquerade as acute abdominal pain.
- Radiographs of the renal tract for renal calculi are no longer commonly performed but when necessary, should have more lateral coning.
- A fizzy drink may be used to distend the stomach with air, thus displacing residue in the transverse colon and better demonstrating the renal areas.
- Collimation is as for adults, but babies' and infants' abdomens tend to be rounder with less anterior abdominal wall adipose tissue; therefore, slightly wider lateral collimation is required.

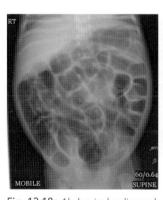

Fig. 13.18c Abdominal radiograph of 1-week-old female neonate with non-specific gaseous bowel distension down to the rectum.

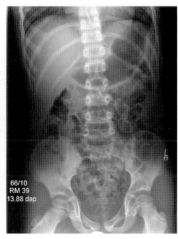

Fig. 13.18d AP supine abdominal radiograph of an 8-year-old male child with suspected gastroenteritis. Normal appearances. Note use of antiscatter grid and gonad protection.

13 Abdomen

Antero-posterior (cont.)

Essential image characteristics

AP projection for whole abdomen:

- Abdomen to include diaphragm, lateral abdominal walls and ischial tuberosities.
- Pelvis and spine should be straight, with no rotation.
- Reproduction of properitoneal fat lines consistent with age.
- Visualisation of kidney and psoas outlines consistent with age and bowel content.
- Visually sharp reproduction of the bones.

Common faults and solutions

- Usually inadequate coning but occasionally too tight coning excludes the diaphragms.
- Male gonads not appropriately protected.
- Artefacts from clothing. All underwear needs to be inspected and removed as modern underwear often has metallic threads or glitter. The child should be covered with a paper towel, cotton pillowcase or a child's gown.

Radiation protection

- An antiscatter grid is not used routinely in children below 5–7 years.
- Optimisation of abdominal radiographs includes using a lower-dose technique, e.g. excluding an antiscatter grid and using a very fast image acquisition system, in the assessment of conditions such as chronic constipation and swallowed foreign body. Repeat images in the latter should not be performed unless there are specific symptoms that might suggest complications such as pain or vomiting.
- All boys should have testicular protection.
- If radiographs are performed for suspected ureteric calculi then they can be more collimated laterally and the diaphragms excluded.
- Although it has been demonstrated that a PA abdominal technique results in a lower dose,[40] a supine technique with male gonad protection is preferred in children.
- In supine neonates who cannot be moved, a horizontal beam lateral should be taken with the neonate's right side nearest the cassette (to reduce the dose to the liver).

Radiological considerations (Figs 13.19a–13.19d, 13.20a)

- Unlike adults, erect images are rarely required or justified.
- Left lateral or ventral decubitus images may be required in cases of suspected necrotising enterocolitis. In the former projection, with the patient lying on the left side, free gas will rise to be located between the lateral margin of the liver and the right abdominal wall.
- Lateral projections may demonstrate Hirschsprung's disease or a retroperitoneal tumour in some rare cases.

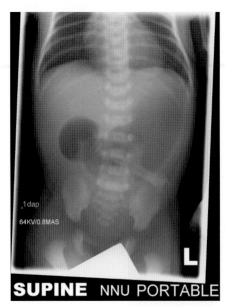

Fig. 13.19a AP supine abdominal radiograph of a 1-day-old male neonate with typical double bubble appearance of duodenal aAtresia. Coning should have been limited to the lung bases only. Gonad protection in situ.

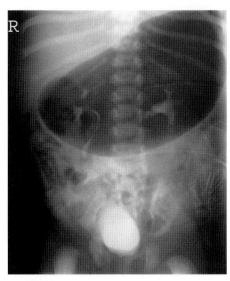

Fig. 13.19b AP supine abdominal radiograph demonstrating the effect of fizzy drink as part of an IVU series.

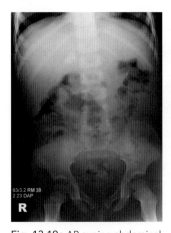

Fig. 13.19c AP supine abdominal radiograph of a 4-year-old male child demonstrating right adrenal calcification. Gonad protection coned off. No antiscatter grid used.

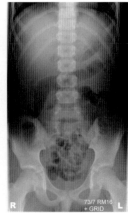

Fig. 13.19d AP supine abdominal radiograph of a10-year-old female with abdominal pain, demonstrating mucosal oedema of the transverse colon due to ulcerative colitis. Note at this age a grid is necessary.

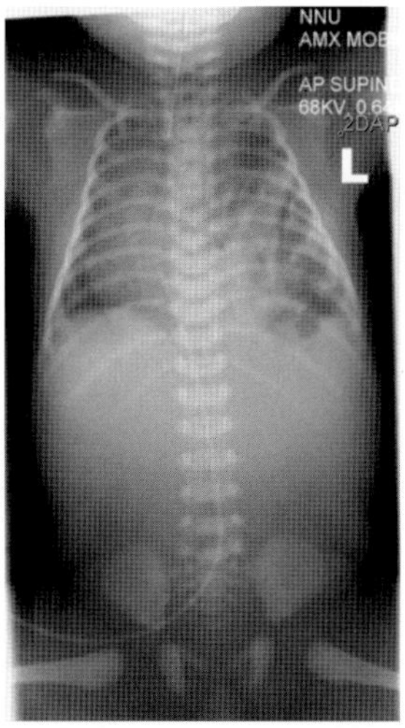

Abdomen 13

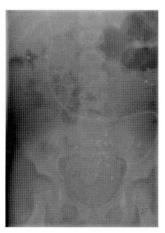

Fig. 13.20a AP supine chest and abdominal radiograph of 1-day-old female with a left diaphragmatic hernia. These patients are intubated early to avoid excessive gas in bowel loops causing mediastinal compression. A straight radiograph is required. Tip of the endotracheal tube is in a satisfactory position in a slightly deviated trachea. Tip of umbilical venous catheter is in a satisfactory position overlying the right atrium.

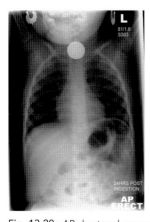

Fig. 13.20b AP supine fluoroscopic, frame grab image of the abdomen of an 8-year-old boy with a ventriculoperitoneal shunt and chronic constipation. Radio-opaque pellets distributed throughout the colon on the 5th day are consistent with slow colonic transit. Coning to the colon; the diaphragms can be excluded. Such low dose technique can also be used for checking position of tubes such as naso jejunal tubes and suspected, asymptomatic swallowed foreign bodies.

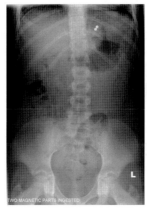

Fig. 13.20c AP chest and upper abdominal radiograph of a 2-year-old child demonstrating a coin-shaped foreign body in the upper oesophagus. Its shape suggests an intraoesophageal position.

Fig. 13.20d AP abdominal radiograph from a 12-year-old boy who had ingested two parts of a magnet. This can be a surgical emergency as bowel wall trapped between the two magnets can undergo necrosis and lead to bowel perforation

Modifications in technique

Constipation (Fig. 13.20b)

- A fast image acquisition system should be used in chronic cases. A study of colonic transit time may also be requested.
- The patient swallows 30 radio-opaque plastic pellets (10 each day for 3 consecutive days) and an AP radiograph with the child in the supine position is performed at 'day five' following ingestion. If on the 5th day, pellets are not present, this is normal. If there is a general delay in colonic transit, the pellets will be distributed throughout the colon. Pellets grouped in the rectum indicate poor evacuation.
- A good quality, higher-resolution image should be obtained in children under 2 years when Hirschsprung's disease is suspected. This is to allow assessment of the bowel that may be complicated by colitis.

Suspected swallowed foreign body (Figs 13.20c, 13.20d)

- The radiograph should demonstrate from below the mandible to the iliac crests and can be either undertaken supine or erect.
- The most likely sites of hold-up are the neck, mid-oesophagus where the left main bronchus crosses the oesophagus, and at the gastro-oesophageal junction. FBs including open pins and needles normally pass unhindered if they are beyond the oesophagus and do not need further radiographs.
- If a FB is demonstrated in the neck or chest, a lateral radiograph should be taken to confirm position. If the child is unable to swallow saliva due to oesophageal obstruction, urgent referral for removal of FB is advised.
- If the history is less than 4 hours and the FB is in the distal oesophagus, the child can be given a fizzy drink, kept erect and an AP radiograph repeated in 30 minutes to see whether the FB has been dislodged. If history is greater than 4hours, the patient should be kept nil by mouth and referred for consideration of physical/endoscopic removal. If no FB is demonstrated, no further radiographs are required in an asymptomatic child.
- Batteries and magnets: in cases of lead, lithium or mercury batteries, the same radiographs are acquired. If the FB is unknown, batteries should be identified by their double rims. If a battery is in the oesophagus urgent endoscopic removal is required. If the battery is in the stomach, then it can react with gastric acid, and referral for surgical opinion is advised.

  The presence of two or more magnets/batteries in the abdomen is also a surgical emergency as if apposed they can cause necrosis and perforation of the intervening bowel wall.

- If a swallowed FB is suspected to be radiolucent and in the oesophagus, then a contrast study may be needed.

Note

- The use of a metal detector in determining the presence of a metal object in the abdomen may reduce the need for unnecessary irradiation of a child.[41]

13 Abdomen

Modifications in technique (cont.)

Suspected necrotising enterocolitis (Fig. 13.21b)

- An AP supine abdominal radiograph is obtained with the legs and arms held in a similar position to that described for the neonatal CXR in a non-sleeping infant (see page 435).
- The abdomen is normally distended in these cases, care must be taken not to collimate within the margins of the abdomen.
- If a perforation is suspected, an AP (left lateral decubitus) projection is selected using a horizontal beam with the child lying on the left side. The right side of the patient is positioned uppermost as it is easier to demonstrate free air around the liver. The patient should be kept in this position for a few minutes before the radiograph is taken (Fig. 13.21a).
- If the infant is too ill to be moved, then a lateral (dorsal decubitus) projection is selected, using a horizontal beam, with the tube directed to the left side of the abdomen to reduce dose to the liver (Fig. 13.21c).
- Lead protection should be used to protect male gonads.

Suspected diaphragmatic hernia, for position of tubes and lines and infants under 1 kg

- A combined AP chest and abdomen on one radiographic image is recommended.

Imperforate anus (prone invertogram) (Figs 13.21d–13.21f)

- Ultrasound is the investigation of choice but radiography can be performed as below.
- A lateral (ventral decubitus) radiograph using a horizontal beam is used. This allows intraluminal air to rise and fill the most distal bowel to assess the level of atresia. Radiography should not be performed <24 hours after birth.

Position of patient and image receptor

- The infant should be placed in the prone position, with the pelvis and buttocks raised on a triangular covered foam pad or rolled-up nappy.
- The infant should be kept in this position for approximately 10–15 minutes.
- The CR cassette is supported vertically against the lateral aspect of the infant's pelvis, and adjusted parallel to the median sagittal plane.

Direction and location of the X-ray beam

- The collimated horizontal beam is directed at right-angles and centred to the middle of the image receptor.

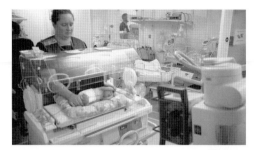

Fig. 13.21a Neonate in left lateral decubitus position. For minimal handling of a sick neonate, a dorsal decubitus is an alternative.

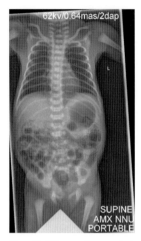 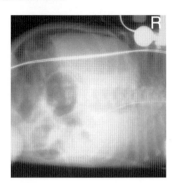

Fig. 13.21c Left lateral decubitus abdomen demonstrating free air around the liver.

Fig. 13.21b AP chest and abdomen image of a 1-week-old male neonate. Intramural air in the bowel wall consistent with necrotising enterocolitis. Note arms slightly away from the chest to avoid skin crease artifacts and infant's head excluded from the imaged area. Gonad protection in position.

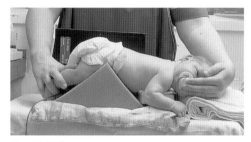

Fig. 13.21d Baby positioned for lateral abdomen – ventral decubitus.

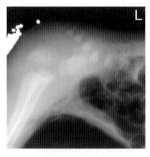 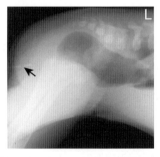

Figs 13.21e and f Radiographs of lateral abdomen, ventral decubitus in imperforate anus. Lower limit of air-filled bowel is demonstrated in relation to the pubo-coccygeal line. Left: high obstruction with lead pellets at anatomical position of anus; right: low obstruction with barium-filled tube tip at level of anus.

Notes

- A lead marker is taped to the skin in the anatomical area where the anus would normally be sited. The distance between this and the most distal air-filled bowel can then be measured.

Skull 13

Obtaining diagnostic quality radiographs of the skull in small children is probably one of the most difficult challenges to any radiographer. The technique described for adults is not so straightforward when the patient is a screaming, red faced, determined toddler accompanied by anxious parents!

Young children may be wrapped in cotton blankets for immobilisation and the use of shaped foam pads is strongly recommended.

A feed or use of a pacifier is very beneficial. All clothing, fasteners, hair clips or beads and sometimes extra stiff hair gel need to be removed. The carer accompanying the child, provided not pregnant, should be encouraged to remain and distract the child with a toy for the exposure.

Children's head sizes are variable and are also of variable density depending on skeletal maturation and various congenital malformations. Below the age of 1 year, there are no visible vascular markings and only the range of additional sutures, which can cause confusion with fractures. Grids are not routinely used in skull radiography of children under the age 3–5 years, thus exposure times and patient dose are reduced.

Referral criteria

Trauma

Serious intracranial injury can occur in the absence of a skull fracture and the use of radiographs has now been superseded by optimised low dose CT, as recommended by the National Institute of Health and Care Excellence (NICE) guidelines on the management of head injury (latest update Jan 2014) (Figs 13.22a, 13.22b).[42]

The indications for the performance of CT within 1 hour of injury include:

- Glasgow coma scale (GCS) score of <14 (<15 for under 1 y).
- Evidence of an open, depressed or base of skull fracture.
- Tense fontanelle.
- Focal neurological deficit or seizure.
- Presence of a bruise.
- Swelling or laceration over 5 cm on the head in those under 1 year.

Various recommendations are given as to when post-trauma scans need to be performed within 1 hour, 4 hours or 8 hours and what clinical observation is required. However, skull radiographs are still indicated for head injury in those under 2 years of age as the head injury could be non-accidental. The possibility of the maltreatment of children should always be considered. In the absence of significant indications for CT and when CT is not available, radiographs can be performed but combined with a period of neurological observation. If there is any deterioration, prompt timely transfer to a specialist neurosurgical centre is paramount.

Other

- Suspected craniosynostosis, abnormally shaped or sized head: see modification of technique.
- Palpable lump or suspected depressed fracture: ultrasound is first investigation of choice. May require tangential radiographic view.
- Integrity of ventriculo-atrial or peritoneal shunt.
- Part of syndrome assessment.
- Headache or epilepsy: a skull radiograph is not indicated.

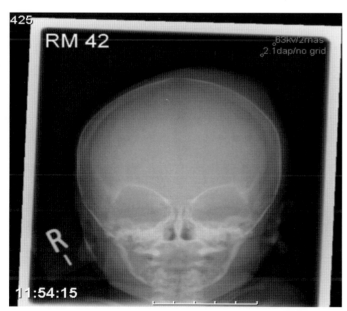

Fig. 13.22a Fronto-occipital radiograph of a 4 day old neonate with subgaleal haematoma over left parietal bone. Note no use of a grid.

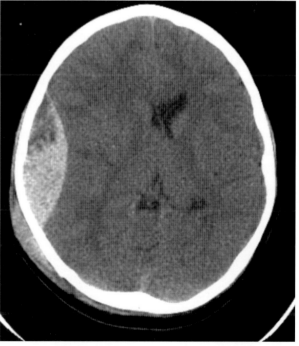

Fig. 13.22b Axial CT of 9-year-old male with large, acute, right extradural haematoma causing midline shift requiring urgent surgery.

13 Skull

Recommended projections

Examination is performed by means of the following:

Basic	OF
	FO – 30° caudal
	Lateral
Alternative	FO
	Tangential

FO, fronto-occipital; OF, occipito-frontal.

Modifications of technique are recommended (according to the referral) as follows, in cases of trauma and when CT is not available:

Condition	Projections
If not knocked unconscious and specific frontal injury	OF/FO Lateral of affected side
If not knocked unconscious and specific occipital injury	FO –30° caudal Lateral of affected side
If knocked unconscious or showing signs of fracture	OF/FO FO – 30° caudal Lateral of affected side

Trauma

- The lateral projection should include the first three cervical vertebrae.
- A horizontal beam lateral is usually performed but is not considered essential before the age of 6 years, as the sphenoid sinus is not pneumatised before this age. After this, air–fluid levels might indicate a base of skull fracture.
- All trauma images should adequately demonstrate the soft tissues.

Craniosynostosis

- For assessment of craniosynostosis, a lateral and under tilted FO – 20° caudal projection will demonstrate all the sutures adequately in most children (Figs 13.23a, 13.23b).
- Ultrasound can confirm suture patency in simple plagiocephaly.

- Tangential projections may be required in some cases of a bony lump.
- Low dose CT with 3D reconstruction is used for more complex deformity.

Radiographic technique

The technique used for adult skull radiography can be readily adopted for older children. The projections described in the following pages are for a 1-year-old child:

- FO.
- FO – 30° caudal.
- Lateral of affected side with horizontal beam.

Radiological considerations

As skull X-rays involve a moderately high dose in terms of plain images (often including a series of projections), justification is essential. Good clinico-radiological co-operation, agreed referral criteria and audit are essential in keeping the number of unnecessary radiographs to a minimum.[6] Studies suggest that over 1/3 of requests following trauma are unnecessary[7] and many have reported that absence of a fracture does not alter management.[43–46] CT to exclude intracranial injury, when indicated, is now the first imaging of choice.

Radiation protection

Justification, optimisation and careful technique are the best ways of conforming to radiation protection guidelines.

- Avoidance of the use of a grid in children under the age of 3–5 years is an important dose-saving measure.
- A short exposure time is particularly important in performing skull radiography to avoid movement unsharpness. The maximum exposure time should be less than 40 ms.
- Children's skulls are almost fully grown by the age of 7 years and therefore children over the age of 7 need almost as much exposure as an adult.
- Holder's hands should not be visible on the radiograph.
- Tight collimation with circular cones of variable size is best suited for the shape of the cranium. In this way unnecessary thyroid radiation can also be avoided in non-trauma cases.
- Occipito-frontal (OF) projections, where possible, will reduce the dose to the eyes.[47]

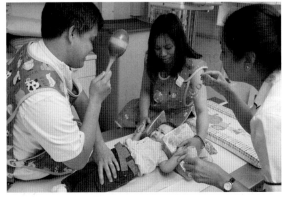

Fig. 13.23a Infant positioned for FO 20° radiography of the skull for craniosynostosis.

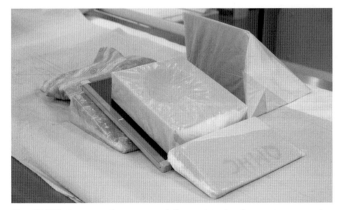

Fig. 13.23b Position of sponge pads for positioning for craniosynostosis.

Skull 13

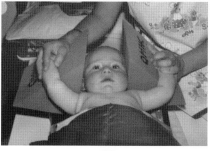

Fig. 13.24a Position of infant for fronto-posterior skull with triangular sponges supporting the head on either side.

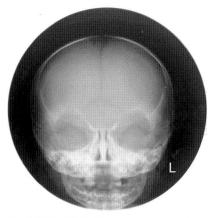

Fig. 13.24b FO skull image – patient supine with normal appearances.

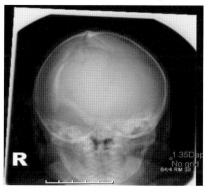

Fig. 13.24c FO skull of a 4-day-old neonate with significant hemifacial and cranial abnormality. Harlequin skull appearance due to premature fusion of right coronal suture.

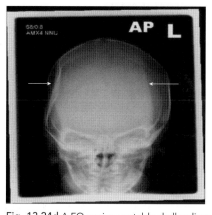

Fig. 13.24d A FO supine portable skull radiograph on Neonatal unit. Newborn with large ping-pong fracture of the right parietal bone. Petrous bones overlie the orbits as a result of the chin being positioned too low. Head sponge support artefact should be avoided if possible.

Fronto-occipital (Figs 13.24a–13.24d)

A 24 × 30 cm or 18 × 24 cm CR cassette is selected, depending on the size of the cranium.

Position of patient and image receptor

- The child is positioned carefully in the supine position with the head resting on a pre-formed skull foam pad positioned on top of the cassette.
- The head is adjusted to bring the median sagittal plane at right-angles to, and in the midline of the receptor.
- The external auditory meati (EAMS) should be equidistant from the film.
- The child is immobilised in this position with the assistance of a carer who is asked to hold two 45° foam pads on either side of the skull during the exposure. The carer usually stands at the head end of the imaging table to undertake this procedure. Occasionally a second carer is required to assist in immobilising the trunk.

Direction and location of the X-ray beam

- The collimated vertical beam is centred to the naison at the necessary angle to allow it to pass along the orbito-meatal plane.
- If it is required that the orbits are shown clear of the petrous bone, the central ray should be angled cranially so that it makes an angle of 20° to the orbito-meatal plane and centred to the naison.

Essential image characteristics

- Whole cranial vault, orbits and petrous bones should be present on the radiograph and symmetrical and the petrous bones projected over the lower orbital margins.
- Lambdoid and coronal sutures should be symmetrical.
- Visually sharp reproduction of the outer and inner tables of the cranial vault according to age.
- Reproduction of sinuses and temporal bones consistent with age with visualisation of the sutures consistent with age.
- Reproduction of soft tissues of the scalp.

Common faults and solutions

The following should be avoided:

- Holder's hands around the face.
- Rotated patient with respect to the receptor.
- Use of wide cones. Whole cervical spine or upper chest should not be on the radiograph.

The following can be helpful:

- Use of a feeding bottle or pacifier often allows the correct position to be maintained and obtaining the child's confidence.
- Use of bubbles and musical toys as distraction aids.
- Giving clear instructions to parents regarding immobilisation.

13 Skull

Fronto-occipital 30° caudal

Position of patient and image receptor
- The child is positioned in a similar way to that described for the FO position. The chin however, is depressed so that the orbito-meatal line is at right-angles to the table.
- The carer will immobilise the head using foam pads positioned gently but firmly either side of the head.
- The image receptor is positioned longitudinally on the table-top with its upper edge at the level of the vertex of the skull.

Direction and location of the X-ray beam
- The collimated beam central ray is angled caudally so that it makes an angle of 30° to the orbito-meatal plane with the central ray coincident with the median sagittal plane.
- If the child's chin cannot be sufficiently depressed to bring the orbito-meatal line at right-angles to the table it will be necessary to angle the central ray more than 30° to the vertical so that it makes the necessary angle of 30° to the orbito-meatal plane.

Essential image characteristics
- The arch of the atlas should be projected through the foramen magnum.
- Lambdoid and coronal sutures should be symmetrical.
- Inner and outer table, soft tissues and sutures as for FO.

Notes (Figs 13.25a–13.25d)
- The technique can be adapted, i.e. 'under tilted Towne's' to enable the coronal and lambdoid sutures to be shown on one image.
- To avoid irradiating the eyes, Denton has suggested a 25° caudal angulation and a collimation field is set such that the lower border is coincident with the upper orbital margin and the upper border includes the skull vertex. Laterally the skin margins should also be included within the field (see adult section page 280).

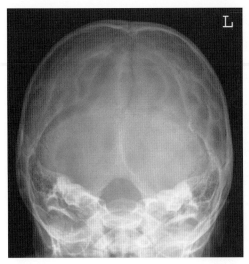

Fig. 13.25b Correctly positioned FO – 25° caudal radiograph of skull as in Denton technique.[48]

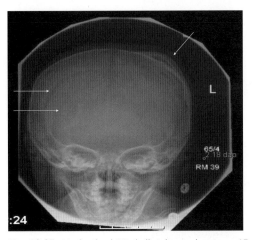

Fig. 13.25c Undertilted FO skull radiograph using a 15 pad under the skull and with a 10° caudal tube angle for optimal demonstration of coronal and lambdoid sutures (arrows) on a single image. 1-year-old infant with a calcified cephalhaematoma of the left parietal bone. Sutures are patent. Note no grid used. (See Figs on page 450.)

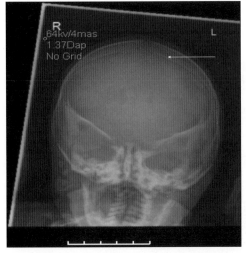

Fig. 13.25d FO, 20° caudal radiograph of a 1-day-old neonate with craniosynostosis of the coronal sutures (arrowed) resulting in abnormal shape of the orbits. Note head could have been tilted down a little more to ensure that the coronal sutures were projected more over the middle of the cranium.

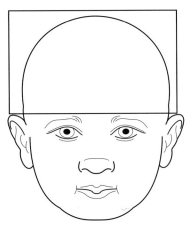

Fig. 13.25a Frontal diagram of skull showing light beam collimation.

Skull 13

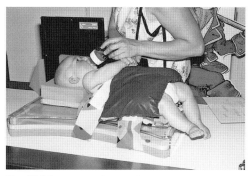

Fig. 13.26a A 6-month-old infant for lateral skull using a horizontal beam technique. Patient supine demonstrating immobilisation and distraction with a feeding bottle.

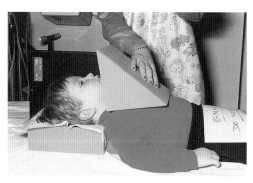

Fig. 13.26b A 3-year-old child positioned for lateral skull, patient supine showing use of a foam pad to immobilise the head.

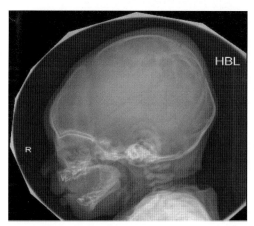

Fig. 13.26c Lateral skull radiograph of a 1-month-old neonate with marked convolutional markings (sometimes associated with spina bifida or vitamin D deficiency) and left parietal fracture. Note no grid used.

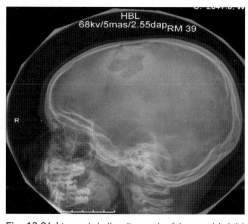

Fig. 13.26d Lateral skull radiograph of 4-year-old child with an eosinophilic granuloma of the right parietal bone.

Lateral – supine (Figs 13.26a–13.26d)

Position of patient and image receptor

- With the patient supine on the Bucky table, a pre-formed foam pad is placed under the head so that the occiput is included on the radiograph.
- The patient's head is now adjusted to bring the median sagittal plane of the head at right-angles to the table by ensuring that the EAMs are equidistant from the table.
- The head is immobilised with the aid of a carer (see photographs opposite for technique according to age).
- An image receptor is supported vertically against the lateral aspect of the head, parallel to the median sagittal plane with its long edge 5 cm above the vertex of the skull.
- A small slim rectangular foam pad may be placed between the image receptor and the cheek for comfort. This also assists in obtaining a true lateral position.

Direction and location of the X-ray beam

- The collimated horizontal beam is directed parallel to the interorbital line so that it is at right-angles to the median plane and the image receptor.
- The beam is directed at right-angles and centred midway between the glabella and the external occipital protuberance.

Essential image characteristics

- The whole cranial vault and base of the skull should be present and symmetrical.
- The floor of the pituitary fossa should be a single line.
- The floors of the anterior cranial fossa should be superimposed.
- The mandibular condyles should be superimposed.
- First three cervical vertebrae should be included for trauma and be lateral.
- Visually sharp reproduction of the outer and inner tables and floor of the sella, consistent with age.
- Visually sharp reproduction of the vascular channels and trabecular structure, consistent with age.
- Reproduction of the sutures and fontanelles, consistent with age.
- Reproduction of the soft tissues and nasal bones, consistent with age.

13 Sinuses

Occipito-mental – erect

An occipito-mental (OM) projection of the sinuses is performed erect in a similar way to that described for adults (see page 306). However, in children the patient's nose and mouth are both placed in contact with the midline of the vertical Bucky and then the head is adjusted to bring the orbito-meatal line at 35° to the horizontal at the centre of the Bucky/DDR detector system with the grid removed.

Maxillary antra are not well pneumatised before the age of 3 years and the frontal sinuses are not developed before the age of 6 years. Sinus X-rays are therefore rarely justified in children below this age, with the trend being to avoid doing sinus X-rays in all children. Sinus radiographs are not required for acute sinusitis and MRI or very low dose CT is recommended for chronic cases that may require surgery (Fig. 13.27a).

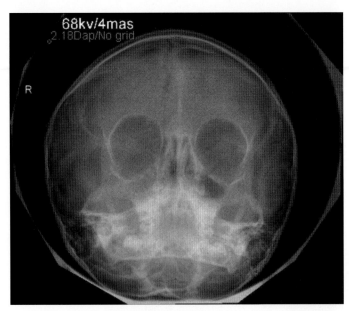

Fig. 13.27a Occipito-mental projection of facial bones of a 7-year-old boy with opaque right maxillary sinus due to sinusitis. Frontal sinuses not yet developed at this age. Note no grid used.

Referral criteria

- Suspected chronic or complicated sinusitis and trauma (Fig. 13.27b).

Essential image characteristics

- The X-ray beam should be well-collimated and should include the frontal sinuses (when pneumatised) and the bases of the maxillary sinuses and upper maxillary teeth.
- Petrous bones should lie at the base of the antra.
- Orbits, sinuses and petrous bones should be symmetrical.
- Bony detail should have visually sharp reproduction.
- Soft tissues and mucosa of sinuses should be visible.

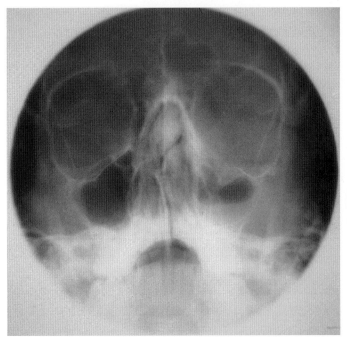

Fig. 13.27b Image of OM projection of a 13-year-old boy demonstrating a blow out fracture of the left inferior orbital margin with fluid levels in the left maxillary and left frontal sinus.

Post-nasal space 13

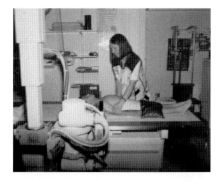

Fig. 13.27c Child positioned for lateral projection of post-nasal space (PNS).

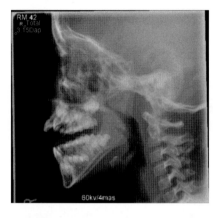

Fig. 13.27d Lateral radiograph of PNS of an 8-year-old boy showing a large adenoidal pad narrowing the PNS.

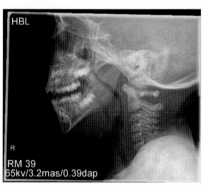

Fig. 13.27e Lateral radiograph of PNS of a 3-year-old boy demonstrating large adenoids and large tonsils. Shoulders should have been excluded.

Lateral supine (Figs 13.27c–13.27e)

A lateral projection (taken supine to minimise patient movement) of the PNS is performed to demonstrate enlarged adenoids; hence the PNS must be air-filled to be radiographically visible.

Referral criteria

Adenoidal speech, chronic cough, suspected postnasal drip; nasal discharge, suspected FB, halitosis and sleep apnoea.

Position of patient and image receptor (Fig. 13.27c)

- The child lies supine, with the lateral aspect of the head in contact with the receptor supported vertically. The medial sagittal plane is parallel to the image receptor.
- The jaw is raised slightly so that the angles of the mandible are separated from the bodies of the upper cervical spine.
- The image should be taken with mouth closed and if PNS is obliterated, the examination should be repeated with the child sniffing.

Direction and location of the X-ray beam

- The collimated horizontal beam is directed at right-angles to the image receptor and is centred to the ramus of the mandible to include the maxillary sinuses to the 3rd cervical vertebrae and the posterior pharynx.

Essential image characteristics (Figs 13.27d, 13.27e)

Inferior orbits to C5 should be included with the condyles of the mandible superimposed. Bony detail should have visually sharp reproduction and soft tissue of adenoidal pads should be reproduced.

13 Dental radiography

Cephalometric radiography and dental panoramic tomography (DPT) are now the most commonly requested imaging techniques in teenagers due to the increasing requirement for orthodontic treatment. These types of radiographs should not be performed routinely in children under the age of 7 years for orthodontic assessment alone. However, paediatric dentists may request DPT on children from 3 years onward to demonstrate 'state of teeth' before dental treatment. This should be performed only if extensive caries are present. Special attention must be given to justification of exposure and optimisation, collimation and avoiding unnecessary repeats (Figs 13.28a, 13.28b).

A detailed description of the radiographic techniques in adults is given in Section 9.

- For lateral cephalometry, in addition to the graduated filter, a triangular coning device is recommended to avoid irradiating the back of the skull and the thyroid (Figs 13.28c, 13.28d).
- The whole skull will need to be demonstrated in craniofacial deformity.
- CT lateral cephalometry can also be considered as a low-dose alternative (Figs 13.28e–13.28g).
- For DPT, eye shields are also recommended in addition to the lateral collimation, where only a fixed aperture is present. Where available, the selection of the paediatric setting is also recommended to reduce radiation exposure to the cervical spine (Fig. 13.28a).

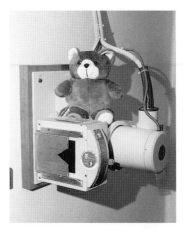

Fig. 13.28c Additional triangular coning device on the X-ray tube assembly for lateral cephalograph.

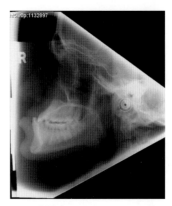

Fig. 13.28d Lateral cephalograph of a 9-year-old boy with overbite. Use of triangular coning device and graduated filter.

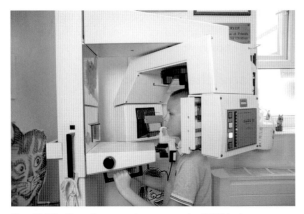

Fig. 13.28a Dental panoramic tomography (DPT) (orthopantomogram, OPG) machine with eye shield positioned for DPT.

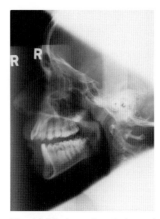

Fig. 13.28e Lateral cephalograph showing teeth not being apposed.

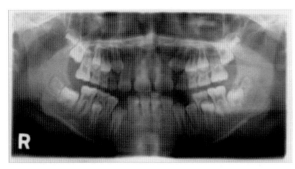

Fig. 13.28b DPT (OPG) image of 10-year-old boy – cervical spine excluded.

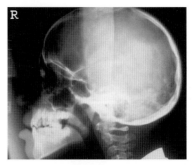 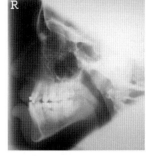

Figs 13.28f and g Lateral cephalograph images of a 9-year-old girl, with (left) and without (right) triangular coning or filter device with unnecessary inclusion of the base of the skull and thyroid. Latter only required for craniofacial deformity.

Referral criteria

- Irritable hip causing pain and limp (most likely aetiologies are transient synovitis, Perthes' disease, slipped upper femoral epiphysis, osteomyelitis and septic arthritis): ultrasound is the first investigation of choice and if an effusion is confirmed, suspected to be due to transient synovitis, with no adverse clinical features then ultrasound alone is sufficient. If the patient remains symptomatic or a hip effusion persists, radiography is indicated. Older children (>9 years) suspected to have a slipped upper femoral epiphysis require initial radiography in addition to ultrasound.
- Development dysplasia of the hip (DDH) for follow-up post treatment or in older children (over 18–24 months depending on size of child); (ultrasound is the first investigation of choice before this age).
- Trauma.
- Post surgery.
- Focal bone pain.
- Knee pain if suspected to be referred from the hip.
- Pelvic tilt.
- Part of a skeletal survey for NAI or suspected syndrome.
- Suspected congenital abnormality, e.g. sacral agenesis in infants of diabetic mothers.

Notes

- Initial pelvic and hip radiography is normally performed in conjunction with ultrasound.
- Radiography may be performed before or during treatment, when a child may present wearing a special splint or plaster cast
- Follow-up radiography of chronic disease should not normally be performed in less than 6 months.
- All follow-up radiographs should have appropriate gonad protection.
- In follow-up DDH radiographs, where patient is pain-free and avascular necrosis is not suspected, use of an antiscatter grid can be minimised.

Pelvis/hips 13

Recommended projections

The AP projection is the most commonly requested projection for children of all ages.

Examination is performed by means of the following:

DDH/CDH	AP – supine AP – erect
Irritable hips, all causes	AP Lateral – frog view (Lauenstein projection)
Post operative for slipped epiphysis	AP – supine Turned lateral
Trauma	AP – supine Lateral – HB
Acetabulo femoral impingement	Ganz view

AP, antero-posterior; CDH, congenital dislocation of the hip; DDH, developmental dysplasia of the hip; HB, horizontal beam.

Gonad shields (Figs 13.29a, 13.29b)

A variety of gonad protection is available: individual male, female or window protection. These can be made of lead-rubber placed on the patient or made of lead and inserted below the light beam diaphragm. A variety of sizes and shapes should be available. Gonad protection can result in a 95% reduction in testicular dose and a >50% reduction in ovarian dose.[9]

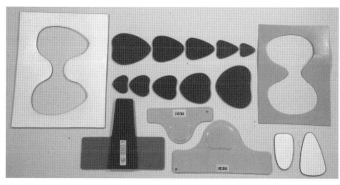

Fig. 13.29a Selection of pelvic gonad protection.

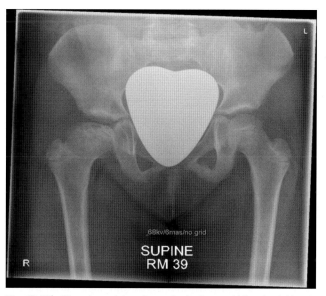

Fig. 13.29b AP supine pelvic radiograph of a 9-year-old female child with Perthes' disease of the right hip showing use of a gonad shield. No grid used.

13 Pelvis/hips

Antero-posterior

The following describes the technique adopted for a 3-month-old baby. A CR 24 × 30 cm or 18 × 24 cm cassette is selected, large enough to include the pelvis and upper femora; alternatively, a DDR system is employed without the use of a grid.

Position of patient and image receptor

- The child lies supine on the X-ray table, on top of the image receptor or a specially designed imaging plate holder, which is placed at the end of the table, with the median sagittal plane of the trunk at right-angles to the middle of the cassette.
- To maintain this position, a sandbag is placed on either side of the baby's trunk, with the child's arms left unrestrained. A Velcro belt may be fastened around the baby's waist to prevent rotation.
- The baby's legs are held straight together, with the holder's hands positioned firmly around each leg, the holder's fingers under the baby's calves and the holder's thumbs on the knees (Fig. 13.32a).
- If using the cassette holder at the end of the table, the knees should be held together and flexed (Fig. 13.6).
- For the older child, positioning is similar to that described for the adult (see page 176).

Direction and location of the X-ray beam

- The collimated vertical beam is centred to the middle of the image receptor.

Note

- Following surgery, low-dose CT may be used to demonstrate the position of the femoral head in patients treated with the use of a long-term plaster cast.

Radiation protection

- Gonad protection is not used for the initial examination.
- Subsequent examinations require the use of gonad protection. If erect position is required, gonad protection can be taped into position; alternatively, a window-shaped coning device can be inserted beneath the light beam diaphragm (Figs 13.30a, 13.30b).

Radiological considerations

- Hip radiographs are a common request in children but the value of initial ultrasound examination should always be considered.
- A line drawn from the midsacrum through the triradiate cartilage should pass through the medial aspect of the femoral metaphysis to exclude dislocation. Similarly, Shenton's line should be uninterrupted. Lines and angles used for the assessment of acetabular morphology are demonstrated in the line drawing (Figs 13.30c, 13.30d).

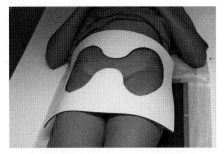

Fig. 13.30a Male child with window gonad protection for AP supine pelvis.

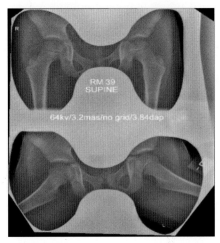

Fig. 13.30b AP and frog lateral radiograph of both hips of a 6-year-old male patient with window protection. No grid. (Combined dose–area product is an overestimate as it does not take into account the lead protection on the patient.)

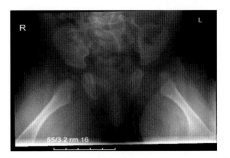

Fig. 13.30c 4-month-old female, presented with frankly dislocated left hip. Attempted treatment with harness. Follow up AP pelvic radiograph shows interruption of Shenton's line on the left due to persistent dislocation. A 30 minute rest is normally instituted after removal of harness, but as in this case it is sometimes difficult to bring the knees together. Shenton's line will still be interrupted as seen here.

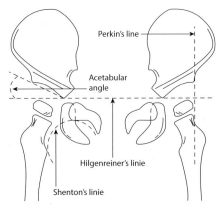

Fig. 13.30d Schematic drawing demonstration of pelvic lines to assess acetabulo-femoral congruity in suspected developmental dysplasia of the hip.

Antero-posterior – erect (weight-bearing) (Figs 13.31a–13.31d)

As soon as a child is able to stand, weight-bearing erect images are frequently performed.

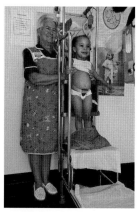

Fig. 13.31a Female child with taped gonad protection for AP pelvis. Gonad protection positioned with inferior margin at pubic symphysis. Sandbag to secure feet. Clothing should be removed if possible. (Underwear used for photograph.)

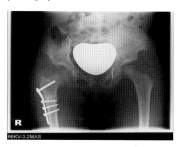

Fig. 13.31b Follow-up AP erect pelvic radiograph of a 6-year-old female following right upper femoral osteotomy. Initially presented with frankly dislocated hips at 2 years of age. No grid. Female gonad protection taped in place.

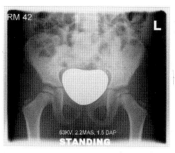

Fig. 13.31c AP erect radiograph of both hips of a 4-year-old female with Meyer's dysplasia of femoral heads. Female gonad protection taped in position. No grid used.

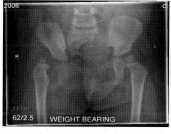

Fig. 13.31d AP erect of both hips of an 8-month-old female with dislocated right hip. No gonad protection for first radiograph and no grid. Note disruption of Shenton's line.

Pelvis/hips 13

Position of patient and image receptor

- The child stands with the posterior aspect of the pelvis against a CR cassette held vertically in the cassette holder.
- The anterior superior iliac spines should be equidistant from the cassette and the median sagittal plane vertical and coincident with the centre of the cassette.
- The ankles should be apart and separated by a small 45° foam pad, with the toes straight and pointing forwards.
- The child is supported above the waist whilst standing on a raised platform, with sandbags secured around the feet. Any pelvic tilt is corrected with the use of a small block.

Essential image characteristics

- Whole pelvis, sacrum and subtrochanteric regions of both femora. (Iliac crests can be excluded in specific hip pathology, e.g. Perthes' disease.)
- Symmetrical, with iliac wings and pubic rami of equal length. Femoral necks should not be foreshortened.
- Visualisation of sacrum and intervertebral foramina depending on bowel content and presence of female protection. Reproduction of sacro-iliac joints according to age, with reproduction of the femoral necks.
- Reproduction of spongiosa and cortex.
- Visualisation of trochanters, consistent with age.
- Visualisation of soft-tissue planes.

Common faults and solutions

- Rotated patient with respect to the image receptor needs careful observation of supine patient and holding technique. Rotation can wrongly suggest dysplasia.
- Gonad protection missing, inadequate, too large or slipped over region of interest. Careful selection of appropriate size and shape is essential. Female protection is the most difficult to select. As the first radiograph of a pelvis is performed without gonad protection, this previous image should be scrutinised to assess the width of the internal bony pelvis compared with the width of the external bony pelvis at the level of the palpable anterior iliac spines. The former is normally <50% of the latter, The approximate interiliac spine distance should be assessed physically for the follow-up radiograph and a suitable size gonad protection selected that has a width of a maximum of 30% of this distance. The inferior margin of the gonad protection is positioned with its tip just above the symphysis pubis. Testicular protection should be below the symphysis pubis. If there is doubt about the selection of size or position, conservative practice is recommended, as the main aim is not to obscure anatomical detail or important pathology. Window protection can be selected similarly with the wider lead section placed over the pelvis for females and the protection inverted for males.

13 Pelvis/hips

Hips – Von Rosen projection

This supplementary projection was sometimes employed to confirm diagnosis of DDH. The disadvantage of the projection is that it produced a number of false positives and negatives and has largely been superseded by hip ultrasound.

The ossification centre of the femoral head tends to be a little eccentric and lateral, particularly following treatment for DDH. This may give the false impression of decentring. Drawing a line through the midsacrum and triradiate cartilage best assesses the degree of dislocation and decentring. This line should pass through the medial aspect of the femoral metaphysis. The use of this line in a straight AP radiograph of the hips is preferred to the Von Rosen projection (Figs 13.32a, 13.32b).

Hips – lateral both hips (frog projection) (Figs 13.32c–13.32e)

This projection may be employed to supplement the AP projection in the investigation of irritable hips.

Position of patient and image receptor

- The child lies supine on the X-ray table with the grid removed or directly on top of the image receptor, i.e. CR cassette. The median sagittal plane of the trunk is at right-angles to the middle of the image receptor.
- To maintain this position, when examining a small infant a sandbag is placed either side of the infant's trunk with the arms left unrestrained.
- The anterior superior iliac spines should be equal distance from the tabletop to ensure that the pelvis is not rotated.
- The hips and knees are flexed and abducted.
- The limbs are then rotated laterally through approximately 60° with the knees separated and the plantar aspects of the feet places in contact with each other.
- A child may be supported in this position with non-opaque 45° foam pads under the knees.

Direction and location of the X-ray beam

- The vertical collimated beam is centred in the midline at the level of the femoral pulse.

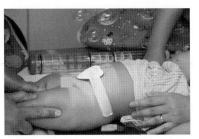

Fig. 13.32a Female infant with gonad protection for AP supine pelvic radiograph.

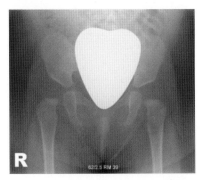

Fig. 13.32b AP supine radiograph of a 6-month-old female with dysplastic right hip. Gonad protection in position. Shenton's line not disrupted. Line from mid-sacrum crosses triradiate cartilages and femoral metaphyses symmetrically, also confirming no dislocation.

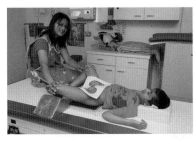

Fig. 13.32c Male child positioned for supine frog lateral both hips, with window protection.

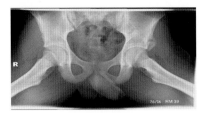

Fig. 13.32d Frog lateral radiograph of both hips of a 9-year-old male child with a healing, chronic avulsion of the origin of the left rectus femoris muscle. Note no gonad protection for first radiograph.

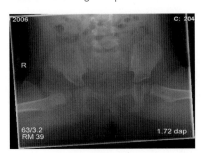

Fig. 13.32e Frog projection of an 8-month-old infant in plaster SPICA post open reduction of dislocated right hip, Gonad protection can be avoided if there is doubt about the positioning, as it is not possible to see anatomical landmarks with the plaster in situ. If convenient a CT scanogram is a lower dose alternative.

Scoliosis is a term for lateral curvature of the vertebral column and it is always accompanied by rotation of the involved vertebrae. The major part of the column is usually involved since the primary curve (often found in the thoracic spine with the convexity to the right) subsequently gives rise to one or two compensatory secondary curves above or below it. Radiography is performed to assess the progression of the disease and to measure the effectiveness of conservative treatment or when surgical treatment is considered.

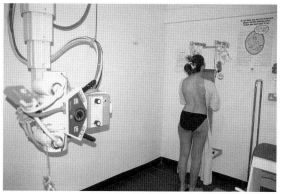

Fig. 13.33a Patient positioned for PA projection of spine for assessment of scoliosis.

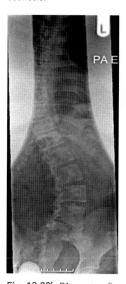

Fig. 13.33b PA erect radiograph of a 17-year-old female with thoraco-lumbar scoliosis and absent hemisacrum. No grid. The right side of the thoracic spine has been coned off by the shaped lateral cones but this does not affect the measurement of a follow-up scoliosis. CR image.

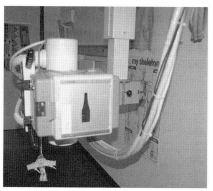

Fig. 13.33c Shaped lateral coning device on the tube housing.

Spine – scoliosis 13

As the curvature will only normally progress whilst the skeleton is growing, it is important to include the iliac crests on PA images so the degree of maturity can be estimated from the degree of apophyseal fusion.

The majority of patients encountered will be children or adolescents most commonly suffering from idiopathic scoliosis. Images will be taken at regular intervals as progression of the disease is monitored. Given the relatively high radiation doses associated with this examination and the heightened radiosensitivity of children, radiation protection considerations are paramount (see below).

Referral criteria

The referral criterion for all types of pathology where a whole spine examination is indicated, rather than a segmental spine, is as follows:

- Idiopathic/congenital/paralytic and post infective scoliosis.
- Spina bifida.
- Suspected syndrome.
- Severe injury.
- Metastatic disease.
- Metabolic disorder.

Radiation protection

- An antiscatter grid can be removed for follow-up examinations to monitor a scoliosis.
- Various systems for 3D surface topographic assessment of a scoliosis have been developed. These avoid the use of any ionising radiation and are based on assessing the degree of distortion that a scoliosis curvature causes on a parallel light fringe pattern projected onto the patient's back. Various techniques have demonstrated a <1% error compared with formal radiographic technique and can be used for some follow-up interval studies with the agreement of the orthopaedic clinician.[49]
- With a radiographic technique additional lateral coning can be used, the grid can be dispensed with, unless the patient is particularly large, and a fast imaging system selected. The iliac crests may not need to be included for every radiograph. The technique and exposure factors employed should be recorded for future reference.
- Developing breast tissue in adolescent females is highly radiosensitive and careful protective measures should be employed to avoid unnecessary irradiation of the breasts (Figs 13.33b, 13.33c).
- The most effective protection measure is to undertake the examination in the PA position (Fig. 13.33a).
- A pre-shaped filter device can be attached to the light beam diaphragm (LBD) when undertaking conventional film radiography or CR to protect the developing breasts, ribs and gonads. For follow up using DDR, this is not possible and the radiographs should be coned to the spine and a separate narrow PA radiograph of the iliac crests taken, according to age (see below).

13 Spine – scoliosis

Referral criteria (cont.)

The projections required will vary depending on the stage of the disease, age of the patient, treatment and the preferences of the orthopaedic surgeon. Close radiologic and orthopaedic liaison is of paramount importance.

Image acquisition may be undertaken using a single exposure technique employing a single CR cassette or DDR imaging receptor. For taller children, a specialised holder for two or three large CR cassettes can be used. Alternatively, specialised DDR equipment similar to that described for leg alignment is used (see page 468).

Both systems will come with automatic switching software and may use a radio-opaque ruler system to aid in the stitching process and facilitate accurate measurements prior to surgery. For DDR systems, using movement of the X-ray tube and DDR detector to acquire a full imaging set requiring multiple exposures, the systems used vary, with some manufacturers requiring confirmation of start and finishing points related to the extent of the spine whilst others simply calculate the exposures required dependent of the initial collimated beam.

A vertical radio-opaque ruler extending the full length of the vertical Perspex platform support may be used with some systems to aid in the electronic stitching process. A ruler is also required for all pre-operative and post-operative radiographs.

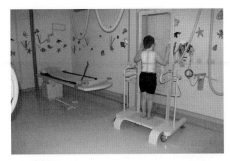

Fig. 13.34a Patient positioned for PA projection using grid and cones fully open.

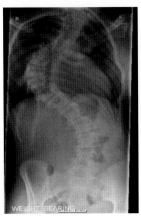

Fig. 13.34b PA erect spine of a 13-year-old patient with severe idiopathic scoliosis. Lateral shaped cones not used because of the severity of the scoliosis. Iliac crests included. Iliac crest apophyses not yet present. Note no grid, CR image.

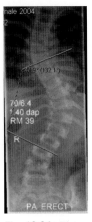

Fig. 13.34c PA erect spine radiograph of a 4-year-old female with infantile scoliosis due to underlying Marfan's syndrome. No grid, CR image.

Recommended projections

- A standing PA is acquired initially and if scoliosis is confirmed at review, a lateral is also performed.
- Prior to surgery recommended routine pre-operative sequences are: PA, lateral, bending left and right in the erect or supine position.
- Images may be required with the patient wearing a brace and repeated with the brace removed in order to monitor its effectiveness and a scoliosis chair can be used to support some children to obtain erect images whilst seated.[50]
- Supine images with or without traction or with the patient lying over a bolster, may also be needed to evaluate postural changes when the patient is unable to stand or sit.
- Evaluation of orthopaedic hardware may require AP and lateral radiography and if necessary tangential projections to look at a focal area of protrusion, i.e. rib humps.

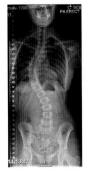
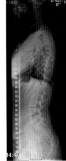

Figs 13.34d and e Radiographs (DDR) of PA and lateral erect spine demonstrating a severe idiopathic scoliosis in a 15-year-old female. Pre-operative radiographs demonstrating position of shoulders, ribs, iliac crests and both hips on PA. Cervical to sacral spine on lateral. Grid used, ruler in place.

Postero-anterior – erect (Figs 13.34a–13.34e)

Positioning of patient and image receptor

- The patient stands fully erect on the patient stand with the anterior aspect of the trunk facing the image receptor.
- The lower edge of the image CR receptor is placed 1.5 cm below the iliac crests with the face resting on the receptor (or with DDR against the Perspex vertical support) to include C7–S1. For those patients with neurological disease, syndromes or pre-operatively, inclusion of the hips would be required. The median sagittal plane should be at right-angles to and coincide with the vertical centre line of the receptor.
- Occasionally a wooden block (height previously determined) is positioned under one foot to correct for pelvic tilt.
- A line joining the highest point of the iliac crests should be horizontal if there is no pathological tilt of the pelvis. For CR imaging the middle of the image receptor should be positioned just above the thoraco-lumbar junction (T11/T12 region).
- For DDR imaging the image receptor will automatically move to the relevant anatomical position dependent on the imaging sequence to capture the full length of the spine.

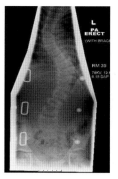

Fig. 13.35a Patient in a brace positioned for PA erect of whole spine for assessment of scoliosis.

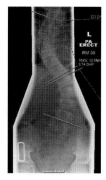

Fig. 13.35b PA erect spine of a 6-year-old female with infantile scoliosis in a brace. Shaped lateral cones and no grid used, CR image.

Fig. 13.35c PA erect spine of a 12-year-old female with idiopathic scoliosis in a brace. Shaped lateral cones and no grid used, CR image.

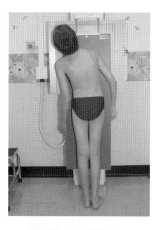

Fig. 13.35d An erect patient bending to the left.

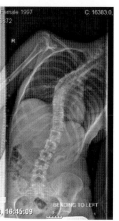
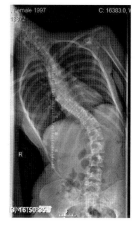

Figs 13.35e and f PA radiographs (DDR) of 16-year-old patient with idiopathic scoliosis, bending to the right and left, demonstrating correction of the compensatory lumbar curve and no significant correction of the primary thoracic curve.

Spine – scoliosis 13

Postero-anterior – erect (cont.) (Figs 13.35a–13.35f)

Direction and location of the X-ray beam

- The technique will vary depending on whether a CR method or DDR technique is employed. The guidance given immediately below is applicable for CR systems.
- The collimated horizontal beam is directed at right-angles to the image receptor/s and centred to include the whole spinal column.
- The lower collimation border positioned at the level of the anterior superior iliac spines thus ensuring inclusion of the 1st sacral segment. The upper border should be at the level of the spinous process of C7.
- An increased FRD is used to ensure the correct image receptor coverage, to reduce dose and magnification) (>180 cm).

DDR systems

- For DDR systems using movement of the X-ray tube and DDR detector to acquire a full imaging set with multiple exposures, the systems used vary: some manufacturers require selection of start and finishing locations with others requiring the collimated beam to be centred over the trunk to include the full extent of the spinal region selected. The extent of the start and finishing locations or collimation selected dictates the number of exposures taken.
- A vertical radio-opaque ruler extending the full length of the vertical Perspex stand may be used with some systems to aid in the electronic stitching process.
- A large FRD is selected, e.g.180–260 cm as per instructions.

Notes

- If there is clinical suspicion of a structural abnormality then the cervical spine, ribs and hips may need to be included on the initial radiograph.
- It is important that the medial aspects of the iliac crests are not excluded to enable the assessment of spinal maturity from apophyseal growth (Risser sign).

Essential image characteristics

- The first image should demonstrate the spine to include above and below the curvature, ribs and iliac crests (latter for girls aged 10–18 years, and in boys aged 13–20 years). For an idiopathic scoliosis, C7 to sacrum is adequate; prior to surgery the cervical spine from C3 should also be included.
- If a structural abnormality is demonstrated, an AP cervical spine and additional coned views may be required.
- Follow-up images should be coned to the spinal curvature and iliac crests as above.
- The image should give good reproduction of vertebral bodies and pedicles, visualisation of posterior facet joints and reproduction of spinous processes and transverse processes, consistent with age.

13 Spine – scoliosis

Lateral

Position of patient and image receptor (Fig. 13.36a)

- The patient stands fully erect on the patient stand with their bare feet, slightly apart with the side of the convexity of the primary curve against the vertical detector mechanism.
- Care is taken to ensure that the patient does not lean towards the image detector.
- The lower edge of the CR image receptor is placed 1.5 cm below the iliac crests.
- The mid-axillary line is centred to the image receptor and the coronal plane should be at right-angles to the receptor.
- The latter may be assessed by palpating the anterior iliac spines and rotating the patient so that a line joining the two sides is at right-angles to the image receptor.
- Similarly a line joining the lateral end of the clavicles should be at right-angles to the image receptor.
- It is important to maintain the spine in a neutral position; this may be achieved by the patient holding their arms in a 'mummy' position with elbows brought forward and fingertips touching clavicles.

Direction and location of the X-ray beam

- For CR imaging the collimated horizontal beam is directed at right-angles to the image receptor and centred to include the whole spinal column (Figs 13.36b, 13.36c).
- The lower collimation border is positioned at the level of the anterior superior iliac spines, thus ensuring inclusion of the 1st sacral segment.
- The upper border should be at the level of the spinous process of C7 for assessment of idiopathic scoliosis and C3 for prior to surgery.
- An increased FRD is used to ensure the correct image receptor coverage (180–200 cm).
- For DDR systems using movement of the X-ray tube and DDR detector to acquire a full imaging set with multiple exposures, the systems used vary: some manufacturers require selection of start and finishing locations with others requiring the collimated beam to be centred over the trunk to include the full extent of the spinal region selected. The extent of the start and finishing locations or collimation selected dictates the number of exposures taken (Figs 13.36d, 13.36e).

Notes

- For CR imaging, using a single exposure technique, care should be taken to ensure that the beam is well-collimated to exclude the breast tissues especially in follow-up radiographs.

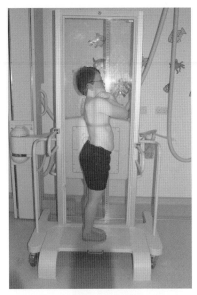

Fig. 13.36a Photograph of patient positioned for lateral projection of the spine.

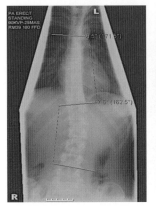 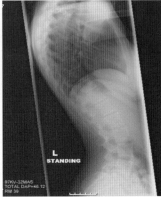

Figs 13.36b and c PA erect and lateral erect images with a grid using CR, of a 14-year-old girl with idiopathic scoliosis. Shaped lateral cones used for PA. Iliac crest apophyses not yet appeared. Usual collimation used to avoid unnecessary breast radiation for lateral.

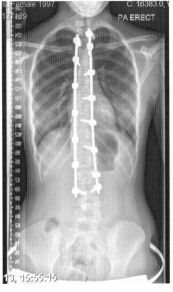 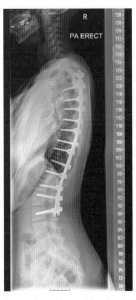

Figs 13.36d and e PA and lateral erect radiographs with a grid using DDR, of a 16-year-old female post spinal fusion. Shoulders and iliac crests required to assess any abnormal tilt. Gonad protection partly protects the pelvic organs. Breasts coned as much as possible on the lateral projection. Use of shaped lateral cones not possible with DDR. Ruler in place.

Spine – scoliosis 13

Lateral (cont.)

Radiological considerations (Figs 13.37a–13.37f)

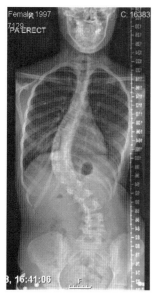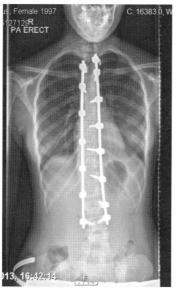

Fig. 13.37a and b PA erect radiographs (DDR) of a 16-year-old patient. Pre- and post-operative radiographs demonstrating correction of curvature. Gonad protection used for latter.

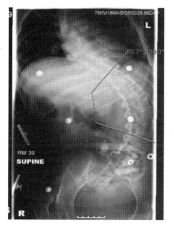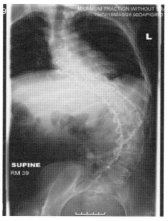

Figs 13.37c and d AP supine images of a 14-year-old female patient with scoliosis due to cerebral palsy. (c) in a brace; (d) with traction. Use of grid, no lateral shaped cones.

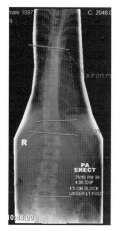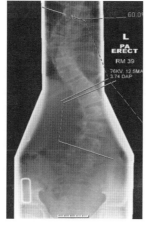

Fig. 13.37e PA erect spine of a 14-year-old patient with a scoliosis showing degree of correction after insertion of 1.5 cm block under left foot. Pelvis and sacrum now horizontal with correction of the lumbar curve. CR images no grid, lateral shaped cones. Iliac crest apophyses not yet present.

Fig. 13.37f PA erect spine of a 12-year-old female with idiopathic scoliosis in a brace. Lateral shaped cones, no grid, CR image.

- The most common referral for scoliosis is now idiopathic scoliosis. The children affected are otherwise completely normal with a normal life expectancy. Multiple radiographs for monitoring are required and therefore dose-saving measures are important.

- There are three main types: infantile scoliosis is a simple C-shaped long curve and 90% undergo spontaneous resolution by the age of 5 years (10% progress). Juvenile scoliosis occurs at 5–6 years and by far the most common is adolescent scoliosis, which occurs at 10–12 years.

- Secondary spinal scoliosis is now less common in most centres. The main causes being: congenital (including hemivertebrae), neuromuscular disorders and neurofibromatosis. Scoliosis secondary to polio and kyphosis due to TB are very uncommon. However, it is extremely important to exclude underlying disease and MRI of the spine is advised in all patients with atypical 'idiopathic' scoliosis or painful scoliosis. MRI should also be considered pre-operatively.

- When a secondary scoliosis is suspected due to abnormalities seen on the first thoraco-lumbar spine film, cervical spine and pelvic radiographs can be considered for additional assessment.

- In idiopathic scoliosis any part of the thoraco-lumbar spine may be affected. There is a primary curve with secondary compensatory curves.

- The lateral curvature is accompanied by rotation of the vertebrae on a vertical axis. This thrusts the ribs backwards in the thoracic area and increases the prominence of the deformity. The rotary component makes the disease more complex than a cosmetic deformity and rotation of the thorax can lead to compression of the heart and lungs, whereas lumbar curves can predispose to later degenerative changes.

- The goal of therapy is to keep the primary curve less than 40° at the end of growth and small curves of less than 15° are usually not treated. Curves of 20–40° are managed in a body brace and curves of more than 40° usually have spinal fusion (e.g. a metal Harrington rod). Follow-up images of patients with a Harrington rod will need to show any breakage of the rods or surrounding luque wiring.

- An assessment of skeletal age is required so that appropriate treatment can be planned. The development of the iliac apophyses (Risser's sign) correlates well with skeletal maturity as determined by assessing bone age of the hand and wrist.[51] The iliac apophyses first appear laterally and anteriorly on the crest of the ilium. Growth develops posteriorly and medially, followed by fusion to the iliac crests.

13 Spine – cervical, thoracic and lumbar

Referral criteria

This section addresses modifications in technique for the cervical spine for those patients aged 4 years and under. Readers are referred to Section 6 Vertebral Column, for guidance in the technique for the adult spine.

Referral criteria for the spine as a whole are slightly different and include:

- Persistent low back pain (any back pain is abnormal in a child). Unlike adults, all children require AP and lateral radiographs performed promptly with coned L4/L5 if necessary. Spondylolysis is relatively common in adolescents with chronic low back pain and can be confirmed with MRI.
- Scoliosis (the whole spine should be performed as described for whole spine).
- Lower motor neuron signs in legs/neuropathic bladder.
- Congenital anomaly of spine or lower limbs.
- Suspected infection (isotope bone scan/MRI may also be indicated).
- Tethered cord (lumbar region) suspected because of skin changes (ultrasound is normally undertaken first, from age 0 to approximately 8 months).
- Trauma (however, this is not routine, since spine fractures are uncommon in children but indicated when significant injury).

Cervical spine (Figs 13.38a–13.38c)

Traumatic injury to the cervical spine in children is very uncommon. The indications for cervical spine radiography in paediatric trauma are:

- GCS <15.
- Neck pain.
- Focal neck tenderness.
- Torticollis.
- Focal neurological deficit.
- Paraesthesia in the peripheries.
- Strong clinical suspicion of cervical spine injury due to the severity of the described accident.

Every effort must be made to obtain the highest quality radiographs despite the presence of immobilisation collars so that CT can be avoided where possible. The aim is to obtain diagnostic quality at the first attempt but, if not achieved, some well-chosen additional projections would still offer less overall dose than CT. If necessary adequate pain relief should be given in order to obtain diagnostic radiography rather than perform an unjustified CT.

Children have flatter facet joints than adults, giving more mobility of the cervical spine and are susceptible to spinal cord injury without radiological bony injury (SCIWORA). MRI is indicated in these cases and for all those with focal neurology.

There are a variety of normal variants in the paediatric cervical spine which include loss of the normal cervical lordosis, pseudosubluxation predominantly at C2/C3, physiological wedging of mid-cervical vertebral bodies, particularly C3 vertebra, widening of the soft tissues in the pre-vertebral space (particularly during expiration or crying), intervertebral disc space widening and a 'pseudo–Jefferson fracture'. There are also variations of the secondary ossification centres.

The odontoid peg has a small secondary ossification centre at its tip (os terminale) and this is visible between 3 and 6 years of age. It fuses by 12 years. The body of C2 fuses with the odontoid process also by 3–6 years of age. However, in some, this fusion line (a cartilaginous synchondrosis) variably persists until about 11 years and can be mistaken for a fracture. The posterior neural arches fuse by 2–3 years of age and the posterior arch of C2 fuses to the body at 3–6 years.

The ring apophyses of the vertebral bodies appear at about 14 years and fuse at about 17 years. During this period, they can be confused with avulsion injuries of the anterior longitudinal ligament.

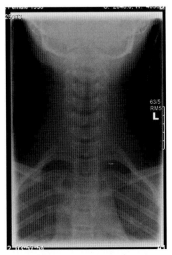
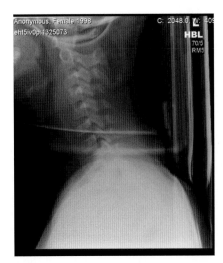
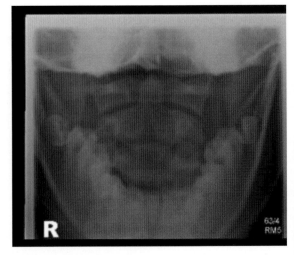

Fig. 13.38a–c AP, lateral and peg cervical spine radiographs of a 14-year-old female in a neck collar post trauma. Normal appearances. Inferior aspect of mandible and occiput should be superimposed on the AP radiograph to maximise visualisation of the whole cervical spine.

Spine 13

Cervical spine (cont.) (Figs 13.39a–13.39e)

The technique is as in adults but it is a difficult area to image in children. The odontoid peg has a separate ossification centre before 7 years. Peg projections are not routinely indicated in trauma below 10 years of age. Lateral projections require the patient to be as straight as possible to allow optimal evaluation, particularly in cases of trauma.

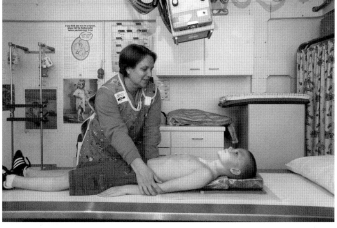

Fig. 13.39a Child positioned for AP supine radiograph of the cervical spine.

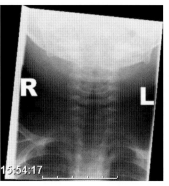
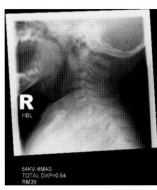

Figs 13.39b and c AP and lateral cervical spine radiographs of a 6-month-old infant. Occiput and mandible are well-superimposed on the AP to allow full demonstration of the cervical spine. Physiological wedging of C3 on the lateral.

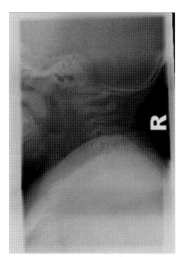
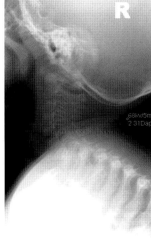

Figs 13.39d and e Lateral cervical spine radiographs of a 7-month-old infant. The first radiograph shows anterior bowing of the pharynx and trachea due to neck flexion or crying. Normal pre-vertebral soft tissues demonstrated on the second radiograph.

Age under 4 years

AP projection

- An image receptor (no grid) is placed longitudinally on the table.
- The child is positioned supine, with the upper chest lying on a 15° foam pad to lift the chin. The head rests in the hollow of a skull foam pad to maintain a straight position.
- To aid positioning and immobilisation, a Velcro band may be secured over the trunk.
- The carer is asked to stand by the side of the table and to hold the child's arms gently by the side of the child's body.

Lateral projection

- The child is maintained in the same position for the AP projection with a horizontal beam used to acquire the image.
- The carer is asked to pull the arms downwards to avoid the shoulders overlying the C7/T1 junction.
- A pacifier or drink in a bottle may be employed to distract or calm an infant.

Notes

- A FRD of 100 cm may be employed for lateral projections to reduce the dose as the object-to-receptor distance of the spine is much reduced compared with the adult distance.
- For the investigation of spondylolisthesis in the older child, both right and left PA oblique projections may be requested.

Essential image characteristics

AP projection

- The inferior border of the mandible should overlie the inferior margin of the occiput (this will allow a maximum number of cervical spine vertebral bodies to be demonstrated).
- Minimum of C3 to T2 should be visible.
- Mandible and occiput should be straight.
- Transverse processes of the vertebral bodies should be symmetrical.
- Posterior spinous processes, when ossified should be in the midline.
- Reproduction of vertebral bodies, transverse processes and posterior elements.

13 Leg length assessment

Leg length images are used to assess discrepancy in leg length that has been confirmed to be real rather than as a result of pelvic tilt due to scoliosis. Assessment with the patient erect or supine, depending on the age of the child, can be undertaken by means of the following:

- Image acquisition undertaken using a single exposure technique employing a multiple CR cassette combination imaging method using a specialised device to secure and join/overlap two or three large CR cassettes, which is dependent on the height of the patient. This is similar to that described for spinal assessment on page 462. CR suppliers offer different ways in their approach to join/overlap the CR cassettes and the manufacturer's instructions should be carefully followed to ensure that the cassettes are correctly aligned. A software package will provide automatic stitching of the acquire images before they are sent to PACS.

- Alternatively, motorised DDR equipment using either a large field vertical detector or similar size table detector and an electronically linked X-ray tube/gantry is selected. Such electronically linked equipment provides multiple exposures of the region concerned employing a single focus imaging technique, which minimise stitching distortions rather than a series of straight multiple exposures of the region, which introduces parallax error (Figs 13.40a, 13.40b). During this process the X-ray tube and detector are electronically linked to provide separate images of the region selected, with the X-ray tube rotating and centring to the DDR detector as it moves to track the full extent of the anatomical region selected. (See diagrams opposite for the principle involved.)

- Localised exposure method. Where none of the above methods are available, i.e. a large DDR (i.e. 43 × 43 cm) detector or a single CR 35 × 43 cm cassette employing radio-opaque graduated rulers using three separate exposures can be employed to acquire images of the joints.

- CT scanogram of both legs.

- MRI scanogram of both legs

CR and DDR methods, which are now most common, are described along with the localised exposure technique.

The reader is directed to manufacturers' instruction manuals for more detailed instruction of CT and MRI scanogram methods.

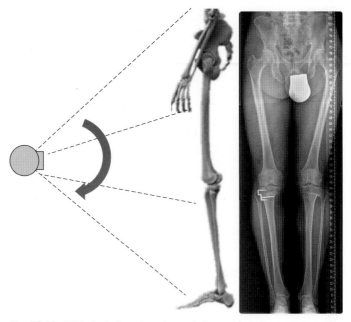

Fig. 13.40a DDR single focus imaging technique with more accurate overlap areas and minimal stitching distortions.

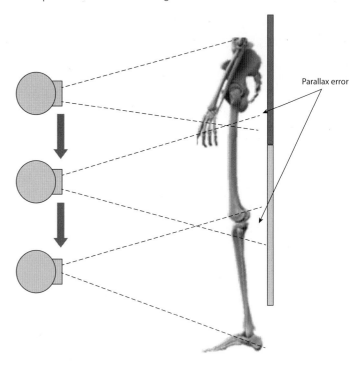

Fig. 13.40b Multiple focus imaging technique with big distortions in overlap areas.

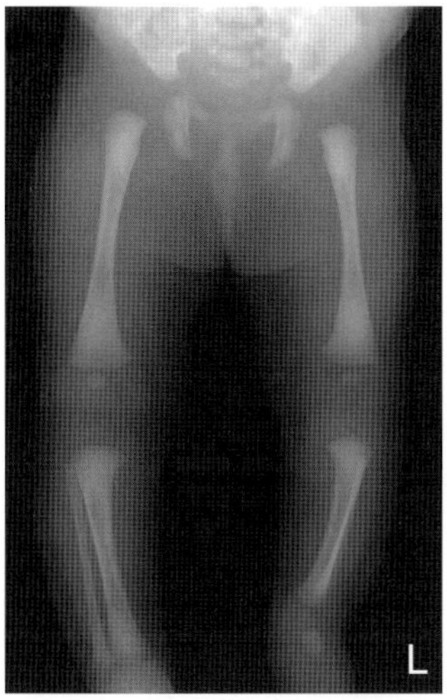

Leg length assessment 13

Radiological considerations (Figs 13.41a–13.41e)

- Differences in limb length can occur as a result of a variety of congenital conditions or as a result of infection or trauma to the growth plates. Successful surgical correction depends on accurate radiographic measurement of the limbs.
- There are two main methods of equalising limb length. One is to fuse the growth plates at one end of a long bone. Alternatively, one can increase the length of the shorter limb by performing a transverse osteotomy and using a device and frame outside the limb to separate the cut ends to allow healing.
- External fixators, Ilizarov device or Taylor spatial frame can be used. The latter devices result in less movement at the osteotomy sites and therefore fewer post-operative radiographs are required compared with lengthening using external fixators.

Essential image characteristics

The following characteristics are essential:

- Pelvis, knees and ankles should be straight.
- Density of the pelvis, knees and ankles should be appropriate for radiological assessment.
- Reproduction of hip, knee and subtalar joints with careful collimation.
- Reproduction of spongiosa and cortex.
- Visualisation of soft-tissue planes.
- When ruler technique is employed the ruler(s) should be straight and visible on the image at each of the joints.

Radiation protection

- Children having such procedures performed often need multiple radiographs and it is important to use gonad protection whenever appropriate and practical.
- Reminder that last menstrual period needs to be ascertained for those of childbearing age and consent obtained.

Ilizarov device (Fig. 13.41d)

When undertaking radiography it is important to note that the main problem is making sure that none of the frame obscures the osteotomy sites. Care should be taken to adopt the radiographic technique in order that the acquired images display any premature union, non-union or delayed union of the distracted segments and any abnormal subluxation or dislocation of the joints on either side. It is also important to demonstrate the pins and screws, which can become loose or infected.

Fig. 13.41a AP supine radiographs of both limbs in a neonate with a short left leg due to hypoplastic tibia, fibula and foot (hemimelia).

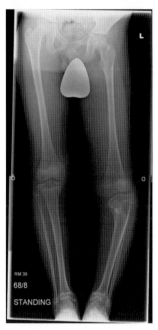

Fig. 13.41b AP erect leg length radiograph of 10-year-old male with previous meningococcal septicaemia and growth plate injury, resulting in shortening and varus deformity of left tibia. CR image, stitched image.

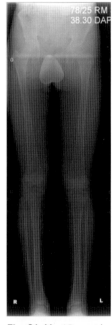

Fig. 31.41c AP erect both legs of 14-year-old boy with leg length discrepancy. CR image, stitched image.

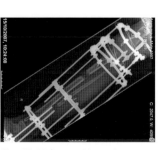

Fig. 13.41d Turned lateral radiograph of right lower leg in an Ilizarov frame. Distraction at the osteotomy sites is demonstrated.

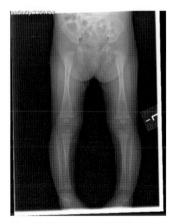

Fig. 13.41e AP erect both legs. 1-year-old boy with intoeing gait. First radiograph, therefore gonad protection not used.

13 Leg length assessment

Single exposure CR method (Figs 13.42a–13.42c)

CR cassettes (two or three dependent on the height of the child) are mounted vertically in a special holder to facilitate radiography in the erect position. Alternatively, depending on the CR cassette combination arrangement, the joined cassettes (two or three combined as one flat image receptor) are placed on the floor with the child examined in the supine position.

With this technique the divergent beam will magnify the limbs; however, the inaccuracy of the measurement of the difference in length due to magnification will probably be less than 5%, i.e. an inaccuracy of less than 2.5 mm when the difference in actual length is 50 mm. This degree of inaccuracy may be considered surgically insignificant.

Alternatively when examining a baby or small child, especially when they cannot stand and may be unco-operative, a smaller image receptor is selected to match the length of the limbs and if possible the child is examined on the imaging table provided a large enough FRD can be obtained (see Fig. 13.43d).

Position of patient and image receptor

- The patient stands on a low platform off the floor with the posterior aspect of the legs against the long image receptor with the arms extended by the side of the trunk.
- The anterior superior iliac spines should be equidistant from the image receptor and the medial sagittal plane should be vertical and coincident with the central longitudinal axis of the cassette.
- The legs should be, as far as possible, in a similar relationship to the pelvis with the feet separated so that the distance between the ankle joints is similar to the distance between the hip joints, with the patella of each knee facing forward.
- Foam pads and sandbags are used to stabilise the legs and ensure that they are straight.
- If necessary a wooden block of appropriate thickness is positioned below the shortened leg to ensure there is no pelvic tilt and that the limbs are adequately aligned.
- A ruler is required for any pre- or post-operative radiographs.

Direction and location of the X-ray beam

- The collimated horizontal beam is centred towards a point midway between the knee joints.
- The X-ray beam is collimated to include both lower limbs from hip joints to ankle joints.

Common faults and solutions

- Reduce magnification and improve image sharpness by placing body parts as close as possible to the image receptor and increasing the FRD to the maximum distance (180–260 cm).
- Maximum FRD also reduces dose.

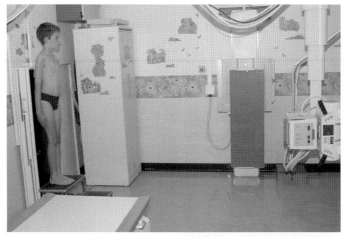

Fig. 13.42a Position of X ray tube for erect leg length radiographs, single exposure, CR cassette.

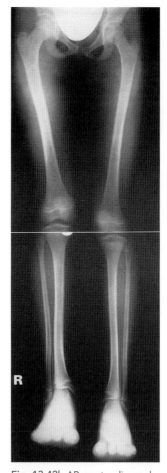

Fig. 13.42b AP erect radiographs of both legs with wooden block under right foot to correct pelvic tilt. Note female gonad protection in position.

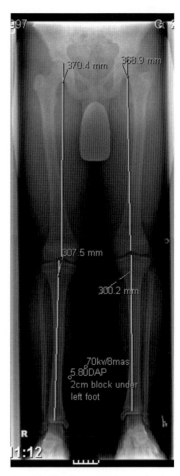

Fig. 13.42c AP erect radiograph of both legs of a 13-year-old boy with leg length discrepancy, 2 cm block inserted under left foot. Gonad protection in situ. CR image.

Notes

- For leg alignment studies the legs from hips to ankles should be included and any clinical defect should not be corrected.
- Automatic stitching of the images and any corrections is undertaken on the CR workstation before being sent to PACS.

Position of patient and image receptor

- Positioning is similar to that described for the CR method but with the patient erect and facing the X-ray tube on the dedicated patient stand. The vertical Perspex support is positioned immediately in front of the DDR detector with sufficient distance to allow it to travel vertically without being impeded.

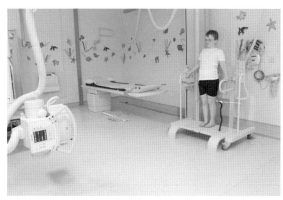

Fig. 13.43a Child positioned for APerect radiograph for leg length DRR. Note sphere for calibration.

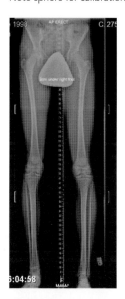

Fig. 13.43b AP erect radiograph of both legs of a 15-year-old boy with leg length discrepancy. Ruler and gonad protection in situ. DDR image.

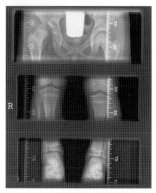

Fig. 13.43c AP erect radiograph of both legs for leg length discrepancy using localised exposure technique.

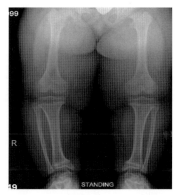

Fig. 13.43d AP erect both legs of an 8-year-old girl with achondroplasia. Additional deformity of bowed legs suspected. Femoral heads not visible. Full demonstration of each leg is normally necessary but radiograph not repeated in this case as only assessment of alignment required.

Leg length assessment 13

DDR method (Figs 13.43a, 13.43b)

Direction and location of the X-ray beam

- The method of determining the image acquisition field with such DDR systems vary: some manufacturers require confirmation of a start and finishing points related to the extent of the image field whilst others simply calculate the exposures required dependent of the collimated beam selected coincident with the anatomical area.
- A large FRD is selected consistent with the manufacturers' recommendation, e.g. 180–260 cm.

Notes

- A vertical radio-opaque ruler extending the full length of the vertical Perspex platform support may be used with some systems to aid in the electronic stitching process.
- A calibration tool may also be used to aid surgical planning, i.e. a sphere/ruler of known dimensions placed between the knees at the level of the knee joints.

Localised exposure method (Fig. 13.43c)

- Assessment is made using three separate exposures, using a 35 × 43 cm CR cassette placed lengthwise in the Bucky tray. The procedure is undertaken with the use of two 100 cm plastic rulers, each with an opaque scale at 1 cm intervals that produce an image on the receptor, which is necessary for drawing lines on the image and obtaining the required measurements.
- The rulers are placed longitudinally on the X-ray tabletop in such a fashion that they are parallel to each other with their scales corresponding and separated approximately 20 cm apart, so that they will be visible on the image. The rulers are secured in position by use of Velcro.
- The patient lies between the rulers with the hips, knees and ankles adopting the AP position with the legs straight and the hips positioned at the top end of the rulers' scales.
- Three separate exposures are made, with the X-ray beam collimated and centred midway between the hip joints, knee joints and ankle joints, starting first at the hips so that their image is recorded on the top 1/3 of the receptor. The process is repeated so that the knees occupy the middle 1/3 and the ankles the lower 1/3 of the receptor.
- Inaccuracy of the measurement due to using the technique is insignificant since the central ray is perpendicular to the film at the appropriate level of each joint.
- The exposure is adjusted accordingly at each of the joints to ensure that the density and contrast at each joint is similar. The dose may be reduces accordingly by removing the grid from the Bucky mechanism.

13 Elbow

The elbow can be one of the most difficult examinations to interpret in children and excellent technique is required. The most common injury in children is a fracture of the lower end of the humerus just above the condyles (supracondylar fracture). Not only is the injury very painful but also careless handling of the limb can aggravate the injury causing further damage to the adjacent nerves and blood vessels.

The arm should not be forcibly extended and rotation of the limb should be avoided. A radiograph is often also undertaken with the elbow flexed in a plaster or supporting sling. The latter should not be removed in an acute injury.

Referral criteria include: trauma, focal pain, deformity and suspected FB.

As with the adult, a radiograph is undertaken using AP and lateral projections with an additional AP oblique used to detect a fracture of the radial head. However, children are sometimes reluctant to extend their elbow for the AP projection. Modification of the basic technique is necessary with images acquired with the child erect or supine so that the child may be able to extend the arm more easily.

Both AP and lateral images are acquired with all three joints in the same plane in order to demonstrate any displacement.

Lateral (alternative positioning)

Child supine/prone (Fig. 13.44a)

- When X-raying a baby it is preferable to lay the patient prone on a soft pillow or pad as shown opposite.
- The side of the trunk places the unaffected arm with the head turned towards the affected side with the affected elbow flexed and gently raised onto the cassette.
- The carer immobilises the patient by holding the wrist on the affected side with the other hand firmly across the patients back.
- It may be necessary to angle the X-ray tube to direct the central ray perpendicular to the shaft of the humerus, centring on the lateral epicondyle.
- If co-operative the child may be seated on the holder's lap with the elbow flexed and placed on a cassette.

Child standing (Figs 13.44b–13.44d)

- This projection should be undertaken such that any supporting sling is not removed.
- The image receptor is supported vertically in a holder.
- The child is stood sideways with the elbow flexed and the lateral aspect of the injured elbow in contact with the cassette. The arm is gently extended backwards from the shoulder. The child is then rotated forwards until the elbow is clear of the rib cage, but still in contact with the cassette, with the line joining the epicondyles of the humerus at right-angles to the cassette.
- The horizontal central ray is directed to the medial epicondyle and the beam collimated to the elbow.

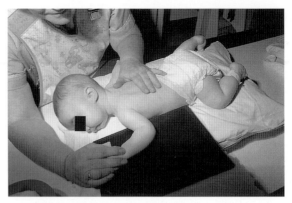

Fig. 13.44a Baby positioned for lateral projection of the elbow in prone position.

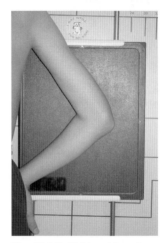

Fig. 13.44b Child positioned erect for lateral projection

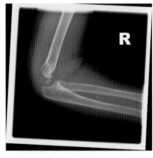

Fig. 13.44c Lateral elbow radiograph showing subtle posterior displacement of anterior humeral line due to a supracondylar fracture and an effusion.

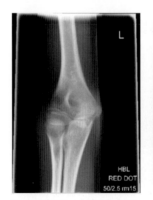 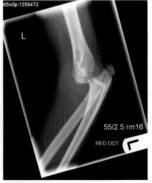

Figs 13.44d and e AP and lateral radiographs of the left elbow demonstrating dislocation. The lateral should be undertaken first and the AP taken with a horizontal beam without moving the patient's elbow to avoid any damage to the neurovascular bundle. If the patient is in great pain, further imaging can be performed under sedation or anaesthetic in theatre.

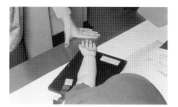 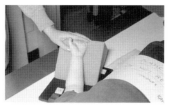

Figs 13.45a and b Child positioned supine for AP projection: (top) elbow extended, (bottom) elbow flexed.

Elbow 13

Antero-posterior (alternative positioning)

Child supine (Figs 13.45a–13.45d)

- The patient lies supine on the imaging couch or patient trolley with the shoulder and hip of the unaffected side raised to bring the side being examined into contact with the image receptor, i.e. 18 × 24 cm CR cassette.
- The arm is slightly abducted and when possible fully extended with the medial and lateral epicondyles equidistant from the film.
- The vertical central ray is directed midway between the epicondyles.
- Specific oblique views of the radial head can also be performed if there is significant clinical suspicion.

Child standing (Figs 13.45e–13.45g)

- For the AP projection a CR cassette is supported vertically in a cassette holder.
- The patient can either stand or sit with the back to the cassette. The arm is slightly abducted and the trunk rotated until the posterior aspect of the upper arm is in contact with the cassette with the epicondyles of the humerus equidistant from the cassette.
- If the elbow is fully flexed the central ray is directed at right-angles to the humerus to pass through the forearm to a point midway between the epicondyles.
- If there is less flexion at the elbow, it should be possible to direct the horizontal central ray to the midpoint between the epicondyles without the X-ray beam having to pass through the forearm.

Radiation protection

- Patients should sit with the affected arm nearest to the X-ray table and not with their legs under the table.
- Avoid holder's hands in the X-ray beam.
- All holders must wear a lead apron.
- Accurate coning with the LBD is essential.

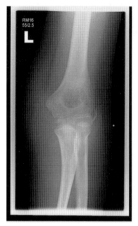 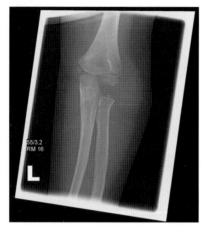

Figs 13.45c and d Comparison of AP images of a 10-year-old child with an avulsed medial epicondyle (normal curvilinear ossification centre of the lateral epicondyle) and 6-year-old child with fracture of the lateral condyle. It is important to demonstrate the soft tissues as the significant soft-tissue swelling focuses attention on the underlying bony injury. The patient with the medial epicondyle avulsion is unable to extend the arm fully and the radius overlaps the capitellum. An AP elbow with the forearm parallel to the cassette or a modified radial head view could have been performed if a radial fracture had been suspected.

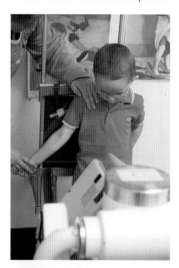

Fig. 13.45e Photograph of child positioned for AP projection of elbow erect.

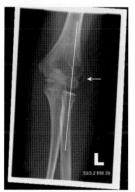 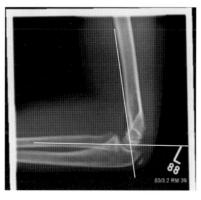

Figs 13.45f and g AP and lateral radiographs of the left elbow of a 9-year-old female. Normal appearances of the lateral epicondyle at this age, which should not be confused with an avulsion fracture. Normal alignment of anterior humeral and radiocapitellar lines.

473

13 Elbow

Antero-posterior (alternative positioning) (cont.) (Figs 13.46a–13.46f)

Essential image characteristics

AP projection

- Distal end of humerus should be straight with no rotation or foreshortening.
- Radius and ulna should be parallel and aligned with the humerus allowing for the carrying angle.
- Radial head should not overlap the capitellum.
- Coning should include distal 1/3 of the humerus and proximal 1/3 of the radius and ulna.
- Cortex and trabecular structures should be visually sharp.
- Reproduction of muscle/fat planes.

Lateral projection

- Humerus should be in true lateral position with superimposition of the condyles.
- Humerus should be at right-angles to the radius and ulna.
- Coning should include distal 1/3 of humerus and proximal 1/3 of radius and ulna.
- Soft-tissue detail should demonstrate the displacement of coronoid and olecranon fat pads.
- Cortex and trabecular structures should be visually sharp.
- Reproduction of muscle/fat planes.

Common faults and solutions

- Sub-optimal view of humerus and radial head due to child being unable to extend the elbow and radiograph has been taken with point of elbow balanced on the cassette. See positioning to avoid this.
- If the child is unable to extend the elbow (or where the elbow is flexed in a plaster) initially the humerus should be placed parallel to the cassette to best demonstrate a supracondylar fracture. If in acute trauma no fracture is evident on this radiograph, a repeat image is acquired with the forearm parallel to the cassette to demonstrate the proximal radius and ulna.
- Forearm pronated instead of correct supination.
- Rotated joint. The joints of the shoulder, elbow and wrist should be in the same plane to obtain best positioning.

Radiological considerations

- A good knowledge of ossification centres around the elbow is required with suitable reference texts being available to avoid necessity for comparison views.
- The radio-capitellar line should pass through the radius and mid-capitellum on any or all projections.
- The anterior humeral line should pass through the anterior 1/3 of the capitellum on the lateral projection.

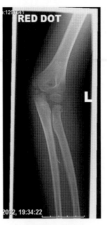
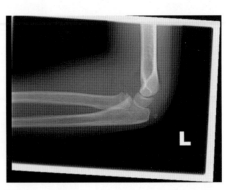

Figs 13.46a and b AP and lateral radiographs of the left elbow of an 8-year-old female demonstrating a transverse fracture of the neck of the radius and a joint effusion. AP slightly rotated to best demonstrate the suspected radial neck fracture.

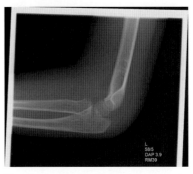

Fig. 13.46c Lateral elbow radiograph of an 11-year-old child showing a large effusion due to an occult supracondylar fracture.

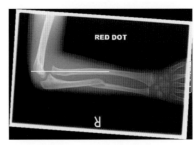

Fig. 13.46d A 7-year-old girl with an ulnar diaphyseal fracture and a dislocated radial head at the elbow described as a Monteggia injury. Any radiograph of a diaaphyseal injury of the forearm should include the wrist and elbow.

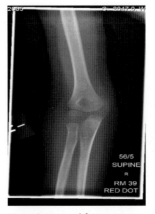
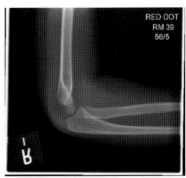

Figs 13.46e and f AP and lateral right elbow images of a 4-year-old male demonstrating an undisplaced supracondylar fracture with a large joint effusion. Note right lateral lead marker partly coned off the AP radiograph; therefore, digital annotations added. Lead markers preferred where possible.

Bone age 13

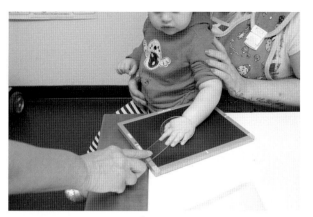

Fig. 13.47a Plexiglass device used to immobilise fingers for dorsi-palmar (DP) projection of the hand of a younger child.

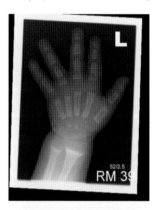

Fig. 13.47b DP radiograph of the left hand for bone age of a 1-year-old male infant with failure to thrive. Irregular and expanded metaphyses due to rickets demonstrated. Bone age is delayed.

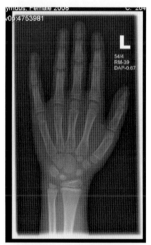

Fig. 13.47c DP radiograph of the left hand for bone age of a 5-year-old child with congenital adrenal hyperplasia and advanced bone age.

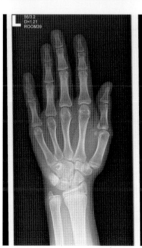

Fig. 13.47d DP image of the left hand of an 11-year-old girl with congenital adrenal hyperplasia demonstrating advanced bone age.

Referral criteria

Bone age is normally required in patients suspected of having an underlying endocrine abnormality and is commonly requested in patients with precocious puberty. A bone age is also performed in patients with suspected significant nutritional deficiency, chronic disease and possible underlying syndrome. Occasionally the diagnosis of a syndrome can be inferred from the hand radiograph, e.g. Turner's syndrome with such patients having short 4th and 5th metacarpals.

Recommended projections (Figs 13.47a–13.47d)

- Greulich and Pyle method is the most common and easily used assessment of bone age.
- The protocol requires a dorsi-palmar (DP) projection of the whole non-dominant hand including all digits and the wrist joint.
- The fingers should be straight with the metaphyses in profile.
- The determination of osseous maturation is based on the number, size and appearance of the ossification centres and on the width of the growth plate or the degree of fusion present.

Radiological considerations

- Girls are more advanced than boys and separate standards are available. 19/20 children are within 2 standard deviations (SDs) from the mean of their chronological age. The SDs vary with age and any assessment of bone age should include the degree of deviation from the mean and value of 1 SD at that age.
- If there are no ossification centres visible in the carpus an AP of the knee can be taken to demonstrate the presence of the distal femoral and proximal tibial ossification centres, which appear at 36 and 37 weeks respectively.
- Children with delayed or advanced bone ages may be short or tall for their age. Children with advanced bone age may undergo premature fusion of the epiphyses and be short in adult life. A predicted adult height can be obtained from standard tables, which require an assessment of current height and bone age.
- If a child cannot confirm a non-dominant hand, then a radiograph of the left hand and wrist should be performed.

13 Feet – supported/weight-bearing

Referral criteria

- Talipes (congenital foot deformity present at birth).
- Painful flat foot/feet.

Recommended projections

Examination of the affected foot/feet is undertaken both for babies and toddlers using the following projections:

Basic	DP – weight-bearing
	Lateral – weight-bearing
Supplementary	Lateral – with forced dorsiflexion
	DP – oblique

DP, dorsi-plantar.

Dorsi-plantar – weight-bearing (Figs 13.48a–13.48f)

A CR cassette is selected, large enough to include the foot/feet.

Position of patient and image receptor

Babies

- The baby is supported supine on the X-ray table and the knee of the affected side is flexed so that the foot rests on the image receptor.
- The foot is adjusted so that the tibia is perpendicular to the image receptor.
- Both feet may be examined together with the knees held together.
- Pressure should be applied gently to the flexed knees to simulate weight-bearing.

Toddlers

- The toddler is seated in a special seat with both feet resting on the cassette similar to as described above.
- The knees are held firmly to ensure that the soles of the feet remain in close contact with the cassette
- No attempt should be made to correct alignment of forefeet.
- Older children can be examined standing erect.

Direction and location of the X-ray beam

- The collimated vertical beam is centred midway between the malleoli and at right-angles to an imaginary line joining the malleoli.
- The central ray may be angled 10° cranial to avoid the tibiae overlapping the hindfeet.

Essential image characteristics

- The alignment of the talus and calcaneus of the hindfoot should be clearly visible with no overlapping by the shins.
- The tibia should be straight to ensure that there is no technical tilt of the talus.
- Visualisation of the bones of the feet, consistent with age.
- Visualisation of the soft-tissue planes.
- Reproduction of the spongiosa and cortex.

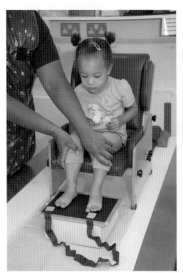 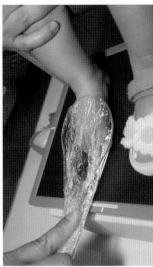

Figs 13.48a and b Baby and child positioned for radiograph of AP foot/feet with lower limbs supported.

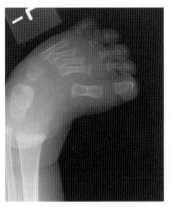 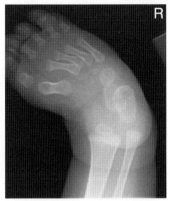

Figs 13.48c and d DP radiographs of both feet in a baby with bilateral talipes equinovarus. Calcaneum and talus are superimposed and parallel.

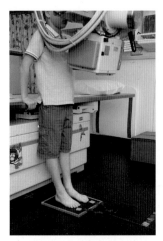 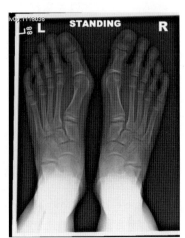

Fig. 13.48e Older child positioned for DP projection of both feet erect. Note slight tube angulation.

Fig. 13.48f DP radiograph of standing both feet of an 11-year-old girl with metatarsus varus primus and secondary hallux valgus. Normal hindfeet.

A CR cassette is selected, large enough to include the foot.

Position of patient and image receptor

Babies

- With the baby supine on the imaging couch the affected leg is preferably internally rotated so that the inner border of the foot is placed against the cassette with the ankle (not forefoot) in the true lateral position. Alternatively the leg is externally rotated with the lateral aspect of the foot against the cassette.

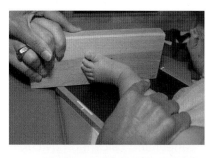

Fig. 13.49a Baby positioned for lateral radiograph of foot. Pressure from carer's hand simulates weight bearing.

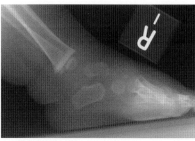

Fig. 13.49b Supported lateral radiograph of right foot in neonate. Talus and calcaneum are parallel.

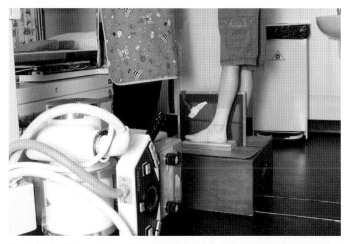

Fig. 13.49c Older child positioned for a lateral weight-bearing projection of the foot. Child standing on wooden block. The receptor should be nearest to the medial side of the foot and ankle.

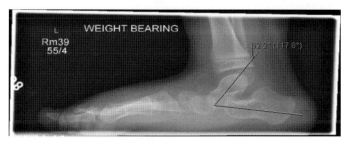

Fig. 13.49d Weight-bearing lateral left foot radiograph of a 3-year-old patient with pes planus and talipes calcaneo valgus. Downward sloping talus with increased talo-calcaneal angle.

Feet – supported/weight-bearing

Lateral – weight bearing (Figs 13.49a–13.49d)

- A wooden block support is positioned beneath the sole of the foot with dorsiflexion pressure applied during exposure, to demonstrate the reducibility of any equinus deformity at the ankle.

Toddlers

- The child is examined standing with a cassette placed in a groove against the inner foot, resting on a wooden block.
- To stop the foot from being inverted, the leg should also not be externally rotated.
- Gentle pressure may be required to produce additional maximum dorsi-/plantar flexion views when assessing the degree of correction of clubfoot after treatment.

Direction and location of the X-ray beam

- The collimated perpendicular beam is centred to the lateral/medial malleolus at right-angles to the axis of the tibia and at right-angles to the image receptor.
- For the toddler the beam is directed horizontally.

Essential image characteristics

- The alignment of the talus and calcaneus in the true lateral position should be clearly visible.
- The sole of the foot should be flat against the block with no elevation of the heel.
- See DP projection characteristics.

Common faults and solutions

- For the DP projection the shins often obscure the hindfeet. Angle the beam 10° cranial to overcome this problem.
- The density of the radiograph should be such that the hind-foot bones are clearly demonstrated, even if this results in some overpenetration of the forefeet.
- For the lateral projection care should be taken to avoid oblique projection of the foot as this could simulate a valgus/varus position.
- Non-weight-bearing views do not demonstrate the malalignment that exists in the functional state and should not be used.

13 Feet – supported/weight-bearing

Radiological considerations

The talus is the only bone in the foot that does not have any direct muscle attachments. Any deformities are due to abnormal rotation or movement of foot bones in relation to the talus. Talipes equinovarus (club foot) is present at birth and is due to malalignment of the hind- and midfoot joints. These become fixed by capsular and ligamentous contractures. Radiographs should allow correct assessment of the alignment of the bones of the hindfoot, midfoot and forefoot. The various positions and terms are described.

Varus

- An axial reference line through the calcaneum is deviated towards the midline of the body. The talo-calcaneal angle on an AP projection is decreased with the two bones being more parallel and sometimes superimposed.
- Parallelism is also seen in the lateral projection.
- Congenital talipes equinovarus is the most common abnormality occurring in 1–4/1000 live births. Males are more commonly affected than females and there is a slight genetic predisposition. It is treated by manipulation and plaster casting (Ponseti technique). Patients may also require tendon release, release of contractures or combined osteotomies and arthrodeses.

Valgus

- An axial reference line though the calcaneum is deviated away from the midline of the body.
- The talo-calcaneal angle on an AP projection of the foot will be increased and similarly on the lateral projection, leading to a more vertical talus.
- This kind of foot (talipes calcaneo valgus) is more commonly seen in children with cerebral palsy.
- The talo-calcaneal angles vary with age and it is to be noted that calculated angles are not always abnormal in abnormal feet.

Metatarsus adductus

- The distal ends of the metatarsals are deviated towards the midline, pivoting at their bases. The hindfoot is normal. This is a more benign condition.

The terms calcaneus and equinus refer to the position of the foot in relation to the ankle. The former indicates dorsiflexion with elevation of the anterior end of the calcaneum and equinus indicates plantar flexion.

The term talipes originates in an old description of a patient walking on his ankle (talus) rather than the foot (pes).

Lateral radiographs allow assessment of the plantar arch. Increased height of the arch (cavum arch) is associated with valgus/varus foot deformities. A flattened arch (pes planus) may be due to a flexible flat foot, tarsal coalition or other congenital conditions.

A convex plantar arch (rocker bottom foot) may be due to a congenital vertical talus or severe cerebral palsy.

Tarsal coalition (talo-calcaneal and calcaneo-navicular)

If a tarsal coalition is suspected because of a painful flat foot, evidence of talar beaking and C-shape of the sustentaculum tali should be sought on the lateral image, which may be due to talo-calcaneal fusion; MRI or CT is required for confirmation. A DP oblique (45°) projection of the foot is necessary for the demonstration of a calcaneo-navicular coalition. It cannot be identified on an AP projection alone. Both forms of coalition can be fibrous/osseous (Fig. 13.50).

Foot deformities need careful positioning and analysis of the derangement pre- and post manipulation and casting or surgery. In a normal patient:

- The mid-talar line should pass through just medial to the 1st metatarsal and the mid-calcaneal line should pass through the base of the 4th metatarsal on the weight-bearing AP radiograph.
- The mid-talar line should pass through or be parallel to the 1st metatarsal and a line drawn along the inferior aspect of the calcaneum should show mild dorsiflexion of the calcaneum on the lateral radiograph.

With successful treatment of hindfoot abnormalities, the calcaneum rotates under the talus into a satisfactory position.

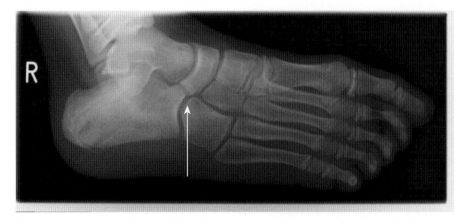

Fig. 13.50 Dorsi-plantar oblique right foot demonstrating calcaneo-navicular coalition, which is not demonstrated on AP and lateral projections.

Feet – supported/weight-bearing 13

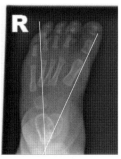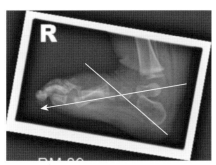

Figs 13.51a and b Simulated dorsi-plantar (DP) and lateral weight-bearing right foot images with radiolucent foam pad in position. 1-month-old infant. Normal hindfoot and forefoot. Radiographic angles demonstrated.
AP: line through the talus extends along 1st metatarsal and calcaneus is aligned with the 4th metatarsal; lateral: talus is aligned with 1st metatarsal with normal talo-calcaneal angle.

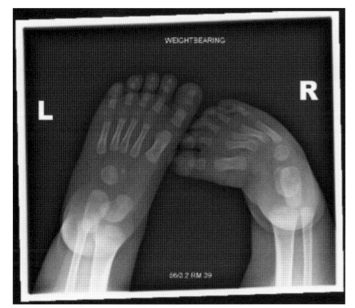

Fig. 13.51c 1-year-old infant, AP weight bearing. Normal left foot. Talipes equinovarus right foot with talus and calcaneum superimposed.

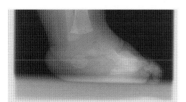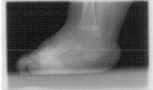

Figs 13.51d and e Lateral feet radiographs of a neonate's feet supported by a wood block. Talipes equinovarus with the talus and calcaneus parallel on each side.

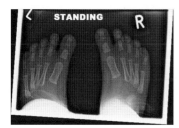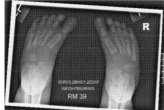

Figs 13.51f and g AP erect radiograph of both feet in a 2-year-old boy with intoeing gait (left). The hindfeet are not demonstrated and it is not possible to distinguish between metatarsus adductus and talipes equinovarus, the latter being more serious. Repeat radiograph (right) confirms metatarsus adductus with normal hindfeet. The patient should lean slightly backwards or the tube should be angled to avoid the shins obscuring the hind feet.

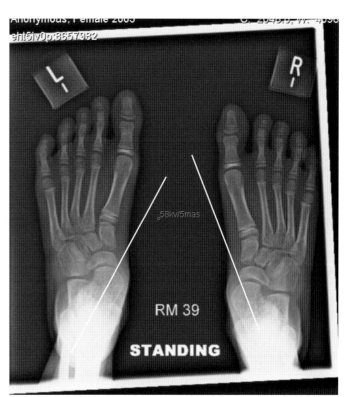

Fig. 13.51h AP erect radiograph of both feet of an 8-year-old girl with pes planus, talo-navicular subluxation and hindfoot valgus. The midline of the talus is medial to the 1st metatarsals.

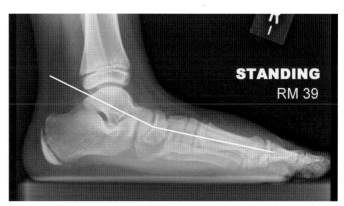

Fig. 13.51i Lateral radiograph of the right foot of a 10-year-old boy with flat feet, pes planus. Patient standing on a wooden block. The mid-talar line extends below the 1st metatarsal line forming an angle.

13 Skeletal survey for non-accidental injury

Rationale for projections

A skeletal survey is the main radiological investigation for non-accidental injury (NAI), and comprises a series of images taken to assess the whole skeleton. NAI to children is seen all too commonly in any department routinely dealing with children. It can result in serious long-term emotional and physical injuries. The latter include serious neurological deficits, mental retardation and in the worst cases, death of the child.

A significant number of skeletal injuries in this condition are diagnostically specific. Posterior rib fractures[52–54] and metaphyseal fractures are almost pathognomonic of NAI. Carefully evaluated, well-collimated, high radiographic detail skeletal radiographs are vital in all cases of suspected infant abuse.[55]

A skeletal survey is needed to demonstrate pathology but it is equally important in dating skeletal injuries, as accurate evaluation and dating of these injuries will be vital in providing legal argument.[56] This may require further projections of certain specific areas and this has to be tailored to the appearances of the initial injuries and to the clinical history given at the time.

Post-mortem skeletal studies may also be required in some cases and can provide useful additional information.[57]

It is rarely, if ever, necessary for a skeletal survey to be performed by inexperienced staff outside normal hours (see Radiological considerations).

Referral criteria

The referral criteria that would justify a skeletal survey in the presence of clinical suspicion, include the following:

Criteria	Examples
Clinical suspicion	• Skin lesions (bites or burns) • Retinal haemorrhage • Torn frenulum under the age of 3 years
Incidental detection of suspicious fractures on radiographs taken for other reasons	• Skull fractures >6 mm wide • Fractures that do not correspond with the history given • Fractures that are older than the history given • More than one fracture of differing age • Metaphyseal fractures • Posterior or anterior rib fractures • Long bone fractures in child <1 year • Abnormal periosteal reactions • Unexplained subdural haematoma
Computed tomography	• Sub-dural haematomas of differing ages

Occult bony injury is rare over 3 years of age, and most NAI surveys are performed on infants under 2 years. They are also indicated in siblings <3 years of age, when the index case is proven NAI.

Recommended projections

The projections advised below are as recommended by the British Society of Paediatric Radiologists and the Royal College of Radiologists in collaboration with the Royal College of Paediatrics and Child Heath.[58]

Fifty percent of rib fractures are occult, compared with 20% of limb fractures, and as they are diagnostically important, oblique rib projections are justified and may be best performed at an interval of 10–14 days when callus formation will be more obvious. Coned projections of any suspicious metaphyses can be undertaken at the same time. A clear explanation for follow-up imaging should be given. Non-attendance is not tolerated and regarded as a further safeguarding issue.

Oblique projections of the hands are preferred as they are more likely to show buckle and subtle cortical fractures.[59] All examinations are performed supine.

The recommended projections are as follows:

AP chest	Chest to show all ribs, clavicles and shoulders
Abdomen to include pelvis	
AP right femur	To include hip and knee joints and upper 2/3 of tibia and fibula
AP left femur	As with right femur
AP right ankle	To include distal 1/3 of tibia and fibula
AP left ankle	As with right ankle
AP right humerus, AP left humerus	
AP right forearm, AP left forearm	
Lateral cervical, lateral thoracic and lumbar spines	
AP skull and lateral skull	
Oblique ribs	May be delayed by up to 10 days in those with no other fractures as this can demonstrate late callus formation
DP oblique of both hands	
DP oblique both feet	

A minimum of 15 radiographs are normally required excluding oblique ribs if they are performed at a 2 week interval and excluding any additional coned views. The practice of imaging the entire body on one radiograph 'babygram' is unacceptable.

Consent

The parent or carer must fully understand the requirements for a skeletal survey. A record of the informed consent obtained by the referring clinician should be in the child's clinical record. Consent is rarely declined but in such a situation a court order would be required before proceeding. The examining radiographer should reaffirm the consent obtained and a minimum of two health care professionals should be present.

A full description of the examination and technique of immobilisation should be given to the parents or guardians. This advice should include use of any accessory immobilisation devices.

A NAI imaging record should be completed that includes the names and positions of the health care workers involved, time and date of the examination, documentation of the examination, consent of the parents or carers and description of the date and extent of any follow-up imaging. A copy of the NAI imaging record, as used at our institution, is enclosed as an appendix.

Infants who may have suffered fractures or soft-tissue injuries may be more fractious and difficult to pacify. If the parents become distressed and perceive undue distress for their child, then the examination should be temporarily suspended and clinical review obtained. Additional pain relief may need to be considered.

Radiation protection

Well-collimated carefully positioned images are required for higher quality and lower radiation dose. Unlike normal paediatric practice, lower kV/higher mAs should be employed for best demonstration of bony detail and soft tissues. It may also be advisable to avoid additional copper filtration as it may have a detrimental effect on image quality when very low kV techniques are used, as in hands and feet.

Skeletal survey for non-accidental injury 13

Radiographic technique (see Figs 13.53c, 13.54a, 13.54g)

Tried and tested immobilisation methods should be employed. The correct name and date of birth of the child should be visible on each image. It is preferable for primary side markers to be used and these should not obscure any anatomical areas. All radiographers, health care workers and witnesses involved should be identified and their role documented in the Radiology information system (RIS) record or equivalent.[60]

A patient, non-judgemental approach is essential. Patient positioning and X-ray beam centring is already described for the individual examinations. Small differences in technique are as outlined below.

Chest (Figs 13.52a, 13.54e, 13.54f)

- Shoulders and all ribs should be included on the image.
- The arms should be abducted from the chest and not raised by the sides of the head.
- A minimum of 400 speed class screen/film combination equivalent is used to reduce movement unsharpness.
- The tube potential should be between 60 and 70 kV to ensure optimum bony detail.

Spine (cervical, thoracic and lumbar) (Fig. 13.52d)

- A minimum of 400 speed class screen/film combination equivalent is used to reduce movement unsharpness.
- A single lateral image is acquired without the use of a grid in a child <3 years.
- Tube potential up to 70 kV.

Skull (Figs 13.52b, 13.52c)

- The AP and lateral images are acquired without the use of a grid for a child under 2 years.
- The lateral image is acquired using a horizontal beam.
- Tube potential up to 70 kV.

Upper and lower limbs (Figs 13.52e, 13.53a, 13.53b, 13.53d, 13.53e, 13.54b–13.54d, 13.54h, 13.54i)

- A 200 speed class screen/film combination equivalent and a lower kV range are used to provide optimum soft tissue and bony detail.
- Separate images of the humerus and radius and ulna are normally acquired after 18 months of age.
- Separate images of the femur and tibia and fibula are acquired. The image of the femur should include the knee joint.

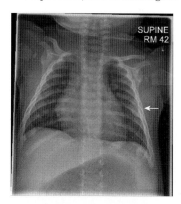

Fig. 13.52a AP supine chest radiograph. of a 5-month-old child. Note callus around healed fractures of the left 6th and 7th ribs.

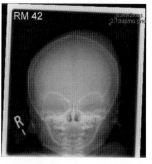 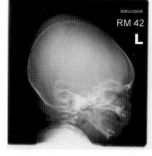

Figs 13.52b and c AP fronto-occipital and lateral supine skull radiographs. Note left parietal fracture and overlying soft-tissue swelling.

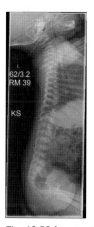 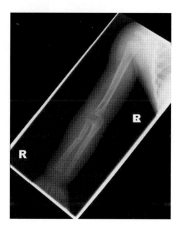

Fig. 13.52d Supine lateral whole spine radiograph of a 6-week-old infant. Normal appearances.

Fig. 13.52e AP supine right whole arm of a 16-month-old infant. Note acute transverse fracture of proximal radial diaphysis.

13 Skeletal survey for non-accidental injury

Essential image characteristics

- General essential characteristics are as described for the individual anatomical areas.
- However, unexplained classic metaphyseal lesions (CMLs), rib fractures and post-traumatic periosteal reactions can be subtle and they are highly suspicious of NAI. Therefore, particular care is required to optimise the skeletal survey images to best demonstrate these injuries.
- Metaphyses should be demonstrated in profile as a single line where anatomically possible.
- Each limb should be demonstrated with as much symmetry as possible to compare metaphyses and periosteal reactions.
- The chest should be as straight as possible to detect any subtle variation in the ribs that might suggest previous or current injury.

Common faults and solutions

- Views of epiphyses and metaphyses in profile are required to show the classical metaphyseal fractures as corner fractures. The fracture occurs right across the metaphysis. If the radiographic beam is angled or the metaphyses are tilted, then the fracture appears as a bucket handle fracture, but this can easily be missed or thought to be due to a normal variation in the appearance of the ossification of the metaphyses. Additional coned images may then be necessary.
- An attempt to radiograph the whole leg together should be avoided; immobilisation can only be provided at the feet and excessive plantar flexion whilst holding can result in the heels obscuring the ankle joints and the metaphyses being tilted.
- Any rotation of the chest or asymmetry of the limbs due to positioning should be avoided.

Radiological considerations

A high index of suspicion is required. However, a skeletal survey should only be requested following discussion between the Consultant Paediatrician and Consultant Radiologist. It requires radiologist involvement to ensure diagnostic quality, to allow additional images of any injury to be taken if necessary and to suggest the timing of any repeat studies. The outcome, whether positive or negative, may have huge implications (for the family especially). Good clinico-radiological co-operation at the highest level is vital, supported by the highest standard of radiography.

Two radiologists are required to provide and corroborate a radiological report on a NAI skeletal survey. This report should be communicated in a timely manner to the referring clinician and should be available to other relevant health and social workers involved in the safeguarding of the child.

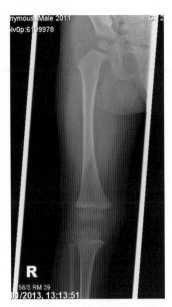
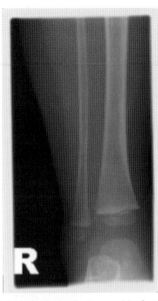

Figs 13.53a and b AP images of the right lower limb of a 2-year-old infant. Separate images to facilitate easier immobilisation, to allow metaphyses to be visualised in profile and to recognise more easily corner metaphyseal fractures. Normal appearances.

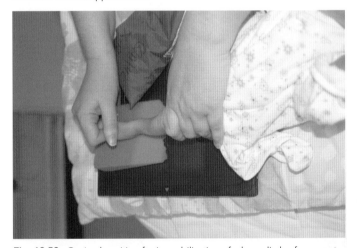

Fig. 13.53c Optimal position for immobilisation of a lower limb of a neonate.

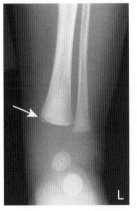

Fig. 13.53d Left ankle radiograph of a neonate with a corner tibial fracture.

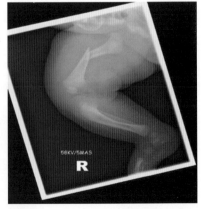

Fig. 13.53e Lateral radiograph of whole right lower limb showing an oblique angulated fracture of mid-femoral diaphysis. When there is obvious deformity or swelling, the first radiograph should be obtained with as little movement of the patient as possible. Whole limbs, AP or lateral are acceptable. Further coned views can then be planned as necessary.

Table of doses for skeletal survey (NAI)

0–6 mo	local DRL 10 cGy cm^2, DRL +20% 12 cGy cm^2
6 mo–1 y	local DRL 14.3, DRL+20% 17.2 cGy cm^2
1 y–18 mo	local DRL 18.1, DRL +20% 21.7 cGy cm^2
18 mo–2 y	local DRL 18.4, DRL+20% 22.1 cGy cm^2

Local DRLs based on mean doses after excluding significantly under- or oversized patients. Level of +20% set as trigger for investigation.

Number of radiographs:

- Minimum 15, excluding oblique ribs performed at 2 weeks
- Older children may have 17–18 if upper limb and lower limbs are radiographed separately or additional coned views are obtained

Skeletal survey for non-accidental injury 13

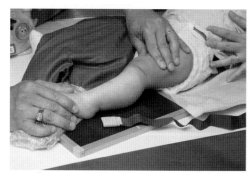

Fig. 13.54a Holding technique for AP radiograph of lower leg in a young infant.

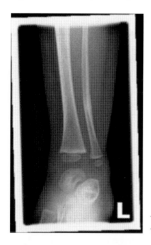

Fig. 13.54b AP left ankle, distal tibia and fibula of a 17-month-old infant. Note healing fracture of the distal fibular diaphysis.

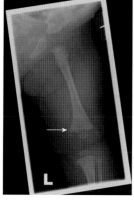

Fig. 13.54c AP radiograph of left femur, knee, upper tibia and fibula of a 6-week-old female infant. Note subtle corner fracture of the medial femoral metaphysis.

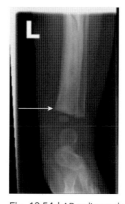

Fig. 13.54d AP radiograph of left ankle, distal tibia and fibula of a 7-month-old infant. Slightly rotated view showing extensive healing and periosteal reaction around an undisplaced spiral fracture of the distal tibia and a corner tibial metaphyseal fracture.

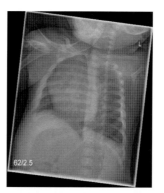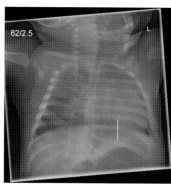

Fig. 13.54e and f Right and left oblique radiographs of the ribs demonstrating the whole chest on each image to allow assessment of the ribs in two projections. Note subtle expansion of mid-left 7th rib due to a healed fracture.

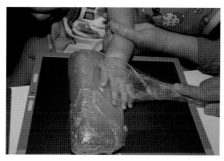

Fig. 13.54g Holding technique to obtain oblique projection of left hand.

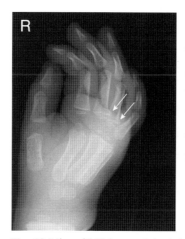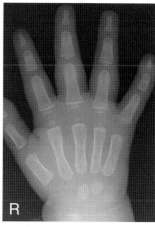

Figs 13.54h and i Oblique and dorsi-plantar (DP) radiographs of right hand. Note fractures of the 3rd and 4th proximal phalanges, seen on oblique but not seen on the DP projection of the same patient.

13 Skeletal survey for syndrome assessment

A similar technique can be used for syndrome assessment. These skeletal surveys are non-urgent and should be performed when a radiologist is available so that the survey can be tailored to the clinical requirements.

The radiographs performed will depend on the suspected syndrome or clinically visible abnormalities.

However, a full syndrome skeletal survey (Figs 13.55a–13.55e, 13.56a–13.56h) will normally include:

Recommended projections include:

- AP skull.
- Lateral skull, including C1 and C2.
- PA/AP chest.
- AP lumbar spine.
- Lateral thoraco-lumbar spine.
- Pelvis.
- AP of one upper limb.
- AP of one lower limb.
- PA of non-dominant hand for bone age.[61]

Notes

- If the patient has already had radiographs performed, these should not be repeated but can be used for the overall assessment.
- A limited skeletal survey would also be appropriate for a patient with a focal abnormality.
- Multi-focal skeletal abnormalities are due to osteochondrodysplasias whose phenotype evolves through life or dysostoses that are due to a defect in foetal development in the first 6 weeks of life and the phenotype is fixed.
- In the former, selected radiographs may be repeated in 1–2 years where the evolution of the appearances may allow a specific diagnosis if the early appearances are less diagnostic.
- Additional radiographs may include coned projections, feet, other limbs and individual radiographs of family members.

The aim of the skeletal survey is to analyse the following:

- Presence, absence, multiplicity and degree of fusion of any bones.
- Bone density and degree of mineralisation.
- Distribution and symmetry of abnormalities (e.g. epiphyseal, metaphyseal, proximal or distal limb shortening).
- Shape of individual bones (e.g. curved, flattened, hooked, scalloped).
- Focal structural abnormalities (e.g. exostoses, enchondromas, striations, bone islands).
- Complications (e.g. fractures, scoliosis, limb length discrepancy and malignancy)
- Identification of classical abnormalities (e.g. tibial pseudoarthrosis in neurofibromatosis Type 1)

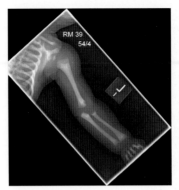
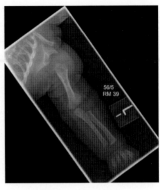

Fig. 13.55a AP radiograph of whole upper limb in a 1-day-old male neonate with short proximal and distal limbs due to osteopetrosis. Note dense bones and metaphyseal lucencies.

Fig. 13.55b AP radiograph of whlole upper limb of a 3-month-old female with achondroplasia demonstrating rhizomelic proximal limb shortening and flaring of the metaphyses.

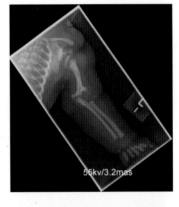

Fig. 13.55c AP radiograph of the whole upper limb of a 1-day-old male infant with chondrodysplasia punctate demonstrating rhizomelic shortening of the humerus with stippled epiphyses.

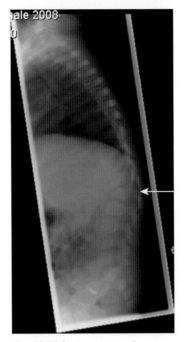
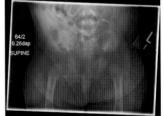

Fig. 13.55d Lateral spine of a 16-month-old girl showing beaked anterior L1 vertebra. Isolated finding in this case but can be present in mucopolysaccharidosis.

Fig. 13.55e AP pelvic radiograph of a 3-month-old girl with achondroplasia showing typical deep sciatic notches.

Skeletal survey for syndrome assessment 13

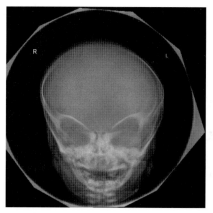

Fig. 13.56a AP skull radiograph of a 1-day-old male neonate with osteopetrosis.

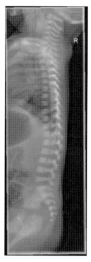

Fig. 13.56e Lateral whole spine of a 1-day-old male neonate with osteopetrosis.

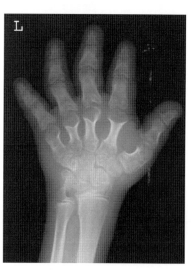

Fig. 13.56f Dorsi-palmar (DP) radiograph of left hand in a child with acrodysostosis.

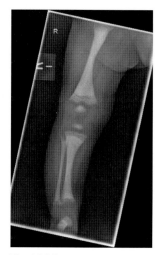

Fig. 13.56b AP radiograph of right lower limb of a 1-day-old neonate with osteopetrosis. Note femoral head had been included on the patient's radiograph of the pelvis and both hips.

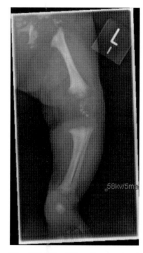

Fig. 13.56c AP radiograph of the whole left lower limb of a 1-day-old male infant with rhizomelic chondrodysplasia punctata. Note radiograph should be straight with less overlap of tibia and fibula.

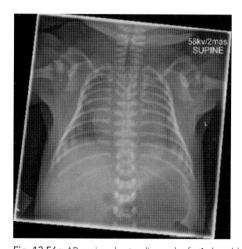

Fig. 13.56g AP supine chest radiograph of a 1-day-old male neonate with rhizomelic proximal limb shortening due to X-linked chondrodysplasia punctata.

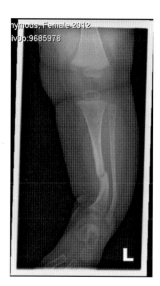

Fig. 13.56d AP radiograph right lower leg. Sometimes only a single radiograph combined with clinical features is required to suggest the diagnosis. Typical deformity with pathological fracture of right distal tibial diaphysis leading to pseudoarthrosis in a patient with multiple café au lait spots consistent with neurofibromatosis Type 1.

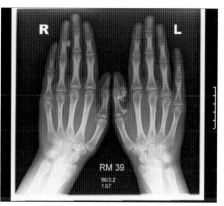

Fig. 13.56h DP radiograph of both hands of a 14-year-old female. If clinical findings are found to be asymmetric, both sides may be required as in this case of inherited tumoral calcinosis, which affected multiple joints, including both hands.

13 Image evaluation

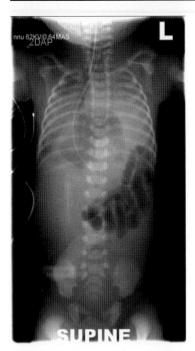

Fig. 13.57a AP supine chest and abdominal radiograph.

IMAGE EVALUATION

AP supine chest and abdominal radiograph (Fig. 13.57a)

The main points to consider are:
- Technical factors are adequate.
- Combined study appropriate for small neonate with relevant suspected pathology. Centring is to the chest.

DIAGNOSIS: left diaphragmatic hernia.

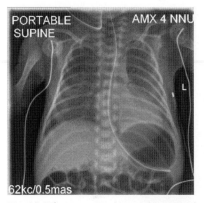

Fig. 13.57b AP supine chest radiograph of a neonate.

IMAGE EVALUATION

AP supine chest radiograph of a neonate (Fig. 13.57b)

The main points to consider are:
- Technical factors are adequate, good collimation and chin excluded.
- Note ECG leads well-positioned on shoulders and not obscuring the lungs.
- Lead side marker preferred for first radiographs of neonates to avoid misdiagnosis of dextrocardia but digital markers can be used for follow up, as in this case.

DIAGNOSIS: chronic lung disease.

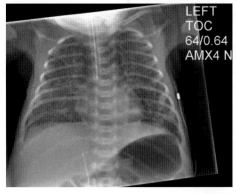

Fig. 13.57c AP supine chest radiograph of a neonate.

IMAGE EVALUATION

AP supine chest radiograph of a neonate (Fig. 13.57c)

The main points to consider are:
- Technical factors are adequate.
- A left skin probe does not obscure the lungs. The UVC is visible and straight, overlying the ductus venosus/inferior vena cava.
- The tip of the ETT is positioned down the right main bronchus and needs to be repositioned.

DIAGNOSIS: meconium aspiration.

Image evaluation 13

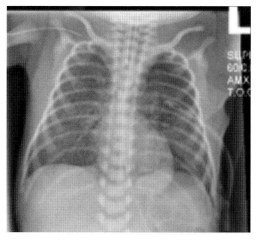

Fig. 13.58a AP supine chest of a neonate.

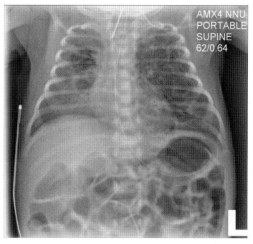

Fig. 13.58c AP supine chest radiograph of a neonate.

IMAGE EVALUATION

AP supine chest of a neonate (Fig. 13.58a)

The main points to consider are:
- Technical factors: adequate.
- Note: tubes and lines well-demonstrated and no extraneous tubing obscuring the lungs. ETT position satisfactory. Tip of right central line overlying the right subclavian vein. Left intercostal drain.

DIAGNOSIS: pulmonary interstitial emphysema and left pneumothorax.

IMAGE EVALUATION

AP supine chest radiograph of a neonate (Fig. 13.58c)

The main points to consider are:
- Technical factors adequate.
- ETT pointing to the right. Nasogastric tube in correct position.
- Care must be taken not to dislodge an ETT when positioning the patient.

DIAGNOSIS: cystic chronic lung disease.

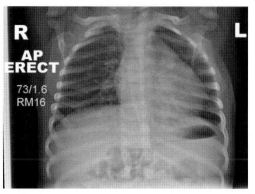

Fig. 13.58b AP erect chest of a 1-year-old child.

IMAGE EVALUATION

AP erect chest of a 1-year-old child (Fig. 13.58b)

The main points to consider are:
- Technical factors: adequate apart from mildly lordotic position of the patient with high clavicles and anterior ribs pointing upwards. This results in the anterior diaphragms obscuring the lung bases.
- Right lung markings are seen overlying the liver. Position can be corrected with a wedge foam pad behind the upper chest.

DIAGNOSIS: left lower lobe pneumonia.

13 Image evaluation

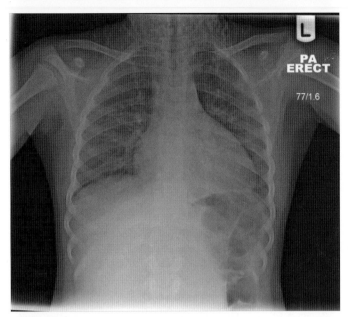

Fig. 13.59a PA erect chest of a 9-year-old female.

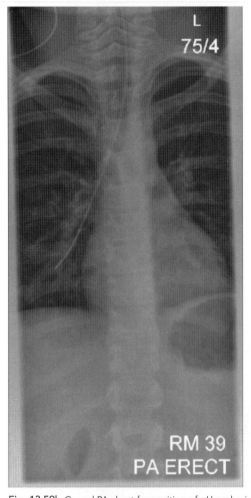

Fig. 13.59b Coned PA chest for position of pH probe in a 10-year-old child.

IMAGE EVALUATION

PA erect chest of a 9-year-old female (Fig. 13.59a)

The main points to consider are:

- Technical factors: there is a wavy artefact over the neck due to hair braids that should have been removed from the field of view.
- There are only eight posterior ribs above the diaphragm and the mild underinspiration is giving a false impression of cardiomegaly.
- The increased clarity of the left heart border is a technical appearance and is not due to a pneumomediastinum in this case.

DIAGNOSIS: normal.

IMAGE EVALUATION

Coned PA chest for position of pH probe in a 10-year-old child (Fig. 13.59b)

The main points to consider are:

- Technical factors: adequate.

DIAGNOSIS: pH probe is down the right main bronchus and should be withdrawn. A satisfactory position of the pH probe is 5 cm proximal to the gastro-oesophageal junction, normally at the level of T7/T8.

Image evaluation 13

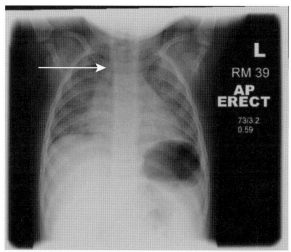

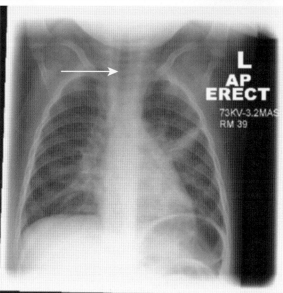

Figs 13.60a and b AP erect chest radiographs of a 2-year-old child.

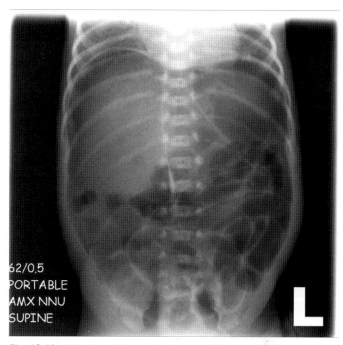

Fig. 13.60c AP supine abdominal radiograph of 1-day-old female neonate.

IMAGE EVALUATION

AP erect chest radiographs of a 2-year-old child (Figs 13.60a, 13.60b)

The main points to consider are:

- Technical factors: radiograph (left) taken in expiration with only 3/4 anterior ribs above the diaphragm and causing physiological bowing of the trachea to the right. Often seen during a child's cry and should be avoided as can be interpreted as due to mediastinal shift.
- Same patient (right) at separate attendance confirming straight trachea.

DIAGNOSIS (right): left upper lobe segmental collapse and right perihilar consolidation.

IMAGE EVALUATION

AP supine abdominal radiograph of 1-day-old female neonate (Fig. 13.60c)

The main points to consider are:

- Technical factors adequate. A neonatal abdomen is physiologically more rounded with less abdominal fat than in older children, particularly in this case with intra-abdominal air.
- Collimation 1 cm wider than the standard abdominal markings is recommended but collimation could have been closer and still adequate in this case.

DIAGNOSIS: extensive free intra-abdominal air due to perforation of an abdominal viscus.

13 Image evaluation

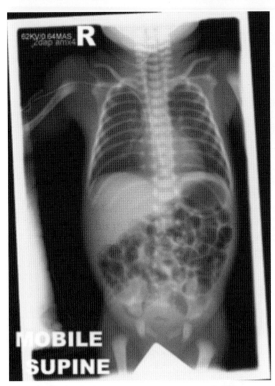

Fig. 13.61a AP supine chest and abdomen of a 1-week-old neonate.

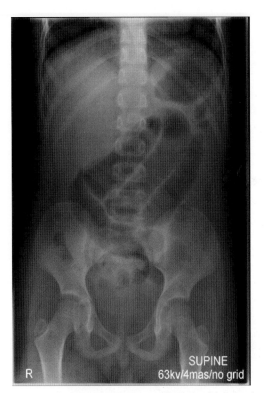

Fig. 13.61b AP supine abdomen of a 7-year-old male.

IMAGE EVALUATION

AP supine chest and abdomen of a 1-week-old neonate (Fig. 13.61a)

The main points to consider are:
- Technical factors: adequate. Combined study on one exposure appropriate for small infants and for position of lines.
- Tip of right central line in a satisfactory position overlying the right atrium.
- Note double sand bag used to immobilise right arm.
- Gonad protection well-positioned.

DIAGNOSIS: normal.

IMAGE EVALUATION

AP supine abdomen of a 7-year-old male (Fig. 13.61b)

The main points to consider are:
- Technical factors: adequate.
- Testes excluded from field of view by collimation but additional gonad protection could have been considered. Diaphragms routinely included to exclude left lower lobe pneumonia as a cause of acute abdominal pain.

DIAGNOSIS: small bowel obstruction due to appendicitis.

Image evaluation 13

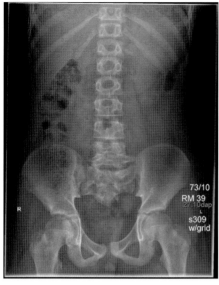

Fig. 13.62a AP supine of the abdomen of a 12-year-old child.

IMAGE EVALUATION

AP supine of the abdomen of a 12-year-old child (Fig. 13.62a)

The main points to consider are:
- Technical factors: adequate: diaphragms can be excluded for radiography of the renal tract.
- Antiscatter grid used at this age.

DIAGNOSIS: partial agenesis of the sacrum.

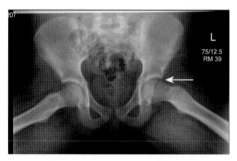

Fig. 13.62b Frog (turned) lateral of both hips of a 12-year-old female child.

IMAGE EVALUATION

Frog (turned) lateral of both hips of a 12-year-old female child (Fig. 13.62b)

The main points to consider are:
- Technical factors: adequate.
- Lateral collimation could have been improved.
- Note no gonad protection for a first radiograph.

DIAGNOSIS: subtle slip of left upper femoral epiphysis. Can be missed if AP hips performed alone.

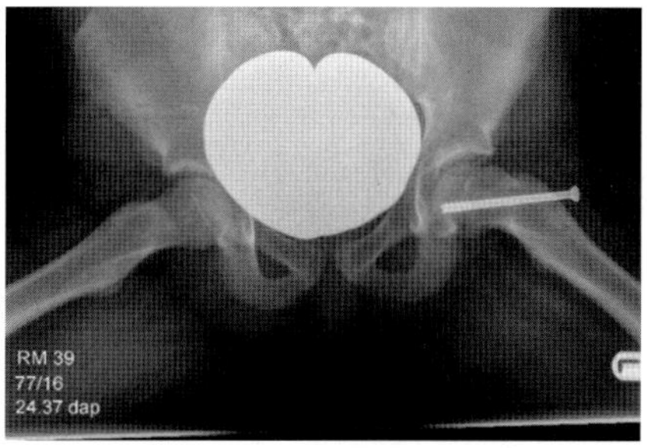

Fig. 13.62c Supine frog lateral radiograph of both hips of a 12-year-old female child, post pinning of left upper femoral epiphysis.

IMAGE EVALUATION

Supine frog lateral radiograph of both hips of a 12-year-old female child, post pinning of left upper femoral epiphysis (Fig. 13.62c)

The main points to consider are:
- Technical factors: well-positioned female gonad protection with inferior margin at pubic symphysis.
- Use of automatic exposure chamber not recommended for children and particularly not when using gonad protection in the field of view as it would effect a significant increase in the dose.

DIAGNOSIS: satisfactory post-operative appearances.

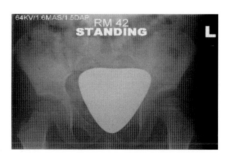

Fig. 13.62d AP erect pelvic radiograph of a 6-year-old female child.

IMAGE EVALUATION

AP erect pelvic radiograph of a 6-year-old female child (Fig. 13.62d)

The main points to consider are:
- Technical factors: adequate. Taped gonad protection well-placed with inferior margin at the top of the pubic symphysis.
- No grid.
- This patient may need multiple follow-up radiographs in the future, so gonad protection and low dose technique should be used.

Diagnosis: minor residual dysplasia of the left hip following treatment for frank late dislocation in infancy.

13 Appendix

NAI consent form

NAI SKELETAL SURVEY RADIOGRAPHY IMAGING RECORD	
PATIENT DETAILS (packet label)	**ADDITIONAL COMMENTS**

RADIOGRAPHER/S	POSITION	SIGNATURE

NURSE/HEALTH CARE STAFF	POSITION	SIGNATURE

OTHER PERSONS PRESENT - PARENT/S/GUARDIAN		

EXAMINATION EXPLAINED BY:		
PARENTS/GUARDIAN CONSENT PRIOR TO PROCEDURE		**SIGNATURE**
*I/we understand & agree to proceed with this examination:		
*I/we understand that in order to minimise movement and radiation it may be necessary to use immobilisation devices such as sandbags, tape, foam pads etc to obtain diagnostic images and therefore give consent:		
*I/we understand that it may be necessary for you and/or another healthcare person to assist in holding the patient to obtain images in the correct anatomical position:		

I/we confirm that the procedure/examination was conducted according to the explanation given.
▫ Appointment for a follow-up chest/rib x-rays has been made:-
On: .... At: ....

Signature: .... Date: ....

Appendix 13

NAI consent form (cont.)

PATIENT DETAILS (address label)	CLINICAL HISTORY (procedure label)

Images Taken	Exposure		Immobilisation Device Used			Reported By
	Kv	mAs	Shaped Perspex Sheet	Clear Adhesive Tape	Foam Pads or Sandbags	
Chest (Supine)						
Skull AP						
Skull Lat						
Left Oblique Ribs (10 day f/up)						
Right Oblique Ribs (10 day f/up)						
Abdomen (to include pelvis)						
Lat Whole Spine						
AP Left Arm (Shoulder – Wrist)< 2yrs						
AP Right Arm (Shoulder – Wrist)< 2yrs						
Oblique Right Hand (DP)						
Oblique Left Hand (DP)						
AP Left Leg (Hip-Lower 1/3 tib & fib)						
AP Right Leg (Hip – Lower 1.3 tib & fib)						
AP Left Ankle (Slight internal rotation)						
AP Right Ankle (Slight internal rotation)						
Oblique Left Foot (DP)						
Oblique Right Foot (DP)						
Total Number of Images			Dose:	Dr's Signature:		
Held by (name in full):					Ward:	
Checked by: (Radiographer/s)	Signature		Signature		Date	
DATE:	Time Commenced:			Time Finished:		

13 Acknowledgements

We would like to thank Mrs Jane Radford for her much-valued support in the typing and layout of the text. We would also like to thank Mr J. Kyriou Radiological Protection Centre, St George's Hospital, London for his generously given advice and for producing our local diagnostic reference levels.

We are also very grateful for the selection of images provided by Mr. Edmond Kinene, Superintendent Radiographer, Royal National Orthopaedic Hospital, Stanmore, Middlesex.

We would also like to thank the Medical Engineering Research Unit (MERU) at QMHC for their assistance and skills in producing the immobilisation device with Perspex top and wooden cassette holder, the chest stand with seat and the various shaped coning devices and filters described in the text. They have all been designed by Kaye Shah and the staff of QMHC.

We would also like to thank the Medical Illustration Department at Queen Mary's Hospital for Children for providing many of the photographic images.

Thanks are also extended to Andrea Hulme, Lead General Radiographer (Children's), Royal Manchester Children's Hospital, and Central Manchester University Hospitals Foundation Trust for her help with the spinal and leg length imaging sections.

We also are very grateful to the models and their parents who willingly gave their time to assist us in producing demonstrative photographs of the various radiographic positions. Our special thanks to Wardray Premise Ltd. for donating the plexiglass immobiliser and the child friendly animal patterned lead screen for our X-ray room.

Section 14
Miscellaneous

CONTENTS

BARIATRIC RADIOGRAPHY	496
Introduction	496
Equipment and imaging considerations	496
TRAUMA RADIOGRAPHY	500
Introduction	500
Equipment and imaging considerations	501
Advanced Trauma and Life Support (ATLS)	506
FOREIGN BODIES	509
Introduction	509
Percutaneous foreign bodies	510
Ingested foreign bodies	511
Inhaled foreign bodies	512
Inserted foreign bodies	513
Transocular foreign bodies	514
SOFT TISSUE	516
Introduction	516
Exposure technique	516
TOMOGRAPHY AND TOMOSYNTHESIS	518
Introduction	518
TOMOGRAPHY	519
Principles	519
Types of tomographic movement	521
Principles	522
Image quality	524
Radiation protection	524
Procedure	525
Kidneys – antero-posterior	526
Larynx – antero-posterior	527
Trachea – antero-posterior	527
TOMOSYNTHESIS	528
Principles	528
Procedure	529
Image quality	530
Applications	531
MACRORADIOGRAPHY	532
Principles	532
Applications	534
SKELETAL SURVEY	535
Introduction	535
Recommended projections	536
FORENSIC RADIOGRAPHY	537
Introduction	537
Classifications of forensic radiography	537
Anatomical terminology	537
Legal issues	538
Equipment and accessories	538
Local radiation rules	538
De-briefing	538
Dental radiography	539
Recommended dental projections	539
General radiography	540
Still born (15–40 weeks)	542
Antero-posterior 'babygram'	542
Lateral 'babygram'	543
Skull – fronto-occipital	543
Lateral skull	544
Post procedure	544
Skeletal survey – out of hours	544
The future	545

14 Bariatric radiography

Introduction

The period between 1993 and 2012 saw an increase in the proportion of adults who were defined as obese in the UK from 13.2% to 24.4% for men and from 16.4% to 25.1% amongst women.[1]

This has an implication for medical imaging in terms of an increase in workload associated with a range co-morbidities, e.g. certain types of cancer and cardiovascular disease, but also from a series of practical and technical challenges when imaging obese patients. These can result in missed diagnoses, non-diagnostic examinations, problems with equipment, embarrassing occurrences for staff and patients, as well as increased radiation doses.[2]

It is important that Radiographers consider and prepare for these challenges before imaging patients who are obese, rather than being reactive to situations when they develop. The latter can result in poor standards of care for the patients concerned and inefficiency and delay in the smooth running of the medical imaging department. Poor preparation can also put staff working within the radiology department at risk of musculoskeletal injuries, due to the use of inappropriate or rushed manual handling techniques.[3]

Psychosocial factors

It is important to gain full co-operation from the patient in order to maximise the likelihood of a successful examination with the minimum chance of a repeat projection or procedure. Obese patients have reported barriers to communication from negative staff attitudes. In one study 80% of patients reported disrespectful treatment.[4] Patients are often blamed for their condition and are stigmatised as a consequence. This can lead to psychological distress in patients who may already have low self-esteem. The consequence of this is a reluctance to engage with healthcare systems due to fears of embarrassment. They may not then get the treatment need that could resolve their condition, which in turn could maintain and increase the divides in health that exist between different groups of the population.

It is important that when a patient suffering from obesity receives care in the medical imaging department they receive an efficient and seamless service free from problems or delays. This will then reduce the frustrations of staff that may give rise to negative attitudes and potential embarrassment for the patient.

Factors include:

- Radiology departments should have a clear and well-rehearsed policy for handling obese patients.
- The policy should be informed by risk analysis and problems solving activities undertaken in each work area.
- Procedures to ensure good communication between hospital departments and with patients should be nurtured to alert the department of situations when special interventions may be required. Ideally, the weight of a patient will be known before they attend for imaging.
- Planning should take place to inform staffing and budget requirements for dealing with situations in both the long and short term.

Equipment and imaging considerations

Legislation requires that all hospital employers provide adequate systems of work and equipment to protect staff from injury during their work. Hospitals could also be at risk of civil proceedings if the correct equipment is not available when caring for bariatric patients.

The following considerations should be borne in mind:

Non-imaging equipment

- The department should have access to suitable wheelchairs. A widened design is required for obese patients; such chairs are useful for patient comfort and will therefore enhance patient compliance when imaging in the chair (Fig. 14.1).
- Departments also need to have access to larger and wider trolleys capable of taking the weight of larger patients.
- Waiting rooms should be designed with bariatric patients in mind, e.g. suitable chairs without arms.
- Imaging department should have access to manual handling equipment that is capable of handling the size of patient under examination. If this is not immediately available then it should be clear where this can be sourced from within the organisation.

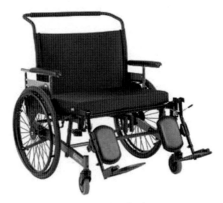

Fig. 14.1 Wide wheelchair for bariatric use.

Imaging equipment

- It is important that all floating top X-ray tables are capable of taking the weight of the patient under examination.
- Weight limits will vary depending on how the patient is positioned on the table. If the patient is at one end of the table, the weight limit will be reduced (see Fig. 14.2a).
- Table weight limits will also reduce when the motors are being used to raise and lower the table. If the limit is exceeded the motors could be damaged.
- If new equipment is being purchased then a limit of 250 kg should be sufficient in all but extreme cases.

Technical factors related to image acquisition

When undertaking plain radiographic imaging of obese patients, image quality will be reduced for two main reasons. Firstly, there will be a low subject contrast due to the increased ratio of soft tissue to bone/target image tissue. Secondly, there will be an increased amount of scattered radiation produced from the greater number of beam interactions with increased amount soft tissue encountered in bariatric patients. Both of these factors will significantly reduce the radiographic contrast within the final image.

The radiographer should focus efforts in maximising the contrast within the image by initially reducing the scatter produced. Efforts should then be made in reducing the remaining scattered radiation that is produced from being detected on the image receptor. This applies for imaging obese and non-obese patients, but is particularly important in imaging patient with a large body habitus.

Bariatric radiography 14

Equipment and imaging considerations (*cont.*)

Strategies for reducing the amount of soft tissue being detected on the image receptor

Use of antiscatter grids: consider using a grid for an obese patient for examinations when a grid may not normally be used, e.g. knee examinations or mobile chest radiographs and antero-posterior (AP) chest examinations undertaken on a chair or trolley (Figs 14.2b–14.2e).

Grid ratio: the grid ratio is the ratio of the height of the lead slats in the grid to the distance they are spaced apart. Typical ratios used in medical imaging are in the range 6:1 to 12:1. The higher ratio grids are more effective in removing scatter from the beam at the cost of a slightly higher radiation dose and an increased risk of reducing image quality due to a grid 'cut off' occurring.

The following points should be considered when imaging obese patients:

- The grid found in a Bucky will have a higher ratio than many of the stationary grids found in imaging departments. If it is safe and practical to image the patient using the Bucky this should be used.
- When reviewing the stock of stationary grids used for trauma imaging, efforts should be made to ensure that at least one of these will have a high ratio (e.g. 10:1) for specific use with obese patients.

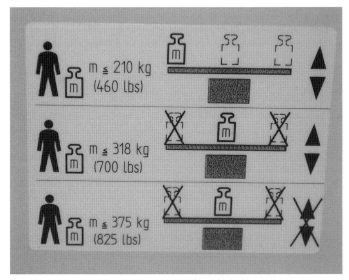

Fig. 14.2a Typical weight limits of an X-ray table. Note how limit changes depending on patient position and if the motors are used.

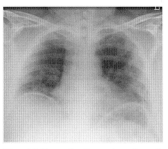 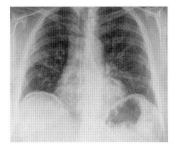

Figs 14.2b and c Examples of an obese patient imaged without a grid (left) and a repeat examination undertaken with a grid (right).

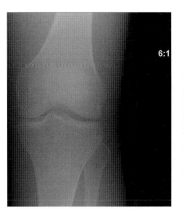 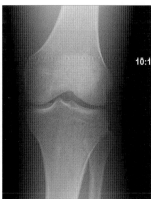

Figs 14.2d and e Two images taken of a phantom, with a 6:1 grid (left) and 10:1 ratio (right) grid.

14 Bariatric radiography

Equipment and imaging considerations (cont.)

Strategies for improving image quality

There are various ways to reduce the amount of soft tissue the beam interacts with which will, in turn, reduce the amount of scatter produced, reduce dose and increase beam quality.

Tissue displacement (Figs 14.3a, 14.3b)

One of the simplest and most effective techniques is to ask the patient to move aside any fat aprons or areas of soft tissue that cover the region of interest. This must be done without causing the patient harm or distress. Communicating this to the patient will obviously entail a degree of tact on the part of the radiographer so the patient is not upset, but if this is done in a professional manner an optimal result will be obtained. Once repositioned the soft tissue can be supported by the patient with pads.

Compression: this is an extremely effective way of displacing soft tissue to either side of the area of interest and thereby reducing the total thickness of tissue that the primary beam traverses. This will in turn reduce the total amount of scatter produced and hence less scatter will be recorded on the image receptor. Compression can be applied using mechanical means via use of the compression device that is attached to the table top. Alternatively 'auto compression' can be used whereby the patient will apply compression themselves either via posture or positioning. A good example of this is when a patient uses the hand rails on a vertical Bucky/detector to pull themselves closer to image receptor during chest radiography, thereby compressing the breasts. This will in turn enhance detail visible in the lung bases.

Collimation and compensation filters

Careful collimation to the region of interest is one of the most effective ways of reducing scatter. This can be challenging though for obese patients as it is difficult to identify bony landmarks or identify surface markings.

Collimation to skin borders should be avoided when this is normally undertaken for a particular examination, e.g. knees. Collimation will generally need to be well within the skin borders for bariatric patients, otherwise an unacceptably large area of soft tissue will be irritated and hence will produce additional scatter.

Compensation filters are a useful method of reducing subject contrast between areas of different patient tissue density (often encountered in obese patients) by introducing a uniform graded attenuator into the beam. This may be useful for shoulder, lateral hip and lateral cervical spine imaging.

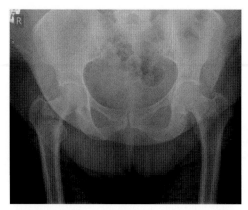

Fig. 14.3a Abdominal fat apron reducing image contrast over the hips.

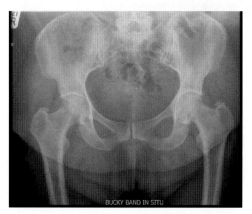

Fig. 14.3b Compression results in improved contrast over hips.

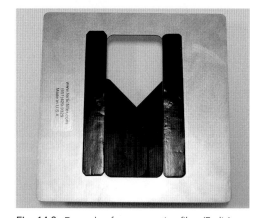

Fig. 14.3c Example of compensation filter (Ferlic).

Combined use of collimation and compensation filters

For collimation to be most effective it needs to be tightly collimated to the region of interest.[5] This is really challenging in obese patients but the use of a well-defined collimation field combined with a compensation filter can be extremely useful in enhancing image quality. An example of such a device is the 'Ferlic Filter', which is inserted onto the front of the light beam diaphragm after the beam is centred. This is extremely effective for reducing scatter by producing a very tightly collimated beam as well as having the additional benefits of the filter (Fig. 14.3c).

Bariatric radiography 14

Equipment and imaging considerations (*cont.*)

Air gaps

The use of air gaps between the body part and the image receptor is a well-recognised technique for reducing the amount of scatter reaching the image receptor in plain radiography. This can be used to good effect in bariatric cases, especially when combined with other techniques, e.g. with a compensation filter and tight collimation for lateral radiography of the hip (Figs 14.4a, 14.4b).

Image receptor size

Standard techniques may need to be adapted for patients with a large body habitus. Abdomen radiographs are often undertaken with the image receptor used in 'portrait' format with the long axis of the image receptor coincident with the sagittal plane. This will often result in the lateral flanks and upper abdomen being excluded from the region of interest. The solution is to undertake two images with the image receptor used in 'landscape format'. At the outset of the examination the radiographer should carefully consider whether two images would be appropriate for the patient concerned, taken using landscape format, rather than taking one image in portrait format and risk repeating the image if the area of interest was not included.

Exposure and centring

Larger patients will need more exposure. Underexposure will result in image noise and non-diagnostic radiographs. It is therefore recommended that the automatic exposure control devices (AEC) should always be employed to determine the mAs for larger patients. It is very difficult to assess the extra exposure required for larger patients using a manual exposure, especially in the case of areas like the abdomen and lumbar spine.

The danger of using the AEC is that if the ionisation chamber is not centred accurately over the area of interest then an incorrect exposure will result. It is important to compensate for extra soft tissue when centring the beam and to make appropriate adaptations for this. In the lumbar spine example given, the beam should have been centred more anteriorly due to extra soft tissue found posteriorly (Figs 14.4c, 14.4d).

It is worth noting that both national and local diagnostic reference levels (DRLs) will be exceeded in bariatric cases. If a very poor image quality is obtained and all strategies for improving the quality have been exhausted, then the radiographer should carefully consider the risks of the examination verses the limited benefits from an image of poor quality.

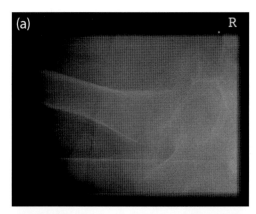
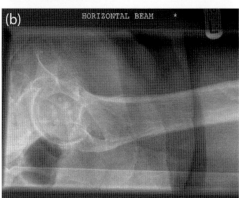

Figs 14.4a and b Image A was taken on a trolley with a stationary grid and no compensation (Ferlic) filter; image B was obtained using an air-gap technique and a compensation filter.

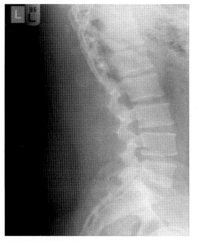

Fig. 14.4c Image was centred too posterior, resulting in automatic exposure control (AEC) error and a 'noisy' image.

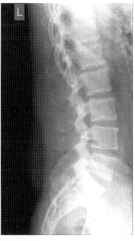

Fig. 14.4d Correctly exposed image as the automatic exposure control (AEC) chamber was positioned directly over the area of interest.

14 Trauma radiography

Introduction

Radiographers are aware that image and thus diagnostic quality is often compromised when examining a patient who has suffered acute trauma, as their mobility and ability to co-operate is often greatly reduced. It is ironic that these patients, who require the quickest diagnosis for any life-threatening injuries, may have a series of images of reduced quality as a result primarily of their inability to co-operate.

Plain radiography of the trauma patient, whether it is undertaken in the emergency room or within the imaging department, should therefore be considered as an imaging speciality in its own right. Radiographers undertaking these examinations need to have particular skills and specialist knowledge that will help them be aware of all the factors that reduce image quality and how to minimise their effects. It is far beyond the scope of this section to give a detailed account of all the relevant imaging factors relevant to trauma radiography. However, it will be possible to provide a series of points that all radiographers should be mindful of when undertaking any radiography of the acutely injured patient.[1]

Assessment of the patient condition

A vital first step in the examination is to justify and assess the referral and most importantly assess the patient condition. A review of the history and mechanism of injury and predicted fracture patterns/possible injuries from the referrer is vital. Also a discussion with the patient (if possible) relating to their condition and capabilities will enable the radiographer to plan the examination for the maximum diagnostic outcome.

Planning the examination (Figs 14.5a, 14.5b)

When the radiographer is presented with a patient requiring multiple examinations, it is important to spend some time planning the examination so that it can be conducted efficiently and fluently, using the most appropriate equipment.

Consider a patient who requires examinations of the whole spine, chest and pelvis. It would be more efficient if all the lateral radiographs were performed in succession before all the AP radiographs.

When examining patients on trauma trolleys, consideration of the side of injury is important to limit movement of the trolley between examinations once in the X-ray room. By doing this the appropriate side of the body can be positioned against

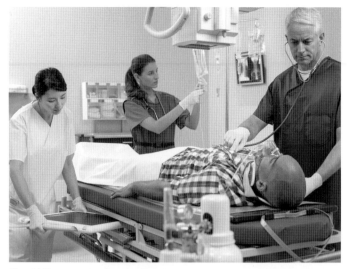

Fig. 14.5a Example of emergency/Resuscitation room equipped with specialist X-ray equipment (courtesy of Philips Healthcare).

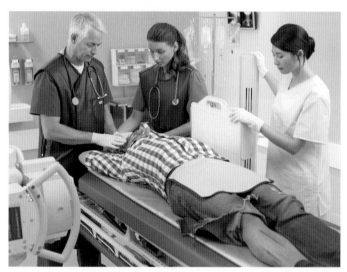

Fig. 14.5b When undertaking trauma examinations involving multiple examinations, it will save time if all the examinations in one plane (e.g. laterals) are undertaken before any others.

the vertical Bucky/detector at this stage, rather than disrupting the examination partway through by moving the trolley.

Good communication with the accident and emergency staff is also of vital importance at the planning stage of any procedure. This will provide the radiographer with valuable information about the patient's condition and ability to co-operate. In addition, if the procedure is being undertaken as a mobile examination, good communication is vital to ensure the radiographer takes the correct equipment to the emergency room and correctly times their arrival in the department.

Trauma radiography 14

Equipment and imaging considerations

Adaptation of technique

Much of the skill of a trauma radiographer stems from an ability to be able to produce images of diagnostic quality in a pressured environment and also when the patient is unable to co-operate to allow standard positioning.

It is far beyond the scope of this section to give a full account of all the common adaptations that are used in trauma radiography. What has been provided are a series of general points and principles that radiographers should consider when presented with a complex trauma case.

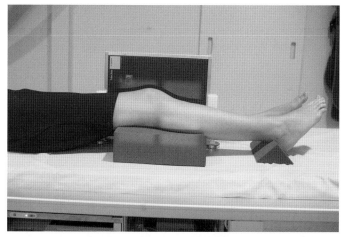

Fig. 14.6a Horizontal beam lateral technique used for a knee examination.

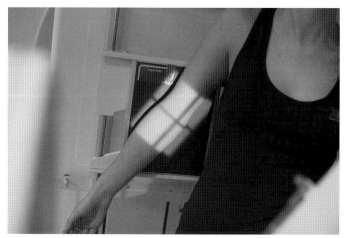

Fig. 14.6b Adaptation of technique commonly used for elbow fractures with patient standing.

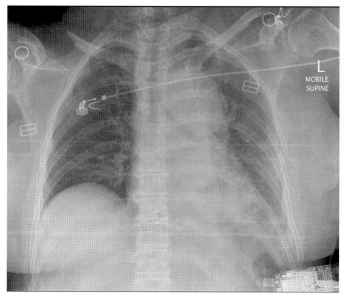

Fig. 14.6c Chest X-ray with grossly displaced fracture to the right clavicle, distended thoracic aorta and pulmonary contusions.

- Horizontal beam laterals. This is an essential adaptation that is used when the patient cannot move/turn into the standard lateral position with a collimated vertical central beam. In the example given opposite, the use of a horizontal beam is actually advantageous to diagnosis. A lipohaemoarthrosis (blood/fat fluid level), which is a soft-tissue indicator of an intra-articular fracture within the knee joint, would not be visible if a standard turned lateral view was performed (Fig. 14.6a).

- Standing up/sitting. Patients may find it difficult to attain the standard positioning when the radiographs are usually undertaken in the seated or supine position. In such cases asking the patient to remain standing (if the condition will allow) to enable a less distressing examination would be beneficial for both parties. A good example of where this is useful is in the case of a suspected supracondylar fracture of the elbow. The patient would not be able to extend the elbow or supinate the forearm to obtain the standard images whilst seated, but may be able to do this when imaged in the erect position (Fig. 14.6b).

- Consider the pathology. An unexperienced radiographer will constantly strive to produce standard projections dictated by departmental protocols; however, in this demanding and yet flexible situation the diagnosing of any serious pathology is of greater priority. This attempt to maintain standardisation could lead to an important diagnosis being overlooked. An example of where this might happen is tight collimation on a chest radiograph (CXR), where visualisation of a gleno-humeral dislocation could be demonstrated, thus allowing for completion of a trauma series with less distress for the patient by ensuring no shoulder distraction is applied for the lateral cervical spine view (Fig. 14.6c).

- Be flexible/teamwork. Radiographers should not become habituated to undertaking examinations only in an exact manner otherwise they will become inflexible and unable to deal with unusual situations. Teamwork is an essential part of being a good trauma radiographer and will be discussed in the ATLS section.

14 Trauma radiography

Equipment and imaging considerations (cont.)

Patient condition (Fig. 14.7a)

It is important to closely supervise trauma patients at all times as their condition can quickly deteriorate. Patients who initially appear quite co-operative and communicative with a high Glasgow Coma Scale (GCS)[2] may suddenly become unstable unless an appropriate intervention takes place.

As has already been discussed, the patient's ability to co-operate will have a strong bearing on the diagnostic quality of the final images. Generally there is little that can be done when a patient is unable to co-operate other than adaptation of the imaging technique. There are some situations when the radiographer may have some control over the patient's ability to co-operate. Some of these are outlined below.

- The intoxicated patient. In the absence of serious trauma, where possible the examination could be delayed until the patient is able to co-operate fully. This is particularly useful for examinations where injuries can be difficult to diagnose. The quality of facial bone radiographs obtained erect with a co-operative patient are far superior to those taken with them supine on a trolley.

- Delaying examinations may also be considered when the patient's ability to co-operate is severely restricted by immobilisation devices or clothing. Once other injuries have been excluded, these devices may be removed and the patient may be more able to co-operate. For example, removing a cervical collar and head blocks to obtain shoulder projections.

Equipment

Several X-ray equipment manufacturers offer a range of dedicated systems for trauma radiography, both direct digital radiography (DDR) and computed radiography (CR). These are useful in terms of time saving and image quality when undertaking multiple procedures. However, it is possible to obtain equally diagnostic images using a general X-ray room equipped with standard equipment and appropriate emergency equipment. One of the most desirable features of a room used for trauma radiography is space. A large X-ray room allows for greater flexibility when adaptations in technique are required and room for additional equipment to monitor and preserve the patient's stability.

Other more specific considerations are considered individually.

- Immobilisation devices. Any room used for trauma radiography should have a generous supply of radiolucent foam pads, sandbags and cassette holders for supporting patients or cassettes. Specialist devices, such as the leg support used for lateral hip radiography, are often invaluable (Figs 14.7b, 14.7c).

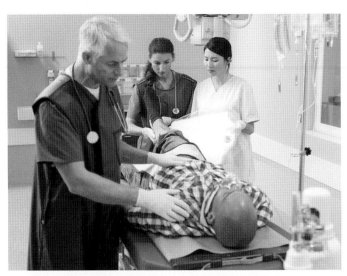

Fig. 14.7a Typical modern style of room used for trauma radiography (courtesy of Philips Healthcare).

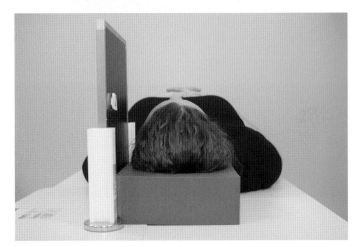

Fig. 14.7b Range of immobilisation devices commonly used in trauma radiography.

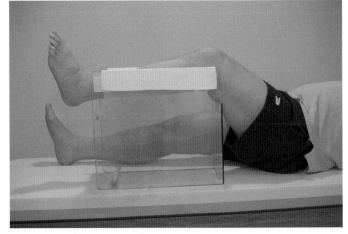

Fig. 14.7c Leg support used for lateral hip radiography.

Trauma radiography 14

Equipment and imaging considerations (cont.)

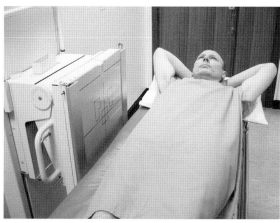

Fig. 14.8a Increase in object-to-receptor distance (ORD) caused by patient position on trolley relative to Bucky.

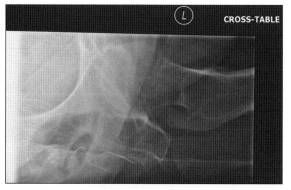

Fig. 14.8b Horizontal beam lateral hip demonstrating detail and contrast due to good collimation.

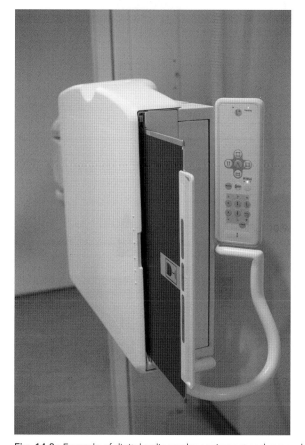

Fig. 14.8c Example of digital radiography equipment and removable grid used for accident and emergency imaging.

- Grids. Adaptations in technique will sometimes result in the use of stationary grids for trauma radiography. These should only be used as a last resort when DDR or a moving grid cannot be utilised, due to the limited efficiency of such grids in terms of scatter attenuation. The stationary grid lattice pattern and relatively low grid ratio, all contribute to a decrease in image quality when stationary grids are used. The type of stationary grid used is also important. If a focussed grid is employed, the radiographer must ensure the correct focus-to-receptor distance (FRD) is used, otherwise 'grid cut-off' artefact can result. Grid cut-off may also occur if the collimated central beam is not perpendicular to the grid and receptor. The use of DDR equipment or CR with built-in moving grid will eliminate these issues (Fig. 14.8c).

- Object-to-receptor distance (ORD). In many cases an increase in ORD will result from the modifications in technique required in trauma radiography. One example is the horizontal beam lateral radiograph of the thoracic or lumbar spine. If the patient is lying in the middle of the trolley, the sagittal plane of the spine will be at an increased distance to the receptor. This would result in an increase in magnification and thus geometric unsharpness upon the image produced. The problem can easily be resolved by increasing the focus-to-object distance (FOD) to compensate. It must be remembered that employment of this strategy without the use of an automatic exposure device would require an increase in the exposure factors (Fig. 14.8a).

- Collimation. Many trauma radiographic examinations are prone to high levels of scattered radiation that dramatically degrade overall image quality. A good example of such an examination would be the horizontal beam lateral lumbar spine as described above. The extra tissue from the abdominal viscera lying either side of the spine increases an amount of tissue irradiated compared with a standard lateral, and there is a corresponding increase in scatter production. In such cases close attention to collimation is important as this will serve to decrease vastly the scatter produced and will significantly improve image quality (Fig. 14.8b).

14 Trauma radiography

Equipment and imaging considerations (cont.)

- Type of trolley. There are many different types of trolley available for use in accident and emergency (A&E) work; therefore, the Imaging department and specifically radiographers should be involved in the trial and decisions regarding new purchases (Fig. 14.9a).
- Receptor cassette holder. The trolley must have either a moveable tray underneath the patient to accommodate cassettes and grids or a wide platform that runs the length and width of the trolley. Whichever method is used to support the cassette underneath the trolley, it is important that the radiographer can easily gain access and view the cassette wherever it is positioned relative to the patient. This is vital for accurate alignment of the cassette to the beam prior to exposure.
- Object/receptor distance. The distance between the trolleytop and the receptor cassette holder underneath should be as small as possible but still allowing reasonable access for the positioning of cassettes. If this distance increases then geometric unsharpness will also increase, thus reducing image quality.
- Uniform trolleytop. The trolleytop should be completely radiolucent (no metal bars or hinges) to reduce artefacts on any images taken using the cassette holder underneath the patient (Fig. 14.9c).
- Vertical cassette holders. Some trolleys come equipped with vertical cassette holders; these may be useful, but not vital, for performing horizontal beam lateral examinations (Fig. 14.9b).

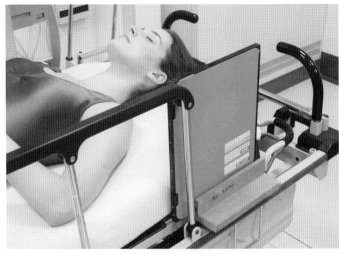

Fig. 14.9b Trolley cassette holder used for horizontal beam imaging.

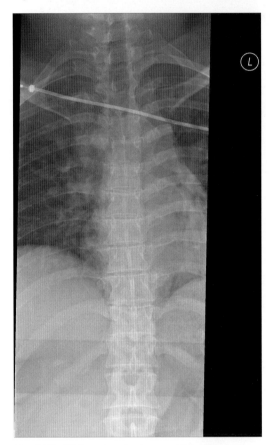

Fig. 14.9c AP thoracic spine image with trolley mattress and electrocardiogram wire artefact.

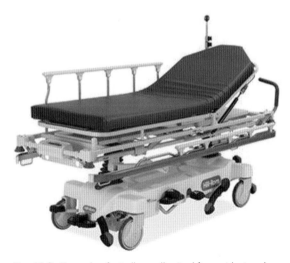

Fig. 14.9a Example of a trolley well suited for accident and emergency imaging.

Trauma radiography 14

Equipment and imaging considerations (cont.)

DDR

The use of modern DDR equipment in the trauma environment is optimum but currently idealistic. The ability for technique adaptation and flexibility of the equipment lends itself to the trauma situation and is currently included in the UK for new plans of Trauma Centres.

- Image artefacts. Artefacts from immobilisation devices applied by paramedical staff are a constant issue for radiographers and the interpretation of trauma radiographs. Jewellery under rigid neck collars may cause problems, as the radiographer may not be aware of their presence until an image is obtained. Again the establishment and maintenance of good communication links between professional groups will allow communication of such problems and raise awareness of the difficulties that arise as a consequence.

With digital imaging low-density artefacts, such as clothing and wound dressings, are easily demonstrated and do detract from image quality. However, trauma imaging is undertaken to stabilise the patient and determine whether any life-threatening pathologies are present and thus some allowances for image quality are accepted (Fig. 14.10a).

Exposure factors

Trauma radiography often requires some modification to the routine exposure factors due to the non-standard imaging conditions encountered. Several methods of reducing exposure time and image optimisation are discussed in the introduction in Section 1 (Fig. 14.10b).

- Automatic exposure devices. These are advantageous for trauma imaging, particularly those located in the erect Bucky, which are used for horizontal beam imaging.

Correct labelling of images

Given the many modifications in technique often employed in trauma radiography, it is important that the final image is correctly labelled (e.g. supine, erect, horizontal beam etc.) so an accurate diagnosis can be made. Also, if the image needs repeating an accurate comparison image can be taken (Fig. 14.10c).

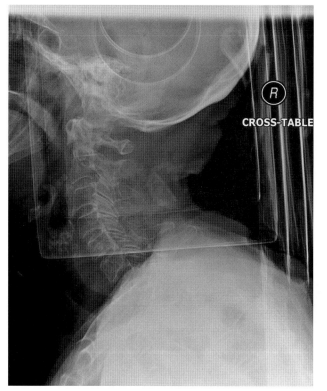

Fig. 14.10a Example of inadequate cervical spine image with artefact obscuring anatomy.

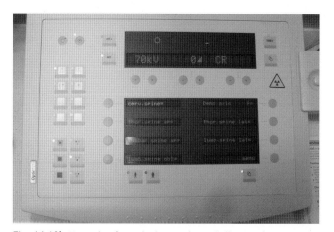

Fig. 14.10b Example of standard control panel allowing the user to review and change exposure factors.

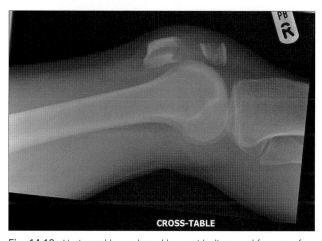

Fig. 14.10c Horizontal beam lateral knee with distracted fracture of the patella and annotation.

14 Trauma radiography

Advanced Trauma and Life Support (ATLS)

The initial assessment and primary management of seriously injured patients is a challenging task and requires a rapid and systematic approach. Injuries causing this mortality occur in predictable patterns and recognition of these patterns led to the development of the ATLS teaching and publications.[3]

This is a comprehensive protocol introduced by the American College of Surgeons to ensure that any patient suffering major trauma would be given adequate emergency care, even remote from a major trauma centre, thus allowing patients to arrive at the centres of excellence in the best possible condition. The ATLS course manual specifies minimum standards of care to all body systems from a variety of viewpoints, including specifications for radiographic examination. It is widely adopted worldwide and is seen as the optimal pathway to limit fatalities and optimise emergency care for trauma patients.

Upon presentation to the A&E department a comprehensive handover will be given by the paramedic/technician who has been caring for the patient whilst in transit. They will give information relative to the patient's stability and vital signs for immediate care but will also impart knowledge and information regarding the mechanism of injury and position/condition the patient was found in. Sometimes the police may also be involved and can give further information on history and mechanism of injury.

An initial assessment the 'Primary survey' is undertaken rapidly upon arrival in the A&E department. The patient is assessed and their treatment priorities are established based on their injuries, vital signs and the injury mechanisms. In severely injured patients logical and sequential treatment priorities must be established based on overall patient assessment.

The Primary survey consists of the ABCDEs:

- Airway maintenance – with cervical spine protection.
- Breathing and ventilation.
- Circulation with haemorrhage control.
- Disability, i.e. neurological status.
- Exposure/Environmental control – patient undressed but with prevention of hypothermia.

The Secondary survey does not begin until the Primary survey is completed and resuscitative efforts are underway and the normalisation of vital functions has been demonstrated.

According to ATLS and local protocols, the initial radiographic assessment of the severely injured patient consists of: lateral cervical spine, CXR and pelvis. NB: skull X-ray (SXR) not included (Figs 14.11a–14.11c).

These are generally performed as part of the secondary assessment and prior to full clinical examination.

The Secondary survey is a head to toe evaluation of the trauma patient and includes a complete (where possible) history and physical examination. This will include a full neurological examination and produce a GCS score.

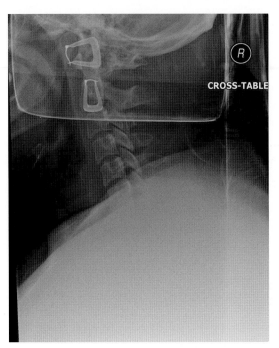

Fig. 14.11a Lateral cervical spine with patient wearing hard collar in head blocks.

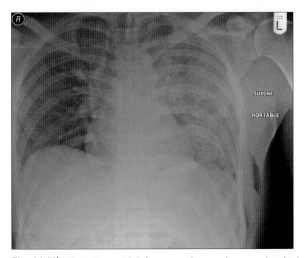

Fig. 14.11b Chest X-ray with left pneumo-haemo thorax and multiple rib fractures.

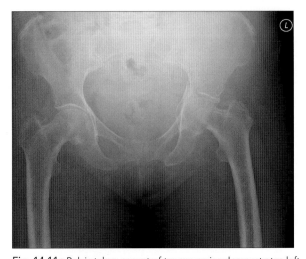

Fig. 14.11c Pelvis taken as part of trauma series demonstrates left acetabular floor fracture.

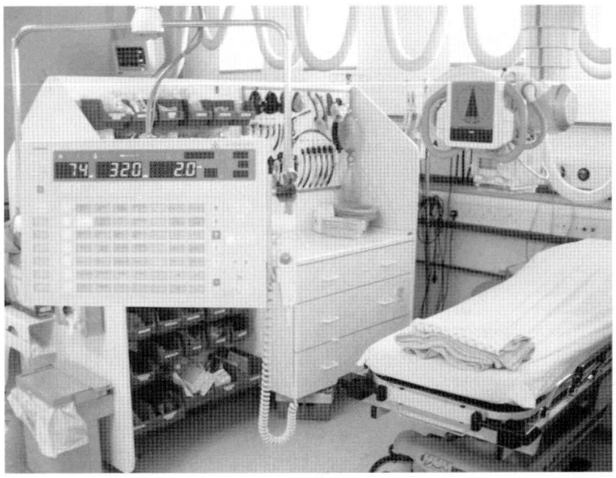

Trauma radiography 14

Advanced Trauma and Life Support (ATLS) (cont.) (Figs 14.12a–14.12c)

The X-rays indicated by this examination will be requested and interspersed into the Secondary survey at an appropriate time.

Complete patient evaluation will require the physical examinations to be repeated multiple times overruling other procedures taking place, such as the radiographic examinations.

Following full clinical evaluation further projections or additional examinations of other areas may be requested. As soon as possible (determined by the patient's clinical priorities), the cervical spine examination must be completed.

If the cervical spine examination does not demonstrate the C7/T1 junction then this is an incomplete exam and further imaging must be undertaken. The choice of projections will be determined by local protocols and may include a swimmer's projection and/or trauma oblique lateral projections. If diagnostic basic projections are not obtained then the use of computed tomography (CT) may become necessary, again as determined by local guidelines.

CT may be the imaging modality of choice in trauma centres depending on patient presentation, stability and obvious injuries. CT can be a relatively quick and thorough examination in the unconscious, ventilated patient but is a high-dose examination. It should not be regarded as an easy alternative to high-quality diagnostic trauma radiography.

Under ATLS guidance, flexion projections of the cervical spine may be requested for patients with spinal soft-tissue injuries only under supervision of an experienced doctor, prior to full 'clearance' of the spine in patients who are alert and neurologically normal but suffering neck pain.

As 7–10% of patients with a confirmed cervical spine fracture will have an associated fracture of the thoracic or lumbar spine, projections of these areas may also be requested.

Significant injury to the thoracic and lumbar spine can occur without local tenderness or pain, especially in the presence of a distracting injury elsewhere. It may therefore be appropriate to perform full spinal projections in patients who have suffered major trauma with a significant mechanism of injury if they have a cervical spine injury, as well as those with depressed level of consciousness.[3]

Fig. 14.12a Typical trauma room in an Accident and emergency department.

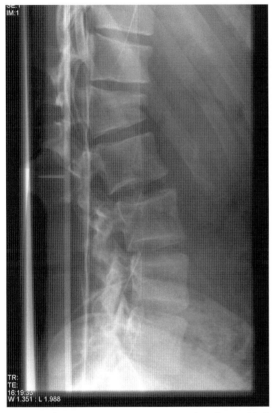

Fig. 14.12b Lateral lumbar spine radiograph with unstable fractures of L1 and L2 vertebral bodies.

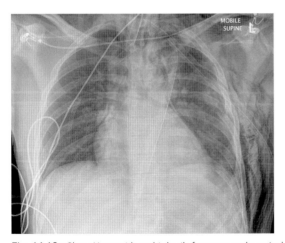

Fig. 14.12c Chest X-ray with multiple rib fractures and surgical emphysema.

14 Trauma radiography

Advanced Trauma and Life Support (ATLS) (*cont.*) (Fig. 14.13)

An essential skill of working in the Radiology department is being able to work as part of a team. An individual's ability to be able to adapt and switch roles within this team from team leader to team member is relevant to current working practices and greatly enhances their skills and the perceptions of others.

The role of the radiographer whether in a major Trauma Centre or District General hospital, is part of the multi-disciplinary trauma team and forms the pathway for the severely injured patient. The team needs to run smoothly and efficiently with each member being aware of others' roles and the procedures that will take place. Quietly observing ATLS procedures in action from patient entry into A&E and possibly attending an accredited ATLS course, again as an observer, can increase confidence and awareness for a radiographer.

However, being a useful team member whilst waiting to undertake the requested X-ray examinations is relatively easy:

- You may be asked to pass equipment and open needles, swabs and so on.
- You may be at hand to operate the suction urgently or be part of the numbers to enable a log roll of the patient in the secondary examination, so be prepared and competent in your handling of these situations and do not volunteer if you are unsure.
- You may also be asked to 'hold or pull' on a limb during a manipulation.
- However, the two tasks you can readily undertake which are well within the radiographers' role are to talk to the patient and give comments on any images you have produced.
- If you feel unsure regarding comments, you could possible get a radiologist/reporting radiographer to look at the images for a 'hot' report and advice for further imaging.

Trauma radiography is fast paced and can be stressful but also very fulfilling and experience in this field produces confident, competent, team-working radiographers.

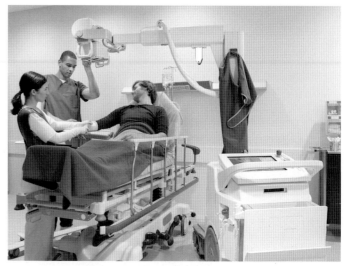

Fig. 14.13 Example of mobile unit used in Accident and emergency departments.

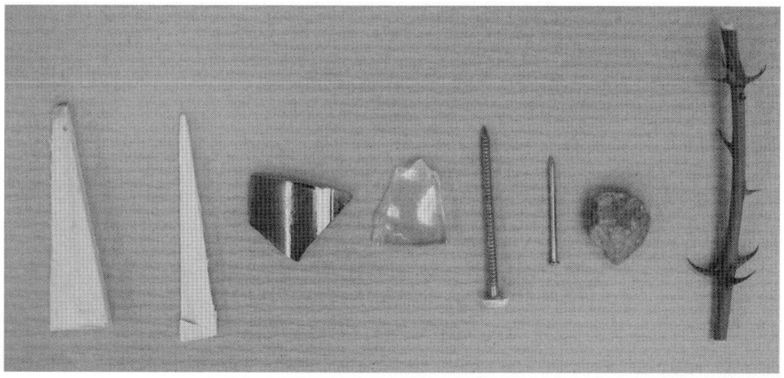

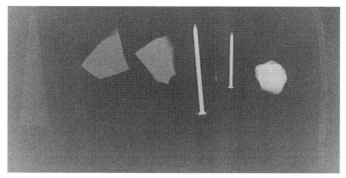

Fig. 14.14a Photograph of samples of wood, glass and objects that may be foreign bodies (FBs)s.

Fig. 14.14b Radiograph of samples of wood, glass and objects that may be FBs.

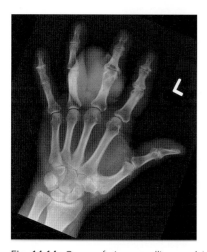

Fig. 14.14c Gross soft tissue swelling overlying and obscuring bone detail.

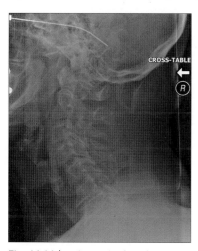

Fig. 14.14d Radiograph of artefacts including hard collar, blocks and glasses overlying detail on lateral cervical spine.

Foreign bodies 14

Introduction (Figs 14.14a–14.14d)

Many different objects may enter body tissues and cavities under a variety of circumstances. The main methods of entry are:

- Percutaneous.
- Ingestion.
- Inhalation.
- Insertion.
- Transocular.

The method adopted to demonstrate the presence and position of a foreign body (FB) is governed by its size and degree of opacity, but also its location. Unless it is radio-opaque, or is in a position where it can be coated with opaque material to render it visible – as, for instance, in the alimentary tract – the FB may not be visualised on a radiograph. Partially opaque FBs such as wood, some types of glass and other low-density materials can usually be demonstrated by suitable adjustment of the kV and image enhancement.

Although the spatial resolution of CR and DDR may be inferior to analogue imaging, the electronic post-processing capabilities of these systems more than compensates. The ability to adjust the image using magnification, edge enhancement and windowing tools make the presence of a FB more easily visualised. Additionally, the contrast resolution of CR and DR is greater than analogue imaging, making it possible to visualise FBs not previously seen on radiographs, for example, splinters of wood.

Removal of bulky and/or soiled dressings from soft-tissue wounds is recommended following local sterile procedure, especially when using CR and DDR, as these artefacts will be seen on the image and can obscure some fine radio-opaque FBs such as glass fragments. Matted blood in the hair can also prevent glass splinters in the scalp from being seen.

Ultrasound is useful in the localisation of non-opaque subcutaneous FBs and in the genital system.

CT or magnetic resonance imaging (MRI) may be used when it is necessary to demonstrate the relationship of a FB relative to internal organs, and any damage to these will be demonstrated.

Notes

- MRI imaging must not be undertaken if there is any possibility that the FB is composed of ferromagnetic material.
- Before commencing any examination it is important to ensure that no confusing opacities are present on clothing, on the skin or in the hair, on the tabletop, receptor, CR cassette or even on the Perspex of the light-beam diaphragm.

14 Foreign bodies

Percutaneous foreign bodies (Figs 14.15a–14.15e)

These are commonly metal, glass or splinters of wood associated with industrial, road and domestic accidents.

Generally two projections at right-angles to each other are required without movement of the patient between exposures, particularly when examining the limbs. The projections will normally be AP or postero-anterior (PA) and a lateral of the area in question as described in the appropriate section of this book.

A radio-opaque marker should be placed adjacent to the site of entry of the FB. The skin surface and a large area surrounding the site of entry should be included on the images since FBs may migrate, for example, along muscle sheaths, and high-velocity FBs may penetrate some distance through the tissues.

Compression must not be applied to the area under examination. Oblique projections may be required to demonstrate the relationship of the FB to adjacent bone. Tangential projections may be required to demonstrate the depth of the FB and are particularly useful in examination of the skull, face, thoracic and abdominal walls.

The exposure technique should demonstrate both bone and soft tissue to facilitate identification of partially opaque foreign bodies and to demonstrate any gas in the tissues associated with the entry of the foreign body or at a late presentation with infective reaction to the foreign body.

The use of digital image acquisition offers significant advantages in the localisation of FBs. CR and DDR both allow soft tissue and bone to be visualised from one exposure using post processing to optimise the image. The use of features such as edge enhancement and windowing enable much better demonstration of FBs that have similar radio-opacity to surrounding tissue. Tools such as black/white invert may also aide in demonstrating a low-opacity FB.

Thus the advanced technology for plain imaging has significantly improved the ability of radiography to demonstrate subcutaneous, low-density FBs.

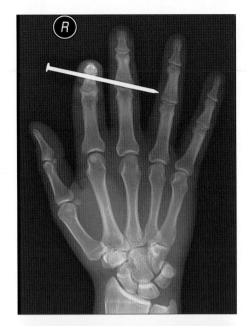
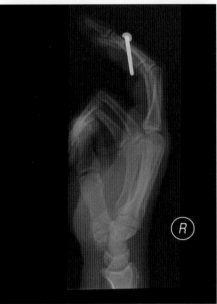

Figs 14.15c and d Dorsi-plantar (left) and lateral (right) images of a hand showing a nail embedded in the distal soft tissues.

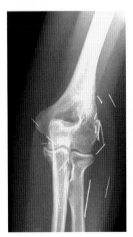
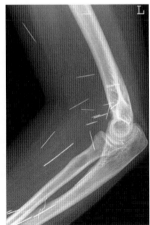

Figs 14.15a and b AP (left) and lateral (right) images of a right elbow demonstrating multiple needle insertions.

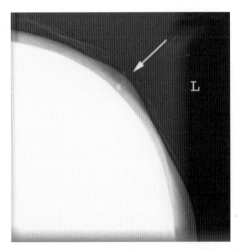

Fig. 14.15e Tangential (profile) projection of the scalp showing glass embedded in the soft tissues.

Foreign bodies 14

Ingested foreign bodies (Figs 14.16a–14.16c)

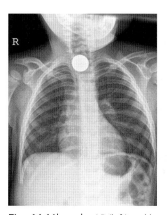

Fig. 14.16a Antero-posterior abdomen image showing multiple condoms filled with drugs lodged in the lower abdomen causing small bowel obstruction.

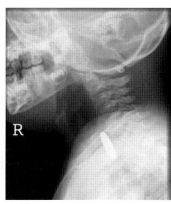

Figs 14.16b and c AP (left) and lateral (right) chest images showing a coin lodged in the upper oesophagus of a child.

A variety of objects, such as coins, beads, needles, dentures and fish bones, may be swallowed accidentally, or occasionally intentionally, by adults but particularly by young children.

A technique used to smuggle drugs through customs (body packing) involves packing the substance into condoms or other low-density compact containers that are subsequently swallowed.

The patient should be asked to undress completely and wear a hospital gown for the examination. The approximate time of swallowing the object and the site of any localised discomfort should be ascertained and noted on the request card along with the time of the examination if the patient is communicative. However, any discomfort may be due to abrasion caused by the passage of the FB. Any rupture of the packaging for the human transportation of drugs can have serious consequences relating to overdose and toxic shock.

It is important to gain the patient's co-operation for this examination, especially young children, since a partially opaque object may be missed if there is any movement during the exposure.

If the patient is a young child the examination is usually restricted to a single AP projection to include the chest and mid to upper abdomen. The lower abdomen is usually excluded to reduce the dose to the gonads, as the examination is performed to confirm the presence of a FB lodged in the stomach unable to pass through the pyloris. Care must be taken to ensure that the exposure selected is sufficient to penetrate the abdomen adequately as well as to visualise the chest.

The examination of older children and adults may require a lateral of the neck to demonstrate the pharynx and upper oesophagus, a right anterior oblique of the thorax to demonstrate the oesphagus and an AP abdomen to demonstrate the remainder of the alimentary tract, exposed in that order. Each image should be inspected before the next is exposed and the examination terminated upon identification of the FB to avoid unnecessary irradiation of the patient. The field size used should be large enough to ensure overlapping areas on adjacent images.

Non-opaque FBs can be outlined with a small amount of barium sulphate; some cases may require a barium swallow examination. However, the routine examination in the UK would be an endoscopy to allow the possibility of removal of the FB once identified.

Note

- The use of a metal detector in determining the presence of a metal object in the abdomen may reduce the need for unnecessary irradiation of a child.[1]

14 Foreign bodies

Inhaled foreign bodies (Figs 14.17a–14.17d)

FBs may be inhaled. For example, infants and young children habitually put objects into their mouths and these may be accidentally inhaled; teeth may be inhaled after a blow to the mouth or during dental surgery. Such FBs may lodge in the larynx, trachea or bronchi.

Bronchoscopy may be used to demonstrate the position of a FB since the FB can also be removed during this procedure.

The patient should be asked to undress completely to the waist and wear a hospital gown for the examination. A PA projection of the chest, including as much of the neck as possible on the image with the head turned laterally, plus a lateral chest projection may be required initially. In the case of a non-opaque inhaled FB, PA projections of the chest in both inspiration and expiration will be required to demonstrate air trapping due to airway obstruction. This may manifest itself as reduced lung attenuation on expiration and/or mediastinal shift. The kV must be sufficiently high to allow penetration and demonstrate a FB which might otherwise be obscured by the mediastinum.

Cross-sectional imaging such as CT and MRI are additional techniques that may provide useful information. (Note: MRI is contra-indicated in cases of suspected ferrous materials as the examination may result in movement of the FB.)

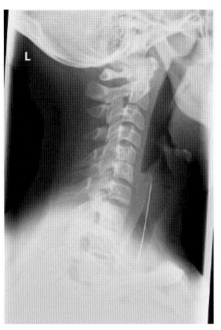

Fig. 14.17b Lateral soft tissue neck showing sewing needle lodged in the larynx.

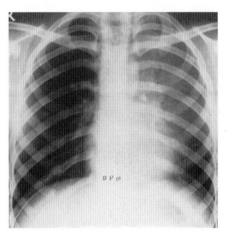

Fig. 14.17c PA chest image demonstrating a tooth in the left superior lobar bronchus and some generalised opacity through the left upper lobe.

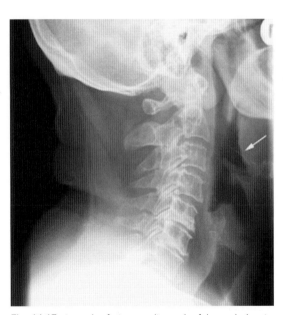

Fig. 14.17a Lateral soft tissue radiograph of the neck showing a fish bone lodged in the larynx.

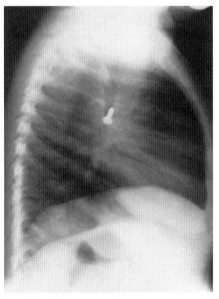

Fig. 14.17d Lateral chest image demonstrating a screw lodged in the right main bronchus.

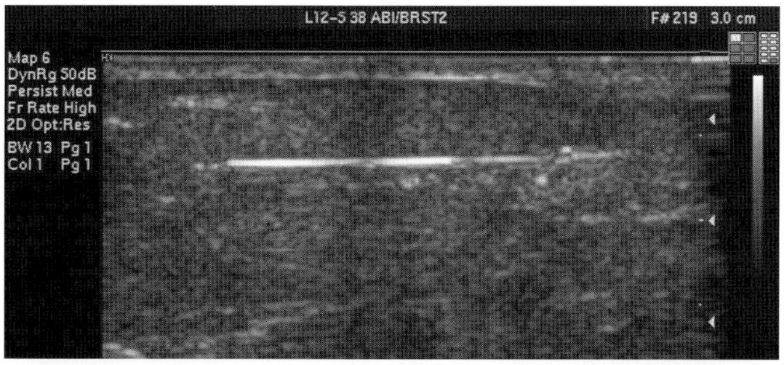

Foreign bodies 14

Inserted foreign bodies (Figs 14.18a–14.18d)

FBs are sometimes inserted into any of the body orifices/cavities. Infants and young children, for example, may insert objects into the nasal passages or an external auditory meatus. In these cases radiography is only occasionally required since most of these objects can be located and removed without referral to radiography.

When radiography is requested, two projections at right-angles to each other of the area concerned will be required.

Swabs may be left in the body following surgery. Such swabs contain a radio-opaque filament consisting of polyvinylchloride impregnated with barium sulphate for radiographic localisation.

It is sometimes necessary to check the position of an intrauterine contraceptive device. In this case ultrasonography should be used to avoid irradiating the gonads.

There have also been incidents where objects, such as sexual aids or even vegetables have been inserted into the anal canal and the patients have been unable to remove them manually. In these cases an AP projection of the abdomen may be required and sometimes a lateral rectum to demonstrate the depth of insertion.

Fig. 14.18a Ultrasound image of a needle in the superficial soft tissue.

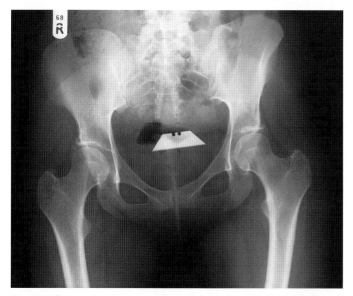

Fig. 14.18b AP pelvis showing a Stanley knife blade inserted into the vagina.

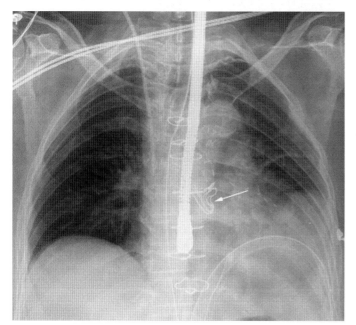

Fig. 14.18c Mobile AP chest taken in theatre to locate a missing swab.

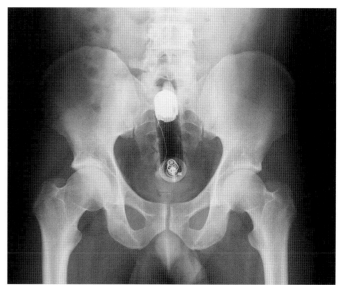

Fig. 14.18d AP pelvis demonstrating a vibrator inserted into the rectum.

14 Foreign bodies

Transocular foreign bodies (Figs 14.19a–14.19c)

FBs that enter the orbital cavity are commonly small fragments of metal, brick, stone or glass associated with industrial, road or domestic accidents, often whilst in the workplace.

Plain imaging is the first modality for investigation of a suspected radio-opaque FB in the orbit due to its availability and low radiation dose. For further investigation, or assessment of a non-opaque FB, CT scanning is the gold standard. CT will give information about damage to the delicate bones of the medial and superior orbital margins, and detail of any brain injury if the orbital roof has been breached. Ultrasound is operator dependent and the expertise is less likely to be immediately available. Also, there is the extra hazard of introducing coupling gel into a wound with the prospect of infection.[2]

Radiographic localisation may be carried out in three stages:

- To confirm the presence of an intraorbital radio-opaque FB.
- To determine whether the FB is intra- or extraocular.
- To determine the precise position of the FB.

Images showing fine detail are essential. A small focal spot (e.g. 0.3 mm^2), should be used to ensure the image detail is optimised.

All imaging equipment used by for this examination needs to be cleaned to ensure there are no artefacts on the receptor/cassette that could be confused with intraorbital FB. If CR is used a nominated cleaned CR cassette that has been erased twice, to remove any latent image due to a previous high exposure, is used specifically for these examinations.[3]

Notes

- MRI must not be undertaken where ferromagnetic FBs are suspected since the magnetic field may cause them to move, resulting in further injury.

Confirmation of a radio-opaque foreign body

This examination is generally undertaken using an erect Bucky/receptor with a moving grid.

An occipito-mental (modified) projection, Waters' view (see page 300) is undertaken due to the shape of the orbital cavity and angulation of the posterior aspect; the projection will demonstrate the complete length of the soft tissue within the orbital cavity. The patient is positioned so that the central ray passes through the centre of the pupil on the side being examined with the eyes level and looking forward and there should be no rotation.

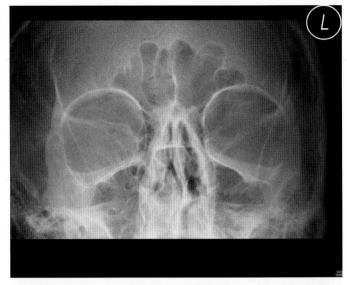

Fig. 14.19a Standard occipito-mental (OM) orbit projection with no foreign body (FB) present.

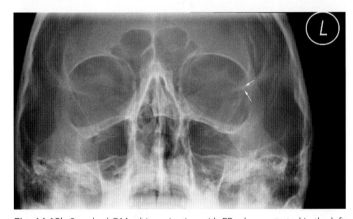

Fig. 14.19b Standard OM orbit projection with FBs demonstrated in the left orbit laterally.

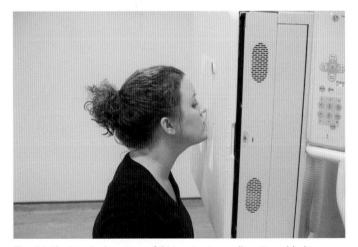

Fig. 14.19c Standard position of OM projection; collimation added to improve contrast and detail specific to the orbits.

Foreign bodies 14

Transocular foreign bodies (cont.) (Figs 14.20a–14.20e)

Localisation of intraorbital foreign body

A lateral projection of the orbit is taken as an additional examination if a radio-opaque FB is demonstrated on the OM projection.

The method described determines the position of the FB relative to the centre of the eye and whether it is intra- or extraocular. It should be ascertained that the patient is able to maintain ocular fixation, i.e. keep the eyes fixed on some given mark, since the exposures are required with the patient looking in different directions.

The examination is preferably carried out using an erect Bucky or skull unit if available. The following projections are required:

- Lateral orbits (see page 298) with the centring adjusted to the outer canthus of the eye.
- Two exposures are made, one with the eyes raised; one with the eyes lowered.
- In each case the patient should look steadily at some pre-determined mark or small object during the exposure. The direction of movement of the FB on the resultant images indicates whether it is located anteriorly or posteriorly in the eye.

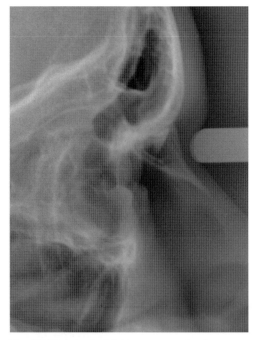

Fig. 14.20a Lateral orbital image – eyes level.

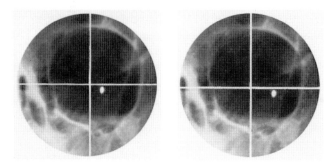

Figs 14.20b and c Occipito-mental images with the eyes level (left) and the left eye adducted (right).

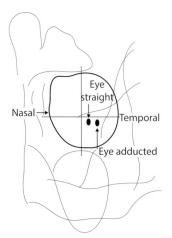

Fig. 14.20d Tracing from occipito-mental projection shows that the foreign body (FB) lies posterior to the centre of the eye.

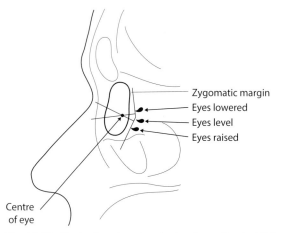

Fig. 14.20e Tracing from lateral projection shows that the FB lies within the orbit.

14 Soft tissue

Introduction

Soft-tissue radiography is the term generally used for radiography of muscle, skin, subcutaneous and glandular tissues without the use of contrast media. There is normally only a small differential attenuation between adjacent structures, which results in a low subject contrast. Fat, however has a lower density than other soft tissue and the attenuation coefficient results in a higher optical density on the image. The fat shadow may therefore delineate adjacent soft tissue structures and is normally demonstrated in subcutaneous tissue, between fascia, muscles and tendons. In order to demonstrate soft tissues successfully, special attention must be given to:

- Radiographic contrast – use of appropriate exposure technique, reduction of scattered radiation.
- Image sharpness – immobilisation, small focal spot.
- Appropriate post processing to optimise detail of contrast required.
- Avoidance of artefacts – scrupulously cleaned receptors, avoidance of dressings, folds in skin or gown/clothing.

Benign skin tumours such as subcutaneous cysts and warts may cause confusing opacities and should be noted on the X-ray referral, along with any other unusual features that may mislead the reporting professional.

Exposure technique

Several different exposure techniques may be used. They may be broadly divided into two categories: those employing a normal kV for the area being examined and those employing a non-standard kV.

Due to the flexibility and ability to manipulate the contrast on digital images the non-standard techniques are rarely used. kV is standardised to optimise detail on radiographic images and when used below 60 kV has been proven to increase the skin dose for the patient being imaged. This is thus a historical chapter with limited current use in the UK.

Normal kV

This category may be divided into three subcategories with the last category having no use in digital imaging and used for 'film' only:

- Use of a normal technique for the area being examined when air shadows or fat pads may delineate abnormalities in adjacent soft tissue structures. Examples of the use of this exposure technique are:
  - Effusion in a synovial cavity causing a filling defect in a fat pad adjacent to a joint.
  - Enlarged adenoids causing a filling defect in the air contained in the naso-pharynx.
- The use of a wedge filter where the thicker part of the wedge attenuates the beam over the soft tissues. An example of the use of this technique is cephalography to demonstrate bony detail of the skull and facial bones along with the soft-tissue outline of the face on one image.
- Analogue imaging only: use two or more films or screen/film combinations to demonstrate both bony detail and soft tissue with one exposure. Examples of the use of this exposure technique are:
  - Facial bones, nasal bones and soft tissues of the face.
  - Calcification of tendons and bony detail of the shoulder joint.

Non-standard kV

This category of exposure technique can also be further divided into three subcategories: subnormal kV, low kV and high kV.

Subnormal kV

This term is used when the kV employed in less than 45 kV, which is the lowest useful kV available on many X-ray units. Modified or special equipment is required that has an X-ray tube with reduced added and inherent filtration along with a small focal spot size. The use of such kV increases differential attenuation of adjacent soft tissues and thus increases subject contrast. Radiographic contrast may be further increased by the use of a film or screen/film combination with a high average gradient, i.e. more than 3. An example of the use of this technique is found in conventional film-based mammography.

Low kV

This term is used when the kV employed is 15–20 kV less than normal for a similar projection of the area being examined. Bony detail is not demonstrated in this case. Examples of the use of this technique are: calcifications in limbs, for example, calcification of arteries or tendons, parasitic calcifications; and superficial tumours, normally demonstrated in a profile projection of the area.

High kV

This term is used when the kV employed is 20 kV or more than is normally used for a similar projection of the same area. The use of such kVs reduces the differential attenuation of soft tissues, decreasing subject contrast thus allowing a greater range of tissues to be demonstrated. When used with CR, edge enhancement (enhancement of the boundaries of different tissues) offsets the reduced contrast.

Soft tissue 14

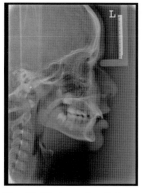

Fig. 14.21a Lateral cephalogram showing both bone and soft tissue outline on a single image to assess for treatment planning.

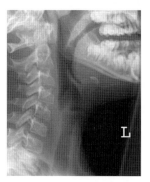

Fig. 14.21b Lateral soft tissue demonstration of the neck.

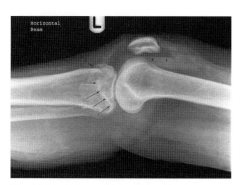

Fig. 14.21c Horizontal beam lateral knee CR image windowed to show soft tissues, showing depressed fracture of tibial plateau (arrows) and lipohaemarthrosis (arrowheads)

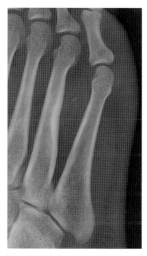

Fig. 14.21d Image of foot with calcification in the soft tissue confirming diagnosis of gout.

Exposure technique (cont.) (Figs 14.21a–14.21d)

Choice of projection

To demonstrate any soft-tissue lesions the most suitable radiographs are those that will project the area under examination clear of the adjacent bone. Normally the projections described in the appropriate section of this book will be used, but occasionally a profile/tangential projection will be required of the area under examination.

Lesions demonstrated by air

Soft-tissue lesions may be demonstrated by air in body cavities, for example, enlarged adenoids encroach on the posterior naso-pharyngeal air space, demonstrated on a lateral projection of the neck. After adenoidectomy there is no longer soft tissue encroachment on the air space. A normal exposure technique for the part being examined is used in these cases.

Air in the soft tissue is known as surgical emphysema and may be caused by trauma, especially a rib fracture, or perforation of an abnormal viscous such as the rectum. A large area must be included on the radiograph.

Lesions demonstrated by fat

Fat has a lower attenuation coefficient than other soft tissue and shows as a higher optical density on the radiograph. Effusion in a synovial cavity may cause a filling effect in a fat pad adjacent to a joint. Haemo-lipid fluid levels may also be demonstrated when a collimated horizontal beam technique is used. It is therefore essential that the kV used to demonstrate joints is sufficient to allow demonstration of both bone and soft tissue structures with the image optimally post processed.

Lipoma is a benign well-defined fatty tumour that is more transradiant than adjacent tissues and therefore appears as a darker area on the radiograph. A standard exposure is used.

Calcifications in soft tissue

Calcifications in limbs, for example, calcifications of arteries, tendons, ligaments and parasitic calcifications with film were usually best demonstrated by using a low kV exposure technique. This is no longer required with digital imaging. Calcifications in the trunk are demonstrated using a normal exposure technique.

Bone and adjacent soft tissues

In conditions such as rheumatoid arthritis, gout, myositis ossificans and osteomyelitis there may be adjacent soft tissue swelling, calcification or crystallisation. It is therefore essential that the kV is sufficient to demonstrate both bone and soft-tissue structures, again with the image optimally post processed.

14 Tomography and tomosynthesis

Introduction (Figs 14.22a–14.22e)

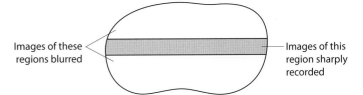

Fig. 14.22a Diagram illustrating tomography theory.

A conventional radiograph is a 2D image formed by the superimposition of images from successive layers of the body in the path of the X-ray beam. The image of a structure in one layer of the body is observed with the superimposition of images of structures in layers above and below it.

Before the introduction and widespread use of CT, a technique known as (conventional) tomography was employed. This uses conventional X-ray equipment, with tomographic attachments, or a dedicated tomographic unit to record images of structures or layers within the patient while images of structures outside the selected layer were made unsharp. Such images are acquired using cassettes fitted with conventional screen/film technology or using CR cassettes. However, tomography is also applied using modern digital imaging equipment with motorised and electronic control of the X-ray tube and DDR detector, which does not require a physical attachment between the X-ray tube and digital detector via a pivot device.

There are several methods of achieving this, all of which involve some form of movement of the patient or equipment during the exposure, but in every case the general principle is the same. Throughout the exposure, movement occurs, causing images from the unwanted layers to move relative to the image receptor and therefore to be unsharp; images from the selected layer are kept stationary relative to the image receptor and are recorded in focus. Tomography involves the synchronised movement of the X-ray tube and the image receptor while the patient remains stationary. If there is movement only of the patient during the exposure, this is called autotomography.

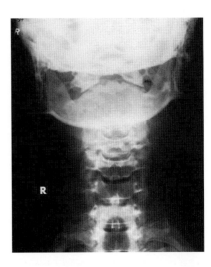

Fig. 14.22b AP conventional image of cervical spine with superimposed mandible on the upper vertebrae.

Autotomography

In this technique, the part to be visualised remains stationary during the exposure while overlying structures produce unsharp images due to some form of patient movement. The part to be visualised should be immobilised. A long exposure time is used to allow sufficient movement and therefore blurring of unwanted images.

The two most common applications of autotomography are as follows. Firstly, an AP projection of the cervical spine, where the patient opens and closes the mouth during the exposure so that the mandible is not recorded as a sharp image obscuring cervical vertebrae. Secondly a lateral projection of the thoracic vertebrae, where the patient continues gentle respiration during the exposure so that images of the ribs and lungs are unsharp, allowing better visualisation of the vertebrae.

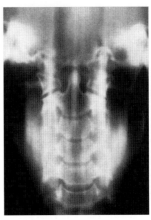

Fig. 14.22c Tomograph – X-ray tube and cassette move during exposure.

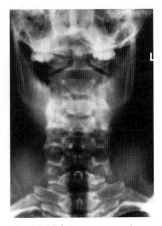

Fig. 14.22d Autotomograph – mandible moving during exposure.

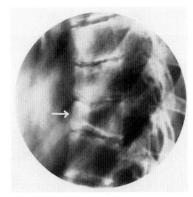

Fig. 14.22e Autotomograph – gentle respiration during long exposure.

Tomosynthesis

Tomosynthesis another method of acquiring images of layers within body structures. This is a volume digital radiography method that enables several multiple planes to be acquired in a single X-ray tube sweep using a multiple exposure technique.

The technique is made possible using DDR detector equipment and specialised software. This modality is described at the end of the chapter.

Tomography 14

Principles (Figs 14.23a–14.23c)

As stated previously, a tomographic image can be produced by relative movement between the patient, the image-recording device and the X-ray tube. In practice, this is normally achieved by the patient remaining stationary while the X-ray tube and the image receptor move.

As the X-ray tube and image receptor move relative to the patient, the projected images of structures at different levels of the body will move with different velocities. The nearer the structure is to the X-ray tube or image receptor, the faster its image will move with greater degree of unsharpness.

With older conventional X-ray equipment the X-ray tube is physically linked to the image receptor tray, such that the cassette moves at the same velocity as images of structures only at the level of the pivot; therefore, only these images are recorded on the same part of the image receptor throughout the movement. Images of structures at or in all other layers move at a different velocity from that of the image receptor and are not recorded on the same part of the image receptor throughout the movement and are therefore blurred. With modern digital imaging equipment a physical link between X-ray tube and image receptor is not necessary as the fulcrum height (sharp layer) is controlled electronically following selection of the required tomographic parameters.

It is therefore possible to record the outlines of structures more sharply on only one layer of the body, free from obscuring images from other layers.

It is an important requirement that throughout the movement there is no change in the magnification of images on the object plane, since this would produce image unsharpness. To ensure constant magnification, the following relationship must be maintained throughout the movement:

$$\frac{\text{Focus-to-image receptor distance}}{\text{Focus-to-pivot distance}} = \text{a constant}$$

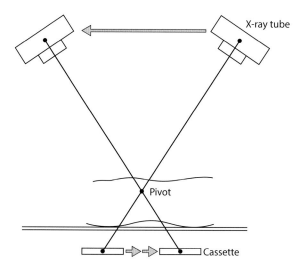

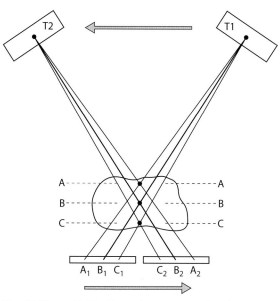

Figs 14.23a and b The X-ray tube is connected to the cassette and pivoted at B. When the X-ray tube moves from T1 to T2 during the exposure, images of layer B move at the same velocity as the image receptor and are recorded on the same part of the image receptor throughout the exposure and the image is sharp; images of layer A move faster than the image receptor and are therefore blurred; images of layer C move slower than the image receptor and are therefore blurred.

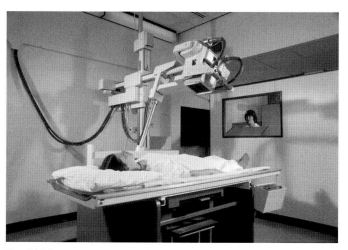

Fig. 14.23c Example of conventional tomography set-up with connecting rod linking X-ray tube and table Bucky tray. (Crown copyright. Reproduced with permission of Public Health England.)

14 Tomography

Principles (*cont.*)
(Figs 14.24a–14.24c)

The layer recorded sharply is called the object plane and it is parallel to the image receptor.

Normally, the image receptor lies parallel to the tabletop and therefore the object plane is parallel to the tabletop at the level of the pivot. If the image receptor lies at an angle to the tabletop, during the movement the layer visualised will be at the same angle. This is called inclined-plane tomography.

Depth of layer – fulcrum/pivot height

The height of the pivot table above the tabletop is variable so that any level in the patient can be selected for tomography. Either the fulcrum/pivot can be raised or lowered above the tabletop to the required level in the patient (variable pivot), or the pivot is in a fixed position and the tabletop can be raised or lowered to bring the required level to the level of the pivot (fixed pivot).

With conventional equipment the height of the fulcrum/pivot above the tabletop is indicated on a scale. If the upper attachment of the connecting rod is at the level of the focal spot and the lower attachment is at the level of the image receptor, then the layer recorded sharply is the layer at the level of the pivot that is parallel to the image receptor. If the image receptor is situated above or below the lower attachment of the connecting rod, then a layer above or below the pivot level will be recorded sharply.

When modern digital equipment is employed the fulcrum/pivot height is set automatically dependent on the organ programme specified. The height, which is also adjustable, will be shown on the control panel display and, if provided, a tomographic height light localiser will mark the position on the patient as well as being able to adjust t the fulcrum height.

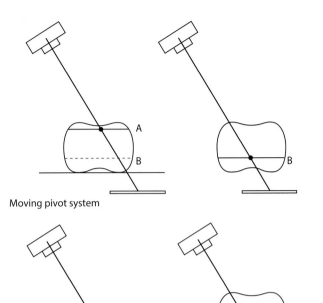

Moving pivot system

Fixed pivot system

Fig. 14.24a Object plane parallel to the image receptor.

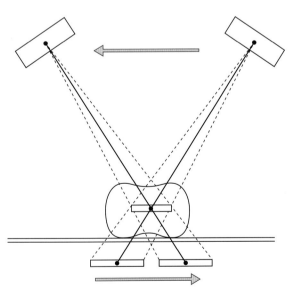

Fig. 14.24b Object plane parallel to the image receptor.

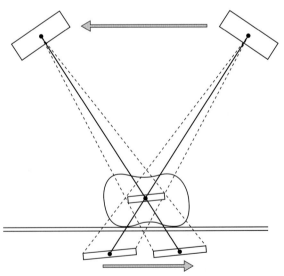

Fig. 14.24c Inclined plane tomography.

Tomography 14

Types of tomographic movement (Figs 14.25a–14.25c)

Before the use of CT, when (conventional) tomography was used more widely, a variety of tube/film movements were employed to produce more effective blurring of unwanted structures, e.g. (in order of increasing complexity):

- Linear.
- Circular.
- Elliptical.
- Spiral.
- Figure-of-eight (Lissajous figure).
- Hypocycloidal.

Dedicated tomographic units were required for all movements other than linear. Since the use of conventional tomography is now limited mainly to imaging the renal tract, linear movement produces adequate blurring and we will only consider this movement in our discussions.

Features of linear movement

This is the simplest form of tomographic movement. The X-ray tube and image receptor move in lines parallel to the tabletop. The FRD changes throughout the movement, being least at the midpoint of the movement. Line-to-line movement is often confined to one direction only, which is along the long axis of the table, but some equipment will allow the linear movement to be in any direction parallel to the tabletop. There are different designs:

- Arc-to-line: the X-ray tube moves in an arc above the table while the image receptor moves below the table in a line parallel to the tabletop. This is typical of the majority of units. Throughout the movement, there is a change in the ratio of the focus-to-receptor/focus-to-pivot distance, resulting in a continual change in the magnification of images in the object layer. This results in some unsharpness, but if the change in magnification is kept to a small value then the image can be accepted by the observer as sharp.
- Arc-to-arc: the X-ray tube and the image receptor move in arcs, the centre of rotation being the pivot. Throughout the movement, the image receptor remains parallel to the tabletop and the FRD is constant.

NB: linear movements have the disadvantage that they produce 'linear streaks'. These are pseudo-shadows caused by structures just outside the layer, which are incompletely blurred out and appear as indistinct linear images superimposed on the sharp image of the selected layer.

Exposure angle

The exposure angle is the angle through which the tube moves during the exposure. It is inversely related to the thickness of layer visualised on the image. For linear tomography, there is usually a choice of exposure angle ranging from about 2° to 40°.

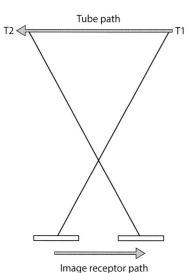

Fig. 14.25a Line-to-line.

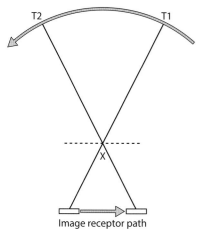

Fig. 14.25b Arc-to-line.

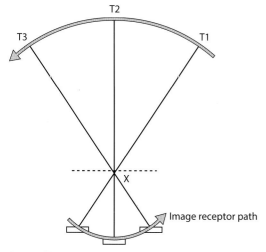

Fig. 14.25c Arc-to-arc.

14 Tomography

Principles (Figs 14.26a–14.26c)

Thickness of layer

Only images of structures at the level of the pivot and parallel to the image receptor are recorded on the same part of the image receptor throughout the movement. This layer is infinitely thin. Images of structures outside this object plane move relative to the image receptor, but if this movement is small (less than about 0.6 mm), they will be recognisable images. Therefore, the visualised layer has some thickness. The amount of relative movement of the image and therefore the thickness of the layer depends on the exposure angle, i.e. the angle through which the X-ray tube moves during the exposure. The greater the exposure angle, the thinner the layer. The layer has no well-defined boundary as there is a progressive deterioration in the sharpness of images of structures with increasing distance from the object plane.

Layer thickness also depends on the distance of the structure above or below the pivot. Images of structures above the pivot are more blurred than those below the pivot, and thus the layer is thinner above the pivot than below it. The practical significance of this is that structures close to the object plane can be 'blurred out' more easily if they are on the tube side of the patient (see the diagram opposite).

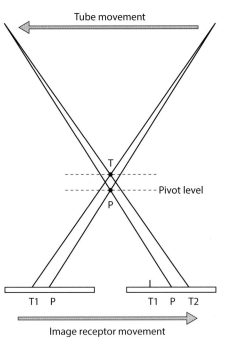

Fig. 14.26a The above diagram demonstrates that during tube movement, the image of P (at the level of the pivot) is recorded on the same part of the image receptor and is a sharp image. T is on a plane higher than the pivot and its image moves on the receptor from T1 to T2, but if this distance is not greater than about 0.6 mm it is still accepted as a sharp image. Therefore, the thickness of the layer extends up to T. There is a similar thickness of the layer below the pivot.

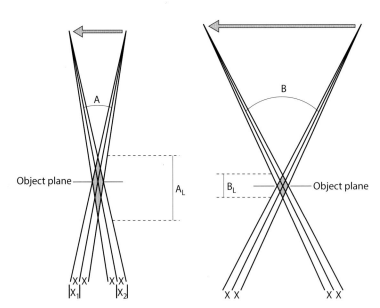

Figs 14.26b and c 2X (e.g. $X_1 + X_2$) represents the amount of image movement (about 0.6 mm) on the image receptor that the observer can still accept as being a sharp image. Therefore, images of objects within the layer A_L are seen as sharp images for exposure angle A, and within the layer B_L for exposure angle B. The larger the exposure angle, the thinner the layer.

Tomography 14

Principles (cont.)
(Figs 14.27a, 14.27b)

The graph below shows how the thickness of the layer varies with exposure angle. At larger angles there is little change in layer thickness with change in exposure angle, whereas at small angles a small change in the exposure angle causes a large change in layer thickness.

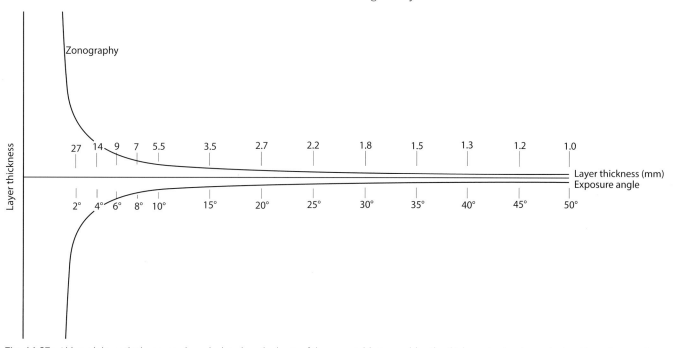

Fig. 14.27a Although layer thickness can be calculated on the basis of the acceptable image blur, the thickness is also dependent on the radio-opacity and shape of structures lying outside the calculated layer. Opaque structures and those lying along the line of the X-ray tube movement are more difficult to 'blur out' and both these factors increase the apparent thickness of the layer.

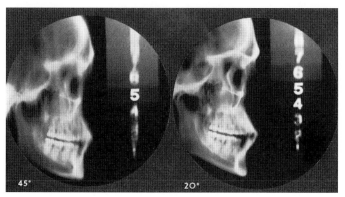

Fig. 14.27b Tomographs illustrating change of layer thickness with exposure angle.

Zonography

This is the term applied to small-angle tomography giving relatively thick layers. There is no fixed exposure angle below which tomography is classified as zonography, but the term is generally reserved for exposure angles of 10° or less.

Thickness of cut and spacing of layers

For zonography, where the layer can be, for example, greater than 2 cm thick, layers at 2 cm intervals can be used. In practice, it is normal to use 10° exposure angles and 1 cm intervals. With wide-angle tomography, spacing of layers should be closer, to ensure that the layers overlap.

Magnification in tomography

As with all projected images, there is some magnification of a tomographic image. The magnification (M) is given by:

$$M = \frac{FRD}{\text{Focus- to- pivot distance}}$$

14 Tomography

Image quality (Figs 14.28a, 14.28b)

Generally, the quality of a tomography image, in terms of its sharpness and contrast, is not as good as that of a standard radiographic image.

Contrast

Because only a thin layer of the body is being recorded, inherent contrast is low, the problem being greater with the larger exposure angles that produce very thin layers. If the region is made up predominantly of soft tissue, then the layer might have to be at least 1 cm thick for contrast to be acceptable.

To improve contrast, particular attention should be paid to the control of scattered radiation by collimating the X-ray beam to the smallest possible field. A further method of improving contrast is to select the lowest kV that will still give optimum penetration (not below 75 kV due to detector sensitivity).

Sharpness

As with a standard radiographic image, unsharpness can be due to patient movement (Um), focal spot size (Ug) and intensifying screens (Us), if used. In addition, the tomographic movement can introduce a source of image unsharpness (Ut).

Particular attention should therefore be paid to the choice of focal spot sizes, immobilisation and intensifying screens to reduce unsharpness to a minimum.

Localisation of the depth of the layer(s) required

The approximate depth may be known from past experience or from records kept of similar examinations. If not, then the depth of the layer can be estimated by studying AP and lateral radiographs.

Clearly, fulcrum/pivot heights will vary from patient to patient. They will also depend on whether the patient lies on a foam mattress and, if so, its thickness.

Radiation protection

The usual steps are taken to reduce the radiation dose to the patient, but there are some additional measures that are particularly applicable to tomography:

- The position and depth of the lesion should be localised accurately, preferably before the examination but if not, then in the early stages of tomography.
- Whenever possible, the patient is positioned so that the structure of interest is parallel to the image receptor, thus reducing the number of layers required.
- In skull tomography, position the patient prone wherever possible to reduce the radiation dose to the lens of the eye.
- The smallest field size compatible with a diagnosis is essential, not only for radiation protection but also to improve radiographic contrast.
- The radiographer must follow an organised procedure for all stages of the examination to avoid the necessity of repeating exposure due to a careless omission.

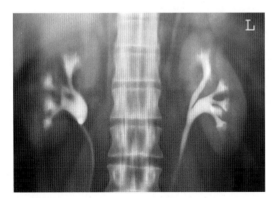

Fig. 14.28a Thick layer (zonogram) required to give contrast in a soft tissue region.

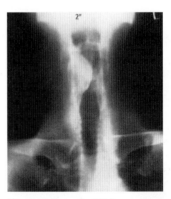 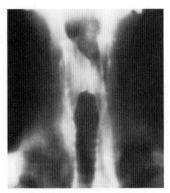

Figs 14.28b and c 30° linear. Contrast can be obtained in a thin layer containing air, bone and soft tissue.

The following procedure should be used as a guide in preparing and undertaking tomography:

- Having read and understood the request card, previous images should be studied for the localisation of the position, extent and depth of the region to be visualised.
- The exposure angle and exposure time combination to be used is selected with reference to the thickness of the zone containing the lesion and the shape of structures to be blurred out.

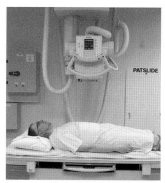

Fig. 14.29a Intravenous urography tomogram – X-ray tube centred over area of interest and correct focus-to-receptor distance.

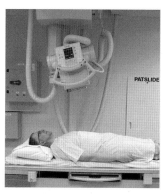

Fig. 14.29b X-ray tube in start position for a 10° exposure angle.

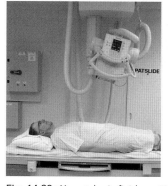

Fig. 14.29c X-ray tube in finish position.

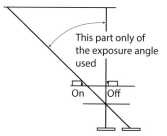

Fig. 14.29d Diagram illustrating asymmetrical exposure angle technique.

Tomography 14

Procedure (Figs 14.29a–14.29d)

- An explanation of the examination is given to the patient. The patient is then positioned and immobilised on the table.
- The vertical central ray is directed to the centre of the region and the X-ray beam is well collimated.
- The fulcrum/pivot height is selected, which should coincide with the height of the structure of interest from the table.
- The image receptor carrying the appropriate radio-opaque legends is placed in position.
- The X-ray tube is moved to the starting position for the movement.
- The patient is given final instructions before the exposure is made.
- The image is reviewed to check for positioning, exposure, contrast and localisation. Further images may be required at different levels to demonstrate the full extent of a lesion.
- The fulcrum/pivot height is changed by a distance that depends on the thickness of the layers being recorded.

Exposure time and exposure angle

For conventional tomography the exposure time selected should be just greater than the time taken for the X-ray tube to complete the entire movement. This ensures that the exposure angle is symmetrical and that the anticipated angle, and hence layer thickness, is obtained. The choice of complex movements that require an exposure time of several seconds may be restricted if patient movement is a problem.

Image acquisition with modern digital equipment is undertaken using the selection of one of a number of programme combinations of exposure angle and exposure time as offered by the equipment manufacturer. This is will be acquired at a pre-determined FRD height, i.e. 102 cm according to the protocol of the manufacturer.

The use of variable-speed equipment allows for a choice of exposure time and mA for a given mAs.

In some examinations, not all of the exposure angle contributes equally to image formation. In such cases, the exposure can be controlled to take place during part of the movement. For example, in linear AP tomography of the larynx (caudal to cranial), the exposure can take place only during the first part of tube movement.

Applications

The widespread availability of CT has resulted in a corresponding decrease in the use of conventional tomography. The main use of conventional tomography is in intravenous urography (IVU) examinations to reduce the effects of superimposed bowel gas. It may still be used for other structures where access to CT is limited or not possible.

Two further applications – larynx and trachea – are included as examples.

14 Tomography

Kidneys – antero-posterior (Figs 14.30a–14.30c)

In this situation, tomography is often used as a simple, cheap and relatively effective method of imaging the renal tract free of overlying structures. Since the structures that are required to be visualised are relatively thick (AP measurement), zonography, or narrow-angle tomography, is used to produce a large layer thickness.

Tomography is used during IVU either at 10–20 minutes after injection, to diffuse the shadows of gas that overlie the calyces preventing their clear visualisation, or immediately on completion of the injection to show the nephrogram stage. This latter method – nephrotomography – was used to differentiate between kidney cysts and tumour and between intra- and extrarenal masses, but has been actively superseded by ultrasound and CT.

Notes

- Although a narrow angle, e.g. 8–10°, can produce a large layer thickness (approximately 5 cm) and may enable the whole of the outline of the kidneys to be shown on one exposure, it will not efficiently 'blur out' overlying bowel shadows in the bowel.
- To 'blur' gas shadows a 20°, 30° or even a 40° angle may have to be used.

Position of patient and image receptor

- The patient is supine on the table, with the median sagittal plane of the body at right-angles to and in the midline of the table.

Direction and location of the X-ray beam

- The collimated vertical beam is centred in the midline, midway between the suprasternal notch and the symphysis pubis.

Pivot height

- 8–11 cm.
- Note: if a mattress is used, then allowance for its thickness must be made when selecting the pivot height.

Tomographic movement

- Linear 10° – zonography.
- Linear 30° – to blur out overlying bowel gas.

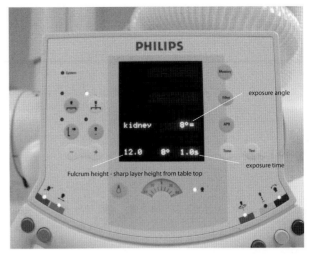

Fig. 14.30a Selection criteria displayed on light beam diaphragm (LBD) for kidney area with an 8° exposure angle and 1 second exposure time.

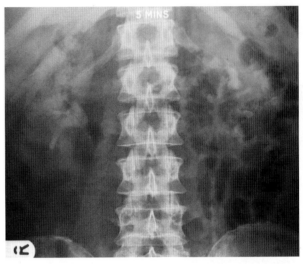

Fig. 14.30b Five-minute post-contrast image with bowel gas obscuring the renal areas.

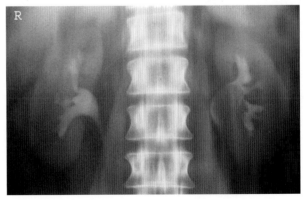

Fig. 14.30c Tomography image showing the renal areas free from gas shadows and a mass in the left renal pelvic region.

Position of patient and image receptor

- The patient lies supine on the table, with the median sagittal plane of the trunk and head at right-angles to and in the midline of the table.
- The patient is located on the table so that a vertical central ray would pass 1 cm inferior to the eminence of the thyroid cartilage.

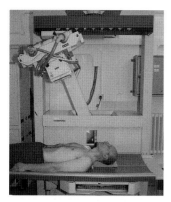

Fig. 14.31a Patient positioning.

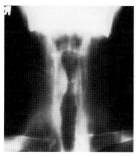

Fig. 14.31b Larynx.

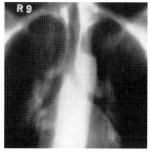

Fig. 14.31c Trachea and bifurcation

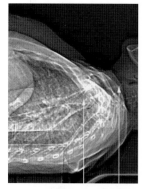

Fig. 14.31d Computed tomography scout image showing the angle of the trachea.

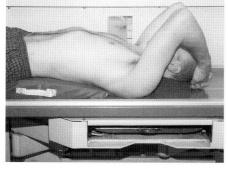

Fig. 14.31e Patient positioning.

Tomography 14

Larynx – antero-posterior (Figs 14.31a, 14.31b)

Pivot height

- From 0.5 cm deep to the skin surface to 4 cm deep to the skin surface.

Tomographic movement

- Linear longitudinal 20°. With the X-ray tube moving in a caudal to cranial direction, the first half of a 40° movement can be used to avoid superimposing the images of the mandible and facial bones on to those of the larynx.
- Because the region is one of inherently high contrast, a high kV (>90 kV) can be used; this reduces the amount of linear streaking recorded.
- Tomography may be taken during quiet breathing and also while the patient is phonating 'ee' to demonstrate an abnormal movement of the vocal cord due to a lesion.

Trachea – antero-posterior (Figs 14.31c–14.31e)

The trachea passes downwards and slightly backwards from its commencement at the lower border of the cricoid cartilage to its bifurcation just below the level of the sternal angle. With the patient supine, the trachea makes an angle of about 20° with the table, its upper end being further from the table than its lower end. To bring the trachea and the image receptor parallel, either the lower trunk is raised on pillows or, if there is sufficient clearance between the cassette tray and the undersurface of the table, the cassette can be inclined about 20° in the cassette tray by raising the edge of the cassette which is under the neck.

Position of patient and image receptor

The patient lies supine on the table with the median sagittal plane of the trunk and head at right-angles to, and in the midline of, the table. The lower trunk is raised as described above, which is essential if the patient has a marked lordosis. The patient is located on the table so that the vertical central ray would pass along the median sagittal plane midway between the cricoid cartilage and the sternal angle.

Pivot height

- 4–5 cm deep to the sternal notch.

Tomographic movement

- Linear transverse 10°; may be followed by large-angle movements if thinner layers are required.

14 Tomosynthesis

Principles (Figs 14.32a, 14.32b)

Conventional radiography is a projection technique. This causes all objects on the path of the X-ray beam to be superimposed on the image. The location of objects in 3D may not be possible to determine and often one object may hide another.

X-Ray Tomosynthesis (GE Healthcare VolumeRAD™) is a technique that can offer access to volume data for many clinical applications, by removing overlying or underlying structures.

- VolumeRAD tomosynthesis acquires multiple projections (exposures). It covers a range of projection angles, and provides multiple image plane reconstructions or 'slices'. The number of reconstructions for a chest exam is typically 61.
- VolumeRAD acquisition technique is controlled via a single energy scout image performed using AEC or manual technique.
- The automated acquisition is a fixed time determined by the scout image.
- The number of acquired projections depends upon the anatomy being examined but is typically 25–60.
- Dose = dose per projection multiplied by the number of projections. Image noise is dependent upon total dose.
- Sweep angle is analogous to the arc in standard tomography.
- The sweep time is dependent on the number of projections and is typically 5–11 seconds.

How does VolumeRAD differ from standard tomography?

With the introduction of modern flat panel digital detectors, experimental work was undertaken to develop a volume acquisition system, which is referred to as tomosynthesis.

The most important attribute of the flat panel detector is the lack of distortion. Because it is laid out in specific rows and columns, the geometry is known exactly and therefore back projection can be utilised for reconstruction of the image.

One bonus with tomosynthesis is that the radiation dose is considerably lower than with CT.

A good detailed review of the workings of digital tomosynthesis can be found in Dobbins et al. (2003).[1]

Standard tomography	Tomosynthesis VolumeRAD
One image plane acquired	Multiple image planes acquired
Single sweep continuous exposure	Single sweep multiple exposures
Moving detector	Stationary detector
No reconstruction	Multiple reconstructed slices

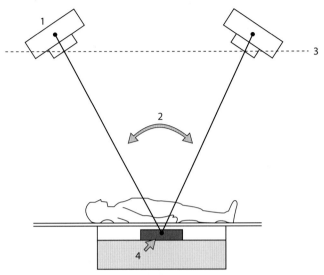

Fig. 14.32a Table configuration.

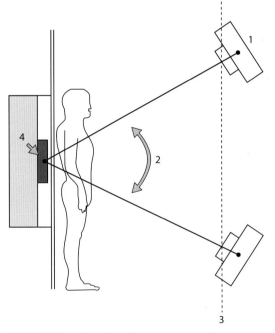

Fig. 14.32b Wall stand configuration – vertical.

Tomosynthesis 14

Principles (cont.) (Figs 14.33a–14.33c)

Radiation protection

The usual steps are taken to reduce the radiation dose to the patient but there are some additional measures which are particularly applicable to tomosynthesis:

- Detailed instructions should be given to the patient regarding breath holding for chest tomosynthesis and control of movement generally, due to the longer exposure times.
- Warn the patient about the tube movement to help prevent anxiety and possible movement.
- The smallest field size compatible with a diagnosis is essential not only for radiation protection but also to minimise scattered radiation.
- The radiographer must follow an organised procedure for all stages of the examination to avoid the necessity of repeating exposure due to a careless omission.

Procedure

- Select appropriate patient demographics from the Worklist or Manual data entry.
- Select appropriate protocol from Protocol Database (VolumeRAD).
- Position patient, tube and image receptor.
- Take VolumeRAD scout acquisition to confirm positioning, collimation and technique. Multiple scouts may be taken for better positioning or improved technical parameters, by selecting 'Retake Scout' button.
- Auto-position the tube to the start position for the VolumeRAD sweep.
- Press and hold the Exposure button, until the sweep has finished and acquisitions are complete.

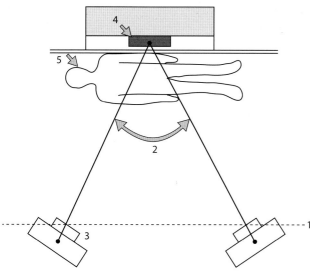

Fig. 14.33a Cross table VolumeRAD lumbar spine exam.

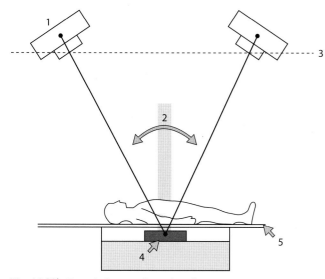

Fig. 14.33b Extended arm wall stand configuration.

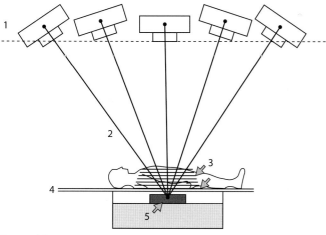

Fig. 14.33c 1, X-ray tube as it moves through the sweep; 2, X-ray emissions as the tube moves through the sweep; 3, reconstructed slices; 4, table; 5, detector.

14 Tomosynthesis

Image quality (Figs 14.34a, 14.34b)

Image quality in VolumeRAD examinations is dependent upon several factors:

- Correct protocol selection.
- Patient positioning and centering (especially for AEC exposures).
- Collimation and selection of correct processing and reconstruction parameters.

Once images are obtained using the VolumeRAD procedure, they can be reprocessed to show different anatomical planes. See images of a head phantom below that illustrate this.

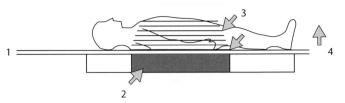

Fig. 14.34a Illustration of slice reconstruction for a table VolumeRAD examination. 1, Table; 2, detector; 3, reconstructed slices; 4, height (distance from table or wall stand surface).

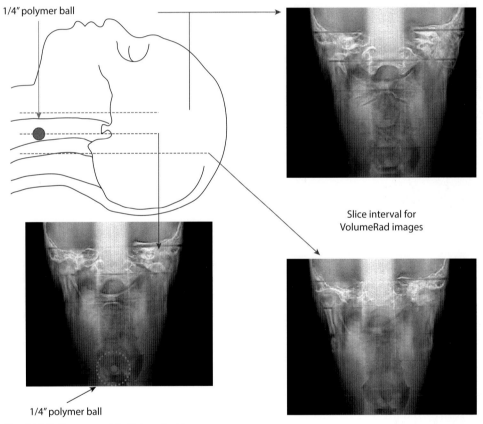

Fig. 14.34b Slice interval for VolumeRad images.

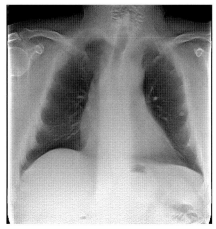

Fig. 14.35a Chest VolumeRAD slice demonstrating lung nodule.

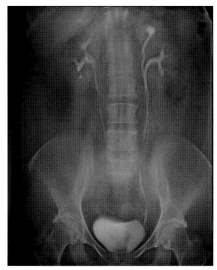

Fig. 14.35b Intravenous urogram VolumeRAD slice demonstrating duplex system.

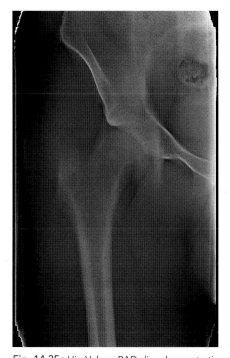

Fig. 14.35c Hip VolumeRAD slice demonstrating acetabulum fracture.

Tomosynthesis 14

Image quality (cont.) (Figs 14.35a–14.35c)

Radiation dose

- As in all radiographic procedures, image quality is dependent on total dose. Chest PA VolumeRAD requires 1.6× the dose of a standard 2-projection chest examination.
- Various studies have shown that tomosynthesis can demonstrate certain anatomies with a lower dose than other imaging modalities.[2,3]

Applications

- Tomosynthesis was initially thought to be helpful for IVU examinations where previously tomography had been used. However, other uses have been found such as spinal exams, scaphoid, pelvis, knee, shoulder and chest.
- The probability of a radiologist detecting small (3–20 mm) lung nodules is 1.6–22.3 times higher with tomosynthesis than with 2-view chest X-ray.[4]

Some images are shown opposite (courtesy of GE Healthcare).

14 Macroradiography

Principles (Figs 14.36a, 14.36b)

In some cases, it is helpful to the person making a diagnosis if the radiographic image can be enlarged, allowing smaller detail to become more obvious. Where digital image recording is used, this magnification can be obtained electronically. Using conventional screen/film technology, an alternative method of producing a magnified image is at the time of exposure, by increasing the ORD; in this case, the X-rays diverging from a point source will produce a directly magnified image.

The magnification (M) can be calculated from:

$$M = \frac{\text{image size}}{\text{object size}} = \frac{\text{FRD}}{\text{FOD}}$$

The FOD (or ORD) is taken from the mid-level of the part or lesion.

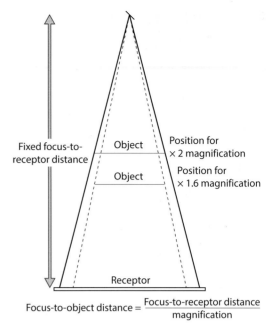

Focus-to-object distance = $\frac{\text{Focus-to-receptor distance}}{\text{magnification}}$

Fig. 14.36a Fixed focus-to-object distance.

Fixed focus-to-receptor distance

For a fixed focus-to-receptor distance (FRD), magnification is increased by bringing the object nearer to the X-ray tube focus. The FOD for a given magnification is calculated from:

$$\text{FOD} = \frac{\text{FRD}}{\text{magnification}}$$

For example, with a fixed FRD of 100 cm, and if a magnification factor of 1.6 is required, then the FOD will be:

$$\text{FOD} = \frac{\text{FRD}}{M} = \frac{100}{1.6} = 62.5$$

Fixed focus-to-object (FOD) distance

So that the skin dose to the patient can be limited, the FOD is kept fixed at, for example, 90 or 100 cm, and the required magnification is obtained by moving the receptor away from the object. The required ORD for a given magnification is than calculated from:

$$\text{ORD} = \text{FOD}\,(M - 1).$$

For example, if a magnification factor of 1.6 is required at an FOD of 100 cm, then the required ORD will be:

$$\text{ORD} = 100*(1.6 - 1) = 60 \text{ cm}$$

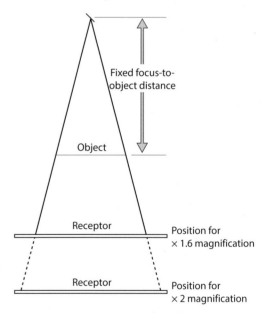

Object-to-receptor distance = Focus-to-object distance × (magnification−1)

Fig. 14.36b Fixed focus-to-object distance.

Similarly, for a magnification factor of 2 at the same FOD, the required ORD will be:

$$\text{ORD} = 100*(2 - 1) = 100 \text{ cm}.$$

Some equipment, e.g. the Orbix, skull unit, has the facility for moving the cassette away from the object along a scale calibrated in magnification factors.

The technique of producing an image by direct magnification is called macroradiography. It has the advantage that although movement and geometrical unsharpness are increased compared with a technique using minimum ORD, there is no increase in photographic unsharpness when using film/screens. However, it must be remembered that such a magnified image will always be less sharp than one taken with the same focal spot with a minimum ORD.

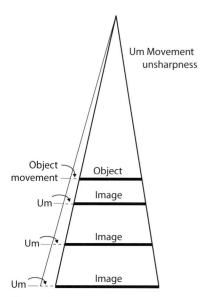

Fig. 14.37a Increasing movement unsharpness (Um) with increase in magnification.

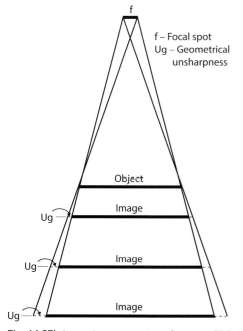

Fig. 14.37b Increasing geometric unsharpness (Ug) with increase in magnification.

Macroradiography 14

Principles (cont.) (Figs 14.37a, 14.37b)

A magnified image of acceptable sharpness will be produced only if movement unsharpness and geometrical unsharpness are kept to a minimum.

Movement unsharpness

Direct magnification by increased ORD can be carried out only if there is complete immobilisation of the patient, because any movement of the patient, be it due to lack of immobilisation or involuntary movement, will be magnified on the radiograph due to the increased ORD. The technique, therefore, lends itself to producing magnified images of bony structures or structures contained within bone, e.g. the lacrimal ducts. For macroradiography, immobilisation devices should be used, e.g. supports, binders, sandbags and pads, and the instructions should be given to the patient to remain still.

Geometrical unsharpness

Geometrical unsharpness occurs because the source of X-rays is not a point source and any distance between the object and receptor will cause an image penumbra in addition to magnifying the image. Thus, for a given focal spot size, there is a limit to the magnification of the image beyond which the geometrical unsharpness is so great that significant detail is lost. The smaller the focal spot size, the greater the possible magnification of the image while still retaining acceptable image quality.

The relationship between image magnification (M) and focal spot size (f) with the corresponding geometrical unsharpness (Ug) is given by:

$$Ug = f*(M - 1).$$

For example, if geometrical unsharpness is to be limited to 0.3 mm, then the maximum obtainable with the corresponding focal spot size is as follows:

Focal spot size (mm)	Maximum magnification
0.1	4.0
0.2	2.5
0.3	2.0
0.6	1.5
1.0	1.3

14 Macroradiography

Principles (*cont.*)
(Figs 14.38a–14.38d)

Scattered radiation

With macroradiography, there is usually an increase in FRD/FFD that requires a corresponding increase in mAs. Because an ultra-fine focus must be used, the permissible mA values will be reduced and hence a longer than normal exposure time is required. Immobilisation is, therefore, essential. To reduce the mAs, and therefore the exposure time required, a secondary radiation grid may not used. It is possible to dispense with the grid because the amount of scatter reaching the receptor is reduced due to the air gap between the patient and the cassette. Scattered radiation leaving the patient diverges through the intervening gap and although it would have been incident on a receptor in contact with the patient, some of it is now scattered outside the area of the receptor.

Additionally, the smallest possible field is used in order to reduce the amount of scatter produced originally.

CR cassette support

A method of supporting the cassette a known distance from the patient is required. An isocentric skull unit is ideal for this purpose, as the distance of the cassette holder from the body part under examination, and hence the magnification, can be varied precisely.

Applications

- Because of the increased radiation dose in macroradiography and the increasing use of CR and DDR, the use of macroradiography is limited mainly to radiography of the skull in dacrocystography.
- Macroradiography can also be used for imaging the carpal bones in cases of suspected fracture of scaphoid.

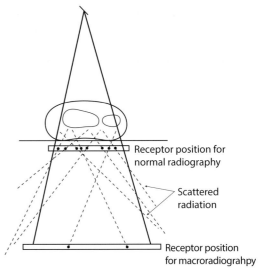

Fig. 14.38a Receptor position for macroradiology.

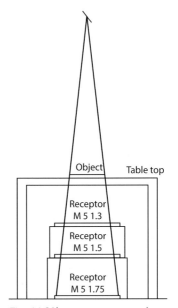

Fig. 14.38b Receptor position for macroradiology.

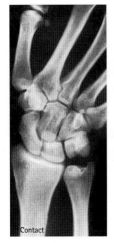
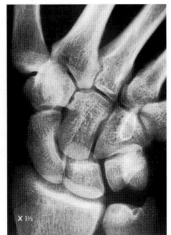
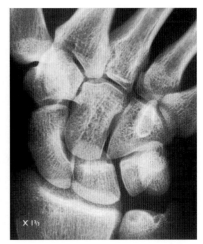

Figs 14.38c–d Examples of macroradiology imaging.

Skeletal survey 14

The commonest application of radiographic survey of the skeletal system is in suspected cases of 'non-accidental injury' (NAI) in children, when it is necessary to demonstrate the presence, multiplicity, and age of any bone injury. The technique and imaging protocols required are described in detail in Section 13 Paediatric Radiography (see page 480).

Prior to the advent of modern radionuclide imaging, plain image radiographic skeletal surveys were used as a primary means of diagnosing and assessing bony involvement in various pathological conditions, especially metastatic disease and some metabolic disorders.

Plain image radiography may have a limited role to play in some of these pathological conditions, and to assess the response to therapy (see table). However, biochemical tests for metabolic and endocrine conditions mean that these are frequently detected and treated before radiographic changes become diagnostic.

The development of disease-modifying drugs for rheumatoid arthritis and other inflammatory arthritides has led to very sensitive protocols for the detection and follow up of erosions and other bone changes using ultrasound and/or MRI. The role of plain radiographs is therefore more restricted than was previously, to the assessment of advanced disease, monitoring of established erosions and peri-operative assessment. Plain radiographs may still be requested for individual areas, such as assessment of suspected atlanto-axial subluxation.

Diseases affecting the skeletal system may affect bones, joints or both together. Different diseases preferentially affect different areas of the skeleton and it therefore follows that if a skeletal survey is required, the projections should be selected according to the likelihood of a positive result. There may be local variations in the projections preferred, for example in imaging of multiple myeloma, so the recommended projections below should be adapted according to local protocols.

Reference has been made to radionuclide imaging as a primary imaging technique for diffuse skeletal disease but other imaging methods, such as CT and MRI scanning are used increasingly for detection and characterisation of bone lesions in malignancy. In particular MRI is the primary investigation in patients with suspected spinal cord compression due to metastatic disease, as its sensitivity and specificity excels over that of radionuclide imaging. In addition, the soft-tissue resolution of MRI allows the level of compression of the cord to be clearly seen, and will show if more than one level is affected, which is vital in planning surgery or radiotherapy. In cord compression MRI should be performed as soon as possible and in any case within 24 hours of onset of symptoms.

CT is increasingly used for staging malignancy (such as breast cancer) as it can assess soft tissue deposits throughout the body as well as in the axial skeleton.

Introduction

Multiple myeloma produces lytic bone lesions that are frequently not detectable on a radionuclide bone scan due to lack of osteoblastic response by the bone. Radiography still has a role in this condition, though MRI is also useful in cases of doubt.[1]

Indications for skeletal system survey

The choice of regions of the skeleton to be included in a survey of a particular patient depends upon the possible diagnoses which are under consideration.

The primary conditions that may radiographic skeletal survey can be grouped as follows:

Type of disease	Examples
Trauma	Non-accidental injury
Malignant	Prostatic
Reticuloses	Myeloma Lymphoma
Metabolic	Scurvy Rickets
Endocrine	Hyperparathyroidism Cushing's syndrome
Inflammatory	Rheumatoid arthritis

Examples of X-ray projection requested

Indication	Projections
Myeloma and metabolic disease	PA and lateral skull PA chest AP and lateral whole spine Pelvis (to include upper femora) AP and lateral left humerus AP and lateral right humerus
Rheumatoid arthritis	PA chest AP and lateral thoraco-lumbar spine AP pelvis, sacro-iliac joints, cervical spine (flexion and extension) DP both hands (to include wrists) AP both knees, DP both feet

AP, antero-posterior; DP, dorsi-palmar; PA, postero-anterior.

14 Skeletal survey

Recommended projections

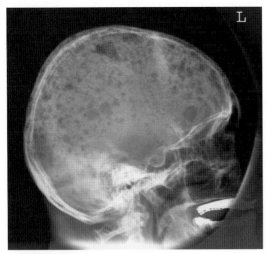

Fig. 14.39a Lateral radiograph of skull showing multiple lytic deposits typical of myeloma.

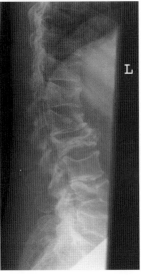

Fig. 14.39b Lateral radiograph of lumbar spine showing multiple areas of vertebral collapse, of varying age, due to myeloma. Excessive collimation has partially obscured the lower two lumbar vertebrae.

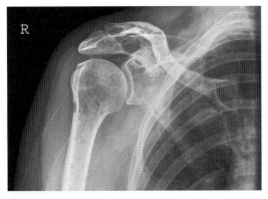

Fig. 14.39c AP radiograph of shoulder showing multiple lytic deposits of myeloma in the humerus, scapula, clavicle and ribs.

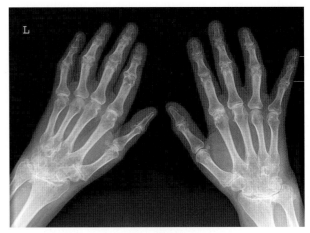

Fig. 14.39d Dorsi-palmar radiograph of both hands and wrists in a patient with seronegative arthritis.

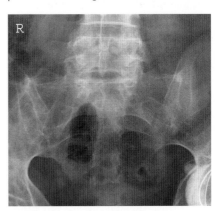

Fig. 14.39e AP radiograph of the sacrum of the same patient shown above, demonstrating fusion of the sacro-iliac joints sometimes seen in this condition.

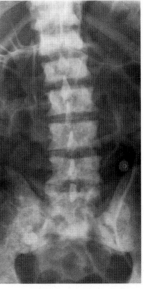

Fig. 14.39f AP radiograph of the lumbar spine in a patient with diffuse sclerotic metastases from carcinoma of the prostate.

Forensic radiography 14

Introduction (Figs 14.40a–14.40c)

Forensic medicine is defined as the use of medical knowledge, especially pathology, to the purposes of the law, as in determining the cause of death.

Forensic radiography is the use of radiographic knowledge to aid in the implication of forensic medicine. The word forensic comes from the Latin word 'forensic', meaning 'to the forum'. The forum was the basis of Roman law and was a place of public discussion and debate pertinent to the law.

Forensic radiography is the production of images (analogue or digital) utilising radiological techniques to assist pathologists in matters pertaining to the law. Forensic radiology is the interpretation of these images.

This area of radiography is seen as specialism and is undertaken by volunteers, but change has been forced in the last decade due to demand and experience. Lessons have been learnt in the UK to undertake imaging for mass fatalities and recent incidents have ensured a change in practice and highlighted the need for standards in forensic radiographic technique.

It is now deemed a necessity in investigations of mass fatalities, primarily as a means of identification but also as an investigative procedure, to ascertain both cause of death and further information with regard to the logistics of the incident.

Imaging is also required in the identification of individuals whose remains may be badly decomposed or only skeletal. Such identification may be associated with war victims or civil atrocities with victims found in mass graves.

Classifications of forensic radiography

Radiography of a cadaver is undertaken for several different medical purposes:

- Foetal and neonatal.
- Identification.
- Cause of death.

All of these investigations are usually requested under the direction of the Coroner and the attending pathologist will request specific areas to be examined radiographically. Post-mortem imaging may also be requested to identify any previous disease processes or trauma the deceased has suffered from, which may or may not have contributed to their death.

Another area of forensic radiography in either the live or deceased patient is in the assessment of NAI. This is usually confined to paediatrics but also now includes the elderly.

- For elderly abuse queries, the areas to be imaged will be identified by the pathologist but may include a skeletal survey.
- For paediatric abuse queries, the protocol authorised within the place of work must be used for either live or deceased patients.

The foremost pitfall in the radiological diagnosis of abuse is suboptimal radiological imaging, radiographic underexposure or overexposure and poor positioning. A protocol will specify the projections required, the high technical image quality needed to identify the fine changes and disruption of normal bone patterns and exposure parameters to maximise soft-tissue detail and range of contrasts.

Imaging of different regions, alternative/additional projections may also be requested by the pathologist/police surgeon to ascertain the maximum amount of information from the X-ray examination.

There may also be a requirement for ante-mortem forensic radiography to assess suspects who may be carrying drug packages stored in body cavities or ingested. These examinations may be requested by the Police surgeon to detect suspected carriers (mules/traffickers) with ingested packages of drugs who may also be in danger if a package should leak. Such examination may be carried out referred by the A&E department or at airport medical centres. An A&E patient must be treated as a routine referral, whereas the Police surgeon referral is a true forensic examination.

Anatomical terminology

There are few clinical words or terms, which are used purely in this scenario.

Anatomical references are generic whether the patient is live or post mortem.

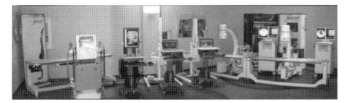

Fig. 14.40a X-ray equipment used for Home Office forensic services.

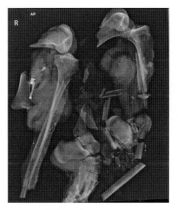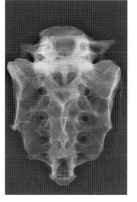

Figs 14.40b and c Radiographs of a forensic anthropology survey.

14 Forensic radiography

Legal issues

The Society and College of Radiographers have recently revised their document *Guidelines for Forensic Radiography*, which was re-issued in Sept 2009.

To ensure parity for all forensic examinations, certain guidelines and methods of recording evidence are necessary. Although the vast majority of forensic radiography will be undertaken using CR/DDR technology producing a digital image, in some more remote sites the examinations may still produce analogue images.

Analogue protocol will include:

- All radiographs taken must be signed by the radiographer.
- Date and identity to be photographed onto the film.
- Number of films and all projections taken to be to be formally noted and signed by the radiographer and a witness.
- No copies made of the original images.

Digital imaging protocols will include:

- All images to include side marker at time of X-ray.
- Two radiographers identified and recorded on Radiology information system (RIS) as operators and practitioners.
- All documents relating to examination scanned into patient file on RIS.
- All images must be saved as taken (i.e. unenhanced) to Trust patient administration system (PACS) and request for copies/CD of images to be authorised appropriate to local policy.[1]

Equipment and accessories

The X-ray equipment required for forensic radiography is variable and dependent on what is available and whether the imaging is to take place off site. It may include:

- Mobile X-ray machine.
- Dental radiographic equipment.
- Fluoroscopy equipment.
- Digital radiographic equipment including image storage facilities.
- CT (on-site or mobile).
- MRI (on-site or mobile).
- Film processing facilities with darkroom (if analogue).
- If standard mobile X-ray machines are to be used then cassettes, grids, film and processing equipment will also be required.
- Cassette size and intensifying screen type is dependent upon the area been examined.

An electricity and water supply will also be required if working off-site with analogue imaging.

Using fluoroscopy or any other digital method of imaging also gives the option of digital storage of the images produced.

Accessories required may include:

- Protective clothing inc. gown/suit, gloves, mask.
- Plastic bags to protect cassettes.
- Cleaning materials.
- Pads and sandbags.
- Radio-opaque markers.
- Stationary.

Local radiation rules

If forensic radiography is undertaken on-site, i.e. on hospital property, then departmental Local Radiation Rules with regard to radiation protection for all radiographic examinations must be adhered to.

Separate local rules will need to be drawn up when working in an emergency mortuary situation. These must include the identification of:

- Radiation Protection Supervisor (RPS).
- Radiation Protection Advisor (RPA); the RPA is the radiographer's employer's (i.e. the hospital's) RPA.
- The definition of a 'controlled area' must be stated including marking boundaries and the erection of warning signs.
- The controlled area must be at least a 2 metre radius from the X-ray tube (vertical beam).
- All personnel within this area must wear protective equipment.
- Monitoring devices must be placed at the boundary of the controlled area.
- For horizontal beam radiography the primary beam, where possible, must be directed towards a primary shield and the controlled area is extended to 6 metres from the X-ray tube.

De-briefing

This structured method of reflective analysis of both the procedures/techniques used and the psychological effects of being involved in any forensic radiography is essential for the welfare and support of those professionals involved. A support mechanism must be provided for these professional volunteers and access to specialist support available if required.

Radiographers must be made aware of the signs and symptoms of stress, and strategies identified to help them cope with this stress.

A de-briefing session after a major incident is standard procedure in the police force and any radiographers involved in these incidents should, where available, participate in these sessions. Hospital support may be offered via Occupational Health to radiographer employees whether the forensic experience was local or not.

The Society and College of Radiographers state that forensic radiography should only be undertaken by *volunteer* radiographers.[2]

Forensic radiography 14

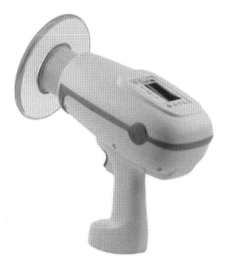

Fig. 14.41a Example of hand held dental X-ray unit.

Dental radiography (Figs 14.41a–14.41d)

The primary radiographic technique used in the identification of a cadaver is the comparison of dental records pre and post mortem. Dental X-rays may be requested and taken at any stage of tissue decomposition. An odontologist/dental surgeon will initially examine the cadaver's dentition to record a plan. In addition to this visual and clinical assessment by the specialist, dental X-rays may also be requested.

The images produced can be evidential proof of cadaver identification when matched to previous dental records. Radiographic detail evaluated includes:

- Fillings and dental intervention.
- Root morphology.
- Unerupted teeth.
- Dental patterns.
- Previous dental surgery will aid the odontologist in the final identification of a cadaver.

Recommended dental projections

The odontologist may request several standard radiographic dental and facial projections.

The primary projections taken to produce maximum information are:

- Intraoral radiographs.
- Lower standard occlusals.
- Upper standard occlusals.
- Mandibular projections.

The technique used, either bisecting angles or paralleling, will be dependent upon that used in the pre-mortem images to ensure reproducibility to aid in comparison of pre-/post-mortem radiological appearances.

The radiographic technique for these projections can be found in the appropriate dental/facial sections of this book (Sections 8 and 9).

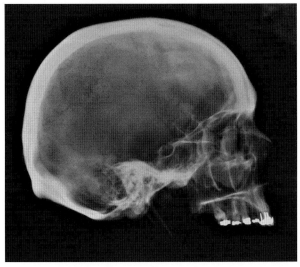

Fig. 14.41b Radiograph of a lateral skull showing extensive dental work.

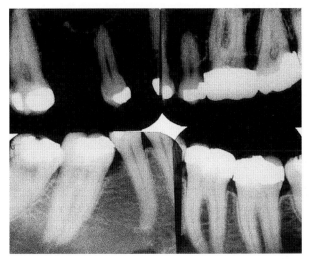

Fig. 14.41c Post-mortem bite-wing radiographs of teeth.

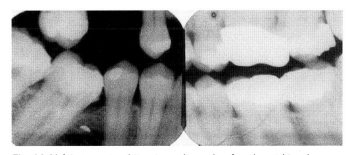

Fig. 14.41d Ante-mortem bite-wing radiographs of teeth matching the post-mortem radiographs seen in the adjacent images.

14 Forensic radiography

General radiography (Figs 14.42a–14.42d)

Adaptation of technique

Several changes to normal radiographic technique for both dental and general forensic radiography examinations may be required. The majority of forensic radiography is carried out distant from the Imaging department, using mobile radiographic equipment and is usually undertaken in either a permanent or temporary mortuary.

The physical state of the cadaver will determine the number and type of projections that will be acquired and the technique that can be employed. The cadaver may be contained (e.g. 'body bag'); whilst this is advantageous with regard to Health and Safety and cross infection, it does limit any changes to be made in positioning of the cadaver for X-ray examination.

Care must be taken to ensure that no sharp or dangerous objects are present in the body or body bag. The radiographer needs to be aware of these potential dangers of injury to himself/herself and others. Thus no protocol can be formalised for forensic imaging as the examination is dependent on many variables.

Adaptations will be required to all standard radiographic techniques for each examination taken. Imaging may be undertaken using a selection of cassettes/DDR systems in order to provide full coverage of the body. Alternatively, imaging may be undertaken using a mobile C-arm fluoroscopic system enabling full screening of the body to identify specific abnormalities. Such systems will incorporate an imaging recording system in order to record and catalogue forensic images and features.

When using such equipment to image a body bag it is important that a fluoroscopic technique is adopted that allows for overlapping of areas of the body, to ensure that no area of the body is left unimaged. The C-arm should be moved in a set pattern; the use of floor markings will aid the radiographer to ensure overlapping of the image intensifier field.

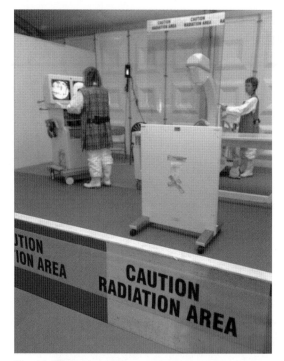

Fig. 14.42b Temporary mortuary set up.

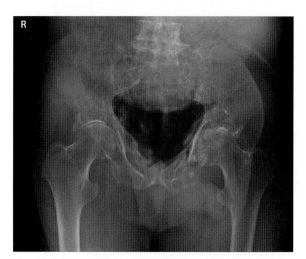

Fig. 14.42c Pelvic image taken mid-post mortem.

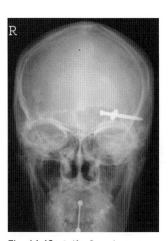

Fig. 14.42a Self-inflicted injury using a nail gun at point blank range.

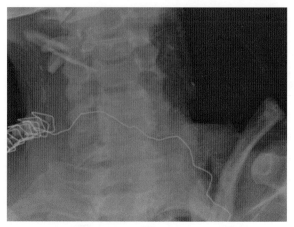

Fig. 14.42d Road traffic fatality seeking cause of death.

Mobile image intensifier fluoroscopic technique to image a body bag for screening purposes

The Primary survey using an image intensifier (II) is generally undertaken whilst the cadaver is sealed in a body bag and a precise technique must be used to ensure every region of the bag has been covered and imaged. The following imaging technique can be employed:

- The mobile II base and patient trolley positions are marked longitudinally on the floor and the II arm is fully extended to cover the most distal aspect of the trolley upon which the body bag is placed. The II is then moved longitudinally with all locks positive except the lateral base movement to traverse the length of the trolley.
- When one length is completed the II arm extension is decreased by 20–25 cm dependent on field size, which in itself is dependent on ORD and hence any image magnification.
- The length of the trolley is traversed again ensuring overlap with the previous path, and when the end of the trolley is reached the arm extension is again reduced and the II returns longitudinally along the length of the trolley.

If at any point the fluoroscopy needs to be stopped then the region in view can simply be marked with forceps placed on the bag or by drawing directly on the bag and imaging resumed when possible (ensuring there is no movement of the body bag in between). The II base may be required to be moved depending on trolley size and length of intensifier arm extension; any changes can again be marked on the flooring to ensure parity between examinations.

Whilst one radiographer is undertaking the fluoroscopy using a technique that verifies all regions are covered, another team

Forensic radiography 14

General radiography (*cont.*) (Figs 14.43a, 14.43b)

member is acting as scribe using a four quadrant map to identify any specific features requiring further investigation.

Often this Primary survey can highlight personal items that can help to identify the deceased such as MP3 players, mobile phones, wallets/purses containing bank/credit cards, etc. The scribe will identify the position of these items on the map using a key code to categorise them.

The Primary survey may also demonstrate any injuries or misplacement of limbs/body parts and can easily demonstrate joint replacements, which are all serial coded and hence a positive aid in victim identification.

The pathologist in charge of the case may be present during the Primary survey or called to witness any particularly interesting or puzzling items demonstrated radiographically. Images can be taken of the items noted on the plan and all information should be passed on and signed off as evidence to the team working with the pathologist.

The Primary survey is pre post-mortem examination.

Where necessary two projections are taken at right-angles of a specific area. This may be required to provide further information on the nature and extent of a sustained injury.

Images may also be required of sections of the body that have been removed by the pathologist for more detailed forensic examination.

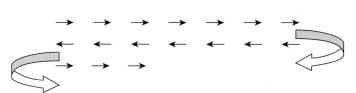

Fig. 14.43a Diagram showing imaging technique.

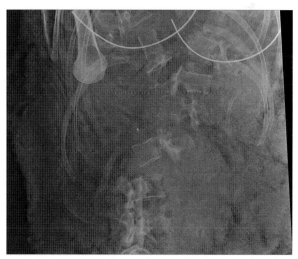

Fig. 14.43b Forensic image of a disarticulated decomposing subject.

14 Forensic radiography

Still born (15–40 weeks)

General comments

- A skeletal survey is undertaken, at the request of the Coroner for the pathologist.
- Identification is by referral card and is cross checked with the identification bands on the limbs of the foetus.
- The technique, normally employed is that of a full skeletal survey as per departmental protocol. Alternatively whole body AP and lateral 'babygrams' may be acquired but most departments have updated in keeping with forensic and pathological guidelines.
- Dependent upon the gestational age of the foetus, additional fronto-occipital and lateral skull images may be taken.
- Images are acquired using a CR/DDR system or occasionally using a 400 speed screen/film system in a standard cassette.
- Images should be shown to a specialist paediatric radiologist.
- Further images may be requested dependent upon any abnormalities that are identified at the time of imaging

Imaging technique

- As health and safety of the staff is imperative and the images/examination may be used as forensic evidence, the standard recommendation is that two radiographers perform the examination.
- The X-ray room is prepared if the examination is in the Imaging department, otherwise adequate additional equipment and accessories should be taken to the mortuary.

Antero-posterior 'babygram' (Figs 14.44a, 14.44b)

- The foetus is placed onto the covered CR cassette in the supine position.
- The limbs are positioned AP where possible. It may be necessary to support these in place by using plastic strips taped down over the limbs or covered sandbags.
- The X-ray tube is centred and collimated to include all the relevant anatomy. (Specific techniques are detailed in Section 13.)
- Lead markers are placed into the collimated area.
- Exposure factors should be selected consistent with size of the foetus.

Notes

Normally X-ray rooms and mobiles used for this purpose have a detailed exposure chart consistent with foetal size (e.g. 60 kV, 2.5 mAs, without a grid for a 25-week-old foetus).

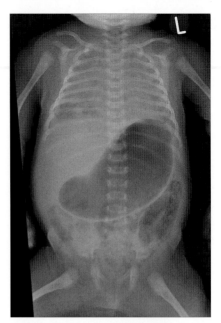

Fig. 14.44a Part of skeletal survey investigation.

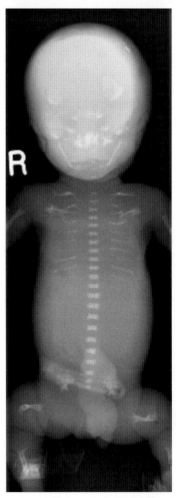

Fig. 14.44b Example of antero-posterior whole body image of foetus.

Identification

The imaging CR cassette is processed immediately ensuring the correct information and orientation is on the image including date and identification number.

Lateral 'babygram' (Fig. 14.45a)

- The foetus is placed onto the CR covered cassette in the lateral position. The cassette size is dependent upon the size of the foetus.
- The limbs are positioned lateral where possible. It may be necessary to support these in place by using plastic strips taped down over the limbs/covered sandbags or soft roll.
- The X-ray tube is centred and collimated to include all the relevant anatomy. (Specific techniques are detailed in Section 13.)
- Lead markers are placed into the collimated area. It may be necessary to mark individual limbs to ensure correct identification.
- Exposure factors should be selected consistent with size of the foetus.

Notes

Normally X-ray rooms used for this purpose have a detailed exposure chart (example 60 kV, 1.6 mAs, without a grid for a 25-week-old foetus).

Identification

The imaging CR cassette is processed immediately ensuring the correct information is on the image including the date, patient identification number and radiographer identity.

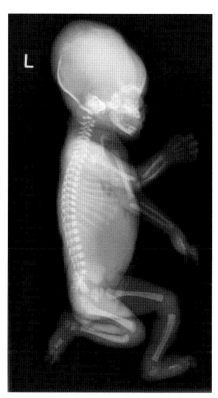

Fig. 14.45a Example of lateral whole body image of foetus.

Forensic radiography 14

Still born (15–40 weeks) (cont.)

Skull – fronto-occipital (Figs 14.45b, 14.45c)

- The foetus is placed onto the covered 18 × 24 cm CR cassette in the supine position.
- The head is normally flexed forward at presentation but a covered 15° wedge may be placed under the shoulders to bring the orbito-meatal line at right-angles to the receptor.
- Soft rolls or covered pads are used to immobilise the skull and prevent rotation.
- The remainder of the technique is as described in Section 13.
- Normally X-ray rooms used for this purpose have a detailed exposure chart (e.g. 56 kV, 2.5 mAs, without a grid for a 25-week-old foetus).

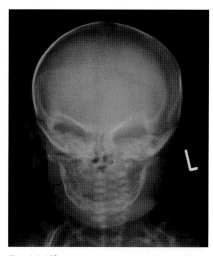

Fig. 14.45b Fronto-occipital skull image for sudden infant death syndrome (SIDS) investigation.

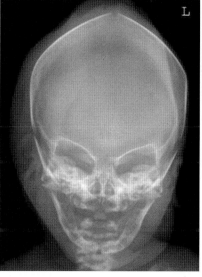

Fig. 14.45c Fronto-occipital image of skull for skeletal survey of a foetus.

14 Forensic radiography

Lateral skull (Fig. 14.46)

- The foetus is turned into the lateral position with the head resting on the covered 18 × 24 cm CR cassette.
- A soft roll or covered pad may be placed to under the face to bring it parallel with the table and cassette.
- The remainder of the technique is as described in Section 13.
- Normally X-ray rooms used for this purpose have a detailed exposure chart (e.g. 60 kV, 2 mAs, without a grid for a 25-week-old foetus).

An alternative technique is to use a horizontal beam lateral. This may be required dependent upon the presentation of the foetus.

Identification

The imaging CR cassettes are processed immediately ensuring the correct orientation and information is on the image, including the date, patient identity number and radiographer identity.

Post procedure

- The X-ray equipment and room are cleaned according to hospital protocol.
- The referral card and images (where appropriate) are presented to the radiologist for report.

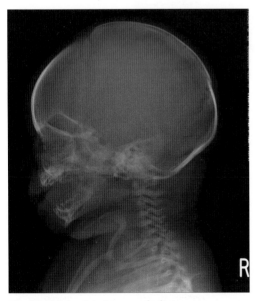

Fig. 14.46 Lateral skull image of a foetus.

Skeletal survey – out of hours

Skeletal survey protocols for cot death and other such fatalities as well as NAI investigations in children are discussed in detail in Section 13. However, in the 'out of hours' situation a protocol should be adopted similar to the one described below, which will assist as a reminder and guide for all those involved in this task. It is often the case that such requests are made infrequently and such a protocol will be helpful in determining the roles and responsibilities of every member of the team. Included on the page are some images for the standard radiography series.

Example protocol

- The accident and emergency sister/mortuary technician to liaise with the on-call radiographer.
- All surveys should be performed in the X-ray department
- A decision is made on the time to perform the survey. (Note that this should be during normal working hours where possible.)
- The lead paediatric radiologist must be informed when the survey is to be performed on a child.
- The on-call radiologist must be informed when the procedure is performed on an adult.
- The entire examination must be witnessed. This may be the sister from A&E, a police officer or coroner officer.
- Witnesses must be present throughout the procedure and not leave the subject unattended at any time.
- The subject must be correctly identified, all images labelled correctly with name and date. Side markers should be present on all projections at the time of the examination.
- At the end of the procedure the digital images are burnt to CD and this with a radiologist report should be handed over to the Coroner's officer.
- In extreme circumstances, i.e. when the Coroner requests to move the body before a radiologist arrives, then it is important to ensure that the referral card is given to the appropriate radiologist for them to issue a report later, as follows:

Compiled by: ....

Name of authoriser: ....

Date of protocol: ....

Review date: ....

Forensic radiography 14

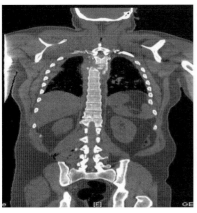
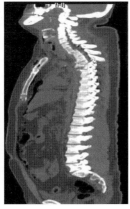

Fig. 14.47a and b Post-mortem CT scan of male involved in fatal road traffic accident.

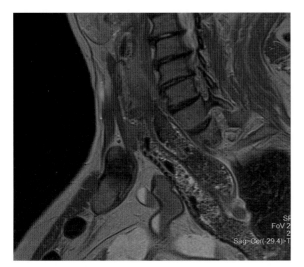

Fig. 14.47c Choking incident resulting in sudden death.

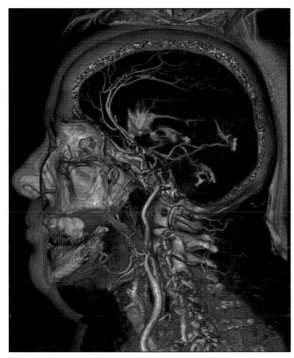

Fig. 14.47d Example of virtopsy image demonstrating detail of imaging.

The future (Figs 14.47a–14.47e)

Forensic radiography has developed dramatically in the last 30 years due to equipment and software changes and the experiences of radiographers and healthcare professionals involved in forensic radiographic examinations.

Due to the increased requirement of imaging as part of the standard post-mortem investigative procedures in specific cases of suspicious death or victim identification, local agreements within Trusts may include CT and even MRI examinations.[3]

It is a possibility that CT may replace other modalities in forensic radiology and potentially some autopsies, mainly those on trauma patients. However, further research is still needed in this area to prove the validity of CT as the prime modality in forensic radiology work.

One method of post-mortem imaging that is currently evolving with continuing research is 'virtopsy'. This is a non-invasive method of 'virtual autopsy' of the deceased.

Virtopsy is a multi-disciplinary, applied research project that uses laser surface scanning, 3D-photogrammetry, CT, and MRI to document forensic evidence in a non-invasive and observer-independent manner in both living and deceased subjects. The information obtained via this combination of imaging techniques is permanent and can be used for review at a later stage if required, whereas tissue will decompose and information/evidence will be lost.

The aim of virtopsy is to combine the advantages of cutting edge imaging technology with the time-tested traditional knowledge of forensic autopsy, in order to develop best practice in forensic investigations.[4]

Another new method of forensic radiology is CT angiography, used primarily to demonstrate coronary artery disease, stroke and pulmonary embolus. These are best visualised by CT with the enhancement of contrast media. Contrast-enhanced CT is also crucial in the investigation of trauma victims. However, both of these investigations rely on cardiovascular function and blood circulation, therefore an alternative method using a heart/lung machine to introduce the contrast medium is currently being researched.[5]

These new methods of cadaveric imaging are dependent upon expertise, cost and availability and are still under research. At present the basic radiography and fluoroscopy procedures that have been used remain a standard.[6]

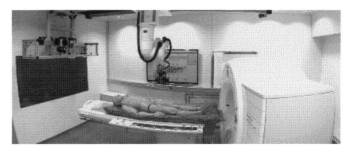

Fig. 14.47e Example of a Virtopsy imaging laboratory.

References/Further reading

Section 1 Basic principles of radiography and digital technology

1. Ionising Radiation (Medical Exposure) Regulations (2000) IRMER.
2. The Ionising Radiations Regulations (1999) Statutory Instrument 1999 No. 3232. Available at http://www.opsi.gov.uk/si/si1999/19993232.htm.
3. The Society and College of Radiographers (2014). Use of anatomical markers. London.
4. Hardy M, Snaith B (2011) The impact of radiographer immediate reporting on patient outcomes and service delivery within the emergency department: designing a randomized controlled trial. *Radiography* 17:275–279.
5. Royal College of Radiologists (2010) Medical image interpretation by radiographers: Guidance for radiologists and healthcare providers. http://www.rcr.ac.uk/docs/radiology/pdf/BFCR(10)3_Medical_interpretation.pdf.
6. Donovan N (2013) McGrigor's lines. http://www.skullandface.info/skullfacial/mcgrigors_lines.html. (Accessed 16/09/2014)
7. Williams IJ (2013) Appendicular skeleton: ABCs image interpretation search strategy. *The South African Radiographer* 51(2):9–14.
8. Sloane *et al.* (2010) Clark's Pocket Handbook for Radiographers. Hodder Education pp. 24–27.
9. Control of Substances Hazardous to Health Regulations 2002. HSE, UK.
10. Royal College of Radiologists (RCR) (2008) Electronic Remote Requesting. [Online]. Available from: http://www.rcr.ac.uk/docs/radiology/pdf/ITguidance_Electronic_Remote_Requesting.pdf. (Accessed 01/10/2013.)
11. National Electrical Manufacturers Association (2013) The DICOM Standard – 2013. [Online]. Available from: http://medical.nema.org/standard.html. (Accessed 01/10/2013.)
12. National Electrical Manufacturers Association (2013) About DICOM. [Online]. Available from: http://medical.nema.org/Dicom/about-DICOM.html. (Accessed 01/10/2013).
13. International Organization for Standardization (1994) Information Technology – Open Systems Interconnection – Basic Reference Model: The Basic Model. [Online]. http://standards.iso.org/ittf/PubliclyAvailableStandards/s020269_ISO_IEC_7498-1_1994(E).zip. (Accessed 01/10/2013.)
14. Health Level 7 (2013) Standards 2013. [Online]. Available from: http://www.hl7.org/implement/standards/ (Accessed 01/10/2013.)
15. Hiles P, Mackenzie A, Scally A, Wall B (2005) IPEM Report 91: Recommended standards for the routine performance testing of diagnostic x-ray imaging systems.
16. Honey ID, Mackenzie A (2009) Artifacts found during quality assurance testing of computed radiography and digital radiography detectors. *Journal of Digital Imaging* 22(4): 383–392.
17. Shetty CM, Barthur A, Kambadakone A, Narayanan N, Kv R (2011) Computed radiography image artifacts revisited. *American Journal of Roentgenology* 196(1):W37–W47.
18. Holmes K, Elkington M, Harris P (2014) *Clark's Essential Physics for Radiographers*. CRC Press.
19. International Atomic Energy Agency (2014) Radiation Protection in Diagnostic and Interventional Radiology. Available from: https://rpop.iaea.org/RPOP/RPoP/Content/AdditionalResources/Training/1_TrainingMaterial/Radiology.htm. (Accessed 16/09/2014.)
20. X-rays; How safe are they? Health Protection Agency UK (archived).
21. HPA–CRCE-034 – Doses to Patients from Radiographic and Fluoroscopic X-ray Imaging Procedures in the UK – 2010 Review. Hart D, Hiller MC, Shrimpton PC.
22. The Basic Safety Standards (BSS) Directive (2013/59/Euratom).

Section 3 Shoulder

1. Goud A, Segal D, Hedayati P, Pan JJ, Weissman BN (2008) Radiographic evaluation of the shoulder. *European Journal of Radiology* 68:2–15.
2. Sanders G, Jersey S (2005) Conventional radiography of the shoulder. *Seminars in Roentgenology* 40(3):207–22.
3. Garth WP, Slappey CE, Ochs CW (1984) Roentgenographic demonstration of instability of the shoulder: the apical oblique projection; a technical note. *The Journal of Bone and Joint Surgery* 66(9):1450–3.
4. Kornguth P, Salazar A (1987) The apical oblique view of the shoulder: its usefullness in acute trauma. *American Journal of Roentgenology* 149:113–16.
5. Richardson JB, Ramsay A, Davidson JK, Kelly IG (1988) Radiographs in shoulder trauma. *The Journal of Bone and Joint Surgery* 70(3):457–60.
6. Manaster BJ (1997) *Handbook of Skeletal Radiology*, 2nd edn. St Louis: Mosby.

Section 4 Lower limb

1. Gupta RT, Wadhwa RP, Learch TJ, Herwick SM (2008) Lisfranc injury: imaging fndings for this important but often-missed diagnosis. *Current Problems In Diagnostic Radiology* 37(3):115–26.
2. Bachmann LM, Kolb E, Koller MT, Steurer J, ter Riet G (2003) Accuracy of Ottawa ankle rules to exclude fractures of the ankle and mid-foot: systematic review. *British Medical Journal* 326(7386):417–19.
3. Raby N, Berman L, de Lacey G (2005) *Accident & Emergency Radiology: A Survival Guide*, 2nd edn. Elsevier Saunders.
4. Varich L, Bancroft L (2010) Radiologic case study: talocalcaneal coalition. *Orthopedics* 33(6):374–452.
5. Taweel NR, Raikin SM, Karanjia HN, Ahmad J (2013) The proximal fibula should be examined in all patients with ankle injury: a case series of missed maisonneuve fractures. *Journal of Emergency Medicine* 44(2):251–5.
6. Shagam JY (2011) Medical imaging and osteoarthritis of the knee. *Radiologic Technology* 83(1):37–56.
7. Hu YL, Je FG, Ji AY, Qiao GX, Liu HF (2009) Three-dimensional computed tomography imaging increases the reliability of classification systems for tibial plateau fractures. *Injury* 40(12):1282–5.
8. Hall FM (1975) Radiographic diagnosis and accuracy in knee joint effusions. *Radiology* 115(1):49–54.
9. Furguson, J, Knottenbelt, JD (1994) Lipohaemarthrosis in knee trauma: an experience of 907 cases. *Injury* 25(5):311–2.
10. Paley D, Tetsworth K (1992) Mechanical axis deviation of the lower limbs. Preoperative planning of uniapical angular deformities of the tibia or femur. *Clinical Orthopedics and Related Research* 280:65–71.
11. Krackow KA (2008) Measurement and analysis of axial deformity of the knee. http://www.ubortho.buffalo.edu/axialdeformity.pdf (Accessed 19/12/2014.)

Section 5 Hip, pelvis and sacro-iliac joints

1. Blain H, Chavassieux P, Portero-Muzy N, *et al.* (2008) Cortical and trabecular bone distribution in the femoral neck in osteoporosis and osteoarthritis. *Bone* 43(5):862–8.
2. Smithsonian National Museum of Natural History (2014) http://anthropology.si.edu/writteninbone/male_female.html (Accessed 19/12/2014.)
3. Tannast M, Siebenrock KA, Anderson SE (2007) Femoroacetabular impingement: radiographic diagnosis– what the radiologist should know. *American Journal of Roentgenology* 188:1540–52. www.ajronline.org/doi/abs/10.2214/AJR.06.0921 (Accessed Jan 2015.)
4. Obaid AK, Barleben A, Porral D, Lush S, Cinat M (2006) Utility of plain film pelvic radiographs in blunt trauma patients in the emergency department. *The American Surgeon* 72(10):951–4. Published Online: March 05, 2014.
5. Barral T (2004) Lateral air gap technique. *Synergy* Jan:20–3.
6. Foster K (2014) The limping child, BIR. FRCR, Birmingham Children's Hospital. Published Online March 05, 2014: DOI: http://dx.doi.org/10.1259/imaging/46032468.

Section 6 Vertebral column

1. Powell JN, Waddell JP, Tucker WS, Transfeldt EE (1989) Multiple-level non-contiguous spinal fractures. *Journal of Trauma* 29:1146–51.

Section 7 Thorax and upper airways

1. European Guidelines on quality criteria for diagnostic radiographic images – EUR 16260 EN http://www.sprmn.pt/legislacao/ficheiros/EuropeanGuidelineseur16260.pdf (Accessed December 2014.)
2. Galea A, Durran A, Adlan T, *et al.* (2014) Practical applications of digital tomosynthesis of the chest. *Clinical Radiology* 69:424–30.
3. Unett EM, Carver BJ (2001) The chest X-ray: centring points and central rays – can we stop confusing our students and ourselves? *Synergy* November:16.
4. HPA-CRCE-034 – Doses to patients from radiographic and fluoroscopic X-ray imaging procedures in the UK – 2010 Review.
5. AP Chest positioning landmarks http://www.bing.com/videos/search?q=AP+CHEST+X-RAY&docid=608052637940254409&mid=E948E8B2D4FA9EE31C32E948E8B2D4FA9EE31C32&view=detail&FORM=VIRE5#view=detail&mid=E948E8B2D4FA9EE31C32E948E8B2D4FA9EE31C32 (Accessed December 2014.)
6. Collins J, Stern EJ (2007) *Chest Radiology, the Essentials*. Lippincott Williams & Wilkins, ISBN:0781763142.
7. Novelline RA (2004) *Squire's Fundamentals of Radiology*. Harvard University Press, ISBN:0674012798.

Section 8 Skull, facial bones and sinuses

1. Clements, R Ponsford, A (1991) A modified view of the facial bones in the seriously injured. *Radiography Today* 57(646):10–12.
2. NICE (2014) www.nice.org.uk/guidance/CG176 2014
3. www.nice.org.uk/guidance/CG176/chapter/introduction
4. www.headway.org.uk/glasgow-coma-scale.aspx

5 Denton BK (1998) Improving plain radiography of the skull: the half-axial projection re-described. *Synergy* August:9–11.

6 UW Medicine, Department of Radiology. Improving Patient Care Today and Leading to the Future of Imaging Science and Healthcare, Facial & Mandibular Fractures.

7 www.imageinterpretation.co.uk/face.html (Accessed Aug 2014.)

8 http://bestpractice.bmj.com/best-practice/monograph/398/resources/images/print/16.html (Accessed October 2014.)

9 www.rad.washington.edu/academics/academic-sections/msk/teaching-materials/online-musculoskeletal-radiology-book/facial-and-mandibular-fractures (Accessed August 2014.)

10 European Commisson *European Guidelines on Quality Criteria for Diagnostic Radiography Images.* EUR 16260 EN.

Section 9 Dental radiography

Brettle DS (2001) A digital frame of reference for viewing digital images. *British Journal of Radiology* 74:69–72.

European Commission (2004) Radiation Protection 136. *European Guidelines on Radiation Protection in Dental Radiology.* The safe use of radiographs in dental practice.

European Commission (2012) Radiation Protection 172. *Cone beam CT for Dental and Maxillofacial Radiology* (Evidence-based Guidelines).

Faculty of General Dental Practitioners (2004) *Selection Criteria for Dental Radiography*, 2nd edn.

Hart D, Wall BF (2002) *Radiation Exposure of the UK Population from Medical and Dental X-ray Examinations.* NRPB-W4. ISBN 0-85951-468-4.

Hart D, Wall BF, Hillier MC, Shrimpton PC (2010) HPA-CRCE-012 *Frequency and Collective Dose for Medical and Dental X-ray Examinations in the UK.* ISBN: 978-0-85951-684-6.

Horner K, Jacobs R, Schulze R (2013) Dental CBCT equipment and performance issues. *Radiation Protection Dosimetry* 153:212–8.

HPA-CRCE -010 – Prepared by the HPA Working Party on Dental Cone Beam CT Equipment http://www.hpa.org.uk/webc/HPAwebFile/HPAweb_C/1287143862981. (Accessed 04/01/2015.)

Isaacson KG, Thom AR, Horner K, Whaites E (2008) *Guidelines for the Use of Radiographs in Clinical Orthodontics*, 3rd edn.

National Radiological Protection Board (2001) *Guidance Notes for Dental Practitioners on the Safe Use of X-ray Equipment.* Department of Health.

Nemtoi A, (2013) Cone beam CT: a current overview of devices. *Dentomaxillofacial Radiology* 42: 20120443.

Rushton, VE, Horner, KA (1994) Comparative study of five periapical radiographic techniques in general dental practice. *Dentomaxillofacial Radiology* 23:37–45, 96.

Rushton VE, Horner K, Worthington H (1999) The quality of panoramic radiographs in a sample of general dental practices. *British Dentistry Journal* 186:630–3.

Report of a Joint Working Party for the Study of Orthodontics and the British Society of Dental and Maxillofacial Radiology (1985) The reduction of the dose to patients during lateral cephalometric radiography. *British Journal of Orthodontics* 12:176–8.

Semple J, Gibb D (1982) The postero-anterior lower occlusal view – a routine projection for the submandibular gland. *Radiography* 48:122–4.

Specialised textbooks on dental radiography

Horner K, Drage N, Brettle D (2008) *21st Century Imaging. Quintessentials of Dental Practice.* ISBN 9781850970972.

Horner K, Rout J, Rushton VE (2002) *Interpreting Dental Radiographs. Quintessentials of Dental Practice.* ISBN 1850970521.

Rushton VE, Rout J (2006) *Panoramic Radiography. Quintessentials of Dental Practice.* ISBN 1850970807.

Section 10 Abdomen and pelvic cavity

1 Standring S (2008) *Grays Anatomy.* Elsevier/Churchill Livingstone.

2 IRefer Making the best use of clinical radiology: http://www.rcr.ac.uk/content.aspx?PageID=995.

3 European Commission (1996) European Guidelines on Quality Criteria for Diagnostic Radiographic Images– EUR 16260 EN http://www.sprmn.pt/legislacao/ficheiros/EuropeanGuidelineseur16260.pdf. (Accessed 05/01/2015.)

4 Bontranger K, Lampignano J (2014) *Textbook of Radiographic Positioning and Related Anatomy*, 8th Edition. Elsevier Health Sciences.

5 MRCP (2013) http://mrcpstudy.com/renal stones/ (Accessed 05/01/2015.)

6 Miller RE (1973) The technical approach to the acute abdomen. *Seminars in Roentgenology* 8:267–9.

7 NHS Abdominal Aortic Aneurysm Screening Programme 2014. http://aaa.screening.nhs.uk/ (Accessed 05/01/2015.)

8 http://www.bing.com/images/search?q=oblique+kidney+x-ray&view=detailv2&&&id=56C59EB90801A3F6E116622 3E83C381CC45CA450&selectedIndex=0&ccid=cxxEEBt g&simid=607995459362489831&thid=JN.aorwHD5Xv1 %2bNy1ztc2xetA&ajaxhist=0 (Last Accessed 25/6/2015.)

9 Bortoff G, Chen M (2000) *Gallbladder Stones: Imaging and Intervention.* RadioGraphics RSNA Education.

https://www.google.co.uk/search?q=oblique+x-ray+abdomen&client=safari&hl=en-gb&tbm=isch&tbo=u&source= univ&fir=QSZzofXSCgTMUM%253A%252CL_pzfg3 FSYQZxM%252C_%253B1bM0rBNanmFtJM%253A %252CL_pzfg3FSYQZxM%252C_%253B4xILZxy0w

Vc0lM%253A%252CGqGPa2IeavicLM%252C_%253BG2T_MT2_hgde7M%253A%252C0VFFiWCAyxQ-TM%252C_%253BtEbi-ZJXVZOQeM%253A%252CEDBr7lGLLjAFZM%252C_&usg=__7n4uCEmk0SGRebWcJ2ISTVPK3Ck%3D&sa=X&ei=MDGKVYjdL6Ka7gbI4IGQCQ&ved=0CDEQ7Ak"\l"imgrc=4xILZxy0wVc0lM%253A%3BGqGPa2IeavicLM%3Bhttp%253A%252F%252Fimages.radiopaedia.org%252Fimages%252F1709692%252Fd3cacdc3c23526c71d715ed354f9cb_big_gallery.jpg%3Bhttp%253A%252F%252Fradiopaedia.org%252Fcases%252Fureteric-calculus-1%3B490%3B630&usg=__7n4uC https://www.google.co.uk/search?q=oblique+x-ray+abdomen&client=safari&hl=en-gb&tbm=isch&tbo=u&source=univ&fir=QSZzofXSCgTMUM%253A%252CL_pzfg3FSYQZxM%252C_%253B1bM0rBNanmFtJM%253A%252CL_pzfg3FSYQZxM%252C_%253B4xILZxy0wVc0lM%253A%252CGqGPa2IeavicLM%252C_%253BG2T_MT2_hgde7M%253A%252C0VFFiWCAyxQ-TM%252C_%253BtEbi-ZJXVZOQeM%253A%252CEDBr7lGLLjAFZM%252C_&usg=__7n4uCEmk0SGRebWcJ2ISTVPK3Ck%3D&sa=X&ei=MDGKVYjdL6Ka7gbI4IGQCQ&ved=0CDEQ7Ak#imgrc=4xILZxy0wVc0lM%253A%3BGqGPa2IeavicLM%3Bhttp%253A%252F%252Fimages.radiopaedia.org%252Fimages%252F1709692%252Fd3cacdc3c23526c71d715ed354f9cb_big_gallery.jpg%3Bhttp%253A%252F%252Fradiopaedia.org%252Fcases%252Fureteric-calculus-1%3B490%3B630&usg=__7n4uCEmk0SGRebWcJ2ISTVPK3Ck%3D (Last Accessed 25/6/2015).

Section 11 Ward radiography

1. Society and College of Radiographers (2006) *Health Care Associated Infections (HCAIs). Practical Guidance and Advice.* London.
2. http://www.nhs.uk/conditions/clostridium-difficile/pages/introduction.aspx (Accessd 05/01/2015.)
3. http://wardray-premise.com/xray/equipment/positioning_and_scaling.html#lateral_cassette_holders (Accessed 06/01/2015.)
4. http://www.npsa.nhs.uk/corporate/news/reducing-the-harm-caused-by-misplaced-nasogastric-feeding-tubes-in-adults-children-and-infants/ (Accessed 12/01/2015.)
5. Law RL, Pullyblank AM, Eveleigh M, et al. (2013) Avoiding never events: improving nasogastric intubation practice and standards. *Clinical Radiology* 68:239–44.
6. National Patient Safety Agency (2010) Nasogastric tube audit of junior doctors. Available at: http://www.nrls.npsa.nhs.uk/resources/search-by-audience/junior-doctor/junior-doctor-audit. (Accessed 06/01/2015.)

Section 12 Theatre radiography

1. Holmes K (2011) Key radiographic skills in the operating theatre. ECR Refresher Course Programme March (Invited review).
2. World Health Organization (WHO) (2009) Guidelines for Safe Surgery: Safe Surgery Saves Lives. (WHO/IER/PSP/2008.08-1E).
3. The Ionising Radiations Regulations (1999) Statutory Instrument 1999 No. 3232. Available at http://www.opsi.gov.uk/si/si1999/19993232.htm
4. Mettler FA, Huda, Yoshizumi TT, Mahesh M (2008) Effective doses in radiology and diagnostic nuclear medicine: A catalog. *Radiology* 248(1):254–63.
5. Hart A, Wall BF (2002) Radiation exposure of the UK population from medical and dental X-ray examinations. NRPB-W4.
6. Whitley S, Alsop C, Moore A (1999) *Clark's Special Procedures in Diagnostic Imaging*, 11th and 12th edn. Oxford: Butterworth–Heinemann.

Section 13 Paediatric radiography

1. Unscear (2008) Report: *Sources, Effects and Risks of Ionizing Radiation* (www.uncrear.org).
2. UK Government (1974) ALARP, As low as reasonably practical. Risk assessment. Health and Safety at Work Act (www.hse.gov.uk).
3. Council Directive (1994) 84/466 Euratom, Official Journal L 265/1 5.10.1994. Basic Safety Standards 2013/59/Euratom. eur-lex.europa.eu.
4. CEC (1996) European Guidelines on Quality Criteria for Diagnostic Radiographic Images in Paediatrics (EUR 16261). ISBN 92-827-7843-6.
5. Health Protection Agency, UK (2000) Recommended national reference doses for individual radiographs on paediatric patients, review, updated 2009 (www.hpa.org.uk).
6. IPEM (2004) Guidance on the establishment and use of diagnostic reference levels for medical X-ray examinations. Report. www.ipem.ac.uk.
7. The Ionising Radiation (Medical Exposure) Regulations (2000) European Directive 97/43/Euratom, www.dh.gov.uk.
8. Hart D, Wall BF, Shrimpton PC, Bungay DR, Dance DR (2000) NRPB -R318- Reference doses and patient size in paediatric radiology. www.hpa.org.uk.
9. Radiation and Nuclear Safety Authority, Finland. www.stuk.fi.
10. ICRP (2007) The 2007 Recommendations of the International Commission on Radiological Protection, ICRP Publication 103, Ann, ICRP 37 (2-4) and ICRP publication 34 ICRP 1982, 9(2–3). www.icrp.org.
11. The Royal College of Radiologists (2012) iRefer: Making the best use of clinical radiology. www.rcr.org.uk.
12. Children's Act (2004) www.legislation.gov.uk.
13. Royal College of Radiologists and Royal College of Paediatrics and Child Health (2008) Standards for Radiological Investigations of suspected NAI, BFCR (08) 1. www.rcr.ac.uk and www.rcpch.ac.uk.
14. Society of Radiographers. www.sor.org.

15 Korner M, Weber CH, Wirth S, Pfeifer KJ, Reiser MF, Treitl M (2007) Advances in digital radiography: physical principles and system overview. *Radiographics* 27:675–86.

16 Brosi P, Stuessi A, Verdun FR, Vock P, Wolf R (2011) Copper filtration in paediatric digital X-ray imaging: its impact on image quality and dose. *Radiological Physics and Technology* 4(2):148–55.

17 McDaniel DL, Cohen G, Wagner LK, Robinson LH (1984) Relative dose efficiencies of antiscatter grids and air gaps in paediatric radiography. *Medical Physics* 11(4):508–12.

18 Hansen J, Jurik AG, Flirgaard B, Egund N (2003) Optimisation of scoliosis examinations in children. *Paediatric Radiology* 33(11):752–65.

19 Kottamasu SR, Kuhns LR, Stringer DA (1997) Pediatric musculoskeletal computed radiography. *Pediatric Radiology* 27:563–75.

20 Willis CE (2004) Strategies for dose reduction in ordinary radiographic examinations using CR and DR. *Paediatric Radiology* 34(Suppl. 3):S196–S200, DOI: 10.1007/s00247-004-1269-6.

21 Huda W (2004) Assessment of the problem: paediatric doses in screen-film and digital radiography. *Paediatric Radiology* 34(Suppl. 3):S173–S182, DOI: 10.1007/s00247-004-1267-8.

22 Sanchez Jacob R, Vano-Galvan E, Vano E, *et al.* (2009) Optimising the use of computed radiography in pediatric chest imaging. *Journal of Digital Imaging* 22(2):104–13 Epub 2007 Sep13.

23 International Commission on Radiological Protection (2004) *Managing Patient Dose in Digital Radiography*. ICRP Publication 93, ann. ICRP 34(1). www.icrp.org.

24 Hufton AP, Doyle SM, Carty HM (1998) Digital radiography in paediatrics: radiation dose considerations and magnitude of possible dose reduction. *British Journal of Radiology* 71(842):186–99.

25 Willis CE, Slovis TL (2004) The ALARA concept in pediatric CR and DR: dose reduction in pediatric radiographic exams – a white paper conference Executive Summary. *Pediatric Radiology* 34:S162–4.

26 Strauss KJ, Poznauski L (2005) Practical applications of CR in paediatric imaging. *Applied Radiology* (June Suppl) S12–8.

27 Vano E, Martinez D, Fernandez JM, *et al.* (2008) Paediatric entrance doses from exposure index in computed radiography. *Physics in Medicine and Biology* 53(12):3365–80.

28 Almen A, Loof M, Mattsson S (1996) Examination technique, image quality, and patient dose in paediatric radiology. A survey including 19 Swedish hospitals. *Acta Radiologica* 37(3 Pt 1):337–42.

29 Kyriou JC, Fitzgerald M, Pettet A, Cook JV, Pablot SM (1996) A comparison of doses and techniques between specialist and non-specialist centres in the diagnostic X-ray imaging of children. *British Journal of Radiology* 69(821):437–50.

30 Ruiz MJ, Gonzalez L, Vano E, Martinez A (1991) Measurement of radiation doses in the most frequent simple examinations in paediatric radiology and its dependence on patient age. *British Journal of Radiology* 64(766):929–33.

31 McParland BJ, Gorka W, Lee R, Lewall DB, Omojola MF (1996) Radiology in the neonatal intensive care unit: dose reduction and image quality. *British Journal of Radiology* 69(826):929–37.

32 Mooney R, Thomas PS (1998) Dose reduction in a paediatric x-ray department following optimization of radiographic technique. *British Journal of Radiology* 71(848):852–60.

33 Vano E, Oliete S, Guibelalde E, Velasco A, Fernandez JM (1995) Image quality and dose in lumbar spine examinations: results of a 5 year quality control programme following the European quality criteria trial. *British Journal of Radiology* 68(816):1332–35.

34 McDonald S, Martin CJ, Darragh CL, Graham DT (1996) Dose-area product measurements in paediatric radiography. *British Journal of Radiology* 69(820):318–25.

35 Goske MJ, Charkot E, Herrmann T, *et al.* (2011) Image gently: challenges for radiologic technologists when performing digital radiography in children. *Pediatric Radiology* 41:611–9.

36 Kiljunen T, Järvinen H, Savolainen S (2007) Diagnostic reference levels for thorax X-ray examinations of paediatric patients. *British Journal of Radiology* 80(954):452–9.

37 Lowe A, Finch A, Boniface D, Chaudhuri R, Shekhdar J (1999) Diagnostic image quality of mobile neonatal chest x-rays and the radiation exposure incurred. *British Journal of Radiology* 72(853):55–61.

38 Satou, GM, Lacro RV, Chung T, Gauvreau K, Jenkins KJ (2001) Heart size on chest x-ray as a predictor of cardiac enlargement by echocardiography in children. *Paediatric Cardiology* 22(3):218–22.

39 Hochschild TJ, Cremin BJ (1975) Technique in infant chest radiography. *Radiography* 41(481):21–5.

40 Marshall NW, Faulkner K, Busch HP, March DM, Pfenning H (1994) A comparison of radiation dose in examination of the abdomen using different radiological imaging techniques. *British Journal of Radiology* 67(797):478–84.

41 Arena L, Baker SR (1990) Use of a metal detector to identify ingested metallic foreign bodies. *American Journal of Radiology* 155(4):803–4.

42 NICE Guidelines on Head Injury. www.nice.org.uk/guidance/cg176.

43 Boulis ZF, Dick R, Barnes NR (1978) Head injuries in children – aetiology, symptoms, physical findings and x ray wastage. *British Journal of Radiology* 51:851–4.

44 Lloyd DA, Carty H, Patterson M, Butcher CK, Roe D (1997) Predictive value of skull radiography for intracranial injury in children with blunt head injury. *Lancet* 349(9055):821–4.

45 Gasniak A, Feivel M, Hertz M, Tadmor R (1986) Skull X-rays in head trauma: are they still necessary? A Review of 1000 cases. *European Journal of Radiology* 6(2):89–91.

46 Masters SJ, McClean PM, Arcarese JS, *et al.* (1987) Skull X-ray examinations after head trauma. Recommendations by a multi disciplinary panel and validation study. *New England Journal of Medicine* 316(2):84–91.

47 Rosenbaum AE, Arnold BA (1978) Postero-anterior radiography: a method for reduction of eye dose. *Radiology* 129(3):812.

48 Denton BK (1998) Improving plain radiography of the skull: the half-axial projection re-described. *Synergy* August:9–11.

49 Berryman F, Pynsent P, Fairbank J Disney S (2008) Reference: A new system for measuring 3 dimensional back shape in scoliosis. *European Spine Journal* 17(5):663–72.

50 Stanmore scoliosis chair. wardray-premise.com/x-ray/equipment/scoliosis_chair.html.

51 Dhar S, Dangerfield PH, Dorgan JC, Klenerman L (1993) Correlation between bone age and Risser's sign in adolescent idiopathic scoliosis. *Spine* 18(1):14–9.

52 Nimkin K, Kleinman PK (1997) Imaging of child abuse. *Pediatric Clinics of North America* 44(3):615–35.

53 Kleinman PK, Schlesinger AE (1997) Mechanical factors associated with posterior rib fractures: laboratory and case studies. *Pediatric Radiology* 27(1):87–91.

54 Carty H (1997) Non-accidental injury: a review of the radiology. *European Radiology* 7(9):1365–76.

55 Kleinman PK, Blackbourne BD, Marks SC, Karellas A, Belanger PL (1989) Radiologic contributions to the investigation and prosecution of cases of fatal infant abuse. *New England Journal of Medicine* 320(8):507–11.

56 Kleinman PK, Nimkin K, Spevak MR, *et al.* (1996) Follow-up skeletal surveys in suspected child abuse. *American Journal of Roentgenology* 167(4):893–6.

57 Thomsen TK, Elle B, Thomsen JL (1997) Post mortem examination in infants: evidence of child abuse? *Forensic Science International* 90(3):223–30.

58 The Royal College of Paediatrics and Child Health (2008) Standards for Radiological Investigation of Suspected Non Accidental Injury. www.rcr.ac.uk.

59 Nimkin K, Spevak MR, Kleinman PK (1997) Fractures of the hands and feet in child abuse: imaging and pathologic features. *Radiology* 203(1):233–6.

60 Freeman C (2009) Skeletal Survey for Suspected NAI, SIDS and SUDI– Guidance for Radiographers. Society of Radiographers, www.sor.org.

61 Offiah AC, Hall CM (2003) Radiological diagnosis of the constitutional disorders of bone. *Paediatric Radiology* 33:153–61.

Section 14 Miscellaneous

Bariatric radiography

1 Health & Social Care Information Centre (2014) Statistics on obesity, physical activity and diet. Available at: http://www.hscic.gov.uk/catalogue/PUB13648/Obes-phys-acti-diet-eng-2014-rep.pdf (Accessed 10th March 2014.)

2 Buckley O, Ward E, Ryan A, Colin W, Snow A, Torreggiani WC (2009) European obesity and the radiology department. What can we do to help? *European Radiology* 19:298–309.

3 Reynolds A (2011) Obesity and medical imaging challenges. *Radiologic Technology* 82(3):219–42.

4 Puhl R, Brownhill KD (2003) Psychological origins of obesity stigma: towards changing a powerful and pervasive bias. *Obesity Review* 4:213–27.

5 Jeffery D (1997) The effect of collimation of the irradiated field on objectively measured image contrast. *Radiography* 3:165–77.

Trauma radiography

1 Carley S, Driscoll P (2001) Trauma education. *Resuscitation* 48:47–56.

2 https://www.headway.org.uk/glasgow-coma-scale.aspx (Accessed March 2014.)

3 American College of Surgeons (2008) *Advanced Trauma Life Support Course*, 8th edn.

Foreign bodies

1 Arena L, Baker SR (1990) Use of a metal detector to identify ingested metallic foreign bodies. *American Journal of Radiology* 155(4):803–4.

2 www.aao.org/publications/eyenet/200710/pearls.cfm Accessed Feb 2014

3 eyewiki.aao.org/Intraocular_Foreign_Bodies_-_Management (Accessed Feb 2014.)

Tomography and tomosynthesis

1 Dobbins JT, Godfrey DJ (2003) Digital x-ray tomosynthesis: current state of the art and clinical potential. *Physics in Medicine and Biology* 48:R65–106.

2 Machida H, Yuhara T, Tamura M, *et al.* (2012) Radiation dose of digital tomosynthesis for sinonasal examination: comparison with multi-detector CT. *European Journal of Radiology* 81(6):1140–5.

3 Sabol JM (2009) A Monte Carlo estimation of effective dose in chest tomosynthesis. *Medical Physics* 36(12):5480–7.

4 Vikgren J, Zachrisson S, Svalkvist A, *et al.* (2008) Comparison of chest tomosynthesis and chest radiography for detection of pulmonary nodules: human observer study of clinical cases. *Radiology* 249(3):1034–41.

Skeletal survey

1 http://www.bcshguidelines.com/documents/MYELOMA_GUIDELINE_Feb_2014_for_BCSH.pdf

Forensic radiography

1 College of Radiographers (2009) *Guidance for the Provision of Forensic Radiography Services*.

2 Thali MJ, Viner MD, Brogdon BG (eds) (2011) *Brogdon's Forensic Radiology*, 2nd edn.

3 www.virtopsy.com/ (Accessed Sep 2014.)

4 www2.le.ac.uk/departments/emfpu/students/md/the-use-of-injected-contrast-agents-in-cadaveric-ct (Accessed Sep 2014.)

5 www.irm.uzh.ch/forschung/bildgebungvirtopsy.html (Accessed Sep 2014.)

6 http://ing.dk/galleri/virtopsy-skaber-virtuelt-billede-af-afdoede-127453#4 (Accessed Sep 2014.)

Index

ABCDEs, trauma radiography 506
abdomen, paediatric radiography
    abdominal pain, acute 444
    acute conditions 444
    antero-posterior projection 445–6
    constipation 444
    diaphragmatic hernia 448
    imperforate anus 444, 448
    meconium, failure of passage 444
    modifications in technique 447
    necrotising enterocolitis 448
    palpable mass 444
    radiation protection 446
    recommended projections 444
    referral criteria 444
    swallowed foreign body 444, 447
    trauma 444
    urinary tract infection 444
abdomen and pelvic cavity
    antero-posterior – erect projection 374
    antero-posterior – left lateral decubitus 375
    antero-posterior projection 382–3
    antero-posterior – supine projection 372–3
    aortic aneurysm 371
    biliary system 380–1
    bladder 376–8
    children 371
    constipation 371
    fluid collections 370
    image evaluation 382–3
    image parameters 369
    imaging protocols 368
    intestinal obstruction 370
    kidneys 376–8
    lateral – dorsal decubitus (supine) 375
    paediatric care 371
    perforation 371
    planes and regions 366–7
    radiation protection 369
    radiological considerations 370–1
    recommended projections 368
    referral criteria 368
    renal calculi 370
    retroperitoneal disease 371
    ureters 376–8
    urinary tract 376–8
    see also chest/upper abdomen; pelvis
abdominal pain, acute paediatric 444
abduction and rotation effect 175
abduction limb position 16
absorption unsharpness 27
accessories
    forensic radiography 538
    paediatric 430
    skull 272
    theatre radiography 408
    ward radiography 386
acetabulum and hip joint 184
acquisition of images
    acquisition systems 8
    bariatric radiography 497
    dental radiography 320
    film imaging 28
    fluoroscopy/fluorography imaging 28
    lungs 234
    panoramic tomography 351–5
    radiographic images 28–31
    screen/film imaging 28
acromioclavicular joints 97, 111
adaptation of technique, trauma radiography 501
    see also alternative projections and positioning
adequacy, image evaluation 10
Advanced Trauma and Life Support (ATLS) 506–8
aftercare, X-rays 6, 7
air, lesions demonstrated by 517
air gaps and air-gap technique
    bariatric radiography 499
    hip joint and upper third of femur 181
    lungs 235
    radiographic image contrast 24
airway maintenance 506
ALARP principle 50
alignment, equipment and images 10, 320
    see also leg alignment
alternative projections and positioning
    abdomen, paediatric radiography 447
    ankle 139
    cranium 277, 278, 285
    elbows, paediatric 472
    hip joint and upper third of femur 182
    humerus – intertuberous sulcus 90
    knee joint 151
    oblique occlusal of the mandible 345
alternative projections and positioning (continued)
    pelvis 185
    scapula 118
    shoulder trauma 103–5
    sternoclavicular joints 115
    see also positioning; specific projection
amorphous selenium detector 30
anatomy
    ankle 135
    facial bones and sinuses 292
    foot 126
    hand 54
    heart and aorta 250–1
    hips, pelvis and sacro-iliac joints 171–4
    knee joint 149
    lungs 238–9
    paediatric comparison 426
    skull, facial bones and sinuses 267–9
    terminology 13
    variation and pathological appearances 11
    vertebral levels 197
ankle
    alternative projection 139
    anatomy 135
    antero-posterior – mortise projection 136
    antero-posterior projection 138–40
    flexion 125
    image evaluation 138
    lateral projection 136, 138–40
    latero-medial projection 139
    medio-lateral projection 137
    radiation protection and dose 136, 140
    recommended projections 124
    stress projections, subluxation 140
    see also lower limbs
anterior anatomical aspect 13
anterior erect aspect projection 14
anterior oblique occlusal projection 343–4
anterior oblique projection
    acetabulum and hip joint 184
    defined 18
    hand 56–7
    scapula 118
    shoulder trauma 105
    wrists 73

anterior projection 340
anterior teeth positioning errors 356
antero-posterior cervical spine
    projection 205
antero-posterior 15 degree caudal
    projection 379
antero-posterior 15 degree erect
    projections 99
antero-posterior 25 degree
    projection 109
antero-posterior – erect projection
    abdomen and pelvic cavity 374
    chest, paediatric 489
    chest – post-neonatal 440–1, 487
    chest/upper abdomen 397
    heart and lungs 390
    humerus – shaft 88
    lungs 242
    pelvis, paediatric 491
    pelvis/hips, paediatric 459
    scapula 117
antero-posterior – left lateral
    decubitus 375
antero-posterior modified projection
    107–8
antero-posterior – mortise
    projection 136
antero-posterior oblique projection
    both hands 59
    knee joint 160
    proximal tibio-fibular joint 148
    sacro-iliac joints 190
antero-posterior – open mouth
    projection 201–2
antero-posterior projection
    abdomen, paediatric 445–6
    abdomen and pelvic cavity 382–3
    ankle 138–40
    calcified tendons 109, 111
    cervical vertebrae 201–3
    coccyx 226
    cross-kidney projection 377
    defined 17
    elbows 78–9, 85
    elbows, paediatric 473–474
    example 20
    femur – shaft 163, 166
    first and second cervical
        vertebrae 201–2
    fractured lower limbs and
        pelvis 400
    heart and lungs 391
    heart and lungs, special care baby
        unit 403
    hip joint, upper third of femur and
        pelvis 176
    hips 176–8
    hips, pelvis and sacro-iliac joints 178

antero-posterior projection (*continued*)
    humerus 87, 94
    humerus – neck 91
    kidneys 526
    knee joint 153
    larynx 527
    lower ribs 258
    lumbar spine image evaluation 221
    lumbar vertebrae 215
    lumbo-sacral junction 223
    lungs 239
    paediatric (gallows traction) 371
    pelvis 176–7, 191
    pelvis/hips, paediatric 458
    sacro-iliac joints 189
    sacrum 224
    shoulder 120, 121
    single hip 178
    spine – cervical, thoracic and lumbar
        (paediatric) 466
    supracondylar fracture 87
    thoracic vertebrae 211, 214
    thumbs 62
    tibia and fibula 147
    tomography 527
    trachea 527
    urinary tract, ureters, kidneys,
        bladder 376–7
antero-posterior – semi-erect
    projection 244
antero-posterior stress projection 155
antero-posterior – supine projection
    abdomen and pelvic cavity 372–3
    chest and abdominal projection,
        paediatric 486, 489–91
    chest – post-neonatal 442
    chest/upper abdomen 396–7
    clavicle 113
    humerus – shaft 89
    knee joint 151
    lungs 243
    neonate 486–7
antero-posterior – weight-bearing
    projection 150
anthropological baseline 266
anthropological plane 266
antiscatter grid, paediatric care 429
aortic aneurysm 371
apical oblique projection 103
apices 246
applications
    macroradiography 534
    tomography 525
    tomosynthesis 531
aprons, radiation protection 47
area of interest, image evaluation 11
arms *see specific part*
artefacts 11, 38–9

arthroplasty postoperative
    radiography 401
assessment, patient condition 500
assessment tools 293
ATLS *see* Advanced Trauma and
    Life Support
audit and quality assurance 430
auricular plane 266
automatic exposure control (AEC)
    digital imaging 31
    fluoroscopy/fluorography imaging 28
    paediatric radiography 429
autotomography 518
axial plane of body 13
axial projection
    calcaneum 142
    carpal tunnel 69
    coracoid process 119
    elbows 80, 83
    forearm 81
    humerus – intertuberous sulcus 90
    humerus – neck 92
    metatarsal-phalangeal sesamoid
        bones 134
    shoulder 120
    ulnar groove 83
axial – upper cervical vertebrae
    projection 206

babies
    chest, requiring holding 435
    forensic radiography 542–4
    see also paediatric care; paediatric
        radiography
ball catcher's projection 59
bariatric radiography
    air gaps 499
    centring 499
    collimation 498
    compensation filters 498
    equipment 496–9
    exposure 499
    image acquisition 497
    image quality 498
    image receptor size 499
    imaging 496–9
    non-imaging equipment 496
    obese patients 497
    psychosocial factors 496
    soft tissue 497
    tissue displacement 498
base of skull fracture 449
beam angulation projection 17, 270
biliary system 380–1
bimolar projection 349
bisecting angle technique 327–30
bit depth, imaging 31
bitewing radiography 324–6

bladder, urinary 379
　see also urinary tract
bones
　and adjacent soft tissues 517
　age, paediatric 475
　image evaluation 10
　of the thorax 256–7
breathing, trauma radiography 506
bruises, paediatric skull 449
buccal surface 316

cadaveric imaging see forensic
　radiography
calcaneal-navicular, paediatric 478
calcaneum
　axial projection 142
　lateral projection 141
　radiation protection and dose 141
　recommended projections 124
calcifications, soft tissue 517
calcified tendons
　antero-posterior 25 degree projection
　　109, 111
　lateral oblique 15 degree
　　projection 110
　recommended projections 97
cancellous hip screws 412
cardio-thoracic ratio 251
carpal bones
　anterior oblique projection – ulnar
　　deviation 65
　lateral projection 67
　posterior oblique projection 66
　postero-anterior projection – ulnar
　　deviation and 30 degree cranial
　　angle 68
　recommended projections 52
carpal tunnel 52, 69
cartilage, image evaluation 10
cassettes 356, 504, 534
CCD see charge-couple device
central venous line pressure 393
cephalometry
　dental radiography 456
　lateral projection 358
　postero-anterior projection 359
　X-ray equipment features 357
cervical – antero-posterior projection 261
cervical spine
　examination, trauma radiography 507
　lateral supine projection 399
　radiation protection 399
cervical vertebrae
　antero-posterior cervical spine
　　projection 205
　antero-posterior projection 201–3
　axial – upper cervical vertebrae
　　projection 206

cervical vertebrae (continued)
　first and second vertebrae
　　projection 201–2
　image evaluation 204–5
　lateral cervical spine projection 204
　lateral erect projection 198–9
　lateral – flexion and extension
　　projection 207
　lateral supine projection 200
　left posterior oblique projection 208
　left posterior oblique supine
　　projection 209
　open mouth projection 201–2
　right posterior oblique projection 208
　right posterior oblique supine
　　projection 209
　third to seventh vertebrae
　　projection 203
cervico-thoracic vertebrae 210
charge-couple device (CCD) 30
checklist, theatre radiography 406–7
chest, paediatric 481
chest drain insertions 393
chest – neonatal 434–7
chest – post-neonatal
　acute conditions 439
　antero-posterior – erect
　　projection 440–1
　antero-posterior – supine
　　projection 442
　chest infection 439
　Cincinnati filter device 443
　congenital heart disease 438
　cough, recurrent 439
　infection, chest 439
　inhaled foreign body 439
　lateral projection 443
　oesophageal pH probe, reflux study
　　439, 488
　postero-anterior – erect
　　projection 440
　recommended projections 439
　recurrent cough 439
　referral criteria 438–9
　stridor, acute 439
　trauma 439
　wheeze 438
chest/upper abdomen
　abdomen 396
　antero-posterior – erect
　　projection 397
　antero-posterior supine projection
　　396, 397
　lateral dorsal decubitus – supine
　　projection 398
　left lateral decubitus projection 397
　naso-gastric tube positioning 394–5
　radiation protection 398

child development 425
　see also paediatric care
cholangiography, operative 417
Cincinnati filter device 443
circulation, trauma radiography 506
classified persons, designation 50
clavicle
　antero-posterior – supine
　　projection 113
　modified infero-superior
　　(modified axial) projection 114
　postero-anterior projection 112
　recommended projections 97
clinical concerns 360
clinical history 10, 43
coccyx 194, 226
collimation
　bariatric radiography 498
　carpal bones 68
　dental radiography 317, 456
　dorsi-palmar hand projection 55
　fingers 61
　image evaluation 11
　lateral hand projection 57
　lungs 239
　radiographic image contrast 24
　thumbs 63
　trauma radiography 503
　see also specific projection
comments/initial report 10–11
　see also image evaluation
comments on images 508
common faults and solutions
　see specific projection
common paediatric examinations 434
communication
　imaging informatics 35
　theatre radiography 406
　ward radiography 387
compensation filters 498
complete/full mouth survey 337
complex oblique projection, skull 271
components, imaging informatics 32–4
computed radiography (CR)
　cassette support 534
　digital imaging 29
　leg alignment 167
　leg length assessment (paediatric) 167
computed tomography (CT) 507
cone beam computed tomography
　advantages 360
　clinical concerns 360
　disadvantages 360
　image analysis 361–4
　imaging procedure 361
confirmation, radio-opaque foreign
　body 514
congenital heart disease 438

coning devices 431–2
connections, imaging informatics 32–4
consent 480–3
consent form 492–3, 537
constipation 371, 444
contrast
   bitewing radiography 326
   media, subject image 23
   radiographic images 23–4, 43
   tomography 524
conventional screen/film-based imaging 8
coracoid process 97, 119
coronal planes 13, 266
correct projection 11
cough, recurrent 439
CR *see* computed radiography
cranial angle projection, carpal bones 68
cranio-facial deformity 456
craniosynostosis 449, 450
cranium
   frontal-occipital 35 degree caudal projection 286–7
   fronto-occipital projection 278
   half axial, frontal-occipital 30 degree caudal projection 279–80
   jugular foramina – submento-vertical 20 degree caudal projection 285
   lateral erect projection 275
   lateral – supine with horizontal beam projection 274
   mastoid – lateral oblique 25 degree projection 288
   mastoid – profile projection 289
   modified half axial projection 280
   occipto-frontal 30 degree cranial angulation projection 281
   occipto-frontal projection 276–7
   optic foramina and jugular foramina projection 284, 285
   optic foramina – postero-anterior oblique projection 284
   petrous – anterior oblique projection 290
   radiologic technique 274
   reverse Towne's projection 281
   sella turcica – lateral projection 283
   Stenver's projection 290
   submento-vertical projection 282, 287
   temporal bones 286
   Towne's projection 279–80
   see also facial bones and sinuses; skull
cross-infection control 322–3
   see also infection control
cross-kidney projection 377
curvature of spine *see* scoliosis
Cushing's syndrome 535

darkroom facilities 408
data integrity checks 38
data protection 35
DDR *see* direct digital radiography
deciduous dentition, Palmer notation 314
decubitus projection 14
dedicated paediatric areas 428
density, images 22–3, 326
dental formula 314–15
dental radiography
   bimolar projection 349
   bitewing technology 324–6
   buccal surface 316
   cephalometry 357–9
   collimation 317
   cone beam computed tomography 360–4
   cross-infection control 322–3
   deciduous dentition 314
   dental formula 314–15
   dentition 312–13
   digital receptors 319
   direct image receptor 318
   distal surface 316
   extraoral image receptors 318
   extraoral radiography 312
   Federation Dentaire International notation 315
   film mounting and identification of intraoral films 321
   image acquisition 320
   image geometry, optimal 323
   image receptors 317–18
   incisal surface 316
   interoral radiography 312
   intraoral image receptors 318
   kilovoltage range 317
   labial surface 316
   lateral oblique, mandible and maxilla 346–9
   lingual surface 316
   mandible and maxilla – lateral oblique projection 346–9
   mesial surface 316
   non-screen image receptor 318
   occlusal planes 316
   occlusal radiography 338–45
   occlusal surface 316
   paediatric 456
   palatal surface 316
   Palmer notation 314
   panoramic tomography 350–6
   periapical radiography 327–37
   permanent dentition 314
   processing, analogue films 321
   radiation protection 322
   radiograph uses in dentistry 312

dental radiography (*continued*)
   receptor stabilisation 317
   specialised image receptor holders 320
   teeth 313
   terminology 316
   X-ray equipment features 317
dental volumetric tomography *see* cone beam computed tomography
dentition 312–13
depressed paediatric skull fracture 449
depressed zygoma fracture 293
designated areas, radiation protection 50
designation of classified persons 50
development *see* processing/development
diaphragmatic hernia 448
DICOM (Digital Imaging and Communications in Medicine) 35
digital images and imaging
   acquisition systems 8
   amorphous selenium detector 30
   automatic exposure control response 31
   bit depth 31
   capture 23
   charge-couple device 30
   computed radiography technology 29
   digital radiography technologies 30
   direct digital radiography 29
   exposure factors 41
   fill factor 31
   grids 31
   image size 31
   imaging informatics 6, 7, 32–5
   optimisation of image 31
   quality factors 31
   radiation exposure 31
   scanning technology 30
   scintillator detector 30
   thin-film transistor flat-panel detector 30
   tiling 31
   see also images and imaging; radiographic images
digital radiography 30, 430
   see also specific projection
digital receptors, dental radiography 319
direct digital radiography (DDR)
   leg alignment 168
   leg length assessment 471
   spine – scoliosis 463
   trauma radiography 505
   see also specific projection
direct image receptor 318
direct peer-to-peer image transfers 34
disability, trauma radiography 506
dislocation of shoulder 97

distal end radius and ulna 52
distal locking, nailing 412
distal surface 316
distortion, radiographic images 25
dorsal surface, foot 125
dorsi-palmar projection
    both hands 58
    fingers 60
    hand 55
dorsi-plantar – erect projection 131
dorsi-plantar oblique projection
    foot 128–9
    subtalar joints 144
    toes 132
dorsi-plantar projection
    foot 127, 129
    toes 132
dorsi-plantar – weight-bearing
    projection 476
dose
    measurement, paediatric 432
    monitoring 48
    quantities 45
    reduction 353
    see also radiation protection and dose
DRL see diagnostic reference levels (DRLs)
dual-energy subtraction 235
dynamic hip screw insertion
    cancellous hip screws 412
    imaging procedure 413
    surgical procedure 414

edge enhancement, images 44
elbows
    antero-posterior projection 78, 85
    axial projection 80–1
    forearm in contact 79, 81
    full flexion projection 80
    head of radius 82–3
    image evaluation 81, 85
    lateral projection 77, 85
    partial flexion 78
    proximal radio-ulnar joint – oblique projection 83
    radiological considerations 84
    recommended projections 52
    ulnar groove – axial projection 83
    upper arm in contact 79–80
elbows, paediatric
    alternative positioning 472
    antero-posterior projection 473–474
    lateral projection 472, 474
    prone position 472
    radiation protection 473
    referral criteria 472
    standing position 472, 473
    supine position 472, 473

electronic patient record (EPR) 34
emergency peripheral vascular procedures 419
endocrine disease 535
endotracheal tube 393
environmental control 428, 506
epilepsy 449
EPR see electronic patient record
equipment
    bariatric radiography 496–9
    facial bones and sinuses 291
    paediatric radiography 429–30
    theatre radiography 406, 408
    trauma radiography 501–5
    ward radiography 386, 388
erect projection 14
    see also specific projection
eRequesting 34
essential image characteristics
    see specific projection
ethmoid sinuses 291
eversion, foot 125
examinations
    paediatric radiography 434
    timeline 7
    trauma radiography 500
examples see image evaluation
expiration technique 240
exposure
    bariatric radiography 499
    charts, radiation protection 47
    lungs 236
    optimum radiographic image quality 43
    radiographic image contrast 24
    soft tissue 516–17
    tomography 521, 525
exposure, radiation
    aprons and shields 47
    diagnostic reference levels 48
    dose monitoring 48
    dose quantities 45
    exposure charts 47
    immobilisation 47
    investigation and notification of overexposure (IRMER) 48–9
    justification 44
    optimisation 46
    overview 44
    patient holding 47
    risk-benefit analysis 44
    risks 46
    training 47
    X-ray examination benefits 45
exposure factors
    choice of 42–3
    digital imaging 41
    focus-to-receptor distance 41

exposure factors (continued)
    intensifying screens 41
    kilovoltage 40
    millampere seconds 40
    overview 39
    secondary radiation grids 42
    trauma radiography 505
extension limb position 16
external auditory meatus 266
external fixation, trauma orthopaedic surgery 411
external occipital protuberance (inion) 266
extracapsular fractures 410
extraoral image receptors 318
extraoral radiography 312
extremity fractures 410
    see also lower limbs; upper limbs
eyes
    foreign body 293, 514–15
    shields, dental radiography 456

facial bones and sinuses
    anatomy 292
    assessment tools 293
    depressed zygoma fracture 293
    equipment 291
    ethmoid sinuses 291
    foreign body in eye 293
    fracture classifications 293
    frontal sinuses 291
    gross trauma 293
    image evaluation 310
    lateral 30 degree cranial projection 302
    lateral projection 298, 305
    mandible 293, 302–4
    maxillary sinuses 291
    modified mento-occipital projection 295
    modified reverse mento-occipital 30 degree projection 297
    nasal bones – lateral projection 301
    nasal injury 293
    occipito-mental 30 degree caudal projection 296, 310
    occipito-mental projection 294, 310
    orbits – occipito-mental (modified) projection 300
    paediatric 454
    paranasal sinuses 291, 306–8
    postero-anterior oblique projection 304
    postero-anterior projection 303
    radiological considerations 293
    recommended projections 293
    severely injured patient 297
    sphenoid sinus 291

facial bones and sinuses (*continued*)
   suspected depressed zygoma fracture 293
   temporo-mandibular joints 293, 305
   trauma 293
   zygoma fracture, depressed 293
   zygomatic arches – infero superior projection 299
   see also cranium; skull
fat, lesions demonstrated by 517
faults and solutions *see specific projection*
Federation Dentaire International notation 315
feet – supported/weight-bearing, paediatric
   babies 476, 477
   calcaneo-navicular 478
   dorsi-plantar – weight-bearing 476
   lateral – weight-bearing 477–9
   metatarsus adductus 478
   radiological considerations 478
   recommended projections 476
   referral criteria 476
   talo-calcaneal 478
   tarsal coalition 478
   toddlers 476, 477
   valgus 478
   varus 478
   see also foot
femur, fractures 401
femur, hip joint and upper third of
   air gap technique 181
   alternative projection 182
   frog's legs position 183
   lateral projection 181–3
   Lauenstein's projection 179
   posterior oblique projection 179
   radiation protection and dose 178, 181
   true lateral – neck of femur projection 180
femur – shaft
   antero-posterior projection 163, 166
   horizontal beam projection 165
   image evaluation 166
   lateral projection 164–6
   radiation protection and dose 164, 165
   recommended projections 124
fibula *see* tibia and fibula
55 degree left anterior oblique with 35 degree caudal angulation 271
fill factor, digital imaging 31
film fog 24
film imaging 28
film/intensifying screen combinations 237, 430
film mounting and identification of 321

film processing, paediatric radiography 430
filtration, additional 429
fingers
   dorsi-palmar (DP) projection 60
   lateral index and middle fingers projection 60
   lateral ring and little fingers projection 61
   recommended projections 52
   see also hands; thumbs
first and second cervical vertebrae 201–2
first and second upper ribs, antero-posterior projection 261
first and second vertebrae projection 201–2
fixed focus-to-object distance, macroradiography 532
fixed focus-to-receptor distance, macroradiography 532
flexibility, trauma radiography 501
flexion position and projections 16, 125, 507
floor of mouth projection 341
flow charts, patient journey 7
fluid collections, abdomen and pelvic cavity 370
fluoroscopy/fluorography imaging 28, 538
focal neurological deficiency 449
focal spot, paediatric radiography 429
foot
   anatomy 126
   ankle extension 125
   ankle flexion 125
   dorsal surface 125
   dorsi-plantar – erect projection 131
   dorsi-plantar oblique projection 128–9
   dorsi-plantar projection 127, 129
   eversion 125
   flexion of knee joint 125
   image evaluation 129
   inversion 125
   lateral aspect 125
   lateral – erect projection 131
   lateral projection 130
   lateral rotation 125
   medial aspect 125
   medial rotation 125
   plantar aspect 125
   positioning terminology 125
   radiation protection 127, 130
   recommended projections 124
   weight-bearing projection 131
   see also feet – supported/weight-bearing, paediatric; lower limbs; toes

forearm
   antero-posterior projection 75
   axial projection 81
   lateral projection 76
   recommended projections 52
foreign bodies
   confirmation, radio-opaque 514
   in eye 293
   image evaluation 10
   ingested 511
   inhaled 512
   inserted 513
   localisation, intraorbital foreign body 515
   overview 509
   percutaneous type 510
   transocular 514–15
forensic radiography
   accessories 538
   adaptation of technique 540
   analogue protocol 538
   anatomy 537
   body bags 541
   classifications 537
   de-briefing 538
   dental radiography 539
   digital imaging protocol 538
   elder abuse queries 537
   equipment 538
   future directions 545
   legal issues 538
   local radiation rules 538
   mobile intensifier fluoroscopic technique 541
   overview 537
   paediatric abuse queries 537
forensic radiography, foetus
   antero-posterior projection 542
   'babygram' 542–3
   identification 542, 543, 544
   lateral projection 543
   lateral skull projection 544
   post-procedure 544
   skeletal survey – out of hours 544
   skull – fronto-occipital projection 543
   still born 542–3
   see also paediatric radiography
formation, radiographic images 22–3
40 degree left anterior oblique projection 271
fractures 293, 400–1
FRD *see* focus-to-receptor distance
'frog's legs' position 183, 491
frontal-occipital 35 degree caudal projection 286–7
frontal sinuses 291
fronto-occipital 30 degree caudal projection 452

fronto-occipital projection
    cranium 278
    skull 270
    skull, paediatric radiography 451
fulcrum 520–1
full flexion projection 80

gallows traction (paediatric) 402
Garth projection 103
geometric unsharpness
    macroradiography 533
    optimum radiographic image
        quality 43
    radiographic images 26, 27
geometry, bitewing radiography 326
glabella 266
Glasgow Coma Scale (GCS)
    facial bones and sinuses 273
    paediatric radiography 449
glenohumeral joint 108
gonad protection 431–2, 457
    see also specific projection
Grashey projection 108
Greulich method, assessment of
    bone age 475
grids
    digital imaging 31
    lungs 235
    trauma radiography 503
gross trauma 293
    see also trauma

half axial, frontal-occipital 30 degree
    caudal projection 279–80
hands
    anatomy 54
    anterior oblique (DP oblique)
        projection 56–7
    antero-posterior oblique both hands
        projection 59
    dorsi-palmar both hands projection 58
    dorsi-palmar projection 55
    image evaluation 57
    lateral projection 57
    over-rotated hand image
        evaluation 52
    recommended projections 52
    see also fingers; thumbs
hanging protocols, image processing 37
Harrington rod 465
headache, paediatric 449
head of radius, elbows 82–3
heart and aorta
    anatomy 250–1
    cardio-thoracic ratio 251
    left lateral projection 254
    postero-anterior projection 252–3
    right anterior oblique 255

heart and lungs
    antero-posterior – erect projection 390
    antero-posterior projection 391
    central venous line pressure 393
    chest drain insertions 393
    endotracheal tube 393
    lateral decubitus projection 391
    lateral dorsal decubitus
        projection 391
    mobile C-arm fluoroscopy 392
    postero-anterior – erect
        projection 389
    postero-anterior projection 391
    post-operative radiography 393
    special care baby unit 403
    temporary pacemaker 392
heart and lungs, special care baby unit 403
high kilovoltage, soft tissue 516
hip joint, upper third of femur and
    pelvis 176–7
    see also femur; pelvis
hip joint and upper third of femur
    air gap technique 181
    alternative projection 182
    lateral projection 181–2, 192
    Lauenstein's projection 179
    posterior oblique projection 179
    radiation protection and dose 178, 181
    true lateral – neck of femur
        projection 180
hips, pelvis, and sacro-iliac joints
    acetabulum and hip joint 184
    anatomy 171–4
    antero-posterior projection 178
    dynamic hip screw insertion 413–14
    fractures 410
    image appearances 171–4
    image evaluation 191–2
    orthopaedic surgery 410
    pelvis 185–7
    posture 174
    radiation protection and dose 174
    recommended projections 170
    rotation and abduction effect 175
    sacro-iliac joints 188–90
    subject type 174
    and upper third of femur 178–83
    and upper third of femur and
        pelvis 176–7
    see also lower limbs; pelvis/hips, paediatric
HIS *see hospital information system*
HL7 messaging 35
holding/pulling limbs 508
horizontal beam projection
    femur – shaft 165
    knee joint 153–4
    trauma radiography 501

hospital information system (HIS) 34
'hot' report 508
'hot spots' 10
housekeeping tasks 37
hub-and-spoke systems 34
humerus
    bicipital groove 90
    intertuberous sulcus 90
    neck 91–4
    recommended projections 52
    shaft 88–9
    supracondylar fracture 87
hyperparathyroidism 535

identification
    forensic radiography 542, 543
    lungs 237
    trauma radiography 505
idiopathic scoliosis 465
illium 185
image acquisition
    acquisition systems 8
    bariatric radiography 497
    dental panoramic tomography 351–5
    dental radiography 320
    film imaging 28
    fluoroscopy/fluorography imaging 28
    lungs 234
    panoramic tomography 351–5
    radiographic images 28–31
    screen/film imaging 28
image characteristics *see specific
    projection*
image evaluation
    abdomen and pelvic cavity 382–3
    additional images 11
    adequacy 10
    alignment 10
    anatomical variation and pathological
        appearances 11
    ankle 138
    area of interest 11
    artefacts 11
    bones 10
    cartilage 10
    cervical vertebrae 204–5
    collimation 11
    conventional screen/film-based
        imaging 8
    correct projection 11
    defined 8–12
    digital imaging acquisition systems 8
    DP oblique, over-rotated hand 57
    elbows 81, 85
    examples 11–12
    femur – shaft 166
    foot 129
    foreign body 10

image evaluation (*continued*)
  hands 57
  hips 195
  hips, pelvis, and sacro-iliac joints 191–2
  'hot spots' 10
  humerus 94
  image exposure 11
  knee joint 153
  logical system 10
  lumbar vertebrae 221
  lungs 248–9
  markers and legends 11
  optimum definition 11
  oral clinical history 10
  overexposure 8
  over-rotated hand 57
  overview, 8–9
  paediatric radiography 486–91
  patient identification 11
  pattern recognition 10
  pelvis 191
  radiographer comments/initial report 10–11
  sacro-iliac joints 191–2
  satisfaction of search 10
  shoulders 120–1
  skull 308
  soft tissue 10
  suggestions, image assessment/evaluation process 10
  thoracic vertebrae 214
  underexposure 8
  wrists 74
image quality
  bariatric radiography 498
  paediatric radiography 430
  skull, facial bones and sinuses 272
  tomography 524
  tomosynthesis 530–1
  see also quality and quality assurance
image receptors
  bariatric radiography 499
  dental radiography 317–18
  see also specific projection
images and imaging
  abdomen and pelvic cavity 368–9
  artefacts 38–9
  bariatric radiography 496–9
  comments on 508
  cone beam computed tomography 361–4
  dental radiography 323
  examination timeline 7
  exposure factors 39–43
  exposure image evaluation 11
  geometry, optimal 323
  hanging protocols 37

images and imaging (*continued*)
  hips, pelvis and sacro-iliac joints 171–4
  image processing 35–9
  informatics 6, 7
  look-up tables 36
  parameters, lungs 234
  post processing 36
  quality and quality assurance 6, 37–8
  sharing gateways/networks 34
  size 31
  trauma radiography 501–5
  window width/window level 36
  see also digital images and imaging; radiographic images; *specific imaging technique*
imaging equipment *see* equipment; *specific type*
imaging informatics
  communication 35
  components and connections 32–4
  data protection 35
  defined 6, 32
  examination timeline 7
  historical developments 32
  overview 32–5
imaging procedure
  dynamic hip screw insertion 413
  emergency peripheral vascular procedures 419
  operative cholangiography 417
  pain management 418
  percutaneous nephrolithotomy 416
  retrograde pyelography 415
imaging room, paediatric areas 428
immobilisation
  paediatric radiography 430
  radiation protection 47
  trauma radiography 502
imperforate anus 444, 448
impingement, shoulders 97
incisal surface 316
indications, skeletal survey 535–6
  see also justification; referral criteria
infantile scoliosis 465
infection control
  chest – post-neonatal 439
  dental radiography 322–3
  theatre radiography 408
  ward radiography 387
infero-superior modified projection 106
infero-superior projections 158–9
infero-superior (reverse axial) projection 93
inflammatory disease, skeletal survey 535
infraorbital line 266
infraorbital margin/point 266

ingestion, foreign body 511
inhaled foreign body
  chest – post-neonatal 439
  overview 509, 512
initial report 10–11
  see also Image evaluation
insertion, foreign body 513
inspiration, lungs 239
instability/recurrent dislocation 97
intensifying screens 41
intercondylar notch – antero-posterior projection 161–2
interoral radiography 312
interpretation of images, skull 266
interpupillary (interorbital) line 266
interventional procedures 415–17
intestinal obstruction 370
intoxicated patients 502
intracapsular fractures 410
intramedullary nailing 412
intraoral image receptors 318
intraorbital foreign body 515
inversion, foot 125
investigation and notification, radiation overexposure 48–9, 50
Ionising Radiations Regulation (1999) 49–50
IRMER *see* investigation and notification, radiation overexposure
isolation/barrier nursing 387

Judet's projection 184
jugular foramina – submento-vertical 20 degree caudal projection 285
justification
  paediatric radiography 423–4
  for radiation 44
  rationale for projections 480
  skeletal survey 535–6
  skeletal survey, paediatric non-accidental injury 480
  see also referral criteria
juvenile scoliosis 465

key skills 386, 406–7
kidneys 376–8, 526
kilovoltage (kV)
  dental radiography 317
  exposure factors 40
  lungs 235
  soft tissue 516
  subject image contrast 24
knee joint
  alternative projections 151
  anatomy 149
  antero-posterior oblique projection 160
  antero-posterior projection 153

knee joint (*continued*)
  antero-posterior stress projection 155
  antero-posterior – supine projection 151
  antero-posterior – weight-bearing projection 150
  flexion of 125
  horizontal beam projection 153–4
  image evaluation 153
  infero-superior projections 158–9
  intercondylar notch – antero-posterior projection 161–2
  lateral projection 152–4
  patella – infero-superior projection 159
  patella projection 156
  postero-anterior oblique projection 160
  postero-anterior projection 156
  'racing start' projection 162
  radiation protection and dose 151, 155, 158
  recommended projections 124
  skyline projections 157–8
  stress – sublaxation projection 155
  trauma 154
  tunnel – antero-posterior projection 161–2
  turned-rolled projection 152

labelling of images 505
  see also Identification
labial surface 316
lacerations, paediatric skull 449
landmarks 195, 266
larynx *see* pharynx and larynx
lateral – air-gap technique 181
lateral anatomical aspect 13
lateral aspect, foot 125
lateral – basic – hallux projection 133
lateral – both hips ('frog's legs') projection 183
lateral cephalometry 456
lateral cervical spine projection 204
lateral decubitus projection 14, 391
lateral 25 degree caudal projection 305
lateral dorsal decubitus projection 391
lateral dorsal decubitus – supine projection
  abdomen and pelvic cavity 375
  chest/upper abdomen 398
lateral erect projection
  cervical vertebrae 198–9
  cranium 275
  foot 131
  humerus – shaft 88–9
lateral flexion and extension projection 207, 219

lateral horizontal beam projection 218
lateral index and middle fingers 60
lateral oblique 15 degree projection 110
lateral oblique 25 degree projection 288
lateral oblique projection
  calcified tendons 110
  defined 19
  humerus – neck 93
  mandible 346–9
  mastoid 288
  maxilla 346–9
  proximal tibio-fibular joint 148
  ramus of the mandible 348–9
  shoulder 121
  subtalar joints 144
  tibia and fibula 148
lateral projection
  ankle 136, 138–40
  calcaneum 141
  cephalometry 358
  chest – post-neonatal 443
  coccyx 226
  defined 17
  elbows 82–3
  elbows, paediatric 472, 474
  example 21
  facial bones and sinuses 298
  femur – shaft 164–6
  foot 130
  fractured femur 401
  hand 57
  head of radius, elbows 82–3
  hip 192
  hip joint 192
  hip joint and upper third of femur 181–2
  humerus 94
  humerus – supracondylar fracture 86
  knee joint 152–4
  lumbar spine image evaluation 221
  lumbar vertebrae 216–17
  lumbo-sacral junction 222
  lungs 245
  metatarsal-phalangeal sesamoid bones 134
  paediatric (gallows traction) 402
  pelvis 186
  pelvis/hips, paediatric 460
  sacrum 225
  skull 270, 309
  spine – cervical, thoracic and lumbar (paediatric) 466
  sternoclavicular joints 116
  still born 543
  thoracic vertebrae 212–14
  thumbs 62
  tibia and fibula 147
  wrists 71–2, 74

lateral projection with angulation, skull 271
lateral ring and little fingers projection 61
lateral rotation, foot 125
lateral – single hip (alternative) projection 182
lateral supine projection
  cervical spine 399
  cervical vertebrae 200
  post-nasal space, paediatric 455
lateral – supine projection 89, 453
lateral – supine with horizontal beam projection 274
lateral suprine projection 200
lateral swimmers' projection 210
lateral – weight-bearing projection 477–9
latero-medial projection 139
Lauenstein's projection 179
layers, tomography
  cut and spacing 523
  depth of 520–1
  localisation of depth 524
  thickness 522–3
left anterior oblique projection 380
left erect aspect projection 14
left lateral decubitus projection 14, 21, 397
left lateral projection 20, 254
left posterior oblique projection 208
  lower ribs 259
  lumbar vertebrae 220
  lumbo-sacral junction 223
  upper ribs 260
  urinary bladder 379
  urinary tract, kidneys, ureters, bladder 378–9
  see also oblique projection
left posterior oblique supine projection 209
leg alignment
  computed radiography method 167
  direct digital radiography method 168
  recommended projections 124
  see also lower limbs
legends *see* markers and legends
legislation, paediatric radiography 423
leg length assessment
  direct digital radiography method 471
  localised exposure method 471
  overview 468–9
  radiation protection 469
  single exposure CR method 470
lesions, soft tissue 517
limb position 16
  see also lower limbs; *specific limb*; upper limbs

limitations, dental panoramic tomography 353
linear movement features, tomography 521
lines, skull 266
lingual surface 316
localisation
    intraorbital foreign body 515
    of layer depth 524
    leg length assessment 471
    thoracic vertebrae 214
logical system 10
look-up tables 36
lordosis, lungs 239
lordotic technique 247
lower limbs
    ankle 135–40
    calcaneum 141–2
    femur – shaft 163–6
    foot 125–31
    fractures 400
    knee joint 149–62
    leg alignment 167–8
    metatarsal-phalangeal sesamoid bones 134
    paediatric, non-accidental injury 481
    proximal tibio-fibular joint 148
    radiation protection 59
    recommended projections 124
    rotation and abduction effect 175
    subtalar joints 143–6
    tibia and fibula 147
    toes 132–3
    trauma orthopaedic surgery 410
    see also hips, pelvis and sacro-iliac joints
lower oblique occlusal projection 345
lower ribs 257–9
low kilovoltage, soft tissue 516
lumbar spine 507
lumbar vertebrae
    antero-posterior lumbar spine image evaluation 221
    antero-posterior projection 215
    image evaluation 221
    lateral flexion and extension 219
    lateral horizontal beam projection 218
    lateral lumbar spine image evaluation 221
    lateral projection 216–17
    recommended projections 194
    right or left posterior oblique projection 220
lumbo-sacral junction
    antero-posterior projection 223
    lateral projection 222
    recommended projections 194
    right or left posterior oblique projection 223

lump or mass, palpable 444, 449
lungs
    air-gap technique 235
    anatomy 238–9
    antero-posterior – erect projection 242
    antero-posterior projections 239
    antero-posterior – semi-erect projection 244
    antero-posterior – supine projection 243
    apices 246
    collimation 239
    dual-energy subtraction 235
    expiration technique 240
    exposure time 236
    fields 238
    film/intensifying screen combinations 237
    focus-to-receptor distance 236
    grid use 235
    identification 237
    image acquisition 234
    image evaluation 248–9
    imaging parameters 234
    inspiration 239
    kilovoltage selection 235
    lateral projection 245
    lordosis 239
    lordotic technique 247
    lung fields 238
    magnification 236
    overexposure 239
    postero-anterior chest projection 248–9
    postero-anterior – erect projection 240–1
    radiation protection 237
    radiological considerations 239
    recommended projections 232
    respiration 233
    rotation 239
    semi-erect projection 239
    soft-tissue artefacts 239
    supine position 239
    tomosynthesis 237
    underexposure 239
    uniformity 236
    upper anterior region – lateral projection 247
    see also heart and lungs
lymphoma, skeletal survey 535

macroradiography
    applications 534
    CR cassette support 534
    fixed focus-to-object distance 532
    fixed focus-to-receptor distance 532

macroradiography (continued)
    geometric unsharpness 533
    movement unsharpness 533
    principles 532–4
    scattered radiation 534
magnification
    dental panoramic tomography 351
    lungs 236
    radiographic images 25
    tomography 523
malignant disease, skeletal survey 535
mandible
    facial bones and sinuses 302–4
    lateral oblique projection 346–9
    ramus of the mandible 348–9
    trauma projections 293
mandibular third molars imaging 336
markers and legends 11
mass or lump, palpable 444, 449
master patient index 34
mastoid 288–9
maxilla 346–9
maxillary sinuses 291
maxillary third molars imaging 337
measurements, unsharpness in images 27
meconium, failure of passage 444
medial anatomical aspect 13
medial aspect, foot 125
medial rotation, foot 125
median sagittal plane 13, 266
medical exposure, radiation
    aprons and shields 47
    diagnostic reference levels 48
    dose monitoring 48
    dose quantities 45
    exposure charts 47
    immobilisation 47
    investigation and notification of overexposure 48–9
    justification 44
    optimisation 46
    overview 44
    patient holding 47
    risk-benefit analysis 44
    risks 46
    training 47
    X-ray examination benefits 45
medio-lateral projection 137
mesial surface 316
metabolic disease, skeletal survey 535
metal detector, ingested foreign bodies 511
metatarsal-phalangeal sesamoid bones 124, 134
    see also lower limbs
metatarsus adductus 478
midline projection 340

mid sagittal plane positioning
  errors 356
millampere seconds 40
mobile C-arm equipment
  emergency peripheral vascular
    procedures 419
  heart and lungs 392
  operative cholangiography 417
  pain management 418
modalities, imaging 34
modifications
  half axial projection 280
  infero-superior (modified axial)
    projection 114
  mento-occipital projection 295
  reverse mento-occipital 30 degree
    projection 297
  see also alternative projections and
    positioning; specific projection
Moiré patterns 31
movement
  macroradiography 533
  tomography 521, 526, 527
  unsharpness 26, 27, 43
myeloma, skeletal survey 535–6

NAI consent form 492–3, 537
nasal bones – lateral projection 301
nasal injury 293
nasion 266
naso-gastric tube positioning 394–5
neck of femur projection 180
neck of humerus 52
necrotising enterocolitis 448
neonates see paediatric care
networks, imaging informatics 35
non-accidental injury, paediatric 427
non-imaging equipment 496
non-screen image receptor 318
non-standard kilovoltage, soft tissue 516
non-trauma orthopaedic surgery 409
Norgaard projection 59
notes see specific projection
nursing, isolation/barrier 387

obese patients 497
oblique lateral projection 146
oblique medial projection 145
oblique occlusal projection 342–5
oblique projection 18–19, 271
occipito-mental 30 degree caudal
  projection 296, 310
occipito-mental projection 294, 310
occipto-frontal 30 degree cranial
  anuglation projection 281
occipto-frontal projection
  cranium 276–7
  skull 270, 309

occlusal plane 316, 356
occlusal radiography
  anterior oblique occlusal projection,
    mandible 344
  anterior oblique occlusal projection,
    maxilla 343
  lower oblique occlusal projection,
    mandible 345
  oblique occlusal projection,
    mandible, 344–5
  oblique occlusal projection,
    maxilla 342–3
  posterior oblique occlusal projection,
    maxilla 343
  radiological considerations 338
  recommended projections 338
  terminology 338
  true occlusal projection,
    mandible 340–1
  vertex occlusal projection,
    maxilla 339
occlusal surface 316
occular issues see eyes
occupational radiation exposure 49–50
  see also radiation protection
    and dose
oesophageal pH probe, reflux study
  439, 488
onward transfers 35
open mouth projection 201–2
open skull fracture 449
operative cholangiography 417
optic foramina and jugular foramina
  projection 284, 285
optic foramina – postero-anterior
  oblique projection 284
optimisation
  digital imaging 11, 31
  paediatric radiography 424
  radiation protection 46
oral clinical history 10, 43
orbito-meatal baseline 266
orbits – occipito-mental (modified)
  projection 300
orthopaedic surgery
  corrective operative procedures 409
  distal locking 412
  external fixation 411
  extracapsular fractures 410
  hints and tips 411–12
  hip fractures 410
  intracapsular fractures 410
  intramedullary nailing 412
  non-trauma 409
  proximal locking 412
  radiation doses 412
  Steinmann pin insertions 411
  tension band wirings 411

orthopaedic surgery (continued)
  trauma 410–12
  upper and lower extremity
    fractures 410
outer canthus of the eye 266
outlet projections 109–11
  antero-posterior 25 degree
    projection 109
  lateral oblique 15 degree
    projection 110
  recommended projections 97
overexposure 8, 239
  see also radiation exposure
overlap, adjacent teeth 352
over-rotated hand 52, 57

pacemaker, temporary 392
PACS see picture archiving and
  communication system
paediatric care
  abdomen and pelvic cavity 371
  antero-posterior projection 371
  gallows traction 402
  heart and lungs, special care baby
    unit 403
  lateral projection 402
paediatric radiography
  abdomen 444–8
  accessories 430
  anatomy differences 426
  antiscatter grid 429
  audit and quality assurance 430
  automatic exposure control 429
  bone age 475
  chest – neonatal 434–7
  chest – post-neonatal 438–43
  child development 425
  common examinations 434
  coning devices 431–2
  dental radiography 456
  digital radiography 430
  dose measurement 432
  elbow 472–4
  environment – dedicated paediatric
    areas 428
  feet – supported/weight-bearing
    476–9
  film/intensifying screen
    combinations 430
  film processing and viewing
    conditions 430
  filtration, additional 429
  focal spot 429
  focus-to-receptor distance 429
  gonad protection 431–2
  image characteristics 430
  image evaluation 486–91
  image quality 430

paediatric radiography (*continued*)
   imaging equipment 429–30
   imaging quality 431–3
   imaging room 428
   immobilisation devices 430
   justification 423–4
   legislation 423
   leg length assessment 468–71
   NAI consent form 492–3
   non-accidental injury 427, 480–3
   optimisation 424
   patients 425–8
   pelvis/hips 457–60
   post-nasal space – lateral supine projection 455
   pregnancy 428
   preparation of patient 426
   psychological considerations 425
   quality assurance 430
   radiation protection 431–3
   sedation 426
   sinuses 454
   skeletal surveys 480–5
   skull 449–53
   special needs children 428
   spine – cervical, thoracic and lumbar 466–7
   spine – scoliosis 461–5
   syndrome assessment 484–5
   tube potential selection 429
   waiting area 428
   X-ray generators 429
   see also Forensic radiography, foetus
pain management 418
palatal surface 316
Palmer notation 314
palpable lump/mass 444, 449
panoramic tomography
   anterior teeth positioning errors 356
   benefits 353
   dose reduction 353
   faults and problems 356
   image acquisition 351–5
   limitations 353
   magnification variation 351
   mid sagittal plane positioning errors 356
   occlusal plane positioning error 356
   overlap, adjacent teeth 352
   patient preparation 354
   patient's shoulder interfering with cassette movement 356
   principles 350
   recent advances 353
   secondary shadows 352
   soft tissue, superimposition 352
   spinal column positioning error 356
   tomographic blur 352

paralleling technique 332–5
paranasal sinuses 291, 306–8
patella – infero-superior projection 159
patella projection 156
pathology 23, 501
patient positioning *see specific projection*
patients
   anatomical aspect 13
   condition assessment 500
   dental panoramic tomography 354
   examination timeline 7
   facial bones and sinuses, severely injured 297
   holding, radiation protection 47
   identification 11
   intoxicated 502
   journey 2, 7
   paediatric radiography 425–8
   radiation protection 4
   shoulder interfering with cassette movement 356
   skull, facial bones and sinuses projection preparation 272
   talking to 508
pattern recognition 10
peer-to-peer image transfers 34
pelvis
   alternative projection 185
   antero-posterior projection 191
   fractures 400
   ilium 185
   lateral projection 186
   posterior oblique projection 185
   postero-anterior – erect projection 187
   recommended projections 170
   symphysis pubis 187
   see also abdomen and pelvic cavity; hip joint, upper third of femur and pelvis
pelvis/hips, paediatric
   antero-posterior – erect projection 459
   antero-posterior projection 458
   both hips, lateral projection 460
   gonad shields 457
   lateral projection 460
   radiation protection 458
   recommended projections 457
   referral criteria 457
   Von Rosen projection 460
percutaneous foreign body 510
percutaneous nephrolithotomy 416
perforation, abdomen and pelvic cavity 371
periapical radiography
   bisecting angle technique 327–30
   complete/full mouth survey 337
   examples 331

periapical radiography (*continued*)
   mandibular third molars imaging 336
   maxillary third molars imaging 337
   paralleling technique 332–5
   third molar region 336–7
peripheral vascular emergency procedures 419
peritoneal shunt integrity 449
permanent dentition, Palmer notation 314
petrous – anterior oblique projection 290
pharynx and larynx 228–9, 527
photographic film 23
   see also specific radiography
pH probe, paediatric 439, 488
Picture Archiving and Communication System (PACS) 32, 408
pivot height, tomography
   kidney 526
   larynx 527
   principles 520–1
planes and regions of body
   abdomen and pelvic cavity 366–7
   defined 13
   skull, facial bones and sinuses 266
plantar aspect, foot 125
positioning
   abduction limb 16
   anterior teeth, errors 356
   elbows, paediatric 472–3
   flexion position 16, 125, 507
   foot 125
   frog's legs lateral 183, 491
   lungs 239
   mid sagittal plane, errors 356
   naso-gastric tube 394–5
   occlusal plane, errors 356
   pronation limb position 16
   rotation limb 16
   spinal column, error 356
   supine position 472, 473
   terminology 13–16
   upper limbs 53
   see also alternative projections and positioning; *specific projection*
position of patient *see specific projection*
posterior anatomical aspect 13
posterior erect aspect projection 14
posterior oblique occlusal projection 343
posterior oblique projection
   acetabulum and hip joint 184
   defined 18
   hip joint and upper third of femur 179
   pelvis 185

posterior projection 341
postero-anterior chest projection 248–9
postero-anterior – erect projection
    chest, paediatric 488
    chest – post-neonatal 440
    heart and lungs 389
    lungs 240–1
    pelvis 187
    radiation protection 241
    symphysis pubis 187
postero-anterior oblique projection
    knee joint 160
    mandible 304
    sternoclavicular joints 115
postero-anterior projection
    cephalometry 359
    clavicle 112
    defined 17
    example 20
    heart and aorta 252–3
    heart and lungs 391
    knee joint 156
    mandible 303
    sacro-iliac joints 188
    sacrum 224
    sternoclavicular joints 116
    thumbs 63
    wrists 70–1, 74
post-examination and aftercare, X-ray procedure 6
post-mortem imaging *see* forensic radiography
post-nasal space – lateral supine projection 455
post-operative radiography 393
post processing, images 36
posture 174
pregnancy
    paediatric radiography 428
    radiation protection 5, 369
    urinary tract, ureters, kidneys, bladder 376
    see also paediatric care
preparation of patient
    paediatric radiography 426
    X-ray procedure 2, 7
    see also specific projection
primary survey, trauma radiography 506
problems and faults *see specific projection*
processing
    dental radiography 321
    radiographic image contrast 24
profile projection, mastoid 289
projection
    acromioalavicular joints 97
    and image view 22soft tissue 517
    terminology 17–21
    see also specific projection

prone position 14, 16, 472
prostatic disease, skeletal survey 535, 536
proximal locking 412
proximal radio-ulnar joint 83
proximal tibio-fibular joint
    antero-posterior oblique projection 148
    lateral oblique projection 148
    recommended projections 124
psychological considerations, paediatric radiography 425
psychosocial factors 496
pulling/holding limbs 508
Pyle method, assessment of bone age 475

quality and quality assurance
    bitewing technology 324–6
    defined 6, 7
    factors, digital imaging 31
    image processing 37–8
    optimum 43
    paediatric radiography 430
    radiographic images 24
    see also image quality

'racing start' projection 162
radiation exposure
    digital imaging 31
    forearms 76
    scattered, macroradiography 534
radiation protection and dose
    abdomen 373
    abdomen, paediatric 446
    abdomen and pelvic cavity 369
    ALARP principle 50
    ankle 136, 140
    antero-posterior oblique both hands projection 59
    aprons and shields 47
    bladder 369
    calcaneum 141
    carpal bones 68
    cervical spine 399
    cervical vertebrae 199, 202, 207, 208
    chest – neonatal 437
    chest/upper abdomen 398
    defined 4–5
    dental radiography 322
    designated areas 50
    designation of classified persons 50
    diagnostic reference levels 48
    dorsi-palmar hand projection 55
    dose monitoring 48
    dose quantities 45
    elbows, paediatric 473
    examination timeline 7

radiation protection and dose (*continued*)
    exposure charts 47
    femur – shaft 164, 165
    fingers 61
    first and second cervical vertebrae 201–2
    foot 127, 130
    forearms 75, 76
    fractured lower limbs and pelvis 400
    gonads 59
    heart and aorta 253, 254
    hip joint, upper third of femur and pelvis 176–7
    hip joint and upper third of femur 178, 181, 183
    hips, pelvis, and sacro-iliac joints 174
    humerus – shaft 89
    humerus – neck 91, 92
    immobilisation 47
    investigation and notification of overexposure 48–9, 50
    justification for radiation 44
    kidneys 369
    knee joint 151, 155, 158
    lateral hand projection 57
    leg length assessment 469
    leg length assessment (paediatric) 469
    lower limbs 59
    lower ribs 259
    lumbo-sacral junction 222
    lungs 237, 241, 245
    measurement, paediatric 432
    medical exposure 44–9
    monitoring 48
    occupational exposure 49–50
    optimisation 46
    overview 44
    patient 4
    patient holding 47
    pelvis/hips, paediatric 458
    pharynx and larynx 229
    pregnancy 5, 369
    quantities 45
    reduction 353
    risk-benefit analysis 44
    risks 46
    skeletal survey, paediatric non-accidental injury 481, 483
    skull, facial bones and sinuses 272
    skull, paediatric radiography 450
    staff and personnel 5, 50
    theatre radiography 407, 408
    thumbs 63
    toes 132
    tomography 524
    tomosynthesis 529, 531
    training 47
    trauma orthopaedic surgery 412

radiation protection and dose (*continued*)
  ureters 369
  urinary tract 369
  urinary tract, ureters, kidneys, bladder 376
  ward radiography 387
  X-ray examination benefits 45
radiographer comments/initial report 10–11
  see also image evaluation
radiographic baseline 266
radiographic contrast, radiographic images 23, 24
radiographic images
  acquisition and display 28–9
  contrast 23–4, 43
  digital image capture 23
  distortion 25
  formation and density 22–3
  magnification 25
  photographic film 23
  projection and view 22
  quality 24
  sharpness 26–7, 43
  see also digital images; images
radiography
  technique 481
  uses in dentistry 312
  vertebral curves 195
radiography comments/initial report 57
  see image evaluation
radiological considerations
  abdomen and pelvic cavity 370–1
  elbows 84
  facial bones and sinuses 293
  feet, paediatric 476
  lungs 239
  occlusal radiography 338
  skull, facial bones and sinuses 273
  see also specific projection
radiologic technique, cranium 274
radiology information system (RIS) 34
ramus of the mandible 348–9
rationale for projections 480
  see also justification; referral criteria
razor insertion 513
receptor
  cassette holder 504
  radiographic image contrast 24
  stabilisation 317
recommended projections
  abdomen, paediatric 444
  abdomen and pelvic cavity 368
  ankle 124
  calcaneum 124
  chest – neonatal 434
  chest – post-neonatal 439
  chest/upper abdomen 396

recommended projections (*continued*)
  dental, forensic 539
  facial bones and sinuses 293
  feet, paediatric 476
  femur – shaft 124
  foot 124
  hips, pelvis and sacro-iliac joints 170
  knee joint 124
  lower limbs 124
  lower ribs 257
  lungs 232
  metatarsal-phalangeal sesamoid bones 124
  occlusal radiography 338
  pelvis/hips, paediatric 457
  proximal tibio-fibular joint 124
  sacro-iliac joints 170
  shoulders 97
  skeletal survey, paediatric non-accidental injury 480
  skull, paediatric 450
  sternum 257
  subtalar joints 124, 143
  tibia and fibula 124
  toes 124
  upper limbs 52
  upper ribs 257
  vertebral column 194
rectum, vibrator insertion 513
recurrent cough 439
red flag 387
  see also warning
referral criteria
  abdomen, paediatric 444
  abdomen and pelvic cavity 368
  bone age, paediatric 475
  chest – neonatal 434
  chest – post-neonatal 438–9
  elbows, paediatric 472
  pelvis/hips, paediatric 457
  post-nasal space 455
  sinuses, paediatric 449
  skeletal survey, paediatric non-accidental injury 480
  see also justification
reflux study, post-neonatal 439
remote viewing applications 34
renal calculi 370
respiration, lungs 233
reticuloses, skeletal survey 535
retrograde pyelography 415
retroperitoneal disease 371
reverse Judet's projection 184
reverse Towne's projection 281
rheumatoid arthritis 535
rickets 535
right anterior oblique projection 255, 381

right erect aspect projection 14
right lateral decubitus projection 14
right lateral projection 21
right posterior oblique projection
  biliary system 381
  cervical vertebrae 208
  example 21
  lower ribs 259
  lumbar vertebrae 220
  lumbo-sacral junction 223
  upper ribs 260
  urinary bladder 379
  urinary tract, kidneys, ureters, bladder, 378–9
  see also oblique projection
right posterior oblique supine projection 209
RIS *see* radiology information system
risk-benefit analysis, radiation 44
risks, radiation 46
road-map technique 419
rotation, lungs 239
rotation and abduction effect 175
rotation limb position 16

sacro-iliac joints 170, 188–92
sacrum 194, 224–5
satisfaction of search 10
scanning technology 30
scaphoid *see* carpal bones
scapula 97, 117–18
scattered radiation 534
scintillator detector 30
screen/film imaging 28
screw insertion, hip 413–14
scurvy, skeletal survey 535
search satisfaction 10
secondary radiation grids 24, 42
secondary shadows 352
secondary spinal scoliosis 465
secondary survey, trauma radiography 506
sedation, paediatric radiography 426
seizures, paediatric 449
Seldinger technique 419
sella turcica 283
semi-erect projection 239
semi-prone (alternative) projection 115
semi-recumbent projection 14
seronegative arthritis 536
severely injured patient 297
shadows, secondary 352
sharpness
  radiographic images 26–7, 43
  tomography 524
shields *see* radiation protection and dose

shoulders
- acromioclavicular joints 111
- antero-posterior 15 degree erect projections 99
- antero-posterior erect projections 100
- arm abducted 119
- basic projections 98–102
- calcified tendons 109–11
- clavicle 112–14
- coracoid process 119
- glenohumeral joint 108
- image evaluation 120–1
- infero-superior (reverse axial) projection 102
- instability/recurrent dislocation 97
- outlet projections 109–11
- radiological considerations 96
- scapula 117–18
- sternoclavicular joints 115–16
- Stryker projection 107
- supero-inferior (axial) projection 100–1
- trauma projections 103–5
- West Point projection 106

shunt integrity 449
single exposure CR method 470
sinuses, paediatric 454
  see also facial bones and sinuses
skeletal survey, general
- indications for 535
- paediatric syndrome assessment 484–5
- recommended projections 536

skeletal survey, paediatric
- non-accidental injury
- chest 481
- consent 480–3
- justification 480
- lower limbs 481
- radiation dose 483
- radiation protection 481
- radiographic technique 481
- rationale for projections 480
- recommended projections 480
- referral criteria 480
- skull 481
- spine (cervical, thoracic and lumbar) 481
- upper limbs 481

skull
- accessories 272
- anatomy 267–9
- anthropological baseline 266
- anthropological plane 266
- auricular plane 266
- beam angulation projection 270
- complex oblique projection 271
- coronal planes 266

skull (continued)
- dental radiography 456
- external auditory meatus 266
- external occipital protuberance (inion) 266
- 55 degree left anterior oblique with 35 degree caudal angulation 271
- 40 degree left anterior oblique projection 271
- fronto-occipital projection 270
- glabella 266
- Glasgow Coma Scale 273
- image evaluation 308
- image quality 272
- infraorbital line 266
- infraorbital margin/point 266
- interpretation of images 266
- interpupillary (interorbital) line 266
- landmarks 266
- lateral projection 270, 309
- lateral projection with angulation 271
- lines 266
- median sagittal plane 266
- nasion 266
- oblique projections 271
- occipto-frontal projection 270, 309
- orbito-meatal baseline 266
- outer anthus of the eye 266
- patient preparation 272
- planes 266
- radiation protection 272
- radiographic baseline 266
- radiological considerations 273
- skull units 269
- vertex 266
- warning 270
- see also cranium; facial bones and sinuses

skull, paediatric radiography
- base of skull fracture 449
- bruises 449
- craniosynostosis 449, 450
- depressed skull fracture 449
- epilepsy 449
- focal neurological deficiency 449
- fronto-occipital 30 degree caudal projection 452
- fronto-occipital projection 451
- Glasgow Coma Scale 449
- headache 449
- lacerations 449
- lateral – supine projection 453
- non-accidental injury 481
- open skull fracture 449
- palpable lump 449
- peritoneal shunt integrity 449
- radiation protection 450
- recommended projections 450

skull, paediatric radiography (continued)
- referral criteria 449
- seizures 449
- skeletal survey 481
- suspected craniosynostosis 449, 450
- suspected depressed fracture 449
- swelling 449
- syndrome assessment 449
- tense fontanelle 449
- trauma 449, 450
- ventriculo-atrial integrity 449

skyline projections 157–8
sleeping baby, chest 435
soft tissue
- air, lesions demonstrated by 517
- artefacts, lungs 239
- bariatric radiography 497
- bone and adjacent soft tissues 517
- calcifications 517
- exposure technique 516–17
- fat, lesions demonstrated by 517
- high kilovoltage 516
- image evaluation 10
- kilovoltage 516
- lesions 517
- low kilovoltage 516
- non-standard kilovoltage 516
- projection choice 517
- subnormal kilovoltage 516
- superimposition, dental 352
- see also tissue displacement

solutions to faults see specific projection
spatial resolution, images 27
special care baby unit 403
specialised image receptor holders 320
specialist applications, imaging modalities 34
special needs children
  see also Paediatric radiography
sphenoid sinus 291
spinal column positioning errors 356
spine, paediatric 481
spine – cervical, thoracic and lumbar (paediatric) 466–7
spine – scoliosis (paediatric)
- lateral projection 464–5
- postero-anterior – erect projection 463
- postero-anterior – erect 462
- radiation protection 461
- recommended projections 462
- referral criteria 461

staff and other personnel
- cross-infection control, dental exams 322–3
- radiation protection 5

standards see quality and quality assurance

standing position
    elbows, paediatric 472, 473
    trauma radiography 501
Steinmann pin insertions 411
Stenver's projection 290
sterile areas 408
    see also infection control
sternoclavicular joints
    lateral projection 116
    postero-anterior oblique projection 115
    postero-anterior projection 116
    recommended projections 97
    semi-prone (alternative) projection 115
sternum
    anterior oblique – trunk rotated 263
    anterior oblique – tube-angled projection 262
    lateral projection 264
    recommended projections 257
still born foetus 542–3
stressful situation, trauma radiography 508
stress projections, subluxation 140, 155
stridor, acute 439
Stryker projection 107
subject contrast, radiographic images 23–4
subjective contrast, radiographic images 23, 24
submento-vertical projection 282, 287
subnormal kilovoltage, soft tissue 516
subtalar joints
    dorsi-plantar – oblique projection 144
    lateral oblique projection 144
    oblique lateral projection 146
    oblique medial projection 145
    recommended projections 124, 143
subtraction angiography 419
suggestions, image assessment/evaluation process 10
supero-inferior (axial) projection 92
supero-inferior modified (modified axial) projection 104
supination limb position 16
supine decubitus projection 14
supported feet see feet – supported/weight-bearing, paediatric
suspected conditions 293
suspected paediatric conditions
    craniosynostosis 449, 450
    depressed fracture 449
    diaphragmatic hernia 448
    necrotising enterocolitis 448
    swallowed foreign body 444, 447
swab insertion 513
swallowed foreign body, paediatric 444

swelling, head, paediatric 449
symphysis pubis 187
syndrome assessment, paediatric 449, 484–5
system availability, image quality 38

talking to patient 508
talo-calcaneal 478
tarsal coalition 478
teamwork, trauma radiography 501, 508
teeth see dental radiography
temporal bones 286
temporary pacemaker 392
temporo-mandibular joints (TMJ) 293, 305
10 point plan see image evaluation
tense fontanelle 449
tension band wirings 411
terminology
    anatomy 13
    dental radiography 316
    examination timeline 7
    image evaluation 8–12
    image quality 6, 7
    imaging informatics 6, 7
    patient aspects 6, 7
    patient journey 2, 7
    positioning 13–16
    projection 17–21
    radiation protection 4–5
    10 point plan 8–12
    X-ray stages 3, 7
theatre radiography
    accessories 408
    checklist 406–7
    communication 406
    darkroom facilities 408
    dynamic hip screw insertion 412–14
    emergency peripheral vascular procedures 419
    equipment 406, 408
    infection control 408
    interventional procedures 415–17
    key skills 406–7
    non-trauma orthopaedic surgery 409
    operative cholangiography 417
    PACS connectivity 408
    pain management 418
    radiation protection 407, 408
    sterile areas 408
    time out 407
    trauma orthopaedic surgery 409–12
thickness, tomography layers 522–3
thin-film transistor (TFT) flat-panel detector 30
third molar region 336–7
third to seventh vertebrae projection 203

thoracic and lumbar spine 507
thoracic spine projections 214
thoracic vertebrae
    antero-posterior projection 211, 214
    image evaluation 214
    lateral projection 212–14
    localised projections 214
    recommended projections 194
    thoracic spine projections 214
thorax and upper airway
    bones of the thorax 256–7
    heart and aorta 250–5
    lower ribs 258–9
    lungs 232–49
    pharynx and larynx 228–9
    sternum 262–4
    trachea (including thoracic inlet) 230–1
    upper ribs 260–1
thumbs 52, 62–3
    see also fingers; hands
tibia and fibula 124, 147–8
tiling, digital imaging 31
tilting table – postero-anterior projection 374
time out 407
tissue displacement 498
    see also soft tissue
TMJ see temporo-mandibular joints (TMJ)
toddler feet 476
    see also paediatric care
toes
    dorsi-plantar oblique projection 132
    dorsi-plantar projection 132
    lateral – basic – hallux projection 133
    radiation protection and dose 132
    recommended projections 124
    see also foot; lower limbs
tomography
    antero-posterior projection 527
    applications 525
    autotomography 518
    blur, dental panoramic 352
    contrast 524
    depth of layer 520–1
    exposure angle 521, 525
    exposure time 525
    fulcrum 520–1
    image quality 524
    kidneys 526
    larynx 527
    linear movement features 521
    localisation of layer depth 524
    magnification 523
    movement 521, 526, 527
    overview 518
    pivot height 520–1, 526, 527

tomography (continued)
   principles 519–23
   procedure 525
   radiation protection 524
   sharpness 524
   thickness of cut and spacing of layers 523
   thickness of layer 522–3
   trachea 527
   zonography 523
tomosynthesis
   applications 531
   image quality 530–1
   lungs 237
   principles 528–9
   procedure 529
   radiation protection 529, 531
   VolumeRAD comparison 528
Towne's projection 279–80
trachea 230–1, 527
training, radiation protection 47
transocular foreign body 514–15
transverse plane, planes of body 13
trauma
   abdomen, paediatric radiology 444
   chest – post-neonatal 439
   knee joint 154
   and pathology 293
   shoulders 97, 103–5
   skeletal survey 535
   skull, paediatric radiography 449, 450
trauma orthopaedic surgery
   corrective operative procedures 409
   distal locking 412
   external fixation 411
   extracapsular fractures 410
   hints and tips 411–12
   hip fractures 410
   intracapsular fractures 410
   intramedullary nailing 412
   proximal locking 412
   radiation doses 412
   Steinmann pin insertions 411
   tension band wirings 411
   trauma 410–12
   upper and lower extremity fractures 410
   see also non-trauma orthopaedic surgery
trauma radiography
   ABCDEs 506
   adaptation of technique 501
   Advanced Trauma and Life Support 506–8
   airway maintenance 506
   assessment, patient condition 500
   breathing and ventilation 506

trauma radiography (continued)
   cervical spine examination 507
   circulation 506
   collimation 503
   comments on images produced 508
   computed tomography 507
   direct digital radiography 505
   disability 506
   equipment 501–5
   examination 500
   exposure/environmental control 506
   exposure factors 505
   flexion projections 507
   grids 503
   holding/pulling limbs 508
   'hot' report 508
   identification, images 505
   imaging 501–5
   immobilisation devices/clothing 502
   intoxicated patients 502
   labelling of images 505
   lumbar spine 507
   object/receptor distance 504
   object-to-receptor distance 503
   primary survey 506
   receptor cassette holder 504
   secondary survey 506
   stressful situation 508
   talking to patient 508
   teamwork 508
   thoracic and lumbar spine 507
   trolley type 504
   trolleytop 504
   ventilation 506
   vertical cassette holders 504
true lateral – neck of femur projection 180
true occlusal projection 340–1
tube potential selection 429
tunnel – antero-posterior projection 161–2
turned-rolled projection 152

ulnar deviation, carpal bones 65, 68
ulnar groove – axial projection 83
underexposure
   image evaluation 8
   lungs 239
   optimum radiographic image quality 43
uniformity, lungs 236
upper abdomen see chest/upper abdomen
upper anterior region – lateral projection 247
upper arm in contact 80
upper limbs
   carpal bones 64–9
   carpal tunnel 69

upper limbs (continued)
   elbows 77–85
   fingers 60–1
   forearms 75–6
   hands 54–9
   humerus 86–94
   paediatric 481
   position of patient, image detector 53
   recommended projections 52
   thumbs 62–3
   trauma orthopaedic surgery 410
   wrists 70–4
   see also specific limb
upper ribs
   cervical – antero-posterior projection 261
   first and second, antero-posterior projection 261
   left posterior oblique projection 260
   recommended projections 257
   right posterior oblique projection 260
urinary bladder 379
urinary tract, ureters, kidneys, bladder
   antero-posterior projection 376–7
   cross-kidney projection 377
   left posterior oblique projection 378
   paediatric care 444
   pregnancy 376
   radiation protection 376
   right posterior oblique projection 378
   urinary tract 377

vagina, razor insertion 513
valgus, paediatric 478
varus, paediatric 478
vascular (peripheral) emergency procedures 419
ventilation, trauma radiography 506
ventriculo-atrial integrity 449
vertebral curves 195
vertebral levels 195, 197
vertebral column
   cervical vertebrae 198–209
   cervico-thoracic vertebrae 210
   coccyx 226
   landmarks 196
   lumbar vertebrae 215–21
   lumbo-sacral junction 222–3
   radiography considerations 195
   recommended projections 194
   sacrum 224–5
   thoracic vertebrae 211–14
   vertebral curves 195
   vertebral levels 196–7
vertex 266

vertex occlusal projection 339
vertical cassette holders 504
   see also cassettes
vibrator insertion 513
viewing conditions, paediatric radiography 430
VolumeRAD comparison 528
volumetric tomography see cone beam computed tomography
Von Rosen projection 460

waiting area, paediatric 428
Wallace projection 104
ward radiography
   accessories 386
   cervical spine 399
   chest/upper abdomen 394–8
   communication 387
   equipment 386, 388
   fractured femur 401
   fractured lower limbs and pelvis 400–1
   heart and lungs 388–93
   heart and lungs, paediatric 403

ward radiography (*continued*)
   infection control 387
   isolation/barrier nursing 387
   key skills 386
   paediatric (gallows traction) 402
   radiation protection 387
   red flag 387
   X-ray equipment 388
warning 270
   see also red flag
weight-bearing antero-posterior projection 111
weight-bearing projection 131
   see also feet – supported/weight-bearing, paediatric
West Point projection 106
wheeze 438
window width/window level 36
wrists
   anterior oblique projection 73
   basic projections 70–1
   image evaluation 74
   lateral projections 71–2, 74
   postero-anterior projection 70–1, 74

X-ray aftercare 6–7
X-ray beam direction and location
   see specific projection
X-ray equipment
   cephalometry 357
   dental radiography 317
   forensic radiography 538
   generators, paediatric radiography 429
   operative cholangiography 417
   ward radiography 388
X-ray procedure and room
   automatic exposure control 28
   benefits 45
   examinations 7, 434
   radiation protection 45
   stages 2

'Y' projection 105

zonography 523
zygoma fracture, depressed 293
zygomatic arches – infero superior projection 299